# Immunological Approaches to Contraception and Promotion of Fertility

# REPRODUCTIVE BIOLOGY

Series Editor: Sheldon J. Segal
*The Rockefeller Foundation*
*New York, New York*

---

**THE ANTIPROGESTIN STEROID RU 486 AND HUMAN FERTILITY CONTROL**
Edited by Etienne-Emile Baulieu and Sheldon J. Segal

**GOSSYPOL: A Potential Contraceptive for Men**
Edited by Sheldon J. Segal

**IMMUNOLOGICAL APPROACHES TO CONTRACEPTION AND PROMOTION OF FERTILITY**
Edited by G. P. Talwar

---

# Immunological Approaches to Contraception and Promotion of Fertility

Edited by

G. P. Talwar
*National Institute of Immunology*
*New Delhi, India*

Plenum Press • New York and London

Library of Congress Cataloging in Publication Data

International Symposium on Immunological Approaches to Contraception and Promotion of Fertility (1985: Fogarty International Center)
Immunological approaches to contraception and promotion of fertility.
(Reproductive biology)
"Proceedings of an International Symposium on Immunological Approaches to Contraception and Promotion of Fertility, presented June 5–7, 1985, at the Fogarty International Center in Bethesda, Maryland"—T.p. verso.
Bibliography: p.
Includes index.
1. Contraception, Immunological—Congresses. 2. Fertility, Human—Immunological aspects—Congresses. I. Talwar, G. P., 1926– . II. Title. III. Series.
RG136.8.157 1986 613.9′432 86-8199
ISBN 0-306-42274-3

Proceedings of an International Symposium on Immunological Approaches to Contraception and Promotion of Fertility, presented June 5–7, 1985, at the Fogarty International Center in Bethesda, Maryland


A Division of Plenum Publishing Corporation
233 Spring Street, New York, N.Y. 10013



Printed in the United States of America

# PREFACE

Contraceptive research has entered the new age of vaccines. Realistic prospects exist for the development of an entirely new battery of vaccines for use in human and veterinary medicine. Among them may be anti-fertility vaccines, based on physiological mechanisms applicable to either the female or male. This volume is a comprehensive review - a status report - of the subjects including fundamental work on the search for useful epitopes and ranging to applied vaccinology. One vaccine to prevent pregnancy, for use by women, has already been studied extensively. G.P. Talwar, the volume's editor and his colleagues in New Delhi, India, published in 1976 a landmark series of papers describing the immunological properties of a preparation consisting of the alum-precipitated beta-subunit of human chorionic gonadotropin (hCG) chemically linked to tetanus toxoid. The principle of enhancing antigenicity of a self-protein by linkage of the epitope to a carrier protein was employed and tested clinically. These trials, carried out under the auspices of the Indian Council for Medical Research, were the first application of the carrier protein concept for a vaccine for human use. The encouraging results stimulated a wave of research not only on the use of hCG-based vaccines, but on other antigens as well. Colleagues in Finland, Sweden, Brazil and the United States, working as a team under the International Committee for Contraception Research, joined with

Talwar in confirming his original results (Fertility and Sterility, volume 34; 1980). With World Health Organization leadership, researchers in several countries focussed upon the specificity of the carboxy-terminal chain of the beta unit of hCG. Other investigators explored the potential of antigens derived from other protein hormones involved in the reproductive process - follicle-stimulating-hormone, prolactin, releasing factors, intra-gonadal regulatory factors. Work began, as well, on non-hormonal antigens - zona pellucida and other egg surface proteins; trophoblast-specific substances, and hormone receptors. Meanwhile, possibilities of a vaccine for use by men were not overlooked. This work has concentrated, primarily, on proteins derived from the surface of spermatozoa or from seminal fluid. The objective has been to interfere with the sperm's motility or its fertilizing capacity.

The initial series of eight papers by Talwar and his colleagues appeared in a dedicated issue of the journal Contraception (volume 13, pp. 183-255) in 1976. It is appropriate that now, ten years later, the subject of an anti-fertility vaccine be re-visited, the progress surveyed, and the prospects evaluated.

Sheldon J. Segal

New York City

May, 1986

CONTENTS

## INAUGURAL REMARKS

Craig K. Wallace

Director
Fogarty International Center for
Advanced Study in Health Sciences
National Institutes of Health
Bethesda, Maryland 20205

On behalf of the Fogarty International Center of the National Institutes of Health, it gives me great pleasure to welcome you to this international symposium on "Immunological Approaches to Contraception and Promotion of Fertility."

Apart from its scientific importance, the presentation of this symposium exemplifies for us of the Fogarty Center the fulfillment of some major objectives. It represents in its organization, a cooperative effort of the center with one of our sister agencies, the National Institute of Child Health and Human Development. Secondly, one of the principal purposes of the Fogarty Center is to facilitate bringing international experiences and perspectives to bear on topics of major significance such as this one to the U.S. scientific community. Finally and most specifically in this case, the symposium allows us the privilege and pleasure of sharing with a wider audience the presence among us of Fogarty Scholar-in-Residence, Dr. G.P. Talwar.

Dr. Talwar is Director, National Institute of Immunology, New Delhi. As a "Scholar-in-Residence" Dr. Talwar is among a very small group of eminent scientists, mostly, but not always, from abroad, whom we invite each year to cast aside their burdens at home and spend some months here on the campus of NIH for interaction with the scientific staff of the various institutes and for pursuit of their particular research interests. Occasionally, as now, we allow them to "surface" briefly.

As an internist having served in health services, I am particularly aware of the important role that vaccines have played in control and containment of communicable diseases. However, a vaccine for birth control is a new and intriguing notion. To be able to regulate a vital process such as reproduction by internally induced antibodies has far reaching implications. I note that the symposium intends to discuss both the interception of fertility by immunological methods as well as the promotion of fertility. Indeed the need is for both, to devise additional methods for family planning and to help overcome infertility due to immunological factors. These studies also are relevant to the production of animals of both nutritional and economic importance.

The reproductive system provides a fascinating example where the immunologic responses can be both of a facilitatory or rejection type. The fact that the mother carries to term a conceptus with fifty percent "foreign" paternal genetic information is well recorded, but the intricate mechanisms by which rejection is avoided is a subject of recent research. An interesting feature of research in this area is the possible practical applications. Experimental and clinical studies on prevention of recurrent abortions will no doubt be debated and evaluated by this group. Therapeutic modalities for helping sterility of this type will bring happiness to couples deprived of a child.

A much larger issue with much wider worldwide impact however would be the development, if possible, of vaccines enabling the prevention of unwanted pregnancies. The world population is increasing at a galloping rate, especially in some parts of the world which can ill afford it, and where the economic progress made, is largely decimated by the numbers. By current projections, the world population will cross six billion in the year 2000. This would impose enormous demands for food, shelter, education and jobs. Vaccines with the ability to control fertility will be a valuable supplement to the presently available methods of family planning. Their feasibility has for the time being been only demonstrated in experimental animals including the sub-human primates. However, the field has grown and I am informed that three vaccines are expected to go in for Phase I Clinical Trials this calendar year.

Our symposium is clearly topical. Its aim is to review the current status of research in this area. As is evident from the program, the symposium coverage is comprehensive with scientists from nine countries assembled to present their findings and to exchange experiences.

This symposium is co-sponsored by the National Institute of Child Health and Human Development of NIH and by the World Health Organization. Colateral support has been provided in various ways by the Rockefeller Foundation, the Population Council, U.S. Agency for International Development, the Program for Applied Research on Fertility Regulation (PARFER) and the Family Health International - reflecting in a way the widespread interest of these organizations in the subject of this symposium.

Last but not least I would like to extend my appreciation to the syumposium organizers: Dr. G.P. Talwar, Fogarty Scholar-in-Residence, Drs. Mort Lipsett, John Robbins, Gabe Bially, Jack Spieler, Peter Corfman and Peter Condliffe, members of the organizing committee, and the conference secretariat comprised of Dr. Kenneth Bridbord and Mrs. Nancy Shapiro.

We are very pleased to be able to support this symposium and wish you a pleasant and successful meeting.

## INAUGURAL REMARKS

Duane Alexander

Acting Director
National Institute of Child Health and Human Development
National Institutes of Health
Bethesda, Maryland 20205

It is a pleasure for me to join Dr. Wallace in welcoming you to this international symposium.

The National Institute of Child Health and Human Development is very pleased to join with the Fogarty International Center, NIH, in co-sponsoring this symposium. The N.I.C.H.D., as most of you know, is the world's largest source of support for research in the population sciences. In 1985, this support amounts to approximately $105 million supplied through our Center for Population Research. About $75 million of that support is in the basic reproductive sciences, about $20 million in demographic and behavioral sciences, $7.7 million in applied research in contraceptive development, and about $3.5 million in applied research in contraceptive evaluation. In addition to those figures, about $4 million in our intramural research program is related to reproductive endocrinology, receptorbiology, and infertility research, including immunologic aspects of infertility. Our total program in research related just to contraceptive development within the Institute is about $20 million in size. Despite that size, it is the Institute's feeling that we are not doing enough in contraceptive development research and believe that more support is needed. The world's population problem is well known to you, and some aspects were just outlined by Dr. Wallace. Even in the United States, more than 50% of pregnancies at this time are unwanted, either at the time they occur or at all. About half of those unwanted pregnancies or unintended pregnancies end in abortion. It is clear that we need better contraceptives and more effective use of the contraceptives that we do have. To this end, the Institute this year has developed and proposed to congress, a special initiative in contraceptive development that would begin in fiscal 1986 and would increase by about $20 million in that year the research program related to contraceptive development, growing to an increase of about $30 million by 1988. This research initiative builds upon recent progress in the applied research program in contraceptive development in the Institute, along with some basic discoveries in the reproductive sciences, and targets a research program to exploit these advances for contraceptive development. Among the new leads to be exploited are characterization and isolation of inhibin and folliculosatin and their use as contraceptives, methods to interfere with gamete maturation, characterization of follicular regulating protein and developing it or similar substances to drive all follicles in each cycle to artesia, and contraception by competitive inhibition of receptors for ovulatory hormones. But heading the list of these new initiatives and approaches is expanded research in immuno-contraception.

Thus, for our purposes, this symposium could not be more timely. The work in this area, though still in its relatively early stages, is farther advanced than that in other areas I mentioned, and holds great opportunity and promise, not only for immuno-contraception, but also for application to immunological causes of infertility. We hope that the information and the interaction at this conference will provide further stimulus to research in this field, as well as provide our institute with the guidance that we need on how to encourage work in this field. One of the major needs we perceive is to try to increase the linkage between the immunologist and the reproductive physiologist in these approaches. This is well demonstrated by Dr. Talwar's involvement in this research area. This conference addresses this situation right at the outset with the addresses by Dr. Talwar and Dr. Robbins. Dr. Robbins is one of the world's leaders in new approaches to vaccine development for infectious diseases and I hope that his address and others that you hear will encourage many of you to increase your interactions with immunologists in your work.

Finally, I want to introduce to you Dr. Florence Haseltine, the new director of our Center for Population Research. Dr. Haseltine has just joined the institute on May 12, 1985, succeeding Dr. Phil Corfman as the Director of the Center for Population Research. You know that Dr. Corfman is now with the World Health Organization's special research program in reproduction based in Geneva. We are confident that Dr. Haseltine will continue to provide the leadership for the Center for Population Research within the Institute and on the world scene that Dr. Corfman had provided for us in the Center since its beginning.

I wish you success in this conference, and would encourage your efforts on this very important topic. We appreciate your coming and sharing your research efforts with us during these three days.

# WHENCE THE ANTI HORMONES?

Roy Hertz

Professor Emeritus
Pharmacology and Obstetrics and Gynecology
The George Washington University Medical Center
Washington, D.C.

It is a privilege to be called upon to relate to you some of the early events in the development of the endocrinologist's interest in an immunological approach to fertility control.

It should be appreciated that before our knowledge of the actual chemical nature of the gonadotropic substances an enormous mass of pertinent data had accumulated from experimental and clinical observation.

A key figure in the initial discovery of the role of the anterior pituitary in the activation of the ovary was Dr. Bernhard Zondek (Fig. I). Dr. Zondek showed in 1926 that the subcutaneous implantation of a small fragment of pituitary tissue into a sexually immature mouse would transform the ovary into a morphologically and functionally mature gonad which in turn would cause the uterus and vagina to undergo maturation. Dr. Zondek also discovered the presence of an active gonadotropic substance in the urine of pregnant women which provided the basis for the first biological test for pregnancy. This substance we now know as "human chorionic gonadotropin" or H.C.G. (1).

It should be noted that somewhat earlier, in 1920, Dr. Hirose in Japan, had also observed that extracts of human placenta, decidua, and hydatidiform mole induced extensive luteinization in the rabbit ovary. He thereby foreshadowed Dr. Zondek's demonstration of a similar effect on the mouse ovary of pregnancy urine (1a).

Dr. Zondek summarized his pioneering observations in a classic monograph published in 1931 (Fig. II). He described therein his finding that patients with certain ovarian tumors also excrete a chorionic type of gonadotropin.

Yet a much more significant aspect of these early studies was the penetrating observation that the ovarian response to gonadotropic stimulation consists of two distinct phases, namely follicular stimulation and luteinization (1).

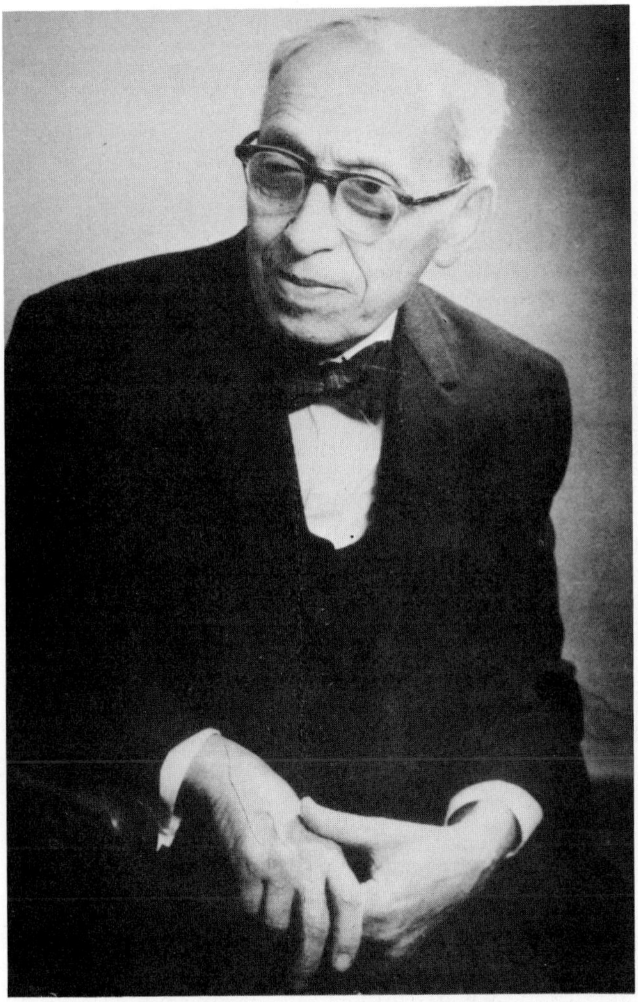

Fig. I: Dr. Bernard Zondek

DIE

# HORMONE DES OVARIUMS

UND DES

# HYPOPHYSENVORDERLAPPENS

UNTERSUCHUNGEN ZUR BIOLOGIE UND KLINIK
DER WEIBLICHEN GENITALFUNKTION

VON

DR. BERNHARD ZONDEK
A. O. PROFESSOR FÜR GEBURTSHILFE UND GYNÄKOLOGIE
AN DER UNIVERSITÄT BERLIN

MIT EINEM ANHANG
DIE HORMONALE SCHWANGERSCHAFTSREAKTION
AUS DEM HARN BEI MENSCH UND TIER

MIT 121 ZUM TEIL FARBIGEN ABBILDUNGEN

BERLIN
VERLAG VON JULIUS SPRINGER
1931



Fig. II: Frontispiece of Dr. B. Zondek's classical monograph on the ovarian and pituitary hormones.

There ensued an intensive controversy as to whether the pituitary provides a single hormone with both follicle stimulating and luteinizing capacity or two distinct gonadotropic substances.

In undertaking to resolve this question my mentor Dr. F.L. Hisaw and his chemical colleague, Dr. H.L. Fevold entered upon extensive studies in the early 1930's at the University of Wisconsin. My first assignment as student assistant to these inspiring teachers was to collect pituitary glands on the killing-floor of the local abattoir. In an hour's time one could recover 20 to 25 glands. These glands were taken back to the laboratory on ice and the anterior lobe dissected free from the posterior lobe and other adherent tissue. The chemical procedures then applied have been well documented in the classic publications from that laboratory (2,3).

It soon became evident that anterior pituitary tissue extracts could be fractionated into preparations which proved in the immature rat test to be primarily follicle-stimulating or luteinizing (2,3). Since these developments came at about the same time that President Roosevelt was creating the alphabetical agencies in Washington such as the W.P.A., the N.Y.A., and the N.R.A., Dr. Hisaw elected to name the one type of extract "F.S.H." and the other "L.H."

It became my assignment to explore the biological effects of these preparations in the immature rabbit in order to extend the prior studies in the rat. In these rabbit studies the observation which is pertinent here was the fact that although we could initially induce with sheep FSH extensive follicular development in the ovary of the immature rabbit, such an effect could not be sustained for more than 10 to 15 days. After this the ovaries involuted to even less than their pre-treatment size and all evidence of follicular stimulation regressed (Fig. III). We characterized this condition as a "refractory state" and were puzzled over the significance of the effect (4).

At this same time Dr. Hans Selye and his colleagues described a similar refractory state to prolonged gonadotropin stimulation with either chorionic gonadotropin or with pituitary extracts in rat (5,6). Moreover, Selye et al. showed that a rat which was refractory to chorionic gonadotropin would still respond to pituitary hormone. Thus, he anticipated the answer to some of our current concerns regarding potential cross-over reactions between HCG and LH.

That this refractory phenomenon was puzzling even to the foremost investigators at that time is shown in a letter received from Dr. Harvey Cushing dated April 16, 1934 (Fig. IV). Therein he describes a similar refractory state in the immature dog after prolonged administration of sheep pituitary gonadotropin.

Meanwhile, Dr. Evelyn Anderson (Fig. V) working in Dr. Collip's laboratory with ovine thyreotropin in the rat observed a similar refractory state to thyreotropic stimulation after prolonged treatment (7). In an inspired series of experiments Dr. Anderson and Dr. Collip showed that the serum of a refractory rat added to an effective dose of thyreotropic extract would completely negate the expected thyreotropic response in a previously untreated animal. She thereby discovered the "antihormones." Shortly thereafter many observers extended these observations to both chorionic and pituitary gonadotropic preparations (8,9).

The problem of the nature of the anti-hormone effect and its biological implications came under extensive study. Dr. Collip viewed the "antihormone" as a physiologically functional factor in the regulation of the reproductive cycle and other normal hormonal functions (10). In this vein Dr. Schafer in 1916 had coined the term "chalone" to define humoral inhibitory agents capable of arresting hormonal effects (11). However, Dr. Collip preferred the term "antihormone" in his attempt to rationalize the role of such an inhibitory agent in normal physiological events.

Other observers postulated a relationship between anti-hormones and classical antibodies. Thus, Meyer and Wolfe (12) studied the temporal relationship between the rise in precipitin titres in the sera of gonadotropin-treated monkeys and their anti-gonadotropin titres. They

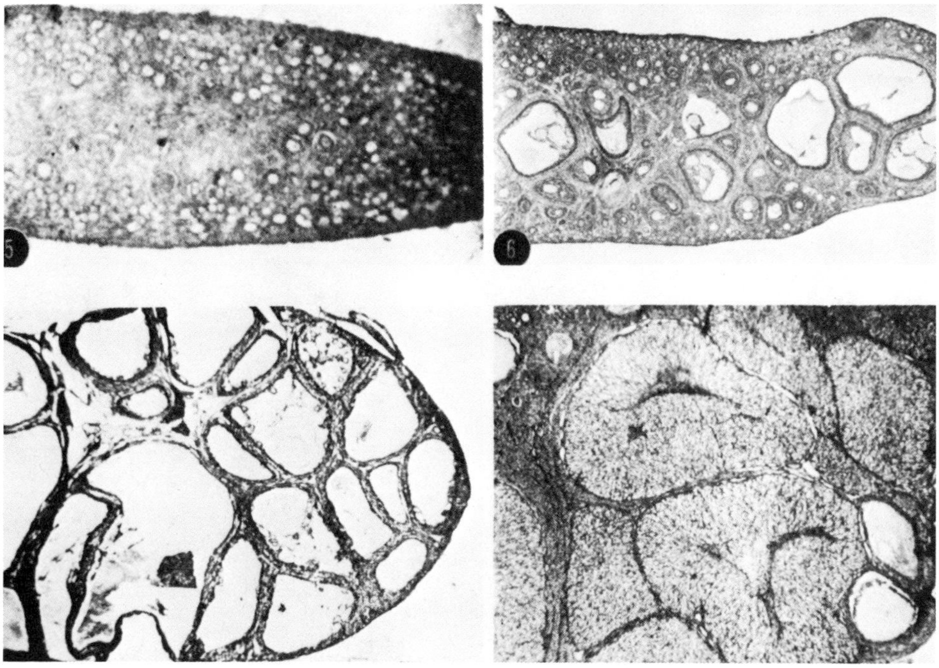


Fig. III: Left Upper - Normal rabbit ovary at 4 weeks of age - not responsive to gonadotropin.
Right Upper - Normal rabbit ovary at 12 weeks of age - responsive to gonadotropin.
Left Lower - Extreme follicular stimulation after 8 days on FSH.
Right Lower - Extensive luteinization after 5 days on unfractionated pituitary extract.

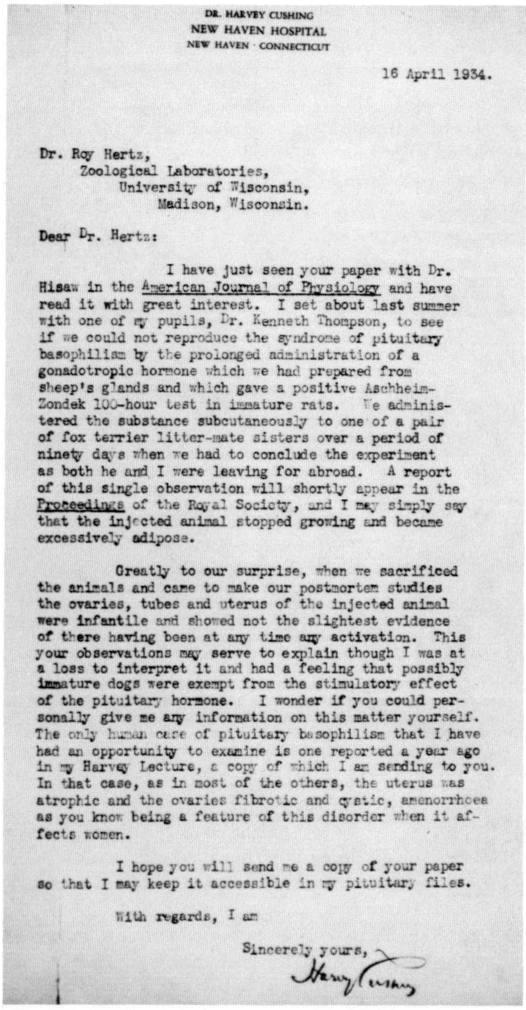

DR. HARVEY CUSHING
NEW HAVEN HOSPITAL
NEW HAVEN · CONNECTICUT

16 April 1934.

Dr. Roy Hertz,
Zoological Laboratories,
University of Wisconsin,
Madison, Wisconsin.

Dear Dr. Hertz:

I have just seen your paper with Dr. Hisaw in the American Journal of Physiology and have read it with great interest. I set about last summer with one of my pupils, Dr. Kenneth Thompson, to see if we could not reproduce the syndrome of pituitary basophilism by the prolonged administration of a gonadotropic hormone which we had prepared from sheep's glands and which gave a positive Aschheim-Zondek 100-hour test in immature rats. We administered the substance subcutaneously to one of a pair of fox terrier litter-mate sisters over a period of ninety days when we had to conclude the experiment as both he and I were leaving for abroad. A report of this single observation will shortly appear in the Proceedings of the Royal Society, and I may simply say that the injected animal stopped growing and became excessively adipose.

Greatly to our surprise, when we sacrificed the animals and came to make our postmortem studies the ovaries, tubes and uterus of the injected animal were infantile and showed not the slightest evidence of there having been at any time any activation. This your observations may serve to explain though I was at a loss to interpret it and had a feeling that possibly immature dogs were exempt from the stimulatory effect of the pituitary hormone. I wonder if you could personally give me any information on this matter yourself. The only human case of pituitary basophilism that I have had an opportunity to examine is one reported a year ago in my Harvey Lecture, a copy of which I am sending to you. In that case, as in most of the others, the uterus was atrophic and the ovaries fibrotic and cystic, amenorrhoea as you know being a feature of this disorder when it affects women.

I hope you will send me a copy of your paper so that I may keep it accessible in my pituitary files.

With regards, I am

Sincerely yours,

Harvey Cushing

Fig. IV.: Letter from Dr. Harvey Cushing, April 18, 1934 regarding refractoriness to gonadotropin stimulation in the dog.

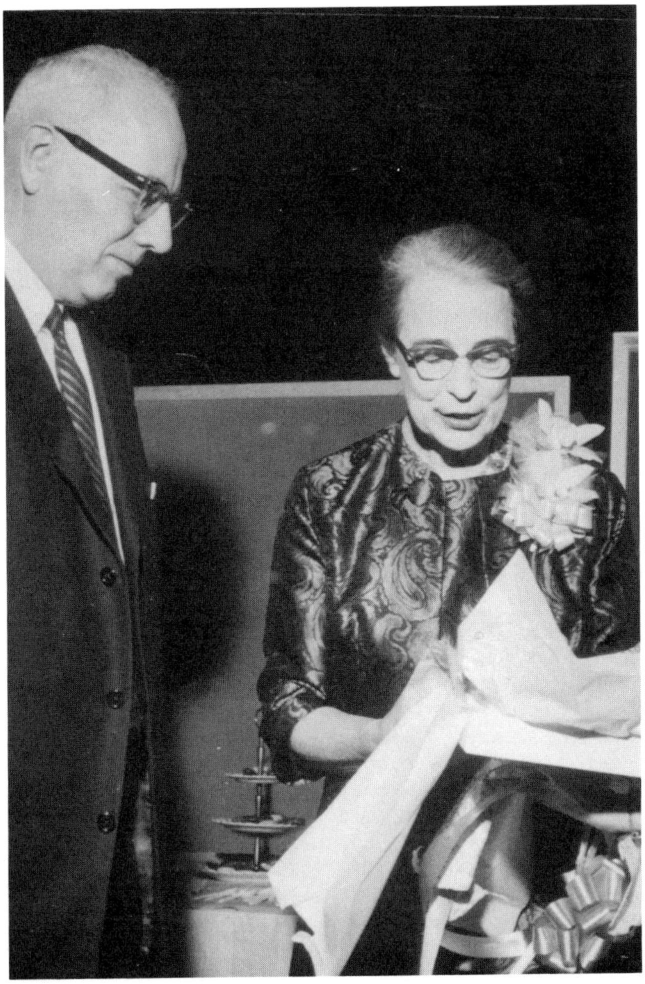

Fig. V.: Dr. Evelyn Anderson receiving an award from Dr. Bates.

found that the precipition titre rose earlier than the anti-gonadotropin titre and inferred that these respective effects may depend on completely different substances.

Further, in order to test the hypothesis that only heterologous hormone would induce anti-hormone activity, Thompson found that ovine gonadotropic extracts failed to induce antihormone in sheep (13). In addition, Drs. DuShane and Witschi showed that when an ovariectomized rat remained in parabiosis with an intact female there resulted persistent ovarian hypertrophy and constant estrus in the intact partner for over a year (14). These and related studies established the principle that one needed a heterologous source of hormone to elicit antihormone formation. These phenomena were interpreted to indicate an analogy between antibody and antihormone.

This analogy was strengthed by the observation that the end-organ in question was not essential for antihormone formation. For it was shown that gonadectomy or thyroidectomy did not affect the antihormone titres produced after protacted administration of the respective hormones involved.

Contrarily, Werner found that highly purified preparations of ovine thyrotropin lacked the capacity to induce antihormone formation, although high titres were produced by less purified extracts (15). Moreover, for both thyrotropic and gonadotropic extracts it was apparent that although these respective hormonal potencies could be greatly concentrated by purification procedures, there was no proportional increment in antihormone induction. This led to the inference that the less pure preparations contained non-hormonal factors which serve to augment the attainable antihormone titres.

Another phenomenon which placed some doubt on the hypothesis that antihormone and antibody were identical was the finding that early in the course of gonadotropin treatment the serum of the treated animal would exhibit a marked "progonadotropic" effect (16,17,18,18a). This phenomenon was observed after administration of heterologous hormone to sheep, horses and dogs. The titre of this "progonadotropic" factor increased over a brief period of time and was soon replaced by an antihormone titre. The significance of this progonadotropic effect remains unclear and the phenomenon has not received notice in recent years.

The question arose early as to whether antihormones could affect the normal response of the ovary to endogenous pituitary gonadotropin. We demonstrated in parabiotic rats that antigonadotropic sera prepared in the rabbit against ovine pituitary extracts could prevent the expected hypertrophy of the ovaries of an intact female joined to a gonadectomized partner (19). Moreover, Kupperman and Meyer showed that daily treatment of rats from birth with antihormonal serum could completely prevent pubertal development of the ovary. However, when such passive immunization was stopped earlier a compensatory response of the previously inhibited pituitary led to the premature onset of pubertal ovarian activity (20). It thus became clear that the peripheral action of endogenous gonadotropin can be blocked by antihormonal sera. Also, cytological study of the pituitaries of rats in which such antihormone treatment had arrested ovarian function exhibited the characteristic cellular evidence of increased hormonal storage in the gonadotropin producing cells of the pituitary (20a).

These effects on endogenous hormone spurred much speculation as to the therapeutic potential of antihormones in controlling hyperhormonal states. A related consideration was the possiblity of antihormonal use for interruption of pregnancy. A most impressive study in this regard was carried out by Dr. K.W. Thompson in 1939 (21). He chose the dog since it had been shown that in the dog pregnancy is interrupted at any stage by hypophysectomy (22). The antiserum used was prepared by adminstering an ovine gonadotropic extract to a dog for 3½ years. A control serum was obtained from a normal adult male dog. The data from this study are presented as originally published in Table I. It will be seen that in 13 of 13 instances prompt abortion was induced by the intravenous administration of from 5 to 10 cc of the antiserm and no abortion occured in three animals treated initially with like amounts of normal serum.

Table I: Induction of abortion in dogs by antigonadotropic serum. See Reference 21.

PROTOCOL[1]

| Experiment No. | Identification of dogs | Stage of pregnancy at time of labor | Treatment given | Day of treatment when labor occurred | State of fetuses |
|---|---|---|---|---|---|
| 1 | 299 | last half | *Antihormone* 5 cc. i.v. 2/d, 3½ d; Total 35 cc. | 3rd and 4th days | 10 dead |
| 2 | 300 | last half | *Antihormone* 5 cc. s.c., 1/d, 3 d; 10 cc. s.c., 1/d, 4 d; 10 cc. i.v., 1/d, 1 d; Total 65 cc. | 9th day | 1 dead, 3 survived and were raised. |
| 3 | 300 and abortion | 49th day | *Antihormone* 5 cc. i.v., 2/d, 2½ d; Total 25 cc. | 3rd day | 4 died soon after birth. |
| 4 | 301 | last half | *Antihormone* 5 cc. i.v., 2/d, 2½ d; Total 25 cc. | 3rd day | 5 found dead. |
| 5 | 301 and abortion | 52nd day | *Antihormone* 5 cc. i.v., 2/d, 3 d; Total 30 cc. | 4th day | Fetuses eaten during night. |
| 6 | 316 | last half | *Antihormone* 5 cc. i.v., 2/d, 3 d; Total 30 cc. | 4th day | 4 seen alive, 4 dead; all died prematurely. |
| 7 | 306 | last half | *Antihormone* 10 cc. i.v., 2/d, 2 d; Total 40 cc. | 3rd day | Fetuses eaten during night. |
| 8 | *Dr. T.'s* dog 1 | 47th day | *Antihormone* 10 cc. i.v., 1/d, 3 d; 7 cc. i.v., 1/d, 1 d; Total 37 cc. | 4½ days | Fetuses eaten during night. |
| 9 | *Dr. T.'s* dog 2 | last half X-ray showed 1 fetus | *Antihormone* 5 cc. i.m., 2/d, 4 d; 10 cc. i.v., 2/d, 6 d; Total 160 cc. | 10th day | 1 fetus died soon after birth. |
| 10 | *Dr. C.'s* dog 1 | last half | *Antihormone* 5 cc. i.v., 2/d, 2½ d; Total 25 cc. | 3rd day | Fetuses eaten. |
| 11 | *Dr. C.'s* dog 2 | last half | *Antihormone* 5 cc. i.v., 2/d, 2 d; Total 20 cc. | 3rd day | Fetuses died, soon after delivery. |
| 12 | *Dr. C.'s* dog 3 | last half | *Normal Serum* 5 cc. i.v., 2/d, 4 d; Total 80 cc. | did not abort; normal delivery 2 wk. later | 2 normal pups at term. |
| 13 | *Cocker spaniel* (pathol.) | 43d day | *Normal Serum* 10 cc. i.v., 2/d, 4 d; Total 80 cc. in 7 days no effect; *Antihormone* 10 cc. i.v., 2/d, 3 d; Total 60 cc. | 4th day after antihormone | Fetuses eaten. |
| 14 | *Tan mongrel* (pathol.) | 54th day | *Normal Serum* 10 cc. i.v., 2/d, 4 d; Total 80 cc. in 7 days no effect; *Antihormone* 10 cc. 2/d, 3 d; Total 60 cc. | 4th day after antihormone | Fetuses eaten. |

[1] The following abbreviations are used: i.v.—intravenously; i.m.—intramuscularly; s.c.—subcutaneously; d—day; /d—per day; cc.—cubic centimeters.

Yet another aspect of the early studies even with admittedly crude preparations merits consideration. In no instance did we observe the persistance of antihormonal titres for prolonged periods of time. In the rabbit, recovery of sensitivity to both endogenous and exogenous gonadotropin occured in from 90 to 120 days in previously refractory animals (23). In the rhesus monkey similar recovery in terms of menstrual function and fertility was regularly observed (23). In fact, in both of these species the maintenance of antihormone titres without constant hormonal administration proved very difficult.

The foregoing studies are cited not only out of historical interest but also for their possible significance for our current efforts in the field of hormonal immunology of contraception.

First, the question of the purity of the antigen with respect to antigenic potential. Of course, it must be fully appreciated that with lesser purity of antigen one should expect to lose specificity of antibody, thereby predisposing the host to potentially unwanted side effects. However, the data cited above indicate no grossly apparent deleterious effects on the immunized animals. Perhaps a cautious experimental study in primates of the response and toxicology to less pure but hopefully more potent antigens, with due emphasis on the problem of non-specific cross-reactions, may prove of practical value in arriving at more effective titres without harm.

The detection of a possible progonadtropic phase during antibody production should be reviewed for both scientific and practical reasons.

Lastly, doubts have been raised concerning the potential reversibility of immunologically induced infertility. The foregoing evidence suggests that rather than irreversibility, a practical problem may prove to be the periodic waning of antihormonal titres over time.

In closing, may I thank the organizers of this symposium for their kind consideration in permitting this brief retrospective but hopefully instructive discourse.

## REFERENCES

1. Zondek, B. Die hormone des ovarioams und des hypophysenvorder lappens. Springer, Berlin, 1931.
2. Hirose, T. Exogenous stimulation of corpus luteum formation in the rabbit; influence of extracts of human placenta, decidua and hydatidiform mole. J. Japanese Gynecological Society, 16:1055, 1920
3. Fevold, H.L., Hisaw, F.L. and Leonard, S.L. The gonad-stimulating and the luteinizing hormones of the anterior lobe of the hypophysis. Am. J. Physiol., 97:291, 1931.
4. Hertz, R. and Hisaw, F.L. Effects of follicule-stimulating and luteinizing pituitary extracts on the ovaries of the infantile and juvenile rabbit. Am. J. Physiol., 108:1, 1934.
5. Selye, H. Collip, J.B., and Thomson, D.L. loss of sensitivity to anterior-pituitary-like hormone of pregnancy urine. Proc. Soc. Exp. Biol. and Med., 31:487, 1934.
6. Selye, H., Collip, J.B., and Thomson, D.L. Loss of sensitivity to the gonadotropic hormone of the hypophysis. Proc. Soc. Exp. Biol. and Med., 31:566, 1934.
7. Collip, J.B. and Anderson, E.M. The production of serum inhibitory to the thyrotropic hormone. Lancet 226:76, 1934.
8. Selye, H., Bachman, C., Thomson, D.L., and Collip, J.B. Further studies on loss of sensitivity to anterior-pituitary-like hormone, Proc. Soc. Exp. Biol. and Med., 31:1113, 1934.
9. Meyer, R.K. and Gustus, E.L. Refractoriness to ovarian stimulation in rhesus monkey. Science, 81:208, 1935.
10. Collip, J.B. Anterior pituitary hormones and anti-hormones. Trans. Am. Neurol. Assn., 1935, p. 7.
11. Schafer, E.A. The endocrine organs. Longmans, Green & Co., London, 1916.
12. Meyer, R.K. and Wolfe, H.R. Gonadotropic inhibitory substance and precipitins in the blood of monkeys receiving gonadotropic hormone preparations. J. Immunol., 37:91, 1939.
13. Thompson, K.W. Inability of sheep to develop antihormone to the gonadotropic hormone from sheep-pituitary glands. Proc. Soc. Exp. Biol., 35:634, 1937.

14. Du Shane et. al. Experimental "constant estrus" and notion of antigonadotropic hormones. Proc. Soc. Exp. Biol., 33:339, 1935.
15. Werner, S.C. Prolonged injection of a thyrotropic extract without development of refractoriness. Proc. Soc. Exp. Biol., 34:390, 1936.
16. Thompson, K.W. The augmentary factor in animal sera after injections of pituitary extract. Proc. Soc. Exp. Biol., 35:640, 1937.
17. Rowlands, I.W. Progonadotropic sera. Proc. Roy. Soc., 13-124:492, 1938.
18. Rowlands, I.W. Further observations on the progonadotropic and antithyrotropic activity of anti sera to extracts of the anterior pituitary gland. J. Endocrinology, 1:177, 1939.
18a. Katzman, P.A., Wade, H.J., and Doisy, E.A. Progonadotropic sera of animals treated with hypophyseal extracts. Endocrinology, 25:554, 1939.
19. Kupperman, H.S., Meyer, R.K., and Hertz, R. The effect of antigonadotropic sera upon gonadotropic secretion in parabiotic rats. Endocrinology, 24:115, 1939.
20. Meyer, R.K. and Kupperman, H.S. Hypersecretion of gonadotropic hormone of pituitary gland of rats resulting from treatment with antigonadotropic serum. Proc. Soc. Exp. Biol., 42:285, 1939.
21. Thompson, K.W. The termination of pregnancy of dogs by gonadotropic antihormone. Endocrinology, 24:613, 1939.
22. Votquenne, M. Hypophysectomy and pregnancy in the dog. Compt. Rend. Soc. de Biol., 122:91, 1936.
23. Hertz, R. Unpublished data.

# IMMUNOLOGICAL APPROACHES TO CONTRACEPTION: THE NEED, BASIC PREMISE, AND OVERVIEW

G.P. Talwar

Scholar-in-Residence
John E. Fogarty International Center
for Advanced Studies in Health Sciences
National Institutes of Health
Bethesda, Maryland

The world population is increasing at a rapid pace. It stood at one billion in 1830, the next billion was attained in 1930, the third in 1957, the fourth in 1979 and at current projections the figure is expected to pass the six billion mark by the year 2000. In the closing two decades of this century, half as many more people will be added to the global habitation as the number accumulated since the origin of man until the year 1980. This rate of expansion is bound to impose considerable strain on resources such as food, housing, jobs, and other social amenities; especially because 90 percent of the increase will be in economically developing countries.

A number of effective methods are available for family planning, and these have been sucessfully employed in many countries. There is need however to develop additional methods for fertility control. Immunological approaches are attractive from several points of view. They require only periodic intake. They are free from user failure risk. They are physiological in the sense that immunological methods mobilize the body's own machinery without the requirement of constant medication with synthetic compounds. Immunization will no doubt require injection of the antigen, but the amount administered is small (microgram or milligram quantities of proteins), and that too at periodic intervals.

## Rationale

The basis of immuno-contraception is to intercept fertility by means of antibodies combining with and inactivating a hormone or a reproductive tract protein important for success of reproduction. Active immunization leads to not only the elicitation of humoral antibody response but also to cell mediated immunity (CMI). CMI may play a part in the overall effect. Critical evidence is however available for the role of antibodies only, by virtue of the demonstration that passive administration of antibodies leads to interception of fertility. Adoptive immunity experiments with cells have not been reported. Antibodies could nonetheless entail cellular participation by mechanisms such as the antibody dependent cellular cytotoxicity (ADCC). Antibodies act by direct binding with the target molecules, as for example anti hormonal antibody neutralizing the bioactivity of a hormone. Antibodies directed against membrane associated antigens may entail complement activation.

## Feasibility

Cases have been described in literature where the cause of infertility was ascribed to immunological factors (for references see (1)). No other clinical abnormality was noted in these cases besides of course those associated with reproductive failure. The mechanism by which these subjects developed antibodies is not clear. The presence of auto-antigens on gametes is recognized. These are normally sequestered in a compartment where sensitization of the immune system does not take place. A breakdown of the barrier could lead to auto-immune response and long term, if not irreversible infertility. For reversible contraception this has to be avoided.

Experimentally, immunization has been carried out with a variety of antigens in laboratory animals and in subhuman primates. With the production of antibodies in adequate amounts it has been repeatedly demonstrated that animals become infertile. Work on these antigens will be reviewed in the present symposium. Immunization against most antigens, especially when these are conjugated to carriers, has given rise to a reversible response. Antibodies decline in course of time and animals regain fertility. Immunological interception is thus conceivable as an approach for fertility regulation.

## Antibody Mediated Control of Fertility

Active immunization of animals leads to statistically significant reduction of fertility. However, a clear proof of the efficacy of antibodies is offered by passive immunization experiments. An example is cited of one of our previous studies (2). Antibodies were raised in monkeys with the vaccine Pr-β-hCG-TT. Regularly cycling baboons were mated with males of proven fertility, the onset of conception was confirmed by appearance of chorionic gonadotropin (CG) in circulation and by rise of blood progesterone. At this stage the monkey anti Pr-β-hCG-TT were injected to baboons, which led to a fall in circulating CG levels and progesterone, followed by termination of pregnancy (2). Immunoglobulins from non-immunized monkeys given in the same amount failed to abort pregnancy. Baboons terminated in a previous cycle by anti Pr-β-hCG-TT antibodies conceived again on mating in a subsequent cycle indicating the reversibility of the procedure. Pregnancy was carried to term and the progeny born was normal in every respect. Follow-up data for over 5 years is available on developmental landmarks of the babies born to baboons previously rendered infertile by active or passive immunization and no significant difference is observable between the progeny born to control and earlier immunized animals. Some baboons in this series have attained or are nearing adulthood. Studies would continue to determine the normalcy or otherwise of their reproductive functions.

Passive termination of pregnancy with anti OLH serum has also been reported in monkeys (3), with anti β-hCG sera in marmosets (4) and baboons (5). Preliminary experiments indicate the efficacy of a monoclonal anti hCG antibody in the chimpanzee. This monoclonal reacts equally well with hCG and β-hCG, it has low ($\leq 2\%$) cross-reaction with hLH but it does not recognize the carboxyterminus peptides of β-hCG (6).

## Safety of Active Immunization

Toxicology studies have been carried out by the Population Council, the Indian Council of Medical Research and by the World Health Organization Task Force on three different vaccines inducing antibodies against hCG and on two vaccines based on immunization with β-OLH and a combination of β-OLH and β-hCG. No contra-indications were given by these studies on safety of the vaccines. One vaccine, Pr-β-hCG-TT has also undergone phase I clinical trials in six centres located in five countries. The anitbody response was reversible in each subject. No side effects were observed on hematological, endocrinological, metabolic and organ functions (7,8,9). These were however studies on a relatively small number of subjects. Side effects of low frequency will not be revealed by these early studies.

## Multiple Birth Control Vaccines Possible

Mammalian reproduction results from the unison of gametes contributed by male and female partners. Both sperm and egg have antigens disposed on membranes and accessible to antibodies. Some of them are unique and serologically specific to the gametes. Conception is followed by the early embryo producing products, some of which like hCG are not only diagnostic markers of pregnancy, but have also a vital role in establishment and progression of early pregnancy. Early embryo has "stage" antigens cross-reactive with some tumours which disappear with further development of embryo. These are also potentially interesting antigens but their workability as target antigens for fertility control has not been demonstrated. The production and maturation of sperm and egg and preparation of accessory reproductive organs is under the control of 3 sets of hormones, the hypothalamic decapeptide GnRH regulating the secretion of pituitary gonadotrophins; the gonatropins FSH and LH and the sex steroid hormones produced by the gonads. The effect of immunization against these hormones will be discussed in the symposium and forms the subject of other papers in this volume (Table 1).

GnRH is theoretically usable in both males and females, being the same molecule in the two cases. Its structure is conserved in the course of evolution. Anti GnRH immunization thus has also potential application in veterinary species, for instance for control of estrus in dogs (10) and for meat raising cattle (11). Medical applications in control of percocious puberty (12) and in hormone dependant cancers(13) are also conceivable as an alternate to treatment with LHRH agonists.

Dr. Moudgil will present his studies showing the lowering of sperm count and fertility in bonnet monkeys on immunization with ovine FSH. Dr. Nieschlag who has not been able to come to the meeting has also carried out long-term studies with FSH in rhesus monkeys. He observes initially a lowering of sperm count, but a return in course of time inspite of circulating FSH neutralizing antibodies. Are the differences between these two studies due to the species of monkeys utilized by them or are there innate mechanisms which release spermatogenesis from dependance on FSH? Further studies are required with this antigen, perferably in another primate species.

It is not long back that immunization against LH was not considered appropriate in the female, as it was expected to lead to impairment of ovulation. The consequences of constant cross-reaction with a physiological hormone and of immune complexes on kidney and pituitary were also of concern. Dr. Rose Marie Thau will describe her work, where a large number of rhesus monkeys were hyperimmunized with β subunit of ovine LH for a period lasting up to 7 years. No pathology of pituitary or other organs

Table 1. Reproductive System Hormones and Constituents under Immunological Investigation for Fertility Regulation

| Category | | Antigen | Remarks |
|---|---|---|---|
| Hormones | | GnRH | Applicable to both sexes Veterinary & Medical Applications |
| | | LH | Partial Neutralization Effective for Female Fertility Control in Primates |
| | | FSH | Usable only for Male |
| | | hCG | Development Most Advanced; Three vaccines going for Phase I Clinical Trials |
| | | Steroids | Promotion of Fertility |
| Gametes | | $LDH-C_4$ | Best Characterized Sperm Antigen |
| | Sperm | About 10-12 Epitopes Specific to Sperm | Recently identified by Monoclonals; several Cross-reactive with other species |
| | Egg | Zona Pellucida | In Rabbits Ovarian Follicular Atresia; in Monkey Reversibility but Hormonal Disturbances |
| Embryo | | Stage Antigens Trophoblast Constituents | Under Study |

was noticed on autopsy. The animals kept ovulating in spite of antibody titres high enough to render the animals infertile. Presumably the antibodies did not scavenge completely LH. Partial interference with hormonal activity produced a deficient corpus luteum with diminished output of progesterone and elevated FSH levels. The actual antifertility action of antibodies turned out to be different than the initial theoretical expectations. Apprehensions of pathological hazards of cross-reactive antibodies against a circulating hormone have been removed to a great extent by these studies. The implications of shortened luteal phase and diminished progesterone output over long periods must however be assessed.

Vaccines against the human chorionic gonadotropin are the most advanced. Four prototypes would be under Phase I clinical trials this year. The immunogen developed by the WHO Task Force is based on a carboxyterminus peptide of 37 amino acids of the beta subunit of hCG, linked to diptheria toxoid. The vaccine requires the use of an MDP derivative, emulsifier and oily vehicle. Dr. David Griffin will present the current status of work on this vaccine on behalf of the WHO Task Force. The International Committee on Contraception Research of the Population Council will renew Phase I clinical trials on βhCG-TT vaccine at different doses and injection schedules. We will start initially in India and later elsewhere, trials on two candidate vaccines which in primates have shown better immunogenicity than our earlier vaccine, β-hCG-TT. The basis for choice of these formulations will be evident from the data that will be presented by Dr. N.C. Sharma and myself. Within the next 18 months information on the relative merits of these vaccines with respect to their ability to induce antibodies in women without disturbance of hormonal profiles, clinical chemistry parameters and tissue reactive antibodies will be available. The decision point however will be the Phase II efficacy trials, which should follow these Phase I studies.

## Take home Lessons from the First Phase I Trial

The first candidate birth control vaccine Pr-β-hCG-TT (immunochemically purified beta subunit of hCG linked to tetanus toxoid) was tested in 63 subjects at a single dose (80 μg equivalent of β-hCG) and injection schedule (4 injections at fortnightly intervals). 61 subjects responded with formation of antibodies against hCG and tetanus toxoid (7,8,9,12). In every case the response was reversible and antibodies declined to near zero levels in course of time. The duration was variable but was of 300-500 days in the case of good responders. Challenge with repeated doses of hCG showed that antibodies recognized and bound with the hormone rendering it inactive in Leydig cell bioassay. Administration of hCG did not lead to a booster effect on antibody titres, for which the carrier conjugated subunit was required. Immunization did not inhibit ovulation. Menstrual cycles remained regular with normal progesterone profiles. Other endocrine and metabolic functions were undisturbed (13,14). No autoimmune or tissue reactive activity was discernible (15). The main limitation of this vaccine given at the dosage and with the adjuvant employed (alum) was the wide variation in antibody titres among the recipients, with the short duration of response in low responders. Given that the antibody is the effective agent, an acceptable birth control vaccine must induce titres above the efficacy threshold. Additional or better adjuvants may be necessary. Genetic influences on immunological responsiveness are recognized, but ways and means will have to be evolved to overcome the variations in antibody titres due to constitutional factors. This problem is particular to antifertility vaccines.

## Adjuvants

Alum has been the adjuvant traditionally employed in communicable diseases vaccines and is approved for human use in all countries. Lipopolysaccharides (LPS) from gram negative bacteria, such as Salmonella, E. coli, are powerful stimulators of antibody response, but are pyrogenic and toxic. Succinyl and pthalyl derivatives of LPS have drastically reduced toxicity and pyrogenicity, but adjuvanticity is retained. A human clinical trial with sodium pthalyl derivative of LPS (SPLPS) has been carried out in USA without ill effects. Muramyl dipeptide (MDP) was identified as the minimal structure in mycobacterial cell wall for adjuvant activity (16). MDP is pyrogenic and also has toxicity problem; however a large number of chemical derivatives of MDP have been synthesized by academic and industrial research laboratories. Many of them have high adjuvanticity. These will be discussed by Dr. Harold Nash and David Griffin in the Symposium. The state of the art in this field enables the inclusion, if necessary, of adjuvants and vehicles which can raise the antibody response by several fold as compared to the titres obtained with alum.

## Improvement of Intrinsic Immunogenicity

Although potent adjuvants are now available, their use in repeated injections may not be devoid of additional side effects. Adjuvant arthritis is a known phenomenon. Some adjuvants are B cell mitogens. Oil, squalene and emulsifiers may produce severe local inflamation. It will be beneficial to "tailor" the antigen in a manner such as to achieve optimum intrinsic immunogencity. One way is to get rid of the "suppressor" determinants in the antigen. These will have to be explored. Another way may be to optimize desirable conformation innate in the molecule. With this idea in mind we annealed the beta subunit of hCG with alpha subunit of ovine LH. This takes place readily, the product has two-fold better steroidogenic potency in Leydig cell system than the homologous complex composed of human alpha and beta subunit of hCG. The gonadotrophins are constituted of two subunits and it is their association that generates the right conformation for binding to the tissue receptors and triggering of the biological effects. Dissociation of the subunits results in loss of the conformation, the alpha subunit has no activity and the β-hCG only 400-fold lower potency than the native hormone (17). The native hormone as an antigen produces better antibodies for bioefficacy, but the alpha subunit common with hTSH and hFSH can produce undesirable cross-reactions. Heterospecies alpha subunit would not have this hazard, hence the reason for taking α OLH-β-hCG. The annealed complex conjugated to tetanus toxoid produced ten-fold higher antibody response than β-hCG-TT in bonnet monkeys. The latent period for appearance of antibodies was also shorter. In rats α OLH-β-hCG-TT was eighteen-fold more immunogenic than β-hCG-TT. The antibodies were devoid of unwanted cross-reaction with hFSH and hTSH.

## Multi Carrier Strategy to Overcome Low Response

Linkage of the hormonal subunit to a carrier has proven to be effective in breaking immunological tolerance to a "self" protein (hCG) as indicated by previous clinical trials. In experimental animals such as mice and monkeys where β-hCG is a "non-self" protein, the immunogenicity of the peptide is enhanced by conjugation to a carrier. Tetanus toxoid is a good carrier, but it cannot be expected to evoke a universally high response from all. This has indeed been the observation in primates. Out of 20 bonnet monkeys immunized with tetanus conjugates, 8 were relative hypo-responders. Immunization of these animals with conjugates made with an alternate carrier, the cholera toxin B chain, resulted in high antibody titres. Use of more than one carrier may help in overcoming the deficient response of the subject to a given carrier. Besides tetanus and cholera toxin chain B, other useful carriers are diptheria toxin and hepatitis B surface protein. By diversifying the carrier, immunoprophylactic benefit can be attained for more than one health hazard enhancing the utility and acceptability of such vaccines. Sporozoite coat protein of P. Falciparum should also be evaluated in this context.

## The Next Generation Vaccines Are Likely To Be Polyvalent

A case has been made for use of more than one carrier. It may also be advantageous to employ more than one hormonal peptide or reproductive system protein to ensure that antibodies are formed in each case intercepting fertility at one or the other point, if not at more than one point. This approach will enhance the efficacy of the vaccines. The second generation vaccines are expected to be multivalent containing more than one reproductive system antigen linked to more than one carrier. Vaccines against gonadotropins may combine determinants of β-hCG and β-OLH linked to tetanus and cholera chain B. A sperm antigen may further be additive. The best characterized sperm antigen at this time is the LDH-$C_4$. Dr. Goldberg will give the latest information on this antigen including the possibility of using a synthetic immunodominant subfragment of this enzyme. A number of other antigens of potential interest have been identified by monoclonal antibodies which will be covered by Dr. Nancy Alexander, Dr. Naz, Dr. Patricia Saling and Dr. Deborah Anderson. The 23 k (or 46 K dimer) of Dr. Naz appears to be of interest with his observation of high anti-fertility effect of antibodies against this glycoprotein. A number of monoclonals have recently been generated in our laboratory against human sperm. Four of them are of particular interest. They are specific, e.g., nonreactive with other cells of the body. Their epitopes are localized on different parts of the sperm; the MoAB $F_{11}G_1$ reacts with the tail only, MoAB $C_1$ with acrosome, MoAb $A_3$ with the equatorial region and tail, and MoAB 65PB$_6$ with all parts of the human sperm. Preliminary studies demonstrate the ability of the monoclonal antibody to block the fertilization of the zona denuded hamster eggs by the human sperm in vitro. Three of these monoclonals are cross-reactive with monkey and baboon sperm, which should enable the carrying out of investigations on the antifertility properites of these antibodies in primates. It is not unlikely that one or a combination of more than one of these sperm antigens may be of interest in the second generation polyvalent vaccines.

## References


1. G.P. Talwar, "Immunology of Contraception," a monograph, Edward Arnold Publishers, London (1980).
2. A. Tandon, C. Das. B.L. Jailkhani, and G.P. Talwar, Efficacy of antibodies generated by Pr-β-hCG-TT to terminate pregnancy in baboons its reversibility and rescue by medroxprogesterone acetate, Contraception, 24:83 (1981).
3. N.R. Moudgil, V.R. Mukku, S. Prahalada, G.S.R.C. Murty, and C.H. Li, Passive immunization with an antibody to the β subunit of ovine luteinizing hormone as a method of early abortion - a feasibility study in monkey (Macaca radiata), Fertil Steril, 30:223 (1978).
4. J.P. Hearn, Immunization against pregnancy, Proc. R. Soc., Lond. B. 195:149 (1976).
5. V.C. Stevens, "Antifertility effects from immunization with intact, subunits and fragments of hCG, in: "Physiological Effects of Immunity Against Reproductive Hormones," R.G. Edwards and M.H. Johnson, eds., Cambridge University Press, Cambridge (1976).

6. S.K. Gupta and G.P. Talwar, Development of hybridomas secreting anti human chorionic gonadotropin antibodies, Ind. J. Exp. Bio. 18:1361 (1980).
7. H. Nash, G.P. Talwar, S. Segal, T. Lukkainen, E.D.B. Johansson, J. Vasquez, E. Coutinho, and K. Sundaram, Observation on the antigenicity and clinical effects of a candidate antipregnancy vaccine: β subunit of human chorionic gonadotropin linked to tetanus toxoid, Fertil Steril, 34:328 (1980).
8. V. Hingorani and S. Kumar, Anti hCG immunization - phase I clinical trials, in: "Recent Advances in Reproduction and Regulation of Fertility," G.P. Talwar, ed., Elsevier North Holland Biomedical Press, Amsterdam (1979).
9. S.M. Shahani, P.P. Kulkarni, K.L. Patel, M. Salahuddin, C. Das, and G.P. Talwar, Clinical and immunological responses with Pr-β-hCG-TT vaccine, Contraception, 25:421 (1982).
10. G.P. Talwar, S.K. Gupta, V. Singh, D. Sahal, K.S.N. Iyer, and O. Singh, Bioeffective monoclonal antibody against the decapeptide gonadotropin releasing hormone: reacting determinant and action on ovulation and estrus suppression, Proc. Natl. Acad. Sci., USA, 82:1228 (1985).
11. H.M. Frazer, This Symposium.
12. G.P. Talwar, N.C. Sharma, S.K. Dubey, M. Salahuddin, C. Das, S. Ramakrishnan, S. Kumar, and V. Hingorani, Isoimmunization against human chorionic gonadotropin with conjugates of processed beta subunit of the hormone and tetanus toxoid, Proc. Natl. Acad. Sci., USA 73:218 (1976).

# LACK OF TOXICOLOGICAL EFFECTS FOLLOWING SEVEN YEARS OF ACTIVE IMMUNIZATION OF RHESUS MONKEYS WITH THE β-SUBUNIT OF OVINE LUTEINIZING HORMONE

R.B. Thau[1], M.G. Bond[2], S.S. Witkin[3], K. Sundaram[1], and Janet K. Sawyer[2]

The Population Council[1] and Cornell University Medical College[3], New York, NY, and Bowman Gray School of Medicine[2], Winston Salem, NC

## ABSTRACT

Immunization of rhesus monkeys against the β-subunit of ovine luteinizing hormone (oLHβ) reduced fertility but did not prevent ovulation or interrupt regular menstrual cycles. The mechanism(s) of antifertility action involves impaired luteal function and/or failure of chorionic gonadotropin to stimulate the corpus luteum. Because of the significant cross reaction of the oLHβ-antibodies with serum LH and a moderate increase in circulating immune complexes, we investigated the effects of immunization on atherosclerotic lesions in ten monkeys which had been immunized for seven years and were fed a diet containing cholesterol (0.33 mg/kcal) during the last year. Ten non-immunized control monkeys were fed the same diet. The diet caused a significant increase in serum cholesterol levels in both groups of animals. Arterial characteristics such as plaque area, which can be used as indicators of the extent and/or severity of atherosclerosis, were measured in coronary and carotid arteries. Statistical analysis showed no significant differences between immunized and non-immunized groups, indicating that long-term immunization against pregnancy had no adverse effects on the extent and severity of atherosclerosis in hypercholesteremic monkeys.

## INTRODUCTION

We have previously shown that active immunization against the β-subunit of ovine luteinizing hormone (oLHβ) prevented pregnancy in rhesus monkeys, but did not interfere with ovulation and regular menstrual cycles (1-3). The anti-oLHβ antibodies showed significant cross reaction with rhesus LH (4). Preliminary observations indicated that long-term immunization against oLHβ was associated with a moderate increase in circulating immune complex (CIC) concentrations and a thickening of the intima in the arteries in some of the animals (5). The possible adverse effects of CICs on the arterial wall and other tissues raise major concerns about the safety of contraceptive methods based on long-term immunization. This prompted us to carry out a more defined study in long-term immunized monkeys and to manipulate the diet to accentuate arterial damage. We now report the effects of immunization on CIC concentrations and on atherosclerotic lesions in ten monkeys which had been immunized for seven years and were fed during the last year a diet moderately high in cholesterol content. Non-immunized, age-matched monkeys were fed the same diet and served as controls.

## MATERIALS AND METHODS

Multiparous female rhesus monkeys (Macaca mulatta) with regular menstrual cycles were housed and maintained as previously described (3). oLHβ (HSN-6-26B2), dissolved in saline and emulsified with an equal volume of Freunds complete adjuvant (FCA), was used as antigen. Incomplete Freunds adjuvant (FIA) was used for booster injections (2) administered once or twice per year (Fig. 1). During the six year period after immunization the monkeys were used in several studies to investigate the immunological and endocrinological effects of the vaccination (4,6-8). Between June and August of 1982 ten immunized monkeys and ten non-immunized controls were placed on a diet high in cholesterol (0.33 mg/kcal) (Bio-Serv, Inc., Frenchtown, NJ).

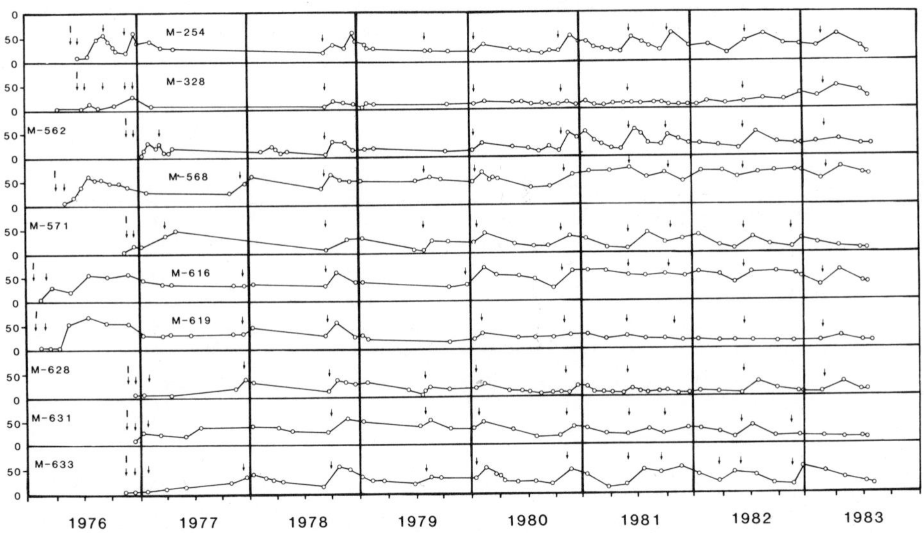


Fig. 1: Antibody titers in 10 rhesus monkeys. Ordinate shows percent of 0.2 ng [$^{125}$I]-hCG bound by 2 µl of serum at 1:400 final dilution. I: primary immunization. Arrows indicate booster injections.

Blood was collected monthly from the saphenous vein for determination of serum antibody titers (2). Serum cholesterol, triglycerides, HDL-cholesterol and CICs were assayed at 3 month intervals. Cholesterol and triglycerides were determined with the Auto Analyzer II as described by Rush et al. (9). HDL-cholesterol was assayed after precipitation of LDL- and VLDL-cholesterol. CICs were analyzed by the Raji cell assay adapted to an enzyme-linked immunosorbent assay (10). The animals were euthanized using an overdose of Nembutal. Tissues for examination of the cardiovascular system (left anterior descending artery: LAD; left circumflex artery: LCX; right coronary artery: RCA; and left and right common carotid arteries: LC and RC) were removed by blunt dissection and treated as previously described (5). Microscopic slide images of the tissue slices were projected on the active surface of a sonic digitizer interfaced with a minicomputer and cross-sectional intimal area was determined by integration.

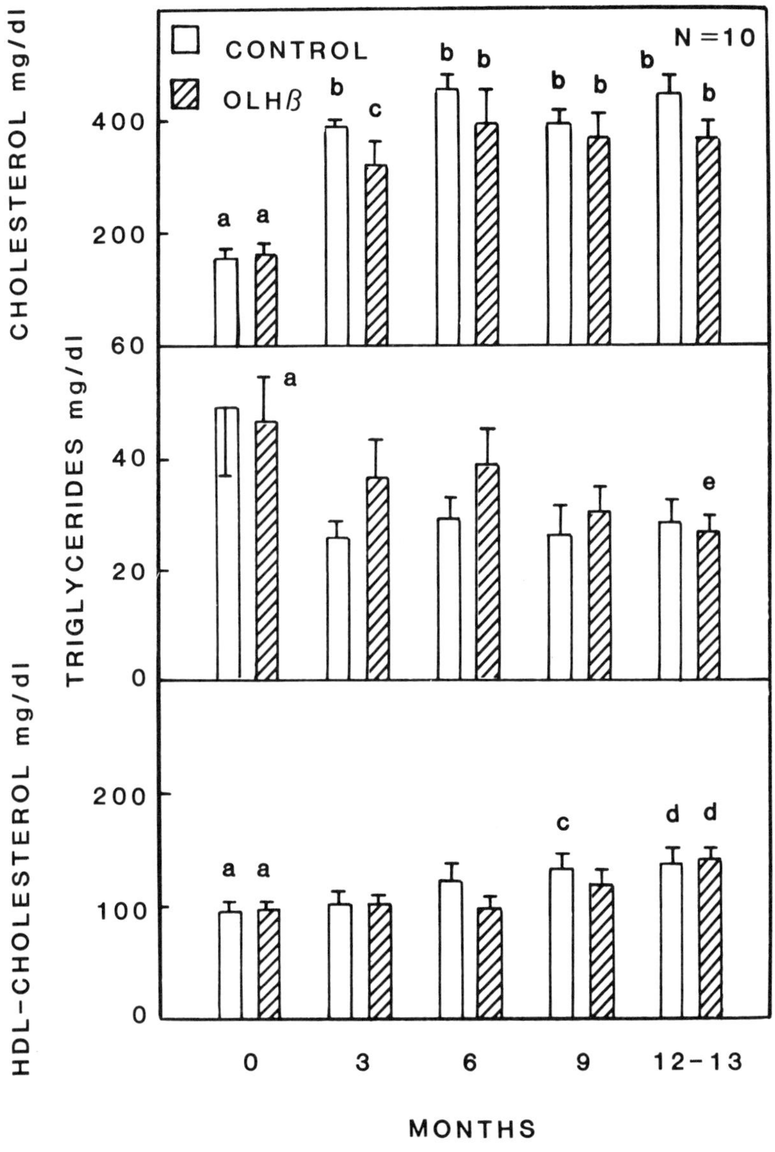


Fig. 2: Serum cholesterol, triglycerides and HDL-cholesterol (mean ± SE) before and during the elevated cholesterol diet. Students t-test: a/b, $p < 0.001$; a/c, $p < 0.005$; a/d, $p < 0.01$; a/e, $p < 0.05$.

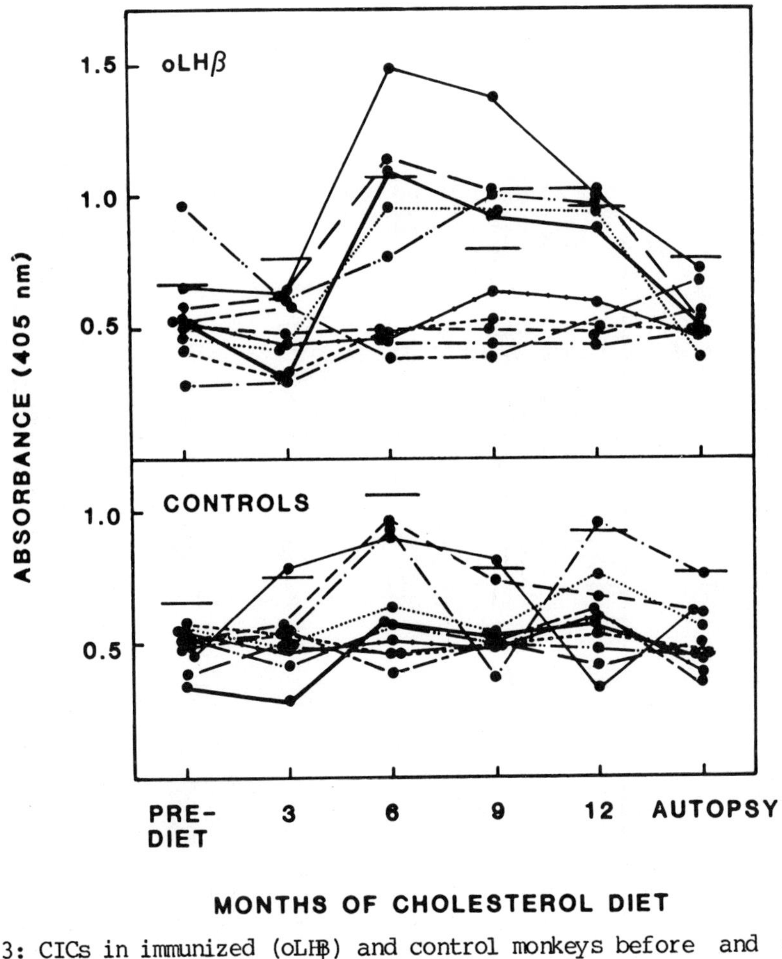


Fig. 3: CICs in immunized (oLHβ) and control monkeys before and during the elevated cholesterol diet. The straight line in the upper and lower panel depicts mean + 2 SD of controls.

Statistical analysis: For comparisons between the two groups (immunized and control), non-parametric methods (Mann-Whitney test) were used. Correlation analysis was carried out using the BMDp6d statistical package (11). Total intimal areas of the three coronary arteries (LAD+LCX+RCA) or of the two carotid arteries (RC+LC) were correlated with the four independent variables which could have caused intimal thickening (antibody titers, CICs, serum cholesterol or age of the monkeys).

RESULTS

Mean serum cholesterol levels were 154 ± 9 mg/dl (mean ± SE, n=10) for controls and 168 ± 12 mg/dl for immunized monkeys before the start of the cholesterol diet. Three, 6, 9, and 12 months later they were significantly increased ($p < 0.005$) in both groups. HDL-cholesterol levels also were significantly higher after 9 to 12 months while serum triglyceride concentration decreased (Fig. 2).

CIC levels varied substantially among monkeys and for individual monkeys throughout the year. Mean values for control and immunized animals did not differ significantly at any time point. If two standard deviations of the mean value obtained from the control monkeys in the CIC assay is defined as the boundary between specific reactivity and background level, then one immunized and no control monkey had CIC levels above normal before initiation of the cholesterol diet. During the diet a total of five immunized and two control animals showed elevated CIC concentrations at sometime, but no monkey had consistently elevated CIC levels. All CICs determined from plasma collected at autopsy were within normal range (Fig. 3). Mean values for CICs and antibody titers for each monkey over the year of the study were used for correlation analysis. No significant correlation between the two variables was observed (Fig. 4).

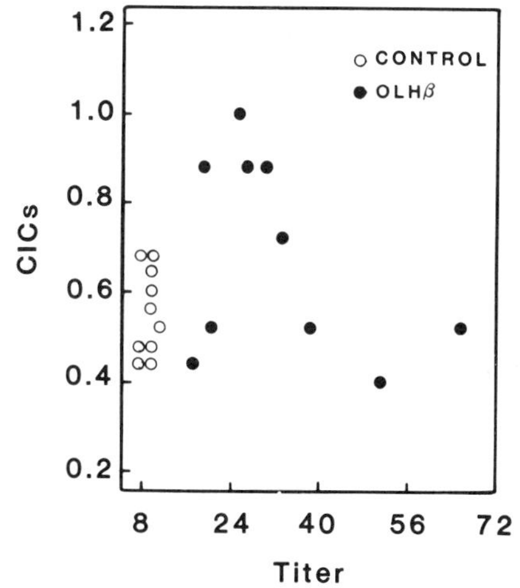


Fig. 4: Scatter plot for mean CIC concentration (absorbance at 405 nm) of each monkey versus mean antibody titer (percent [$^{125}$I]-hCG bound) during the elevated cholesterol diet.

Table 1. Summary of Independent Variables (Age, Titer, Serum Cholesterol, and CIC) and Total Intimal Area of Carotid and Coronary Arteries

| Monkey Number | Age (Years) | Antibody Titers (%) | Mean Serum Cholesterol (mg/dl) | Mean CICs (O.D. 405) | IntCarot[a] ($mm^2$) | IntCoron[b] ($mm^2$) |
|---|---|---|---|---|---|---|
| Controls | | | | | | |
| 425 | 16 | 9 | 360 | 0.497 | 0.01 | 0.01 |
| 572 | 16 | 10 | 352 | 0.480 | 0.01 | 0.02 |
| 579 | 17 | 10 | 407 | 0.667 | 0.10 | 0.08 |
| 670 | 15 | 10 | 721 | 0.669 | 1.04 | 0.11 |
| 680 | 17 | 9 | 467 | 0.587 | 0.08 | 0.01 |
| 687 | 15 | 10 | 407 | 0.569 | 0.06 | 0.03 |
| 696 | 17 | 10 | 432 | 0.455 | 0.02 | 0.18 |
| 698 | 17 | 11 | 362 | 0.512 | 0.00 | 0.01 |
| 706 | 17 | 10 | 290 | 0.458 | 0.21 | 0.07 |
| 723 | 15 | 10 | 469 | 0.649 | 0.02 | 0.00 |
| Immunized | | | | | | |
| 254 | 18 | 39 | 300 | 0.527 | 0.05 | 0.02 |
| 328 | 18 | 25 | 494 | 0.983 | 0.11 | 0.16 |
| 562 | 17 | 34 | 254 | 0.715 | 0.12 | 0.10 |
| 68 | 15 | 66 | 284 | 0.518 | 0.12 | 0.05 |
| 571 | 17 | 18 | 369 | 0.457 | 0.01 | 0.06 |
| 616 | 15 | 51 | 400 | 0.400 | 0.03 | 0.05 |
| 619 | 13 | 20 | 258 | 0.507 | 0.02 | 0.01 |
| 628 | 15 | 19 | 249 | 0.865 | 0.01 | 0.01 |
| 631 | 14 | 27 | 602 | 0.881 | 0.24 | 0.01 |
| 633 | 15 | 31 | 395 | 0.679 | 0.02 | 0.02 |

[a]Intimal area of carotid arteries (RC+LC).

[b]Intimal area of coronary arteries (LAD+LCX+RCA).

The data for intimal areas of the coronary arteries (LCX+LAD+RCA) and of the carotid arteries (RC+LC) are presented in Table 1. Correlation analysis of intimal areas versus antibody titers, CICs, serum cholesterol and age showed that there was no correlation with antibody titers or CICs. However, the size of the intima of the coronary arteries was significantly correlated with the age of the monkeys (Fig. 5), while intimal areas of the carotid arteries showed significant correlation with serum cholesterol levels (Fig. 6).

DISCUSSION

Contraceptive methods based on long-term immunization against hormones are a promising approach to fertility control. The possibility of immunopathological complications raised concerns about the safety of immunological methods of contraception (12,13). We have previously reported that rhesus monkeys immunized against oLHβ for five to six years had moderately elevated CICs, although no significant increase in vascular disease was found (5). We concluded from these results that a longer, more definitive study was necessary in which the diet was manipulated so that plasma cholesterol levels were elevated to accentuate

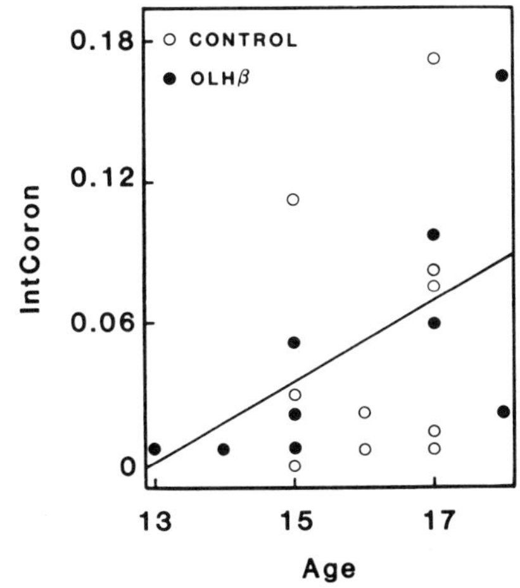


Fig. 5: Scatter plot for intimal areas ($mm^2$) of coronary arteries (LAD+LCX+RCA) versus age (yr) of monkeys. Immunized monkeys (oLHβ): r=0.670, $p < 0.02$; both groups: r=0.459, $p < 0.05$.

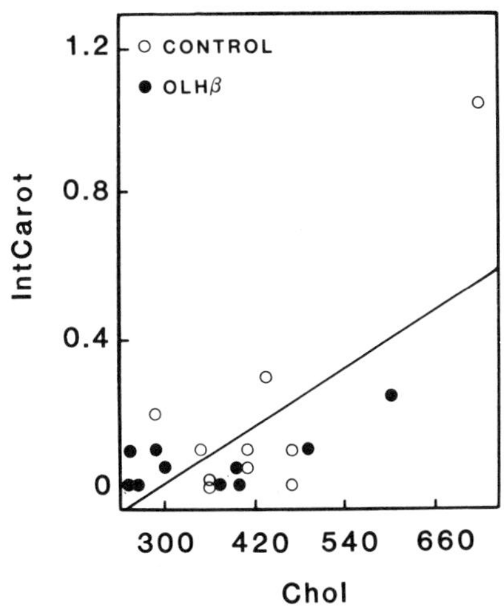


Fig. 6: Scatter plot for intimal areas ($mm^2$) of carotid arteries (LC+RC) versus mean serum cholesterol concentration (mg/dl) during the elevated cholesterol diet. Immunized monkeys (oLHβ): r=0.599, $p < 0.05$; controls: r=0.826, $p < 0.001$; both groups: r=0.693, $p < 0.001$.

the development of atheromatous arterial lesions. We now report that in spite of the fact that several of the ten monkeys immunized for seven years had slightly elevated concentrations of CICs, there was no correlation between antibody titers and CICs. In this study the adjuvants *per se* (FCA and FIA) may have been the cause of the intermittent increases in CICs in some of the monkeys. The animal model described here may constitute the worst possible situation that may arise if an immunological method of contraception is used and, therefore, provides a high probability of observing any adverse effects associated with the use of this method.

Cross-sectional intimal areas were measured at several arterial sites in immunized monkeys and non-immunized controls, maintained on an elevated cholesterol diet for one year. Statistical analyses showed no significant differences between the two experimental groups. Correlation analysis revealed that the plaque area of the coronary arteries correlated significantly with age which accounted for 21 to 45% of total variance. Serum cholesterol was the second most important independent variable. The plaque area of carotid arteries correlated significantly with serum cholesterol which accounted for 68 and 35% of the total variance for the immunized and control groups, respectively. No consistent correlations between arterial characteristics and antibody titers and/or CICs were observed.

We conclude from these findings that long-term immunization against pregnancy had no adverse effects on the extent and severity of atherosclerosis in hypercholesteremic monkeys.

ACKNOWLEDGEMENT

The authors are indebted to Dr. D.N. Ward, Department of Biochemistry, The University of Texas, System Cancer Center, M.D. Anderson Hospital, and Tumor Institute, Houston, Texas, for providing the β-subunit of ovine luteinizing hormone used for immunization, to Ms. Nina Ann Stokes of Bowman Gray Medical Center, Winston-Salem, North Carolina for the lipid analysis, to Dr. Y.Y. Tsong, The Population Council, for the human chorionic gonadotropin used for antibody titer determination, and to Ms. Jean Schweis for her skillful preparation of the manuscript. This work was undertaken as part of the contraceptive development program sponsored and coordinated by the International Committee for Contraception Research of The Population Council, Inc., New York. The financial support provided by the Ford Foundation, the International Development Research Centre of Canada, the U.S. Agency for International Development (Grant AID/pha 1116), the Rockefeller Foundation, and the George J. Hecht Fund is gratefully acknowledged. The content of this report does not necessarily reflect the policy of any of the funding sources.

REFERENCES

1. Thau, R.B. and Sundaram, K. The mechanism of action of an antifertility vaccine in the rhesus monkey: Reversal of the effects of antisera to the β-subunit of ovine luteinizing hormone by medroxyprogesterone acetate. *Fertil. Steril.* 33:317-320 (1980).

2. Thau, R.B., Sundaram, K., Thornton, Y.S., and Seidman, L.S. Effects of immunization with the β-subunit of ovine luteinizing hormone on corpus luteum function in the rhesus monkey. *Fertil. Steril.* 31:200-204 (1979).

3. Sundaram, K., Chang, C.C., Laurence, K.A., Brinson, A.O., Atkinson, L.E., and Segal, S.J. The effectiveness in rhesus monkeys of an antifertility vaccine based on neutralization of chorionic gonadotropin. *Contraception* 14:639-653 (1976).

4. Yamamoto, Y., Gunsalus, G.L., Sundaram, K., and Thau, R.B. Characterization of anti oLHβ-antibodies acting as contraceptives in rhesus monkeys. I. In vitro binding properties. J. Reprod. Immunol. 4:295-311 (1982).

5. Thau, R.B., Witkin, S.S., Bond, M.G., Sawyer, J.K., and Yamamoto, Y. Effects of long-term immunization against the β-subunit of ovine luteinizing hormone on circulating immune complex formation and on arterial changes in rhesus monkeys. Am. J. Reprod. Immunol. 3:83-88 (1983).

6. Spinola, P.G., Seidman, L.S., Sundaram, K., and Thau, R.B. Impaired steroidogenesis in the luteal phase of the reproductive cycle and during pregnancy in rhesus monkeys immunized with the β-subunit of ovine luteinizing hormone. J. Steroid. Biochem. 16:151-156 (1982).

7. Thau, R.B., Yamamoto, Y., Sundaram, K., and Spinola, P.G. Human chorionic gonadotropin stimulates luteal function in rhesus monkeys immunized against the β-subunit of ovine luteinizing hormone. Endocrinology 112:277-283 (1983).

8. Yamamoto, Y., Gunsalus, G.L., Sundaram, K., and Thau, R.B. Antibodies against the β-subunit of ovine luteinizing hormone can decrease the clearance of human chorionic gonadotropin in rhesus monkeys. Am. J. Reprod. Immunol. 5:164-170 (1984).

9. Rush, R.L., Leon, L., and Turrell, J. Automated simultaneous cholesterol and triglyceride determination on the Auto Analyzer III instrument. In: E. Barton (eds) Advances in Automated Analysis and Technicon International Congress. Futura Publishing Co. , Mt. Kisco, NY, pp 503-507 (1971).

10. Witkin, S.S., Zelikovsky, G., Bongiovanni, A.M., Geller, N., Good, G.A., and Day, N.K. Sperm-related antigens, antibodies and circulating immune complexes in sera of recently vasectomized men. J. Clin. Invest. 70:33-40 (1982).

11. Dixon, W.J. BMDP Statistical Software. University of California Press , Berkeley, CA(1983).

12. WHO Steering Committee on Immunological Methods. Clin. Exptl. Immunol. 33:360-375 (1978).

13. Tung, K.S.K. Antifertility vaccines: Considerations of their potential immunopathologic complications. Intl. J. Fertil. 21:197-206 (1976).

# REACTION OF A CHIMPANZEE TO IMMUNIZATION WITH oLHβ

N.R. Moudgal

Center for Advanced Research in Reproductive Biology
Laboratory of Endocrine Biochemistry
Department of Biochemistry
Indian Institute of Science
Bangalore 560 012, India

Based on the experiments of Thau and coworkers in the rhesus monkey, it is currently held that immunization of primates with oLHβ would lead to production of antibodies which would exhibit a greater degree of cross-reactivity with CG rather than LH. This apparently is responsible for oLHβ immunization having no effect on ovulation and luteal function of rhesus monkeys.

The results we have obtained using the bonnet monkey and the chimpanzee are at variance with that reported by Thau. Firstly we reported in 1978 [Moudgal, N.R., Mukku, V.R., Prahalada, S., Murty, G.S.R.C. and Li, C.H.- Passive immunization with an antibody to the β-subunit of ovine luteinizing hormone as a method of early abortion: a feasibility study in monkeys (Macaca radiata), Fert.Sterl. 30:223-229] that antisera (a/s) produced to oLHβ in bonnet monkeys when given to cycling bonnets is capable of blocking ovulation as well as luteinization. More recently, we immunized a chimpanzee with oLHβ and characterized the antiserum so produced for titer and cross-reactivity. The results essentially indicate the following:

- a: The chimpanzee responds to oLHβ immunization in a positive manner producing high titer antibodies.
- b: Using $^{125}$I hCG as the radioligand and the chimpanzee a/s to oLHβ as the source of antibody, it was observed that both hCG and chimpanzee CG cross-react to an equal extent. Perhaps this system could be used very conveniently to measure chimpanzee CG in serum.
- c: The ability of the antiserum to neutralize primate LH action was ascertained by administering 5 ml of a/s to cycling bonnet monkeys on day 18 of cycle. A single injection of the a/s brought about over 70-80% reduction in serum progesterone levels within 2h and this was maintained over the next 24h resulting in termination of cycle.
- d: The same volume of a/s when given to bonnet monkeys during early pregnancy (day 30-31 of cycle) brought about, once again drastic reduction in progesterone levels by 24h and this led to termination of pregnancy by 48-72h.

These results essentially suggest that the chimpanzee, an ape close to man, responds to immunization with oLHβ by producing high titer antibodies capable of neutralizing with equal felicity both LH and CG. In the light of this one would wonder if immunization of women with oLHβ would lead to disruption in their cyclicity due to interference with their luteal function.

# IMPROVED IMMUNOGENIC FORMULATIONS FOR ANTIGONADOTROPIN RESPONSE

N.C. Sharma, Om Singh, Amitabh Gaur, D.N. Rao, Vinod Singh, L.V. Rao, Shobha Sehgal[a], C. Das and G.P. Talwar

National Institute of Immunology, Department of Biochemistry All India Institute of Medical Sciences, New Delhi, and [a]Department of Immunopathology, Postgraduate Institute of Medical Education and Research, Chandigarh, India

## INTRODUCTION

Effective control of fertility by immunization with beta-hCG has been demonstrated in non-human primates (Stevens, 1974;Hearn, 1976; Tandon et al., 1981, 1984) and rats (Hulme et al., 1980). A vaccine consisting of beta subunit of hCG conjugated with tetanus toxoid (TT) was proposed earlier (Talwar et al., 1974,1976). This vaccine induced antibodies to both hCG and TT and thus provided additional immunoprophylactic benefit against tetanus. After initial animal experiments and toxicology studies, Phase I clinical trials were conducted with this vaccine in 63 women of reproductive age in six centres located in five countries. Anti-hCG antibodies were formed in 61 out of 63 recepients without any significant side effects and disturbances (Kumar et al., 1976, Hingorani and Kumar, 1979;Shahani et al., 1979, 1982;Nash et al., 1980). The response was reversible with a duration of 300 to 500 days in good responders. The main limitation of this vaccine was the variability of the antibody response from individual to individual and those with inadequate titres were not protected from pregnancy. This presentation will describe an improved formulation which can generate higher antibody titres in a larger percentage of the recepients.

## VACCINES AND THEIR CONSTITUENTS

Three vaccine formulations consisting of (i). alpha-oLH annealed to beta-hCG conjugated to TT(alpha-oLH-beta-hCG-TT), (ii). equimolar mixture of beta-hCG-TT and beta-oLH-TT and (iii). beta-hCG and beta-oLH linked to the common carrier TT (beta-hCG-TT-beta-oLH) were designed for these studies. Beta-hCG-TT and beta-oLH-TT were simultaneously tested as reference immunogens.

## IMMUNOGENECITY

Five female bonnet monkeys (*Macaca radiata*)of proven fertility were used for immunization with each of the above mentioned formulations. Immunization was carried out by giving three intramuscular injections in the hind limbs of the conjugates containing 0.05 mg equivalent of gonadotropin adsorbed on alum at monthly intervals.

In the first injection, 1.0 mg of sodium phthalylated lipopolysaccharide (SPLPS), prepared as described (Elin et al., 1981) was added. Some animals received a booster injection on day 145 after immunization with 1.0 ml of Liera's basic adjuvant. Anti-hCG titres were determined at regular intervals as described earlier (Shastri et al., 1978) and expressed as hCG binding capacity in ng per ml.

All animals produced anti-hCG antibodies. However, the extent of response varied with the formulations. In general three animals out of five in each group had high anti-hCG titres. Monkeys immunized with alpha-oLH-beta-hCG-TT had the highest antibody titres ranging from 1500 to 5200 ng per ml in three animals attained within 75 days of the first injection. Thereafter titres declined slowly. On day 304,titres ranged from 53 to 400 ng per ml in these monkeys.

Immunization with the mixture of beta-hCG-TT and beta-oLH-TT produced anti-hCG antibodies around 2000-3200 ng per ml in two out of five animals. The response was sustained above 100 ng per ml for about a year in these animals. A booster on day 145 improved the anti-hCG titres, one of the monkey reached a level of 250 ng, but in the other two low responders,the titres did not go beyond 100 ng per ml.

Monkeys immunized with beta-hCG-TT-beta-oLH had titres of 560 to 1100 ng per ml in three of the five animals. The response was sustained above 100 ng per ml in two monkeys for nearly a year.

Anti-hCG response in animals immunized with beta-hCG-TT and beta-oLH-TT was comparatively much lower. The titres were below 350 ng per ml in all the animals. An additional booster injection on day 145 did increase the anti-hCG titres but not beyond 900 ng per ml. It may be pointed out that in all cases, the adjuvant employed was alum.

These studies indicate the superior immunogenècity of alpha-oLH-beta-hCG-TT, beta-hCG-TT + beta-oLH-TT and beta-hCG-TT-beta-oLH to induce anti-hCG response in monkeys in comparison to the previous prototype vaccine beta-hCG-TT, or beta-oLH-TT.

## CHARACTERISTICS OF ANTIBODIES

Association constant(Ka) of the antibodies in monkey sera collected on day 182 or 200 after immunization with the five formulations ranged from $1.0 \times 10^9$ to $2.0 \times 10^{10} M^{-1}$ for binding with hCG. The presence of alpha-oLH as an associated subunit in alpha-oLH-beta-hCG-TT and beta-oLH in beta-hCG-TT-beta-oLH and beta-hCG-TT+beta-oLH-TT mixture did not lead to cross-reactive antibodies to hTSH and hFSH. The cross-reactivity with hLH was of the order of 53-73%.

## ORGAN, METABOLIC FUNCTIONS AND TISSUE AUTO-ANTIBODIES

The conjugates were well tolerated. Animals immunized with these five formulations showed no significant side effects. Acute and subacute toxicology studies revealed no significant abnormality in their behaviour, reflexes, locomotion, food and water intake. No local reactions were noted at the site of injection.

Haematological parameters (Haemoglobin, total and differential leukocyte counts, packed cell volume and erythrocyte sedimentation rate) and blood chemistry parameters (alkaline phosphatase, serum glutamic pyruvate transaminase, cholestrol, glucose, creatinine, urea, total and differential proteins were determined at 6,9,12 and 15 months after immunization. No significant variations in these parameters were observed as compared to the values determined in 66 non-immunized monkeys.

Urine analysis performed one year after immunization (physical, chemical and microscopic) also did not show any significant abnormality.

The antibodies were devoid of smooth muscle, thyroid, microsomal, thyroglobulin, antinuclear, antimitochondrial, anti-DNA, C-reactive protein, rheumatoid factor and islet cell reactivity. In few cases the reaction with parietal cells was positive.

Only one animal(93) in the study died after 171 days of immunization with beta-hCG-TT-beta-oLH. Autopsy of the animal did not show any pathology attributable to immunization. The animal died due to severe diarrhoea.

Beta-oLH was included in two formulations e.g. beta-hCG-TT + beta-oLH-TT and beta-hCG-TT-beta-oLH. Apprehension about the safety of immunization with beta-hCG and beta-oLH due to possible cross-reaction with pituitary LH appears no longer valid. Active immunization of rhesus monkeys against beta-oLH with Freund's complete adjuvant and repeated boosters over several years did not reveal any significant pathology (Thau et al., 1979,1980, 1983). Animals had regular ovulation and menstrual cycles. Only progesterone production during the luteal phase of the cycle was reduced and luteal phase was slightly shortened. Animals had significantly reduced fertility (Sundaram et al., 1976). The partial cross-reaction with pituitary LH may in fact be benefitial.

Anti-hCG titres produced by the three polyvalent vaccines appear adequate for preventing pregnancy. Immunized monkeys were continuously mated in the ovulatory cycles with males of demonstrated fertility. None of the animals became pregnant when the anti-hCG titres were in excess of 140 ng per ml. About 16.7% of the animals became pregnant when anti-hCG titres were between 110-140 ng per ml. Anti-hCG titres lower than 50 ng per ml did not prevent pregnancy. Seven control non-immunized monkeys became pregnant in the first cycle and four in the second cycle. No clear information is available on the titres of anti-hCG antibodies that may prevent pregnancy in humans. At the early post-implantation stages, hCG levels at 4 to 4.5 weeks after last menstrual period are reported to be 353 $\pm$ 89 m I.U. per ml (Braunstein et al., 1976) which would demand 35 to 60 ng per ml of hCG neutralizing antibodies.


## ACKNOWLEDGEMENT

This work was supported by grants from the National Co-ordinated Project of the Indian Council of Medical Research, The International Development Research Center, Canada and the Rockfeller Foundation. Mr. M.G. Sharma and Miss. S. Chawla rendered valuable technical assistance.


## REFERENCES


Braunstein, G.D., Rasor, J., Adler, D., Danzer, M., and Wade, M.E., 1976, Serum human chorionic gonadotropin levels throughout normal pregnancy, Am.J. Obstet. Gynec., 126 : 678.

Elin, R.J., Wolff, S.M.,McAdam, K.P.W.J., Chedid, L., Audibert, F., Bernard, C., and Oberling, F., 1981, Properties of reference Escherichia coli endotoxin and its phthalylated derivative in humans, J.Infect. Diseases, 144 : 329.

Hearn, J.P., 1976, Immunization against pregnancy, Proc. R. Soc. Lond.B., 195 : 149.

Hingorani, V. and Kumar, S., 1979, Anti-hCG immunization-phase I clinical trials, in : "Recent Advances in Reproduction and Regulations of Fertility", G.P. Talwar, ed., Elsevier/North-Holland Biomedical Press, Amesterdam, p. 467.

Hulme, M.J., Fehilly, C.B., and Hearn, J.P., 1980, The immune response to hCG-beta subunit in rats and the effects of active immunization on their fertility, J.Reprod. Immunol., 1 : 329.

Kumar, S., Sharma, N.C., Bajaj, J.S., Talwar, G.P., and Hingorani, V., 1976, Clinical profile and toxicology studies on four women immunized with Pr-β-hCG-TT, Contraception, 13 : 253.

Nash, H., Talwar, G.P., Segal, S., Luukkainen, T., Johannsson, E.D.B., Vasquez, J., Coutinho, E., and Sundaram, K., 1980, Observations on the antigenecity and clinical effects of a candidate àntipregnancy vaccine : Beta subunit of human chorionic gonadotropin linked to tetanus toxoid, Fert.Steril., 34 : 328.

Shahani, S.M., Kulkarni, P.P., and Patel, K.L., 1979, Evaluation of immunological and safety data in women treated with Pr- β -hCG-TT vaccine, In : "Recent Advances in Reproduction and Regulation of Fertility", G.P. Talwar, ed., Elsevier/North-Holland Biomedical Press, Amsterdam, p. 473.

Shahani, S.M., Kulkarni, P.P., Patel, K.L., Salahuddin, M., Das, C., and Talwar, G.P., 1982, Clinical and immunological responses with Pr-β-hCG-TT vaccine, Contraception, 25 : 421.

Shastri, N., Dubey, S.K., Vijay Ragavan, S., and Talwar, G.P.., 1978, Differential affinity of anti-Pr-B-hCG-TT antibodies for hCG and hLH, Contraception, 18 : 23.

Stevens, V., 1974, Fertility control through active immunization using placeta proteins, in "Immunological approaches to Fertility Control", 7th Karolinska Symposium on Research Methods in Reproductive Endocrinology, E. Diczfalusy, ed.,Karolinska Institute, Stockholm, p. 357.

Sundaram, K., Chang, C.C., Laurence, K.A., Brinson, A.O., Atkinson, L.E., Segal, S.J. and Ward, D.N., 1976, The effectiveness in rhesus monkeys of an anti-fertility vaccine based on neutralization of chorionic gonadotropin, Contraception, 14 : 639.

Talwar, G.P., Sharma, N.C., Dubey, S.K., Das, C., Salahuddin, M., Ramakrishnan, S., Nath, I., Kumar, S., Hingorani, V., and Bloom, B., 1974, Immunological studies on human placental trophoblast components of potential utility for fertility regulation, in : "Biological and Clinical Aspects of Reproduction", Excerpta Medica International Congress Series No. 394,Excerpta Medica, Amsterdam p.225.

Talwar, G.P., Sharma, N.C., Dubey, S.K., Salahuddin, M., Das, C., Ramakrishnan, S., Kumar, S., and Hingorani, V., 1976, Isoimmunization against human chorionic gonadotropin with conjugates of processed β-subunit of the hormone and tetanus toxoid, Proc. Nat. Acad. Sci. USA, 73 : 218.

Tandon, A., Das, C., Jailkhani, B.L., and Talwar, G.P., 1981, Efficacy of antibodies generated by Pr-β-hCG-TT to terminate pregnancy in baboons :Its reversibility and rescue by medroxyprogesterone acetate, Contraception, 24 : 83.

Tandon, A., Das, C., Jailkhani, B.L., Gaur, A., Sehgal, S., Gopinath, G., and Talwar, G.P., 1984, Effect on pregnancy in mice of passive immunization against ovine LH and human gonadotrophin, J.Reprod. Fert., 70 : 369.

Thau, R.B., and Sundaram, K., 1980, The mechanism of action of an antifertility vaccine in the rhesus monkey : Reversal of the effects of antisera to the β-subunit of ovine luteinizing hormone by medroxyprogesterone acetate, Fert. Steril., 33 : 317.

Thau, R.B., Sundaram, K., Thornton, Y.S., and Seidman, L.S., 1979, Effects of immunization with the β-subunit of ovine luteinizing hormone on corpus luteum function in the rhesus monkey, Fert. Steril., 31 : 200.

Thau, R.B., Yamamoto, Y., Sundaram, K., and Spinola, P.G., 1983, Human chorionic gonadotropin stimulates luteal function in rhesus monkeys immunized against the β-subunit of ovine luteinizing hormone, Endocrionology, 112 : 277.

# A FERTILITY REGULATING VACCINE BASED ON THE CARBOXYL-TERMINAL PEPTIDE OF THE BETA SUBUNIT OF HUMAN CHORIONIC GONADOTROPHIN

P.D. Griffin

Special Programme of Research, Development
and Research Training in Human Reproduction
World Health Organization, Geneva, Switzerland

## INTRODUCTION

The World Health Organization's Special Programme of Research, Development and Research Training in Human Reproduction was established in 1972 in response to requests from a number of its member states that the Organization take a more active role in family planning research. The methods of birth control available at that time did not, and to a large extent still do not, satisfy all of the varied cultural and service demands of different populations and there was an expressed need to develop a greater variety of methods which would find wide acceptance, particularly in developing countries. One of the principal objectives of the WHO Programme, therefore, is the development of new family planning technology to meet these demands. A safe and effective method which could be administered at infrequent intervals, perhaps by paramedical personnel, and which is independant of active participation by the user to remain effective, is attractive to both the users and providers of family planning services. The acceptability of such a method would be further enhanced if its activity is restricted to the intended target, it is devoid of pharmacological activity and it does not produce undesirable side-effects. A birth control vaccine, eliciting a specific, safe and effective antifertility immune response lasting for 1-2 years is likely, therefore, to have a major impact in family planning programmes.

It was against this background and in consideration of these requirements that the WHO Task Force on Vaccines for Fertility Regulation embarked on its programme to develop a target-specific vaccine based on the beta subunit of human chorionic gonadotrophin (β-hCG). Whilst the complete role of hCG is still not clear, it is known that one of its functions is to maintain the corpus luteum and its production of progesterone until the placental production of this hormone is established. A vaccine directed against hCG, therefore, represents a very attractive approach to birth control. Since, by removing this very early embryonic signal to the mother by immunological means, either by neutralizing hCG in the maternal circulation or by a direct effect on the peri-implantation blastocyst, the corpus luteum will regress, progesterone production will fall and a situation analogous to a non-pregnant cycle will occur and menstruation will ensue at or around the expected time.

Two major problems have to be resolved in the development of this type of iso-vaccine. The first is the need to enhance the immunogenicity of a molecule to which women are normally tolerant (Stevens & Crystle, 1974; Talwar et al. 1976), and the second is the need to generate an immune response specific for the intended target. These criteria of immunogenicity and specificity, relating to efficacy and safety respectively, have governed the Task Force's studies in this area which have now reached the stage at which a Phase I clinical evaluation of a prototype hCG vaccine is planned. This vaccine, developed over the past ten years as a result of collaborative research involving investigators from a variety of scientific disciplines in a number of different countries (WHO, 1984), is a complex preparation consisting of a synthetic peptide of β-hCG coupled to a diphtheria toxoid carrier, mixed with a muramyl dipeptide adjuvant and administered in a oil and water emulsion vehicle. The rationale for the selection of each of these components and the way in which the vaccine has been developed and evaluated is described below.

## SELECTION OF THE PEPTIDE COMPONENT OF THE IMMUNOGEN

HCG is a glycoprotein consisting of two non-covalently linked dissimilar alpha and beta subunits. The alpha subunit of hCG is identical in primary structure to corresponding parts of other glycoprotein hormones, such as hLH, hFSH and hTSH. However the beta subunits of hCG, hLH and, to a greater extent, hFSH and hTSH are dissimilar in structure and it is in the beta subunit of these molecules that their hormone specificity resides.

Not surprisingly, antisera raised to the intact hCG molecule crossreact extensively with these other hormones, particularly hLH. This crossreactivity is greatly reduced when β-hCG is used as the immunogen (Stevens, 1976) although detectable and sometimes substantial levels of crossreactivity with hLH are still observed (Fig. 1). Nevertheless, β-hCG

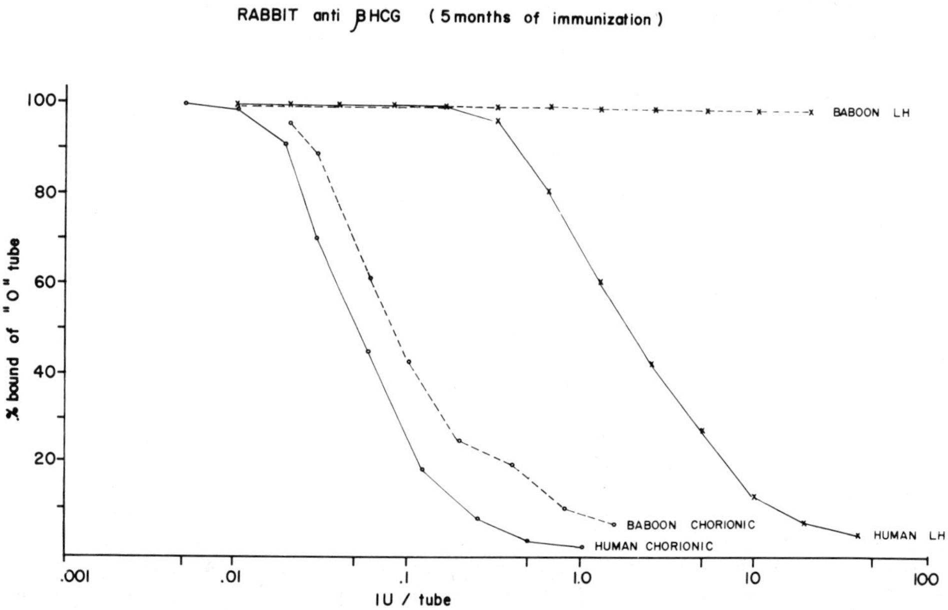


Fig. 1. Relative binding potencies of rabbit anti-β-hCG serum for hCG, bCG, hLH and bLH.

Table 1. Effect on fertility of female baboons of immunization with β-hCG.

| Baboon No. | No. of Matings | Ovulations | Pregnancy |
|---|---|---|---|
| 1 | 3 | 3 | 0 |
| 2 | 3 | 3 | 0 |
| 3 | 3 | 2 | 0 |
| 4 | 3 | 3 | 0 |
| 5 | 3 | 3 | 0 |
| 6 | 3 | 3 | 0 |
| 7 | 3 | 3 | 0 |
| 8 | 3 | 2 | 0 |
| 9 | 3 | 3 | 0 |
| 10 | 3 | 3 | 0 |
| TOTAL 10 | 30 | 28 | 0 |

does represent one possibility for the development of an anti-hCG vaccine and many studies have been carried out with preparations based on this molecule. For example, in earlier studies carried out by the Task Force, a β-hCG preparation, purified by affinity chromatography using an alpha-hCG sepharose column to remove intact hormone, was used to immunize rabbits, sheep and baboons both in its 'native' form and after chemical alteration. High levels of antibodies reacting with hCG were raised in all species although some crossreactivity to hLH was always found. Antisera from the immunized baboons reacted significantly with hCG, baboon CG (bCG) and hLH but not with baboon LH (bLH). The immunized animals continued to ovulate and exhibit normal menstrual cycles however when 10 of these animals were each mated to proven fertile males for 3 consecutive cycles, no pregnancies occurred from these 30 exposures (Table 1). A similar mating schedule carried out in 10 non-immunized control baboons resulted in a total of 24 pregnancies, representing an 80% fertility rate (Stevens, 1974). Although these results were encouraging in terms of antifertility effects, concern was expressed about the unknown risks of the variable levels of crossreactivity to hLH exhibited by the baboon antisera and the Task Force therefore sought a more specific hCG immunogen.

At the same time that these baboon data were being generated, reports appeared in the scientific literature describing the primary structure of hCG (Morgan et al., 1973) and hLH. These reports revealed that, whilst there was extensive homology in the amino terminal regions of the beta subunits of these two hormones, there was a carboxyl terminal extension of approximately 30 amino acids in β-hCG which was not present in β-hLH. In addition, few amino acid residues were identical beyond the last common cysteine residue at position 110 (Fig. 2). This information suggested that part or all of this carboxyl terminal peptide of β-hCG (CTP-β-hCG) might represent a potentially hCG-specific immunogen for vaccine development.

To investigate this possibility, rabbits were immunized with natural CTP-β-hCG, obtained by digesting the purified subunit with trypsin, chymotrypsin or thermolysin. The resulting antisera reacted with hCG but were devoid of crossreactivity with hLH, demonstrating that the CTP-β-hCG did represent a viable candidate for the development of a vaccine specific for hCG (Stevens, 1976). Problems of low yield, high cost and difficulties with quality control of peptides obtained from the natural hormone, necessitated the production of these materials by solid-phase synthesis. Antisera raised to the natural and synthetic peptides exhibited similar titres, affinities and specificities and although they differed in their reactivities with whole hCG these differences were slight and therefore all subsequent vaccine development has been carried out using synthetic peptides (Powell et al., 1980).

Numerous peptides of various lengths within the 105-145 region of β-hCG have been synthesised and evaluated, both in terms of their immunogenicity and the specificity, affinity and hCG-neutralizing ability of the antisera raised to them. In summary, the results of these experiments indicate that peptides of less than 20, or more than 40, amino acids (starting from the C-terminal) elicited low titres of antibodies reacting with intact hCG. In contrast, peptides of 35 and 37 residues, representing the 111-145 and 109-145 regions of β-hCG respectively, elicited antibodies with potent in vitro binding (Fig. 3) and in vivo neutralizing (Fig. 4) activities for hCG. In addition, the 109-145 peptide contains a cysteine residue (at position 110) which offers certain advantages for conjugation to carrier molecules to be described later. The immunogenic profiles of a large number of variants of the 109-145 peptide have been examined and compared (Stevens et al., 1981b). These include peptides in which amino acid substitutions have been made at either the amino or carboxyl terminals to provide different conjugation options at these two positions, as well as those in which poly-proline spacers have

```
        1                                10                          20             25
                                                    (CHO)
β-hCG  H2N-Ser-Lys-Glu-Pro-Leu-Arg-Pro-Arg-Cys-Arg-Pro-Ile-Asn-Ala-Thr-Leu-Ala-Val-Glu-Lys-Glu-Gly-Cys-Pro-Val-
β-hLH  H2N-   -Arg-  -   -   -   -   -Trp-   -His-   -   -   -   -Ile-   -   -   -Gln-   -   -   -   -   -   -   -
        26      30                              40                                          50
               (CHO)
β-hCG  Cys-Ile-Thr-Val-Asn-Thr-Thr-Ile-Cys-Ala-Gly-Tyr-Cys-Pro-Thr-Met-Thr-Arg-Val-Leu-Gln-Gly-Val-Leu-Pro-
β-hLH   -   -   -   -   -   -   -   -   -   -   -   -   -   -   -   -Arg-Met-Leu-   -   -Ala-   -   -   -
        51                              60                                   70  ·          75
β-hCG  Ala-Leu-Pro-Gln-Val-Val-Cys-Asn-Tyr-Arg-Asp-Val-Arg-Phe-Glu-Ser-Ile-Arg-Leu-Pro-Gly-Cys-Pro-Arg-Gly-
β-hLH  Pro-   -   -   -Pro-   -   -Thr-   -   -   -   -   -   -   -   -   -   -   -   -   -   -   -   -   -
        76      80                                  90                                      100
β-hCG  Val-Asn-Pro-Val-Val-Ser-Tyr-Ala-Val-Ala-Leu-Ser-Cys-Gln-Cys-Ala-Leu-Cys-Arg-Arg-Ser-Thr-Thr-Asp-Cys-
β-hLH     -Asp-   -   -   -   -Phe-Pro-   -   -   -   -   -Arg-   -Gly-Pro-   -   -   -   -   -Ser-   -   -
        101                             110                                  120            125
                                                                               (CHO)
β-hCG  Gly-Gly-Pro-Lys-Asp-His-Pro-Leu-Thr-Cys-Asp-Asp-Pro-Arg-Phe-Gln-Asp-Ser-Ser-Ser-Ser-Lys-Ala-Pro-Pro-
β-hLH   -   -   -   -   -   -   -   -   -   -   -   -Pro-Gln-His-Ser-Gly-COOH
        126        130                              140                145
          (CHO)          (CHO)              (CHO)
β-hCG  Pro-Ser-Leu-Pro-Ser-Pro-Ser-Arg-Leu-Pro-Gly-Pro-Ser-Asp-Thr-Pro-Ile-Leu-Pro-Gln-COOH
```

Fig. 2. The amino acid sequences of the beta subunits of hCG (upper letters) and hLH (lower letters) aligned by the position of cysteine residues. Where no residue is indicated on the hLH sequence, it is identical to that of hCG. Carbohydrate groups are indicated by CHO.

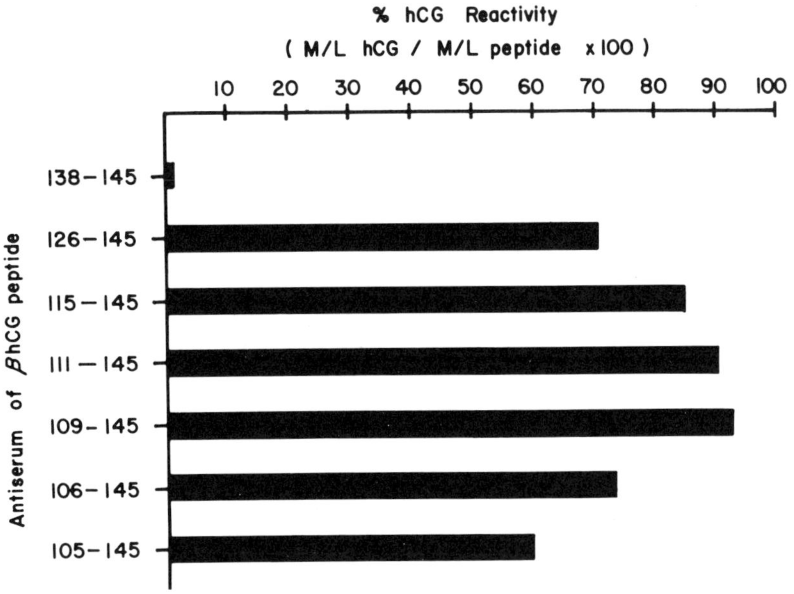


Fig. 3. Relative hCG reactivities of antisera raised to conjugates containing β-hCG carboxyl terminal peptides (CTP) of different lengths.

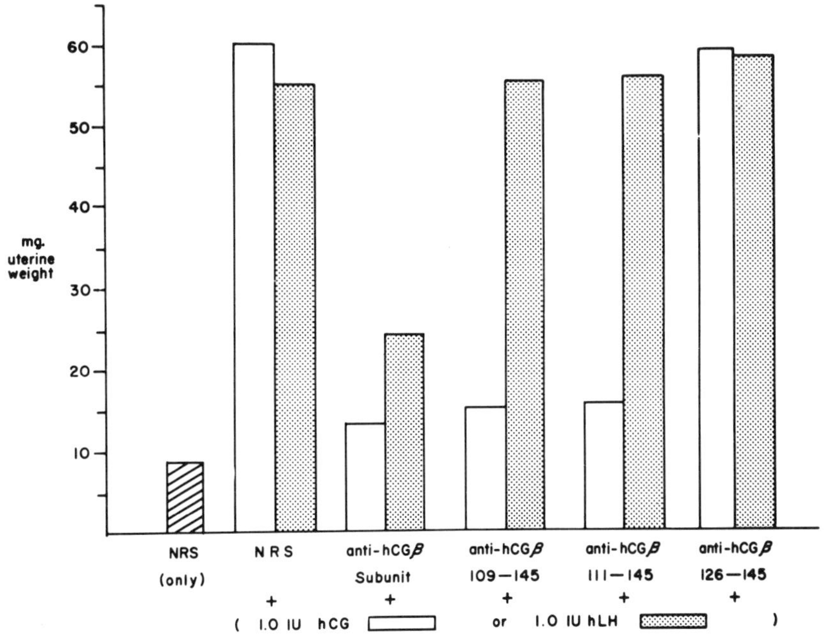


Fig. 4. Comparative evaluation of the ability of antisera raised to β-hCG and antisera raised to three different CTPs of β-hCG to selectively neutralize the biological activities of hCG and hLH.

(native sequence) *

$H_2N$ - ASP ---------------------------- GLN - CYS - COOH

111 145

* (native sequence)

$H_2N$ - CYS - $(PRO)^6$ - ASP ---------------------------- GLN - COOH

111 145

(acm) (native sequence) *

$H_2N$ - THR - CYS ---------------------------- GLN - $(PRO)^6$ - CYS - COOH

109 110 145

Fig. 5. Three variants of the CTP of β-hCG assessed for relative immunogenic potencies. The first represents an option for conjugation through an additional carboxyl terminal cysteine at position 146. The second and third represent peptides with poly-proline spacers at the amino and carboxyl terminals respectively. (* = point of conjugation)

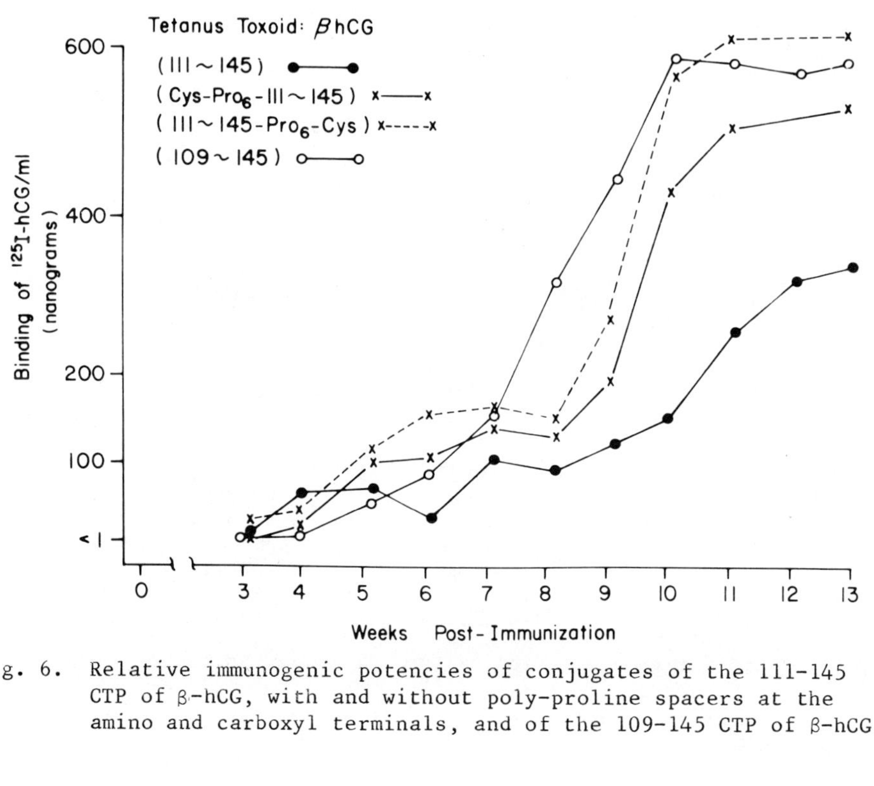


Fig. 6. Relative immunogenic potencies of conjugates of the 111-145 CTP of β-hCG, with and without poly-proline spacers at the amino and carboxyl terminals, and of the 109-145 CTP of β-hCG.

Table 2. Comparison of maximum antibody levels reactive to hCG in rabbits immunized with the 109-145 CTP of β-hCG conjugated to various macromolecular carriers.

| | Mean maximum antigen binding levels [a] | | | |
|---|---|---|---|---|
| | $^{125}$I-hCG | | $^{125}$I-109-145 | |
| hCG-β peptide 109-145 coupled to: | M/L x $10^{-10}$ | SD | M/L x $10^{-10}$ | SD |
| bov GG | 479.2[b] | 402.5 | 552.3[b] | 410.8 |
| Diphtheria toxoid | 365.3[b] | 176.8 | 423.3[b] | 189.3 |
| Tetanus toxoid | 339.3[b] | 95.5 | 417.6[b] | 106.2 |
| C parvum | 215.9 | 121.5 | 255.4 | 131.6 |
| Flagellin | 210.4 | 157.5 | 244.6 | 198.1 |
| Pneumococcus polysaccharide | 135.7 | 102.8 | 153.7 | 113.0 |
| Meningococcal protein | 97.9 | 107.6 | 118.4 | 122.6 |
| TGAL | 29.9 | 22.6 | 37.3 | 35.5 |
| Ficoll | 10.6 | 8.3 | 13.0 | 9.0 |
| Polyalanine | 8.6 | 4.7 | 12.2 | 7.5 |

*Immunization carried out using complete Freund's adjuvant

[a]Four rabbits/group

[b]Not significantly different ($p < 0.05$)

been added at either end of the peptide in an attempt to enhance its presentation to the immune system and thereby increase its immunogenicity (Fig. 5). None of these variants however produced antibody responses significantly better than the 'native' 109-145 peptide (Fig. 6). For these reasons the 109-145 peptide was selected for further vaccine development.

## SELECTION OF THE CARRIER COMPONENT OF THE IMMUNOGEN

In anticipation of poor immunogenicity of the hCG vaccine in the clinical situation, because of partial or complete tolerance to the peptide and its comparatively small molecular size, the Task Force has investigated a number of macromolecules to act as a carrier for the 109-145 CTP-β-hCG peptide and thereby enhance its immunogenicity. These include bovine gamma globulin (BGG), keyhole limpet haemocyanin (KLH), tetanus toxoid (TT), diphtheria toxoid (DT) and others. The best antibody responses were produced to conjugates consisting of the CTP-β-hCG coupled to BGG, TT and DT (Table 2). Because of the risk of inducing crossreactive immunity to human gamma globulin, BGG was not considered a viable carrier candidate. Of the remaining two options, DT was considered the more attractive since it contained a large number of free-$NH_2$ groups to which the CTP-β-hCG could be conjugated and produced less of the delayed type sensitivity reactions observed in preliminary animal studies with conjugates of TT.

## SELECTION OF THE CONJUGATION PROCEDURE

Initially, these carrier-peptide conjugates were prepared using conventional crosslinking reagents such as carbodiimide, glutaraldehyde, and the isocyanates. Although conjugates prepared by these procedures were capable of eliciting high and specific antibody responses, they contained a variable mixture of conjugate and peptide and carrier polymers. The unpredictability and variability of these preparations makes them

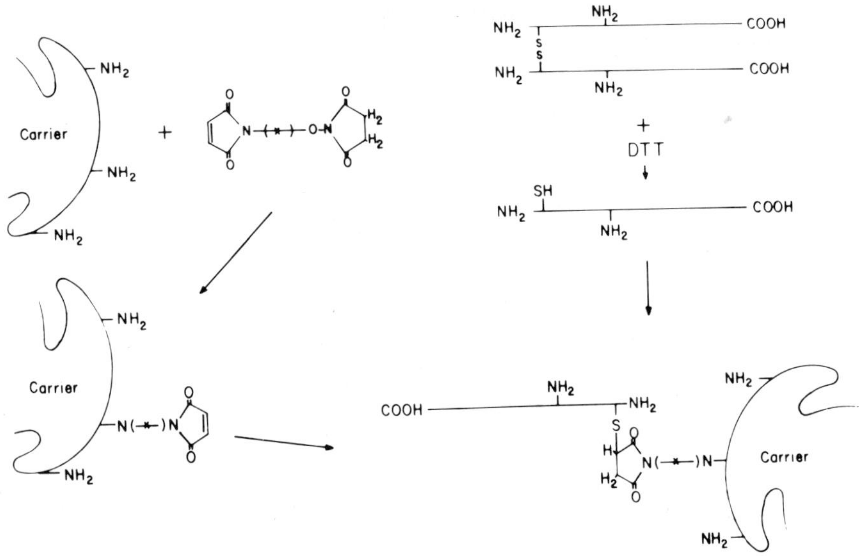


Fig. 7. Conjugation of CTP of β-hCG to diphtheria toxoid carrier using 6-maleimido caproic acyl N-hydroxy succinimide ester.

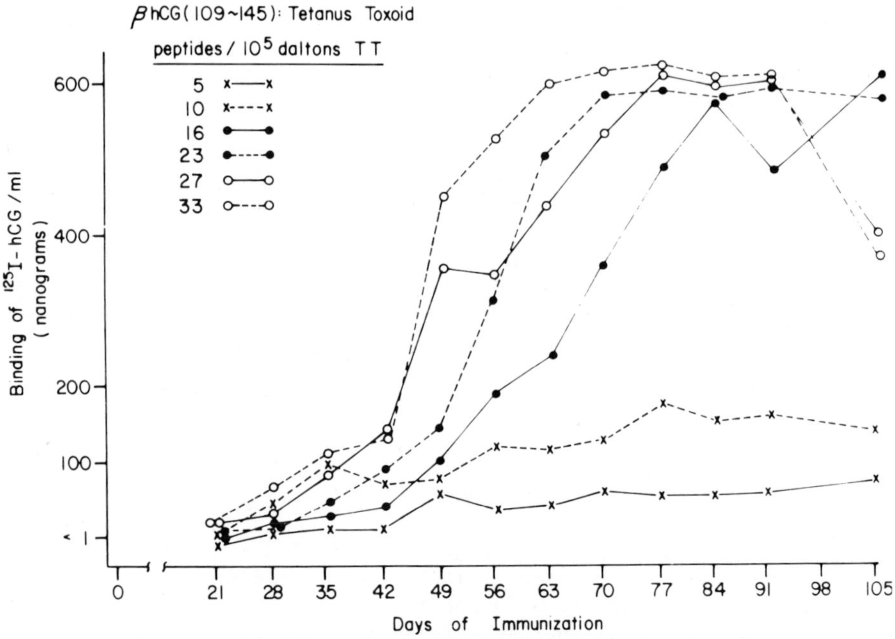


Fig. 8. Comparison of immunogenic potencies of the 109-145 CTP of β-hCG conjugated to diphtheria toxoid in various peptide:carrier ratios.

unsuitable for clinical application and the Task Force therefore initiated a number of studies to identify a conjugation methodology that would permit the production of conjugates of predictable and predetermined composition and characteristics which would satisfy the manufacturing and quality control requirements of drug regulatory authorities.

The bifunctional reagent, 6-maleimido caproic acyl N-hydroxy succinimide ester (MCS) appears to be ideal for this purpose in that conjugation can be effected between the amino groups on the DT carrier and the sulfhydral groups on the N-terminal cysteine of the CTP-β-hCG peptide in a predictable and controlled manner (Fig. 7). The reaction can be controlled to the extent that the number of peptides conjugated per $10^5$ Daltons of carrier can be adjusted within fairly fine limits (Lee et al., 1980). A number of conjugates of different peptide:carrier ratios have been prepared and evaluated for their immunogenic properties. A ratio of $25 \pm 2$ peptides per $10^5$D of carrier was found to give maximal responses (Fig. 8) and there appeared to be no advantage, in terms of antibody production, in increasing the peptide loading beyond this level (Stevens et al., 1981b).

## SELECTION OF A CLINICALLY ACCEPTABLE IMMUNOSTIMULANT

Although Freund's Complete Adjuvant (FCA) has been used in some preliminary animal studies with the hCG vaccine, it is obviously not acceptable for clinical use and the Task Force has therefore evaluated a number of experimental immunostimulants potentially suitable for clinical application (Stevens et al., 1981c). Two preparations were found to be at least as good, and sometimes better, than FCA in eliciting antibodies to the CTP-β-hCG peptide:DT conjugate (Fig. 9). One of these preparations, an analogue of N-acetylmuramyl-L-alanyl-D-isoglutamine (Fig. 10), was selected for further study by the Task Force in connection with the development of the hCG vaccine. This selection was made on the basis of the compound's immunostimulating properties and its potential for clinical acceptance, as deduced from the substantial amount of toxicology carried out on the compound.

## SELECTION OF A SUITABLE VACCINE VEHICLE

Finally, the Task Force was faced with the problem of identifying a suitable vehicle in which the vaccine could be injected. Poor antibody responses were produced by the vaccine administered in saline and water and vegetable oil emulsions, probably as a result of rapid clearance of the injected materials. There was a need therefore for a vehicle that would function as a slow release depot to ensure effective immunization but which would not produce undesirable side-effects. Again several different preparations have been evaluated for this purpose, including oils from a variety of sources and emulsified with water in a number of different formulations (Stevens et al., 1981c). One formulation which provided consistently high antibody responses when used as a vehicle for the CTP-β-hCG peptide:DT conjugate and adjuvant mixtures, was an emulsion of squalene and water, using mannide monooleate as the emulsifying agent (Table 3) and this vehicle was selected for further evaluation.

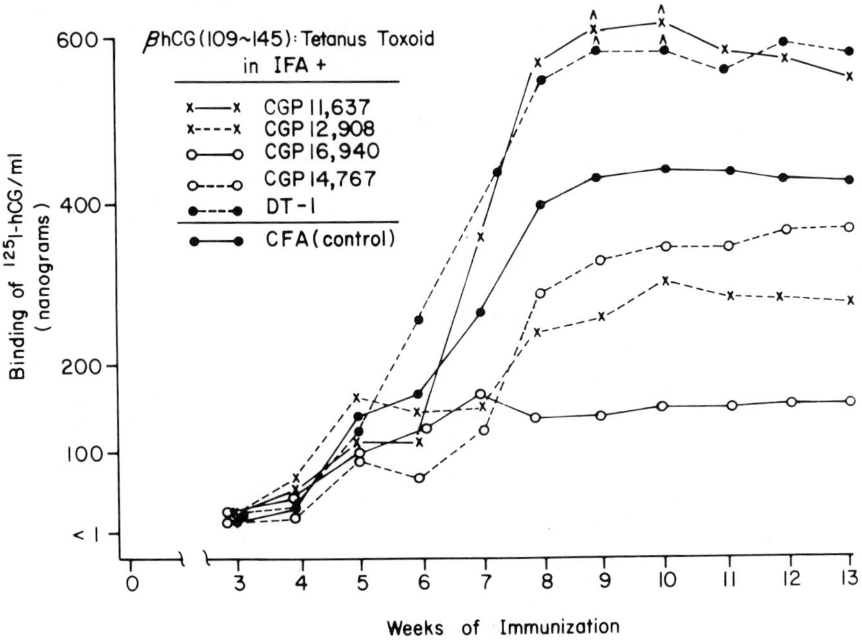


Fig. 9. Relative potencies of different immunostimulants to potentiate the production of antibodies to a conjugate of the 109-145 CTP of β-hCG.

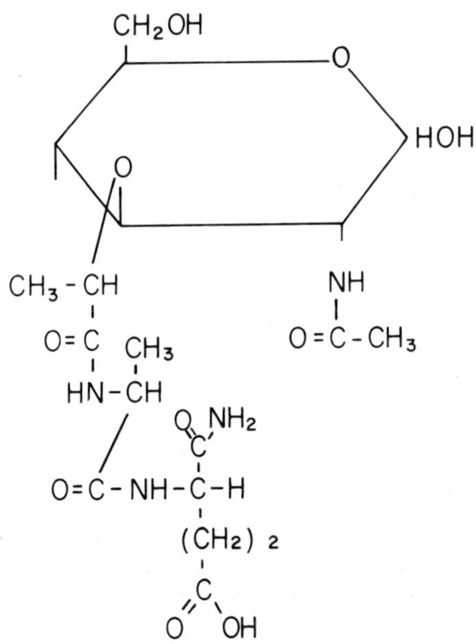


Fig. 10. N-acetyl muramyl-L-alanyl-D-isoglutamine ($MDP_1$).

Table 3. Comparison of antibody levels to hCG in rabbits immunized with a conjugate of the 111-145 CTP of β-hCG with a poly-proline spacer at the amino terminal and administered in different vehicles.

| Vehicle | n | Antibody level M/L x $10^{-10}$ Minimum | Median | Maximum | Mean | 95% CI | SD | p[a] |
|---|---|---|---|---|---|---|---|---|
| CFA | 12 | 52.4 | 150.8 | 320.2 | 161.3 | (101.7-220.9) | 93.7 | |
| Squalene-arlacel | 11 | 189.0 | 312.6 | 833.7 | 400.1 | (225.7-574.4) | 226.7 | 0.01 |
| Squalane-arlacel | 11 | 44.2 | 150.6 | 290.0 | 168.5 | (114.5-222.5) | 80.4 | NS |
| Peanut oil | 9 | 12.5 | 22.5 | 27.1 | 21.3 | ( 17.5-25.1 ) | 4.9 | $<$0.001 |
| Alum precipitate | 12 | 5.8 | 8.4 | 16.1 | 9.9 | ( 7.9-11.9 ) | 3.2 | $<$0.001 |

*Conjugate incorporated into CFA served as reference. Values from the peak antibody levels together with those from one week earlier and one week later were pooled for evaluation.

[a]Probability, compared with CFA. NS= not significant ($p > 0.05$)

ANTIFERTILITY TESTING IN BABOONS

The antifertility activity of this complex vaccine formulation, consisting of the 109-145 CTP-β-hCG:DT conjugate mixed with MDP and administered in a squalene-arlacel-water emulsion, has been evaluated in baboons.

In this study (Stevens et al., 1981a), fifteen female baboons received a total of 6 intramuscular injections of the vaccine at 28 day intervals and were mated with proven fertile males for 3 consecutive cycles, starting with the third cycle after the first injection. All matings were carried out at the peak of sex-skin turgescence during the periovulatory phase of the cycle. The same injection and mating schedule was used for fifteen control animals receiving the DT, MDP and emulsion vehicle. A total of 70% of the control group matings resulted in pregnancies compared to only 4.6% in the group receiving the complete vaccine (Table 4). These results were particularly encouraging in view of the fact that the antibodies raised to the CTP-β-hCG:DT conjugate in these animals crossreacted substantially with whole hCG but only poorly (3-15%) with the bCG target in this heterologous system (Table 5). The high level of antifertility efficacy achieved in these animals suggests that close to 100% protection may occur in the clinical situation where a much higher level of crossreactivity is to be expected.

TOXICITY AND SAFETY STUDIES

A substantial number of toxicity studies have been carried out in rodents, rabbits and baboons with this vaccine and its individual components in order to generate data to form the basis of a request to carry out an initial clinical evaluation of the vaccine. These studies included,

(i) an acute intramuscular tolerance study in mice,
(ii) an acute intramuscular tolerance study in rats,
(iii) a thirteen week intramuscular toxicity study in rats,

Table 4. Fertility rates of baboons immunized with diphtheria toxoid compared to those of baboons immunized with the 109-145 CTP of β-hCG conjugated to diphtheria toxoid.

| Baboons Immunized With | Mating Cycle | | | |
|---|---|---|---|---|
| | 1 | 2 | 3 | TOTALS |
| **Diphtheria Toxoid** | | | | |
| No. Mated | 15 | 4 | 1 | 20 |
| No. Pregnant | 11 | 3 | 0 | 14 |
| Fertility Rate (%) | 73.3 | 75.0 | 0 | 70.0 |
| **Diphtheria Toxoid:β-hCG(109-145)** | | | | |
| No. Mated | 15 | 15 | 14 | 44 |
| No. Pregnant | 0 | 1 | 1 | 2 |
| Fertility Rate (%) | 0 | 6.7 | 7.1 | 4.6 |

(a) Matings commenced during the course of the third menstrual cycle following immunization.

(iv) an intramuscular irritation study in rabbits,
(v) a five month intramuscular toxicity and immunosafety study in baboons,
(vi) a five month hyperimmunization study in baboons.

The results obtained in these and other studies, together with data provided by the suppliers of the various vaccine components and a protocol for a proposed Phase I clinical trial, were submitted as an Investigational New Drug application to the United States Food and Drug Administration in mid-1984. Approval to conduct this Phase I clinical study was obtained from the USFDA in September 1984 and subject to similar approval from the Australian drug regulatory authorities, it is proposed to initiate this study in Australia during 1985.

## PHASE I CLINICAL STUDY

The primary purpose of this clinical study is to evaluate the tolerability of the prototype vaccine although some provisional data on its efficacy also will be obtained by assessing antibody responses. The protocol allows for a five-dose schedule, starting at 50µg of conjugate mixed with 25µg of MDP and administered in 25µl of vehicle, and increasing by approximately doubling doses to lmg of conjugate with 500µg of MDP in 500µl of vehicle. The highest proposed clinical dose being the amount required to elicit effective antibody titres in the baboon fertility studies. There will be six women in each dosage group all of whom will have been previously electively sterilized. They will receive two injections of the same preparation, given 42 days apart, and will be followed up, on both an in-patient and out-patient basis, for a minimum period of 12 months. A large number of clinical and laboratory tests will be carried out to assess a variety of haematological, biochemical, endocrinological and immunological parameters.

Table 5. Relative binding properties of antiserum raised to CTP-β-hCG for the peptide immunogen, bCG and hCG.

| Antibody Reactive To | Antibody level during menstrual cycle | | | | |
|---|---|---|---|---|---|
| | 1 | 2 | 3 | 4 | 5 |
| | MOLES/LITER X $10^{-10}$ | | | | |
| β-hCG(109-145) | | | | | |
| MEAN | 41.4 | 186.0 | 205.6 | 252.0 | 284.1 |
| SD | 28.6 | 84.1 | 67.5 | 118.7 | 99.7 |
| 95% CI | (25.6-57.3) | (139.4-232.5) | (168.3-243.0) | (186.1-317.7) | (226.5-341.7) |
| bCG | | | | | |
| MEAN | 0.7 | 3.7 | 5.5 | 7.7 | 9.0 |
| SD | 0.6 | 3.3 | 3.4 | 4.8 | 4.8 |
| 95% CI | (0.3-1.0) | (1.9-5.6) | (3.6-7.3) | (5.0-10.4) | (6.3-11.8) |
| hCG | | | | | |
| MEAN | 31.9 | 160.0 | 172.1 | 205.5 | 224.8 |
| SD | 23.9 | 77.7 | 55.0 | 108.2 | 89.8 |
| 95% CI | (18.7-45.2) | (117.0-203.1) | (141.6-202.5) | (145.5-265.4) | (172.9-276.6) |
| Number of Cycles | 15 | 15 | 15 | 15 | 14 |

(a) values were determined from serum samples obtained during the early luteal phase of each menstrual cycle.

## FUTURE STUDIES

The Task Force considers the current vaccine to be a prototype only and accepts that further research and development of an improved second generation vaccine is needed, and may be mandatory, prior to the initiation of Phase II clinical trials of vaccine efficacy. Studies are under way to develop smaller peptide immunogens, based on immunodominant epitopes and conformational determinants of the hCG molecule (Puett et al., 1982), as well as peptide polymers which may obviate the need for a macromolecular carrier. New immunostimulants and biodegradable and biocompatible slow release delivery systems are also being evaluated as possible substitutes for the MDP and squalene-arlacel-water emulsion in the existing formulation.

Although the primate CGs are closely related molecules they are not identical and an homologous animal model needs to be used in a definitive preclinical assessment of the safety and efficacy of an hCG vaccine (Fig. 11). The Task Force has been trying for several years to isolate and sequence bCG in order to synthesise a β-bCG peptide, analogous to the 109-145 peptide of β-hCG, for development into a bCG vaccine. These studies have proved very difficult because of the inherent lability of the baboon hormone, its secretion profile and the logistical problems involved in collecting clean urine specimens from this species. Recently, attempts have been made to derive the amino acid sequence from the nucleotide sequence of the gene coding for the hormone. Difficulties have been encountered here also in that it appears there may be several different genes carrying out this function.

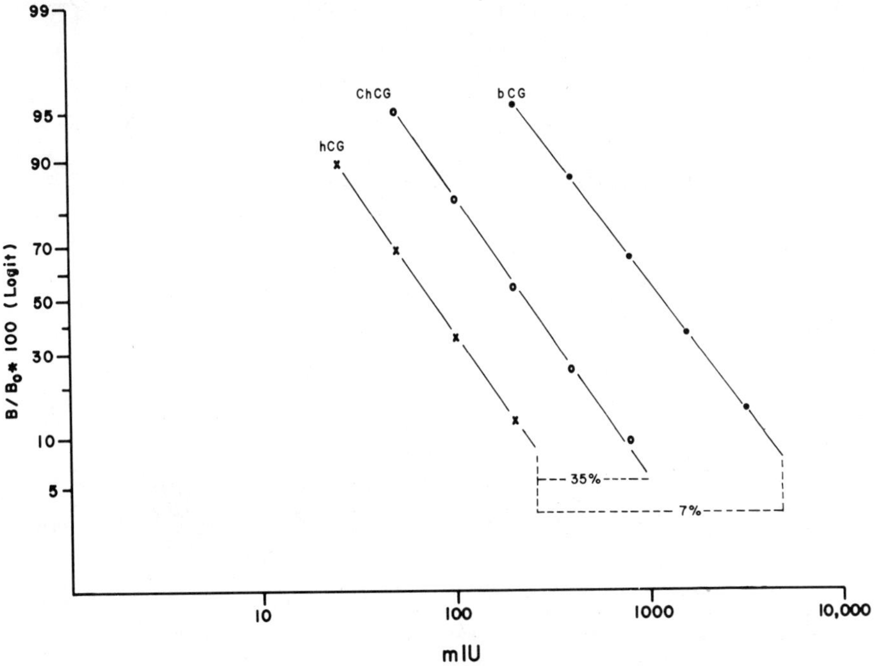


Fig. 11. Relative binding potency for human, chimpanzee and baboon chorionic gonadotrophins of antiserum raised to hCG.

The way in which the hCG vaccine achieves its antifertility effect is not clear and it would be interesting to carry out further research to define the vaccine's mechanism of action. Some preliminary studies have been carried out in this area already and have yielded data to suggest that the antifertility effect may not be due solely to the removal of the endocrine support of the corpus luteum, and its consequent cessation of progesterone production, but may involve a direct effect on the blastocyst. For example, antisera from a baboon immunized with either β-hCG (Fig. 12) or CTP-β-hCG (Fig. 13) will abort a non-immunized pregnant animal but the abortion occurs within 24-36 hours, a significantly shorter period than the 5-6 day operation-to-abortion interval which is observed following ovariectomy in a pregnant baboon. On the other hand, if exogenous progesterone is given at the same time as the antiserum and its administration continued until the luteo-placental shift in progesterone production has occurred, the pregnancy can be maintained and a normal infant produced (Fig. 14). In addition, to suggesting a possible procedure by which the antifertility effect of the vaccine could be reversed, these preliminary observations indicate that further experiments to more precisely describe the functions of hCG and the role it plays in the complex materno-fetal interactions of pregnancy would not only be scientifically interesting but could have practical applications to the development of improved antifertility vaccines.

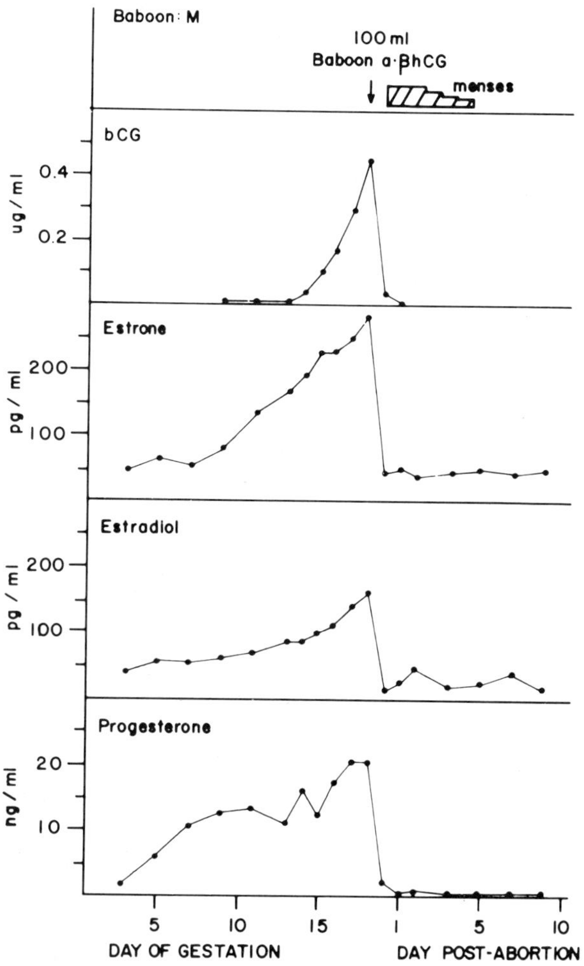


Fig. 12. Effect on the pregnancy of a non-immunized baboon of passive immunization with sera obtained from a baboon previously immunized with β-hCG.

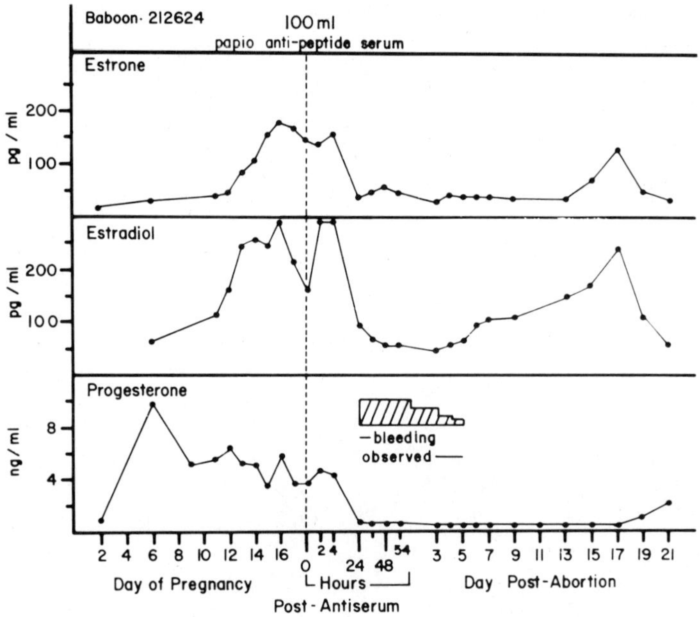


Fig. 13. Effect on the pregnancy of a non-immunized baboon of passive immunization with sera obtained from a baboon previously immunized with a CTP of β-hCG conjugated to diphtheria toxoid.

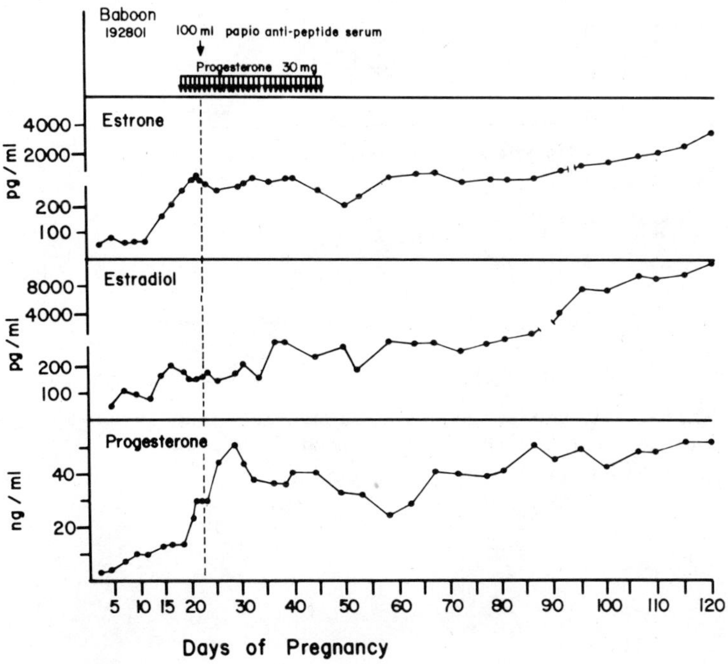


Fig. 14. Effect of exogenous progesterone on the ability of baboon antiserum raised to a conjugate of the CTP of β-hCG to interrupt pregnancy in a non-immunized baboon.

## REFERENCES


Lee, A.C., Powell, J.E., Tregear, G.W., Niall, H.D., Stevens, V.C., 1980, A method for preparing β-hCG COOH peptide-carrier conjugates of predictable composition. Molecular Immunology, 17: 749-755.

Morgan, F.J., Birken, S., Canfield, R.E., 1973, Human chorionic gonadotropin:a proposal for the amino acid sequence. Molecular and Cellular Biochemistry, 2: 97-99.

Powell, J.E., Lee, A.C., Tregear, G.W., Niall, H.D., Stevens, V.C., 1980, Characteristics of antibodies raised to carboxy-terminal peptides of hCG beta subunit. Journal of Reproductive Immunology, 2: 1-13.

Puett, D., Ryan, R.J., Stevens, V.C., 1982, Circular dichroic and immunological properties of human choriogonadotropin-β carboxyl terminal peptides. International Journal of Peptide and Protein Research, 19: 506-513.

Stevens, V.C., Crystle, C.D., 1973, Effects of immunization with hapten-coupled hCG on the human menstrual cycle. Obstetrics and Gynecology, 42: 485-495.

Stevens, V.C., 1974, Fertility control through active immunization using placental proteins, in: Immunological Approaches to Fertility Control, Karolinska Symposium, 7, E. Diczfalusy, ed., Forum, Copenhagen.

Stevens, V.C., 1976, Actions of antisera to hCG-β: In vitro and in vivo assessment, in: Proceedings of the Fifth International Congress of Endocrinology. Vol. 1: 379, Excerpta Medica International Congress Series No. 402, Hamburg.

Stevens, V.C., Powell, J.E., Lee, A.C., Griffin, P.D., 1981a, Antifertility effects from immunization of female baboons with C-terminal peptides of hCG beta subunit. Fertility and Sterility, 36: 98-105.

Stevens, V.C., Cinader, B., Powell, J.E., Lee, A.C., Koh, S.W., 1981b Preparation and formulation of a hCG antifertility vaccine. Selection of peptide immunogen. American Journal of Reproductive Immunology, 6: 307-314.

Stevens, V.C., Cinader, B., Powell, J.E., Lee, A.C., Koh, S.W., 1981c, Preparation and formulation of a hCG antifertility vaccine. Selection of adjuvant and vehicle. American Journal of Reproductive Immunology, 6: 315-321.

Talwar, G.P., Sharma, N.C., Dubey, S.K., Salahuddin, M., Das, C., Ramakrishnan, S., Kumar, S., Hingorani, V., 1976, Isoimmunization against human chorionic gonadotropin with conjugates of processed β-subunit of the hormone and tetanus toxoid. Proceedings of the National Academy of Sciences, USA 73, 218-222.

WHO Special Programme of Research, Development and Research Training in Human Reproduction, 1984, Thirteenth Annual Report.

# ENHANCEMENT OF ANTIBODY RESPONSE TO AN ANTIGONADOTROPIN VACCINE BY USE OF ADJUVANTS

H.A. Nash, C.C. Chang, and Y.Y. Tsong

Center for Biomedical Research, The Population Council
1230 York Avenue, New York, New York 10021

## INTRODUCTION

Initial clinical trials of an antipregnancy vaccine consisting of the β-subunit of human chorionic gonadotropin linked to tetanus toxoid (β-hCG-TT) and adsorbed on $Al(OH)_3$ resulted in low and short-lived antibody titers in some of the women studied (1,2). It was therefore judged necessary to find ways to enhance the antibody response. Approaches explored included the use of other adjuvants to supplement the aluminum hydroxide and the use of modified vehicles. The effectiveness of these expedients was evaluated by vaccinating rabbits and measuring the concentration in serum of antibodies capable of binding labeled hCG. In selected instances, the ability of the antiserum to inhibit stimulation by hCG of uterine growth in immature rats was also measured. Some of the findings have been reported in earlier publications (3,4). They are summarized and extended in the present review.

## MATERIALS

β-hCG was prepared and coupled to tetanus toxoid as described by Tsong *et al.* (5). The coupling was effected by reaction with 1-ethyl-3-)3-dimethylaminopropyl) carbodiimide. The reaction product was adsorbed on $Al(OH)_3$ by adding aluminum potassium sulfate dodecahydrate to a solution of the β-hCG-TT and precipitating by adding sodium bicarbonate solution (5). The precipitate was washed three times with phosphate-buffered saline (PBS) and finally resuspended in PBS.

Supplementary adjuvants used in the studies reported in this paper are listed in Table 1. Muramyl dipeptide (MDP) and its several analogs were incorporated into the vaccine to provide 250 µg in each of the three vaccinations administered to each rabbit. OK 432 was administered in graduated doses to supply 0.5, 1.0, and 2.0 mg per rabbit in the three successive vaccinations.

Five types of formulations were used: (a) aqueous suspensions, (b) water-in-oil emulsions, (c) oil-in-water emulsions, (d) Pluronic formulations, and (e) a liposome preparation. Water-in-oil emulsions were prepared by mixing, in a high speed Waring Blendor, the suspension of β-hCG-TT on $Al(OH)_3$, the MDP analog and an equal volume of 1 part emulsifying agent and 6 parts by weight of peanut oil. Emulsifying agents included Arlacel A, Span 80, Span 85, and a mixture of Span 80 and Tween 80. Arlacel A is a mannide monooleate (purchased from Sigma Chemical).

TABLE 1

IDENTITY OF ADJUVANTS

| | |
|---|---|
| MDP | = N-ACETYLMURAMYL-L-ALANYL-D-ISOGLUTAMINE |
| $A_1$ | = N-HEXANOYLMURAMYL-D-PROPIONYL-L-ALANYL-D-ISOGLUTAMINE |
| $A_2$ | = N-ACETYLMURAMYL-D-PROPIONYL-L-THREONYL-D-ISOGLUTAMINE |
| $A_3$ | = N-GLYCOYLNORMURAMYL-ACETYL-L-α-AMINOGLUTYRYL-D-ISOGLUTAMINE |
| $A_4$ | = N-ACETYLNORMURAMYL-ACETYL-L-α-AMINOBUTYRYL-D-ISOGLUTAMINE |
| $A_5$ | = N-ACETYLNORMURAMYL-L-ALANYL-D-ISOGLUTAMINE |
| $A_6$ | = N-ACETYLMURAMYL-L-THREONYL-D-ISOGLUTAMINE |
| 37923 | = N-ACETYLMURAMYL-D-PROOPIONYL-L-α-AMINOBUTYRYL-D-ISOGLUTAMINE |
| MURABUTIDE | = N-ACETYLMURAMYL-L-ALANYL-D-GLUTAMINE-α-N-BUTYL ESTER |
| OK 432 | = LYOPHYLIZED PREPARATION OF SU STRAIN OF STREPTOCOCCUS PYOGENES |
| SPLPS | = SODIUM PHTHALATED LIPOPOLYSACCHARIDE |
| AVRIDINE | = N.N-DIOCTADECYL-N'.N'-BIS-(2-HYDROXETHYL)PROPANEDIAMINE |

Span 80 and Span 85 are sorbitan monooleate and sorbitan trioleate, respectively (manufactured by ICI). Tween 80 is polyoxyethylene sorbitan monooleate (Sigma Chemical). Oil-in-water emulsions were prepared using equal parts of PBS and Lipomal; or 2.5 parts saline, 0.1 part Tween 80, and 4.6 parts Intralipid; or 1 part PBS, 2 parts peanut oil containing 1 percent Tween 80 and 1 part glycerol. Lipomal is a soy phosphatide emulsion kindly supplied by Huhtamaki Oy/Leiras Pharmaceuticals of Pori, Finland. Intralipid is a fat emulsion manufactured by Cutter Laboratories of Emeryville, California. Pluronic is a BASF-Wyandotte tradename for block copolymers of propylene oxide and ethylene oxide. Our formulations included 2.5 percent Pluronic L121 and 0.2 percent Tween 80 in PBS. Squalane was included at a concentration of 5 percent in some of the Pluronic formulations. Liposomes were prepared using equamolar quantities of DL-α-phosphatidylcholine, dipalmitol, and cholesterol (6).

MDP analogs were tested as adjuvants in each of the formulation types listed earlier (data on liposome formulation not reported). OK 432 was tested only in aqueous suspension, as was SPLPS. Avridine was tested in aqueous suspension, water-in-oil emulsion and a liposome formulation.

## METHODS

Groups of five New Zealand albino rabbits weighing approximately 3 kg at the time of first vaccination were used for assessing antibody response. Animals received three vaccinations, with two-week intervals between vaccinations. Vaccinations were either intradermal or intramuscular, and consisted of 1.6 ml of the vaccine formulation split equally between two sites on the animal's rump. Each vaccine dose contained 100 μg of β-hCG subunit linked to tetanus toxoid. To provide a basis for estimating the contribution of supplementary adjuvants, a group of animals vaccinated with β-hCG-TT on $Al(OH)_3$ in aqueous suspension and without supplementary adjuvant was included in each experiment.

Antibody concentrations were measured by radioimmunoassay using $^{125}$I-labeled hCG as a ligand on samples drawn 2, 4, 6, and 8 weeks after the last vaccination. All samples from a single experiment were assayed in a single titration series. Additional details of the assay are given in a paper by Tsong _et al_. (5). For purposes of comparing antibody concentrations, the dilution of antiserum binding 33 percent of the labeled hCG was interpolated from binding data obtained on four dilutions of each antiserum sample.

The effectiveness of the antisera in neutralizing the biological activity of hCG was determined by comparing the gain in uterine weight of immature rats receiving hCG or hCG mixed with a sample of antiserum (3). Five 19-day-old female Sprague-Dawley rats were used in each experimental and control group. On each of three days they received 0.2 IU of hCG dissolved in saline containing 1 percent bovine serum albumin or a saline dilution of the antiserum. Animals were sacrificed 24 hours after the last injection and the uteri removed and weighed.

The pyrogenicity of the vaccine formulations was assessed by measuring body temperature rectally 40 minutes prevaccination and 1, 2, and 3 hours post-vaccination, using a Yellow Springs Instrument Model 43TF telethermometer.

RESULTS

The effectiveness of MDP analogs in enhancing antibody response when they are added to aqueous suspensions of β-hCG-TT on $Al(OH)_3$ was examined in several experiments. As is apparent from the findings tabulated in Table 2, none of the analogs tested appreciably enhanced the response at the doses tested. Preparing the antigen in a water-in-oil emulsion gave a moderately increased antibody titer in two out of three experiments. Markedly higher responses were, however, attained when the antigen was formulated with an MDP analog in a water-in-oil emulsion.

TABLE 2

MEAN DILUTION OF ANTISERA TAKEN 2, 4, 6, AND 8 WEEKS AFTER FINAL VACCINATION GIVING 33 PERCENT BINDING OF $^{125}$I-HCG. ANTIGEN = β-HCG-TT ON $AI(OH)_3$

| EXPERIMENT | ANTIGEN AQUEOUS SUSPENSION | ANTIGEN + MDP ANALOG AQUEOUS SUSPENSION | ANTIGEN IN WATER-IN-OIL EMULSION | ANTIGEN + MDP ANALOG IN WATER-IN-OIL EMULSION |
|---|---|---|---|---|
| 1 | 1000 | | 3400 | |
| 2 | 4300 | | 900 | |
| 6 | 800 | $1800^A$ | | $7100^A$ |
| 7 | 400 | $400^A$ | | |
| 8 | 800 | $700^A$ | 2900 | $10.000^A$ |
| 8 | 800 | $800^B$ | | $2000^B$ |
| 13 | 2600 | $3000^C$ | | $16.600^C$ |

$^A$ $A_5$

$^B$ 37923

$^C$ MURABUTIDE

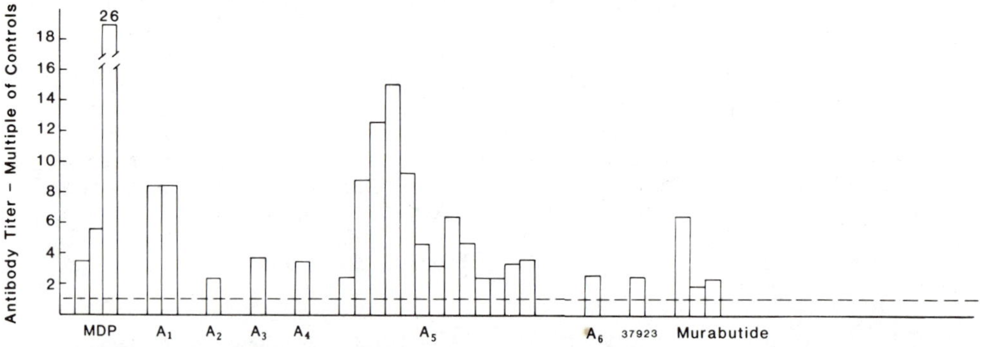


Fig. 1: Comparison of antibody titers attained in rabbits vaccinated with β-hCG-TT on $Al(OH)_3$ in a water-in-oil emulsion containing the indicated MDP analogs against those attained in controls vaccinated with β-hCG-TT on $Al(OH)_3$ in aqueous suspension. The dotted line indicates the response of the control rabbits.

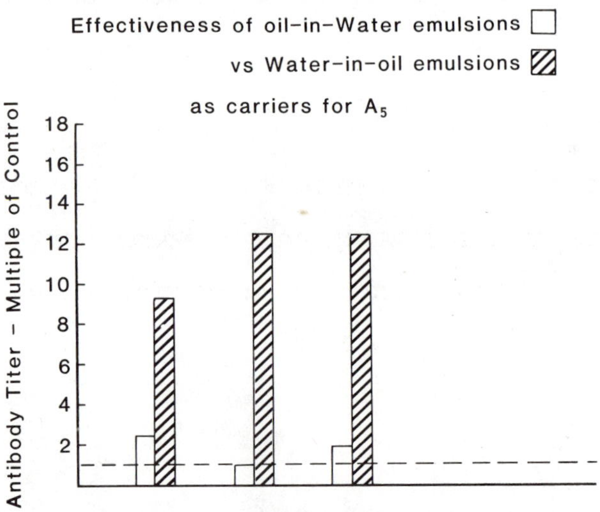


Fig. 2: Antibody titers using oil-in-water emulsions or water-in-oil emulsions as carriers of $A_5$ and β-hCG-TT on $Al(OH)_3$ compared with those of β-hCG-TT on $Al(OH)_3$ in aqueous suspension (dotted line).

TABLE 3

RELATIVE EFFECTIVENESS IN NEUTRALIZING

HCG IN THE RAT UTERINE WEIGHT ASSAY

OF ANTISERA OF VACCINATED RABBITS

| EXPERIMENT | ANTIGEN AQUEOUS SUSPENSION | ANTIGEN + MDP ANALOG AQUEOUS SUSPENSION | ANTIGEN IN WATER-IN-OIL EMULSION | ANTIGEN + MDP ANALOG IN WATER-IN-OIL EMULSION |
|---|---|---|---|---|
| 6 | 1 | $1^A$ | | $>3^A$ |
| 8 | 1 | $0.3^A$ | 0.5 | $4^A$ |
| 8 | 1 | $0.3^B$ | | $0.8^B$ |

$^A$ $A_5$

$^B$ 37923

The effectiveness of the antisera listed in Table 2 in neutralizing the stimulation of uterine growth by hCG is reported in Table 3. Neutralizing capacity generally corresponded to titer (see Table 2 for titers), although the neutralizing capacity of antisera from vaccinations using 37923 in water-in-oil emulsion did not exceed that of antisera from animals receiving antigen without supplementary adjuvant.

The generally high effectiveness of MDP analogs in enhancing antibody response when incorporated in water-in-oil emulsions is shown in Fig. 1. In every experiment, the response was greater than in the control group receiving only β-hCG-TT on $Al(OH)_3$. The increment was from 2- to 26-fold. Because of the differing degree of response relative to controls in different experiments, Fig. 1 cannot be used to judge the relative effectiveness of different MDP analogs. Data from experiments comparing $A_5$, $A_6$, and murabutide are shown in Table 4. All three appear to be equipotent. Two of the MDP series of MDP analogs tested and reported in Table 1 were judged unacceptable because of pyrogenicity. They were MDP itself and analog $A_1$.

Oil-in-water emulsions were also tested as carriers for analog $A_5$. Titers relative to controls receiving β-hCGTT on $Al(OH)_3$ in aqueous suspension are shown in Fig. 2 for three experiments, together with relative titers for animals in the same experiments receiving water-in-oil formulations. The superiority of the water-in-oil emulsions was marked.

Titers observed using Pluronic vehicles as carriers for MDP analogs are compared in Table 5 with those found in the same experiments using water-in-oil emulsions. The titers were comparable. There was no marked advantage in including squalane in the Pluronic formulation.

One experiment was conducted to test the necessity of adsorbing the β-hCG-TT on $Al(OH)_3$ if the antigen is incorporated in a water-in-oil emulsion with analog $A_5$ as an adjuvant. The titers following vaccination with the preparation including $Al(OH)_3$ were 4.7 times greater than those of the controls; those of the group omitting $Al(OH)_3$ were only 1.5 times greater.

## TABLE 4

### RECIPROCAL OF ANTISERUM DILUTION GIVING 33% BINDING OF $^{125}I$-HCG

| EXPT. | ANTIGEN + $A_5$ WATER-IN-OIL EMULSION | ANTIGEN + $A_6$ WATER-IN-OIL EMULSION | ANTIGEN + MURABUTIDE WATER-IN-OIL EMULSION |
|---|---|---|---|
| 15 | 4.100; 4.100 | | 3.100 |
| 13 | 16.300 | | 16.600 |
| 17 | | 8.500 | 7.400 |

ANTIGEN = β-HCG-TT ON $AL(OH)_3$

## TABLE 5

### RECIPROCAL OF ANTISERUM DILUTION GIVING 33% BINDING OF $^{125}I$-HCG

| EXPT. | ANTIGEN + $A_5$ WATER-IN-OIL EMULSION | ANTIGEN + $A_6$ WATER-IN-OIL EMULSION | ANTIGEN + $A_6$ PLURONIC | ANTIGEN + $A_6$ PLURONIC SQUALANE |
|---|---|---|---|---|
| 15 | 5.600 | | | 5.300 |
| 16 | 12.000 | | 8.900 | 9.400 |
| 17 | | 8.500 | 9.200 | 12.200 |

ANTIGEN = β-HCG-TT ON $AL(OH)_3$

TABLE 6

RECIPROCAL OF ANTISERUM DILUTION GIVING 33% BINDING OF $^{125}$I-HCG

| EXPERIMENT | ANTIGEN + $A_5$ WATER-IN-OIL EMULSION | ANTIGEN + OK 432 |
|---|---|---|
| 8 | 10.000; 12.000 | 14.000 |
| 10 | 6.400 | 10.900 |
| 10 | 8.100 | 32.100 |
| 13 | 16.300 | 12.400 |
| 14 | 21.700 | 19.000 |

ANTIGEN = β-HCG-TT ON $AL(OH)_3$

Used as an adjuvant, the streptococcal preparation OK 432 in aqueous suspension gave antibody titers 4- to 17-fold greater than those of the control preparation. Comparisons with the titers attained with MDP analog $A_5$ in water-in-oil emulsion are shown in Table 6. The titers attained with the two adjuvant systems were comparable.

The data presented indicate mean titers for five animals in each group over an eight-week period. Since the perceived need for supplementary adjuvants in an antigonadotropin vaccine based on β-hCG is to increase the antigenic response of those individuals who respond poorly, the distribution of response when supplementary adjuvants are used is of crucial interest. The range of antigenic response among rabbits in the same experimental groups was frequently as great as 4-fold and sometimes as great as 8-fold. Inquiry, therefore, focuses on the effect of supplementary antigen on the low part of the response range. The question is examined in Table 7, where the responses of individual animals in the test and control groups are compared. Eighty-two percent of the test animals receiving the formulations noted in that Table had titers greater than any of the animals in the control group for the experiment that included a given test animal. Ninety-seven percent had titers above the median for the relevant control group.

DISCUSSION

The findings in these studies show that several MDP analogs and the streptococcal preparation OK 432 can consistently increase the antibody response in rabbits to an antigen derived from a gonadotropin. They also emphasize the importance of the vehicle. The MDP analogs were relatively ineffective at the doses used when formulated in aqueous suspensions or in oil-in-water emulsions, but were highly effective in water-in-oil emulsions or in a vehicle containing Pluronic polymer. OK

TABLE 7

DISTRIBUTION OF TITERS VS. THOSE OF CONTROLS OF INDIVIDUAL RABBITS RECEIVING MDP ANALOG[A] IN WATER-IN-OIL EMULSION OR IN PLURONIC FORMULATION[B,C]

CONTROLS, N = 60
ADJUVANT, N = 115

ANTIBODY TITER DISTRIBUTION IN ADJUVANT GROUPS

| | NUMBER | PERCENT |
|---|---|---|
| ABOVE ALL CONTROL ANIMALS[D] | 94 | 82 |
| ABOVE MEDIAN CONTROLS[D] | 112 | 97 |
| ABOVE LOWEST 40% OF CONTROLS | 115 | 100 |

[A]MDP ANALOGS $A_5$, $A_6$ OR MURABUTIDE

[B]ALL ANIMALS RECEIVED β-HCG-TT ON $AL(OH)_3$

[C]MEAN TITERS OF SERUM 2, 4, 6, 8 WEEKS AFTER LAST VACCINATION

[D]COMPARISONS WERE WITH CONTROLS IN SAME EXPERIMENT

432, in contrast, did not require emulsions or polymer for a high level of effectiveness. Avoiding emulsion formulations is of obvious practical advantage from the standpoint of pharmaceutical elegance and physical stability, but we have succeeded in formulating emulsions, using Span and Tween emulsifying agents that are readily redispersed by hand shaking. The formulations used also substitute a biodegradable vegetable oil for the mineral oil of Fruend's adjuvants.

The interaction between adsorption of the antigen on $Al(OH)_3$ and the supplementary adjuvants has not been adequately explored, but in the one experiment directed to this question, omission of the $Al(OH)_3$ led to much lower antibody titers than when it was included. This was despite the inclusion of MDP analog $A_5$ and the use of a water-in-oil emulsion in both formulations.

The degree to which findings in rabbits can be extrapolated to other species is not known. MDP analogs have been found to enhance antibody response in several species (7,8) and Pluronic formulations of an MDP analog have been found to increase antibody response in several test systems (9,10). At the same time, the complexity of the immunological system and its controls is so great that differences in responsiveness to adjuvants among species seem inevitable.

The generality of the response to MDP analogs formulated in water-in-oil emulsions, found in these studies, cannot be taken as evidence of similar potency throughout the series. The analogs tested had been identified as outstanding candidates in other testing programs by those who made them available to us. Neither does lack of antibody-enhancing activity in aqueous suspension indicate that such activity would not have been evidenced if we had tested higher doses.

Several other adjuvants may be promising candidates for use in antigonadotropin vaccines. Some have been preliminarily tested in our experimental series. Modified lipopolysaccharides (SPLPS) have been the subject of considerable interest as adjuvants and have reached human trial (11). In our experiments, SPLPS preparations increased antibody response to 1.6 and 1.7 times that of the control group when administered at non-pyrogenic doses. At a markedly pyrogenic dose, one preparation gave an increase of 7.2-fold. Another candidate that has shown adjuvant effectiveness in a number of systems is Avridine [N',N'-dioctadecyl-N',N'-bis-(20-hydroxyethyl) propanediamine] (12,13). When Avridine and β-hCG-TT on $Al(OH)_3$ were formulated in liposomes, we observed a 4.2-fold increase in titer over the control formulation (4). A number of other substances have been reported to increase titers of circulating antibodies when given at or near the time of antigen administration. Included among them are dextran sulfate (14), dimethyldioctadecyl-ammonium bromide (14), small polysaccharides from gram-negative bacteria (15), and lipoteichoic acids from gram-positive bacteria (15).

The use of adjuvants has not overcome the variation in response among animals. However, as is evident in Table 7, all of the animals receiving the more effective adjuvant preparations have given higher antibody titers than has the lower 40 percent among the controls; 82 percent have given higher responses than any of the controls. These findings give reason to hope that supplementary adjuvants may contribute substantially to the effectiveness of antipregnancy vaccines in humans. Several formulations have been identified that appear to be practical and potentially useful.

ACKNOWLEDGEMENTS

This research was carried out as part of the contraceptive development program of the International Committee for Contraception Research of the Population Council, Inc., New York. The financial support provided by the International Development Research Centre of Canada, The Rockefeller Foundation, The Ford Foundation, The Mellon Foundation, and the George J. Hecht Fund is gratefully acknowledged. The gifts of OK 432 by Chugai Pharmaceutical, various MDP analogs by Syntex Research, murabutide and SPLPS by Institut Pasteur, SPLPS by the National Institute of Immunology (India), and tetanus toxoid from Wyeth Laboratories were crucial to the research. The hCG standard was furnished by the National Pituitary Agency.

REFERENCES

1. Nash, H., Talwar, G.P., Segal, S., Luukkainen, T., Johansson, E.D.B., Vasquez, J., Coutinho, E., and Sundaram, K. Observations on the antigenicity and clinical effects of a candidate antipregnancy vaccine: β-subunit of human chorionic gonadotropin linked to tetanus toxoid. Fertil. Steril. 34:328 (1980).

2. Shahani, S.M., Kulkarni, P.P., Patel, K.L., Salahuddin, M., Das, C., and Talwar, G.P. Clinical and immunological responses with Pr-β-hCG-TT vaccine. Contraception 25:421 (1982).

3. Nash, H.A., Chang, C.C., and Tsong, Y.Y. Formulation of a potential antipregnancy vaccine based on the β-subunit of human chorionic gonadotropin (β-hCG). Use of compounds of the muramyl dipeptide (MDP) family as adjuvants. J. Reprod. Immunol. 7:151 (1985).

4. Chang, C.C., Tsong, Y.Y., and Nash, H.A. Formulation of a potential antipregnancy vaccine based on the β-subunit of human chorionic gonadotropin (β-hCG). III. Evaluation of various vehicles and adjuvants. J. Reprod. Immunol. 7:163 (1985).

5. Tsong, Y.Y., Chang, C.C., and Nash, H.A. Formulation of a potential antipregnancy vaccine based on the β-subunit of human chorionic gonadotropin (β-hCG). I. Alternative macromolecular carriers. J. Reprod. Immunol. 7:139 (1985).

6. Siddiqui, W.A., Taylor, D.W., Kan, S.-C., Kramer, K., Richmond-Crum, S.M., Kotani, S., Shiba, T., and Kusumoto, S. Vaccination of experimental monkeys against *Plasmodium falciparum*; a possible safe adjuvant. Science 201:1237 (1978).

7. Audibert, F., Parant, M., Damais, C., Lefrancier, P., Derrien, M., Choay, J., and Chedid, L. Dissociation of immunostimulant activities of muramyl dipeptide (MDP) by linking amino acids or peptides to the glutaminyl residue. Biochem. Biophys. Res. Commun. 96:915 (1980).

8. Jolivet, M., Sache, E., and Audibert, F. Biological studies of lipophilic MDP derivatives incorporated in liposomes. Immunol Commun. 10:511 (1981).

9. Hunter, R., Strickland, F., and Kezdy, F. The adjuvant activity of nonionic block polymer surfactants. I. The role of hydrophile-lipophile balance. J. Immunol. 127:1244 (1981).

10. Snippe, H., DeReuver, M.J., Strickland, F., Willers, J.M.N., and Hunter, R.L. Adjuvant effect of nonionic block surfactants in humoral and cellular immunity. Int. Arch. Allergy Appl. Immunol. 65:390 (1981).

11. Elin, R.J., Wolff, S.M., McAdam, K.P.W.J, Chedid, L., Audibert, F., Barnard, C., and Aberling, F. Properties of reference Eschrechia coli endotoxin and its phthalylated derivative in humans. J. Infect. Dis. 144:329 (1981).

12. Niblack, J.F., Otterness, I.G., Hemsworth, G.R., Wolff, J.S. III, Hoffman, W.W., and Kraska, A.R. CP-20,961: A structurally novel synthetic adjuvant. J. Reticuloendothel. Soc. 26:655 (1979).

13. Anderson, A.O. and Reynolds, J.A. Adjuvant effects of the lipid amine CP 20,961. J. Reticuloendothel. Soc. 26:667 (1979).

14. Hilgers, A.Th.H, Snippe, H., Jansze, M., and Willers, J.M.N. Immuno-modulating properties of two synthetic adjuvants: Dependence on type of antigen, dose and time of administration. Cellular Immunol. 86:393 (1984).

15. Friedman, H. Immunomodulation by small molecular weight bacterial products. Adv. Exptl. Med. Biol. 166:199 (1983).

**RATIONAL VACCINE DESIGN: OPPORTUNITIES OFFERED BY MOLECULAR GENETICS**

**N.A. Mitchison**

Imperial Cancer Research Fund, Tumour Immunology Unit
Department of Zoology, University College London
Gower Street, London WC1E 6BT

The issue discussed here is how current knowledge of immunoregulation can help design safe and effective birth control vaccines. The principle questions are (i) how to obtain an effective response in terms of magnitude and duration, (ii) how to avoid generating autoimmunity to self-components of the body, (iii) how to avoid anamnastic immunity (avoiding boosting of the response eg by incipient pregnancy, in order to ensure that vaccination is reversible), and (iv) how much new modes of vaccination, such as using vaccinia as a vector, have to offer. This discussion will centre round the two immunological mechanisms which are central to all vaccine development, differentiation of epitopes as suppressors or helpers, and intrastructural antigenic competition.

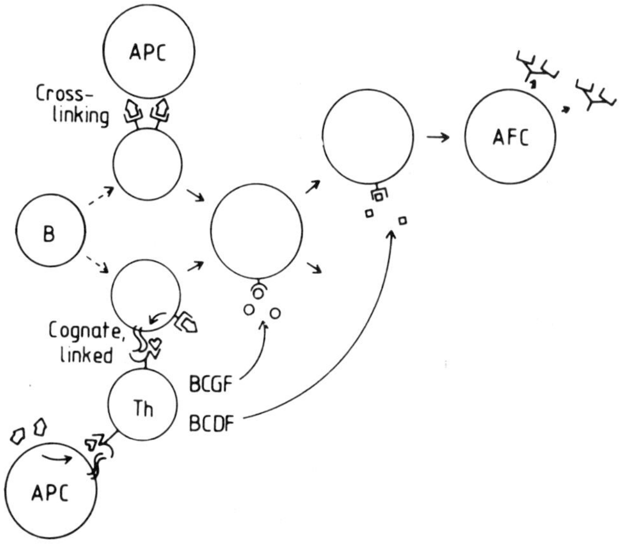


Fig. 1 Regulation of the B-cell responses

Figure 1 illustrates the major features of immunoregulation as they are currently understood (1). It refers only to regulation of B-cells, but cytolytic T cells and other effectors are subject to regulation in much the same way. Antigen (shown in the figure as a broad arrow) enters the immune system by two routes; one is via antigen presenting cells (? follicular dendritic cells) which specialise in presenting a matrix of conformational epitopes able to cross-link receptor immunoglobulin on B-cells; the other is via presenting cells (? tissue and intestitial dendritic cells, MHC Class II-expressing macrophages) which degrade antigen within vesicles in order to expose hydrophobic sites and which then expose the resulting sequence epitopes in association with MHC Class II molecules to regulatory T cells. The principle regulatory T-cells are helper (Th) cells. After being activated in this way they go on to recognise the same sequence epitopes on B-cell, and so activate the B-cells in a cognate (i.e. in association with a self-MHC molecule) and linked (i.e. the T- and B-cells must see epitopes on the same antigenic structure) manner. The B-cell has thus acquired the epitope by processing the antigen in essentially the same way as does the specialized antigen presenting cell first in the chain.

Why have two ways of signalling to B-cells? Modelling experiments have been carried out in which anti-immunoglobulin antibodies mimic the physiological process of receptor cross-linking by antigen, and T-cells reacting with allo-antigens on the B-cell surface mimic the physiological linked, cognate process. In such systems the two processes are found to syngerise strongly. It is a reasonable guess, then, that physiologically they work together by signal storage: probably cross-linking activation comes first, up-regulation of MHC Class II expression comes next (2), and the linked cognate interaction then completes the activation process. In this way B-cells are able to sample two distinct micro-environments for the presence of antigen, and thus respond more accurately to its presence.

Activation of this kind takes the B-cell into G2 of the cell cycle, and there the cell will die in G2 arrest unless further stimulated with growth and differentiation factors, as shown in the Figure (3). This G2 arrest represents another example of signal storage, and the whole process of activation, proliferation, and differentiation can thus be regarded as a step-by-step process which enjoys the same advantages of information storage, signal expansion, and feed-back control as do the classical serum protein cascade systems (complement activation, clotting, fibrinolysis).

From the point of view of vaccine development, five points in this scheme deserve particular comment.

(i) The epitopes recognised or defined by T- and B-cells will generally be different from one another, with T-cells specializing in sequences associated with hydrophobic areas and B-cells specialising in conformational structures. Nevertheless because a 'bridge' in the old sense never forms between T and B cell, i.e. at no point do their receptors bind simultaneously to the same antigenic structure, the epitopes which they recognise do not have to be located on different parts of the antigen. Indeed there is evidence that the receptor immunoglobulin used by the B-cell to pick up antigen remains attached during the processing step within the cell, resulting in protection of the sequences around the B-cell-defined epitope from cleavage. This in turn forces T and B epitopes to occur close to or superimposed on one another (4).

(ii) Immunological memory. As both T- and B-cells participate in most responses (except for T-independent responses, which depend on cross-linking alone), immunological memory depends on priming both populations. This is highly relevant to the β-hCG peptide vaccines, where the T-cell component of the response is directed towards a carrier protein; after immunization with a vaccine of this type a secondary response should not develop against hCG alone, and little danger of irreversible immunization should arise.

To the extent that helper T-cells may be generated against the peptide used in the vaccine this argument will not apply. If and when such helper cells do develop, there is a further problem that the rest of the hCG molecule may get draged into the response. Note however that the behaviour of the immune system towards new epitopes added onto an immunogen after the response has started is complex, and that a new epitope may become a focus of activity for suppressor T cells (5).

The components of immunological memory within each lymphocyte compartment are (i) activation, and (ii) clonal expansion. Circumstantial evidence indicates that the former predominates in the T-cell compartment, and the latter in the B-cell one (6). Consequently repeated immunization tends to boost progressively the B-cell response, whereas that of T-cells rapidly reaches a maximum beyond which there is little benefit from prolonging exposure to the immunogen. T-cells seem, in other words, to be under particularly tight homeostatic constraint.

(iii) Competition. Dual recognition by T-cells, as illustratd in the figure, offers much scope for antigenic competition particularly between epitopes within a single structure. Following internalization of the antigen by a reactive B-cell, stringent competition occurs between the various epitopes for association with MHC Class II molecules (7,8). This by no means implies that they actually bind to these molecules, but rather that they become available for dual recognition by T-cells. The fact that proliferation among T-cells is under tight constraint no doubt makes such competition all the more stringent.

(iv) Immunoregulatory factors. The physiological role of BCDF and BCGF is far from clear (9). They may well represent points at which the immune respone can be most readily manipulated. Certainly these factors currently elicit a great deal of commercial interest, which is predicated on the notion that cloned molecules of this type can be used for therapeutic intervention. If these hopes are fulfilled, they will have a major impact on the design of vaccines. But there is an alternative and less rosey view, that while these molecules are undoubtedly important for keeping lymphocytes happy in vitro, they may not be rate limiting within the intact immune system.

(v) Antigen presenting cells as a rate limiting step. Immunization by means of antigen-encoding genes incorporated into the vaccinia genome represents an exciting new development (10). Its main value is likely to be in eliciting cytotoxic T-cells, a response in which specialized antigen presenting cells are not required (11). In eliciting Th-cells they are required, and as shown in the figure are likely to represent a rate-limiting step. Conventional immunization can probably saturate this step. Consequently the vaccinia approach is likely to prove more valuable in generating protective immunity against viral infection than in developing birth control vaccines.

What has been left out of this scheme is the suppressor cell pathway. This is because suppressor T cells are currently under a cloud. Their troubles in respect of molecular biology are well known - the lack of receptor β chain rearrangement, the failure to find transcription of Class II MHC genes, the lack of a DNA sequence counterpart to I-J, and so on (12). Furthermore in the best studied instance of suppression in an infectious disease, Leishmaniasis, chaos currently reigns. Nevertheless the hope of defining and manipulating suppressor determinants remains one of the great hopes for the second generation of vaccines. I have not changed my opinion over the last year (13,14), and remain convinced that suppressor epitopes do exist, and have a logical basis in the way that intermediate concentration self-proteins manipulate the T-cell repertoires.

REFERENCES


1. M. J. H. Ratcliffe and N. A. Mitchison, Function of Ig receptors in B-cell triggering. Annales D'Immunologie de l'Institut Pasteur 135D:73 (1984).

2. J. A. Ledbetter, P. J. Martin, and E. A. Clark, Mantle Zone in Germinal Center B-cells respond to different activation signals. in: Proc. 16th Leucocyte Culture Conference. N. A. Mitchison and M. Feldman eds.,(1985) (Humana Press - in press).

3. F. Melchers et al, Proc Natl Acad Sci (1985) (in press).

4. J. A. Berzowsky, T-B reciprocity. An Ia-restricted eiptope-specific circuit regulating T-cell-B-cell interaction and antibody specificity, Surv Immunol Res. 2:223 (1983).

5. C. A. Herzenberg, T. Tokuisa, L. A. Herzenberg, Epitope-specific regulation. III Induction of allotype-restricted suppression for IgG antibody responses to individual epitopes on complex antigens. Eur J Immunol. 10:814 (1982).

6. N. A. Mitchison and S. Petersson, Does clonal selection occur among T-cells? Annales d'Immunologie de l'Institut Pasteur. 134D:37 (1983).

7. E. A. Clarke, P. Lake, L. Favila-Castillo, Modulation of Thy-1 alloantibody responses: donor cell associated H-2 inhibition and augmentation without recipient Ir gene control, J Immunol 127:2135. (1981).

8. K. L. Rock, B. Benaccerraf, Inhibition of antigen specific T lymphocyte activaton by structurally related Ir gene-controlled polymers: evidence of specific competition for accesory cell antigen proliferation, J Exp Med 157:1618 (1983).

9. T. Kishimoto, Factors affecting B-cell growth and differentiation, Ann Rev Immunol (1985) (in press).

10. Ed. R. Bell and G. Torrigiani, New approaches to vaccine development, Schwabe, Basel (1984).

11. A. A. Czitrom, G. H. Sunshine, T. Reme, R. Ceredig, A. L. Glasbrook, A. Kelso, H. R. MacDonald. Stimulator cell requirements for allospecific T-cell subsets: specialised accessory cells are

required to activate helper but not cytolytic T lymphocyte precursors, J Immunol 130:546 (1983).

12. S. M. Hedrick, R. N. Germain, M. J. Bevan. Rearrangement and transcription of a T-cell receptor β-chain gene in different T-cell subsets, Proc Natl Acad Sci 82:531 (1985).

13. N. A. Mitchison, Rational design of vaccines. Nature (News and Views) 308:112 (1984).

14. N. A. Mitchison, Four Intermediate Concentration Proteins and Their Message for Self-Tolerance, Autoimmunity and Suppressor Epitopes. Clinical Immunology Newsletter 6:1 12 (1985).

CLONING AND EXPRESSION OF BIOLOGICALLY ACTIVE

HUMAN FERTILITY HORMONES

Vemuri B. Reddy, Anton K. Beck, Vincent Vellucci, Anthony J. Garramone and Edward G. Bernstine

Integrated Genetics, Inc.
31 New York Avenue
Framingham, Massachusetts

## INTRODUCTION

The three human gonadotropins, choriogonadotropin (hCG), luteinizing hormone (hLH) and follicle stimulating hormone (hFSH), are glycoproteins playing a major role in ovulation, spermatogenesis and conception. hCG is secreted by the developing placenta during the first trimester of pregnancy. Both hLH and hFSH are secreted by the pituitary and together play a central role in regulating menstrual cycle and ovulation.

All three hormones are dimeric glycoproteins consisting of two distinct polypeptide chains, an $\alpha$ subunit and a $\beta$ subunit (1,2). While the $\beta$ subunit of each hormone is unique, the $\alpha$ subunit is shared by all three gonadotropins. Glycosylation is a key feature of the gonadotropins. For example, hCG cosists of 30% carbohydrate by weight. The common $\alpha$ subunit is glycosylated at two asparagine residues. The $\beta$hCG chain at two asparagines and four serines, the $\beta$hLH at one asparagine and the $\beta$hFSH at two asparagines (3,4). Although there is no definitive data, it has been suggested that the carbohydrate moieties are involved in secretion and in determining the half-lives of the proteins in circulation.

Amino acid sequence of the purified proteins indicated that the $\alpha$ chain is composed of 92 amino acids and the $\beta$ chains for hCG, hLH, hFSH are 145, 115 and 118 amino acids, respectively (5). DNA sequence data predicts that the $\alpha$ chain consists of 92 amino acids and the $\beta$ chains of hCG, hLH and hFSH consists of 145, 121 and 111 amino acids respectively. Here we report the cloning and expression of the three gonadotropins in biologically active forms in Simian Virus 40 (SV40).

Simian Virus 40 has been used as a vector for the expression of a number of eukaryotic genes in monkey cells (6-8). All the vectors made thus far can be grouped into two categories: late replacement vectors and early replacement vectors. The former make use of the SV40 late promoter, the late splicing and polyadenylation signals. Expression is achieved in CV-1 cells along with the temperature-sensitive helper virus tsA58, which codes for the missing functions (6). The latter group makes use of the SV40 early promoter and the early splicing and poly A signals. Expression is achieved in COS cells which are monkey kidney cells constitutively producing large T antigen needed for the replication of the recombinant SV40 (7,9). The recombinant SV40 vectors are made by replacing either the late or early coding sequences with the genes of interest while keeping the SV40 origin of replication and transcriptional signals intact. Although SV40 has been used commonly as an expression vector because of the ease with which costructions can be made, all applications to date have used only one foreign gene in any one vector. This report describes the construction of vectors in which the SV40 late region has been replaced by two cDNAs coding for $\alpha$ and $\beta$ subunits.

## CLONING OF THE GONADOTROPIN SUBUNITS

First trimester human placental poly A RNA was converted into cDNA and cloned into the Pstl site of pBR322 by GC tailing. $\alpha$ and $\beta$ hCG cDNA clones were isolated from this library by screening with complementary DNA probes. The cDNAs were sequenced using Maxam-Gilbert chemical degradation method (10) and found to agree with the published nucleotide sequence (11,12).

Human pituitary poly A RNA was converted into cDNA using reverse transcriptase and DNA polymerase. The cDNA was cloned into the Pstl site of pBR322 by means of GC tails. Because of the extensive amino acid homology between $\beta$ hCG and $\beta$ hLH (13) the $\beta$ hCG cDNA fragment was used to screen the pituitary library. Analysis of the $\beta$ hLH clone isolated showed it lacked sequences coding for the first six amino acids of the leader pepetide. Taking advantage of the large homologies between $\beta$ hCG and $\beta$ hLH (95% at the nucloetide level), the 5' portion of the $\beta$ hCG leader was ligated to the $\beta$ hLH cDNA to produce a full length $\beta$ hLH cDNA with a hybrid $\beta$ hLH-hCG leader.

To isolate a $\beta$ FSH DNA clone, a human genomic library in Charon 4A phage (14) was screened with a mixture of 45 residue long oligonucleotides in which the third position in each codon was chosen based on codon usage data. Southern blot analysis of this clone using fragments of a porcine FSH cDNA clone as hybridization probes, and subsequent sequencing of the coding region confirmed this DNA for the human $\beta$ FSH peptide. A 18 amino acid signal peptide is followed by the 111 amino acid mature peptide whose coding sequence is separated by a single intron of approximately 1.6kb between the codons for amino acids 35 and 36. The amino acid sequence deduced from the nucleotide sequence differs from the published protein sequences in several positions; most notably the carboxy-terminus is Met-Lys-Glu. The results of Southern blots of human DNA probed with fragments of the genomic clone are consistent with there being one gene coding for beta FSH. A $\beta$ hFSH cDNA equivalent was constructed by removing the intron from the genomic DNA by means of restriction enzymes and filling the coding sequences with synthetic oligonucleotides.

The nucleotide sequences of the engineered cDNAs of the $\alpha$ and the $\beta$ hCG and $\beta$ hLH subunits are shown in the following figure (Figure 1) along with the amino acid sequences. The amino acid sequence of $\beta$ hFSH is shown here and its nucleotide sequence will be published elsewhere.

**a**

```
                                                  31                                          61
AATTCCC ATG GAT TAC TAC AGA AAA TAT GCA GCT ATC TTT CTG GTC ACA TTG TCG GTG TTT
        Met Asp Tyr Tyr Arg Lys Tyr Ala Ala Ile Phe Leu Val Thr Leu Ser Val Phe

                                  91                                          121
CTG CAT GTT CTC CAT TCC↓GCT CCT GAT GTG CAG GAT TGC CCA GAA TGC ACG CTA CAG GAA
Leu His Val Leu His Ser Ala Pro Asp Val Gln Asp Cys Pro Glu Cys Thr Leu Gln Glu

                                  151                                         181
AAC CCA TTC TTC TCC CAG CCG GGT GCC CCA ATA CTT CAG TGC ATG GGC TGC TGC TTC TCT
Asn Pro Phe Phe Ser Gln Pro Gly Ala Pro Ile Leu Gln Cys Met Gly Cys Cys Phe Ser

                                  211                                         241
AGA GCA TAT CCC ACT CCA CTA AGG TCC AAG AAG ACG ATG TTG GTC CAA AAG AAC GTC ACC
Arg Ala Tyr Pro Thr Pro Leu Arg Ser Lys Lys Thr Met Leu Val Gln Lys Asn Val Thr

                                  271                                         301
TCA GAG TCC ACT TGC TGT GTA GCT AAA TCA TAT AAC AGG GTC ACA GTA ATG GGG GGT TTC
Ser Glu Ser Thr Cys Cys Val Ala Lys Ser Tyr Asn Arg Val Thr Val Met Gly Gly Phe

                                  331                                         361
AAA GTG GAG AAC CAC ACG GCG TGC CAC TGC AGT ACT TGT TAT TAT CAC AAA TCT TAA ATG
Lys Val Glu Asn His Thr Ala Cys His Cys Ser Thr Cys Tyr Tyr His Lys Ser End

TTTTACCAAGTGCTGTCTTGATGACTGCTGATTTTCTGGAATGGAAAATTAAGTTGTTTAGTGTTTATGGCTTTGTGAG

ATAAAACTCTCCTTTTCCTTACCATACCACTTTGACACGCTTCAAGGATATACTGCAGCTTTACTGCCTTCCTCCTTAT

CCTACAGTACAATCAGCAGTCTAGTTCTTTTCATTTGGAATGAATACAGCATTAAGCTCGGATC
```

**b**

```
                                                 32                                          62
AATTCCGGATG GAG ATG TTC CAG GGG CTG CTG CTG TTG CTG CTG CTG AGC ATG GGC GGG ACA
            Met Glu Met Phe Gln Gly Leu Leu Leu Leu Leu Leu Leu Ser Met Gly Gly Thr

                                  ·92                                         122
TGG GCA↓TCC AAG GAG CCG CTT CGG CCA CGG TGC CGC CCC ATC AAT GCC ACC CTG GCT GTG
Trp Ala Ser Lys Glu Pro Leu Arg Pro Arg Cys Arg Pro Ile Asn Ala Thr Leu Ala Val

                                  152                                         182
GAG AAG GAG GGC TGC CCC GTG TGC ATC ACC GTC AAC ACC ACC ATC TGT GCC GGC TAC TGC
Glu Lys Glu Gly Cys Pro Val Cys Ile Thr Val Asn Thr Thr Ile Cys Ala Gly Tyr Cys

                                  212                                         242
CCC ACC ATG ACC CGC GTG CTG CAG GGG GTC CTG CCG GCC CTG CCT CAG GTG GTG TGC AAC
Pro Thr Met Thr Arg Val Leu Gln Gly Val Leu Pro Ala Leu Pro Gln Val Val Cys Asn

                                  272                                         302
TAC CGC GAT GTG CGC TTC GAG TCC ATC CGG CTC CCT GGC TGC CCG CGC GGC GTG AAC CCC
Tyr Arg Asp Val Arg Phe Glu Ser Ile Arg Leu Pro Gly Cys Pro Arg Gly Val Asn Pro

                                  332                                         362
GTG GTC TCC TAC GCC GTG GCT CTC AGC TGT CAA TGT GCA CTC TGC CGC CGC AGC ACC ACT
Val Val Ser Tyr Ala Val Ala Leu Ser Cys Gln Cys Ala Leu Cys Arg Arg Ser Thr Thr

                                  392                                         422
GAC TGC GGG GGT CCC AAG GAC CAC CCC TTG ACC TGT GAT GAC CCC CGC TTC CAG GAC TCC
Asp Cys Gly Gly Pro Lys Asp His Pro Leu Thr Cys Asp Asp Pro Arg Phe Gln Asp Ser

                                  452                                         482
TCT TCC TCA AAG GCC CCT CCC CCC AGC CTT CCA AGT CCA TCC CGA CTC CCG GGG CCC TCG
Ser Ser Ser Lys Ala Pro Pro Pro Ser Leu Pro Ser Pro Ser Arg Leu Pro Gly Pro Ser

GAC ACC CCG ATC CTC CCA CAA TAA AGGCTTCTCAATCCGCAAAAAAAAAAAAAAAAAAAAAAAAAAAAAAA
Asp Thr Pro Ile Leu Pro Gln End

AAAAAAAAACAAGCTCGGATC
```

Figure 1: Nucleotide and amino acid sequences of the subunits of human gonadotropins: (a) α hCG, (b) β hCG, (c) β hLH and (d) β hFSH. The nucleotide sequence of β hFSH is not shown here and it wil be published elsewhere. The nucleotide sequences are engineered with EcoR I linkers at the 5' end, and BamH I linkers at the 3' ends. The β hLH leader contains β hCG sequences as explained in the text. The arrows on the amino acid sequences indicate amino terminal ends of the mature peptides.

(continued over leaf)

**c**

```
                                             32                                                62
AATTCCGGATG GAG ATG TTC CAG GGG CTG CTG CTG TTG CTG CTG CTG AGC ATG GGC GGG GCA
            Met Glu Met Phe Gln Gly Leu Leu Leu Leu Leu Leu Leu Ser Met Gly Gly Ala

                                             92                                               122
TGG GCA↓TCC AGG GAG CCG CTT CGG CCA TGG TGC CAC CCC ATC AAT GCC ATC CTG GCT GTG
Trp Ala Ser Arg Glu Pro Leu Arg Pro Trp Cys His Pro Ile Asn Ala Ile Leu Ala Val

                                            152                                               182
GAG AAG GAG GGC TGC CCC GTG TGC ATC ACC GTC AAC ACC ACC ATC TGT GCC GGC TAC TGC
Glu Lys Glu Gly Cys Pro Val Cys Ile Thr Val Asn Thr Thr Ile Cys Ala Gly Tyr Cys

                                            212                                               242
CCC ACC ATG ATG CGC GTG CTG CAG GCG GTC CTG CCG CCC CTG CCT CAG GTG GTG TGC ACC
Pro Thr Met Met Arg Val Leu Gln Ala Val Leu Pro Pro Leu Pro Gln Val Val Cys Thr

                                            272                                               302
TAC CGT GAT GTG CGC TTC GAG TCC ATC CGG CTC CCT GGC TGC CCG CGT GGC GTG GAC CCC
Tyr Arg Asp Val Arg Phe Glu Ser Ile Arg Leu Pro Gly Cys Pro Arg Gly Val Asp Pro

                                            332                                               362
GTG GTC TCC TTC CCT GTG GCT CTC AGC TGT CGC TGT GGA CCC TGC CGC CGC AGC ACC TCT
Val Val Ser Phe Pro Val Ala Leu Ser Cys Arg Cys Gly Pro Cys Arg Arg Ser Thr Ser

                                            392                                               422
GAC TGT GGG GGT CCC AAA GAC CAC CCC TTG ACC TGT GAC CAC CCC CAA CTC TCA GGC CTC
Asp Cys Gly Gly Pro Lys Asp His Pro Leu Thr Cys Asp His Pro Gln Leu Ser Gly Leu

CTC TTC CTC TAA AGACCCTCCCCGCAGCCTTCCAAGTCCATCCCGACTCCTGGAGCCCTGACACCCCGATCCGGA
Leu Phe Leu End

TC
```

**d**

```
                                    10                                      20
Met Lys Thr Leu Gln Phe Phe Phe Leu Phe Cys Cys Trp Lys Ala Ile Cys Cys↓Asn Ser

                                    30                                      40
Cys Glu Leu Thr Asn Ile Thr Ile Ala Ile Glu Lys Glu Glu Cys Arg Phe Cys Ile Ser

                                    50                                      60
Ile Asn Thr Thr Trp Cys Ala Gly Tyr Cys Tyr Thr Arg Asp Leu Val Tyr Lys Asp Pro

                                    70                                      80
Ala Arg Pro Lys Ile Gln Lys Thr Cys Thr Phe Lys Glu Leu Val Tyr Glu Thr Val Arg

                                    90                                     100
Val Pro Gly Cys Ala His His Ala Asp Ser Leu Tyr Thr Tyr Pro Val Ala Thr Gln Cys

                                   110                                     120
His Cys Gly Lys Cys Asp Ser Asp Ser Thr Asp Cys Thr Val Arg Gly Leu Gly Pro Ser

Tyr Cys Ser Phe Gly Glu Met Lys Glu
```

EXPRESSION OF GONADOTROPIN SUBUNITS IN CV-1 CELLS USING SV40 VECTORS

The cDNAs of all the subunits and the genomic DNA of hFSH were engineered by means of restriction enzymes and oligomeric linkers so that they could be inserted suitably in the positions of the coding sequences of VP1 and VP2 of SV40. For this EcoR I linkers at the 5' ends of the cDNAs were placed close to the initiator ATG codon and BamH I linkers placed within the 3' noncoding regions. The α subunit was engineered with Hind III linkers.

The α hCG cDNA which was approximately 700bp long, was engineered by using the single Nco I site (CCATGG) at the 5' end and the Hind III site in the 3'noncoding sequence. The cDNA was cleaved with Nco I and filled in by Klenow polymerase and linked either with Hind III or EcoR I linkers. Restriction with Hind III gave the Hind III α hCG cDNA. The Hind III site at the end of the EcoR I-Hind III fragment was converted into a BamH I site by means of Klenow polymerase and BamH I linkers to yield EcoR I-BamH I α hCG cDNA.

The β hCG cDNA, which is approximately 580bp long, was cloned into pBR322 by means of BamH I linkers. The plasmid was later restricted with Hga 1 ($GACGCN_5 3'N_{10} 5'$), which cuts 2 bp 5' to the ATG, filled in by Klenow polymerase, ligated to EcoR I linkers, cut with EcoR I and BamH I and cloned into pBR322.

The 5' EcoR I-Dde I fragment of β hCG was ligated to the Dde I fragment of β LH. The resulting fragment was then combined with the 3' fragment of β LH at the single Nco I site. the Sau3A I site (GATC) in the 3' untranslated region of β LH was filled in with Klenow polymerase and BamH I linkers were attached to give the β LH cDNA with a hybrid β hCG- β LH leader as EcoR I-BamH I fragment.

The hFSH gene is contained on a 6.8kb EcoR I-BamH I fragment. The distance between the ATG and the TAA codons is approximately 2kb. A Fok I site ($GGATGN_9 3'N_{13} 5'$) containing the ATG intiation codon was used to attach synthetic oligomers replacing the deleted sequences and inserting an EcoR I site 5' of the ATG. A Sau3A I site just 3' of the TAA stop codon was converted into a BamH I site. The approximately 1600bp long intron was removed by cutting the DNA with SfaN I ($GCATCN_5 3'N_9 5'$) in the first exon and Sau3A I at the 5' end of the second exon and joining the two fragments with oligomers containing the deleted coding sequences.

Figure 2 depicts the salient restriction sites in the engineered DNAs.

## Construction of SV40 Expression Vectors

SV40 DNA was linearized by partial Hind III endonuclease digestion, treated with Klenow polymerase in the presence of dNTPs, ligated to EcoR I linkers, cut with EcoR I and BamH I and cloned into pBR322. The plasmid pSVHR which contains SV40 DNA between 0.95 map units (m.u.) and 0.14 m.u. including the origin of replication and the entire early region, was identified by restriction mapping.

pα R/B, containing α hCG cDNA as an EcoR I-BamH I fragment, was methylated by using EcoR I methylase, restricted with Nde I, and EcoR I linkers were added to the ends by filling in with Klenow polymerase. The plasmid was then cut with EcoR I and BamH I and

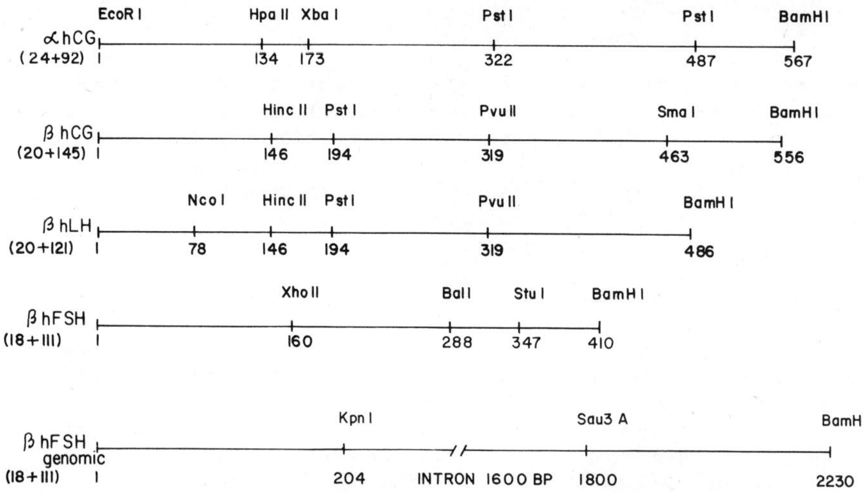


Figure 2: Restriction map of the engineered cDNAs of the gonadotropins. EcoR I linkers are at the 5' ends and BamH I linkers are at the 3' ends. β hFSH genomic DNA has 1600bp intron. The numbers within brackets indicate the number of amino acids in the leader and the mature peptide portions of the subunits.

ligated to EcoR I and BamH I cut pSVHR. Transformation of HB101 and screening the resulting colonies with appropriate restriction enzymes yielded the plasmid pαSVVP1, which was digested with EcoR I, ligated, cut with BamH I and cloned into pBR322 to yield pαSVVP1 Bam. A similar procedure was followed to construct p βSVVP1 Bam starting from pβR/B and pSVHR. The cloning steps are shown below (Figure 3).

SV40 viral DNA was restricted with Avall, filled in with Klenow polymerase and dNTPs. The 682bp long SV40 fragment between 0.64m.u. and 0.77m.u. was isolated, ligated to Hind III linkers, cut with Hind III and Kpn I. The resulting DNA fragments were cloned into a pBR322 derivative (obtained by converting the original EcoR I site to a Kpn 1 site), and the plasmid containing the 266bp long SV40 DNA fragment (0.71 m.u. to 0.77 m.u.) was isolated.

pβSVVP1 Bam was cut with Hind III and BamH I and the hCG-containing fragment was cloned into pSV266K. The resulting plasmid pβVP1266K was cut with Hind III and the αhCG cDNA was inserted as a 574bp HindIII fragment. The plasmid pαβVP1266K was restricted with Kpn I and Sal I and cloned into pαSVVP1Bam to obtain pαβSVVP1. A similar strategy was used to construct vectors for the expression of hLH and hFSH cDNAs. The following figure shows the procedure to construct pαβSVVP1 (Figure 4).

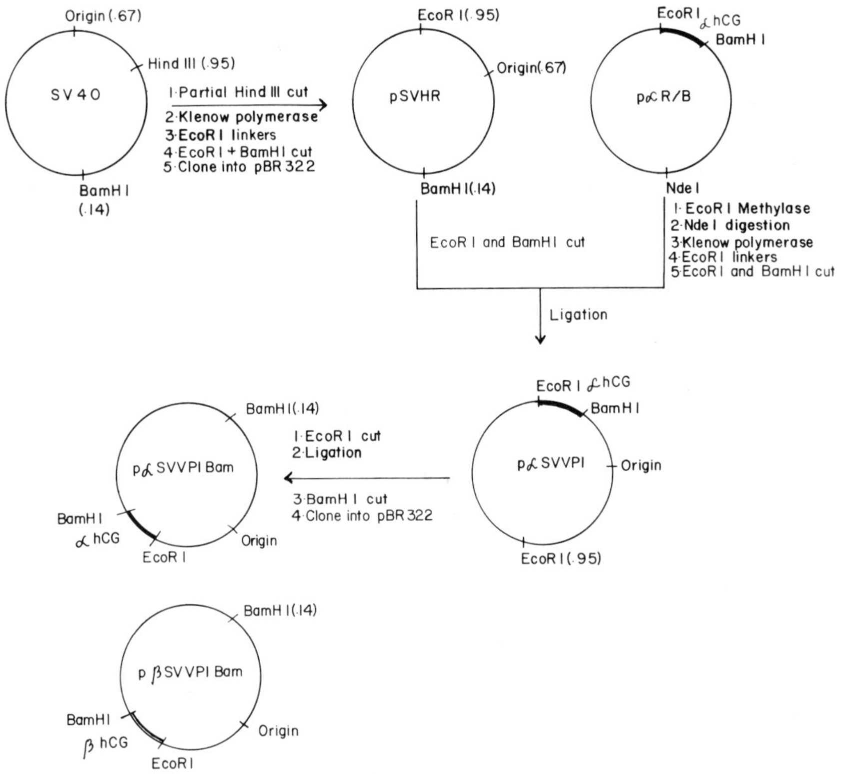


Figure 3: Construction of VP1 replacement vectors, pαSVVP1Bam and pβSVVP1 Bam. These constructions, after transfections into CV-1 cells, give the expression of dimeric hCG. Similar constructions were carried out for βhLH and βhFSH.

For the expression of the FSH genomic clone in a SV40 vector, pRI-E-Bam, containing SV40 DNA between 0.72 m.u. and 0.14 m.u., was digested with EcoR I and BamH I and ligated to EcoR I-BamH I digested pFSHR/B which contains the hFSH genomic DNA with the 1600bp long intron. The ligation mixture was cut with BamH I and cloned into the BamH I site of pBR322 to obtain pFSHSVLP. As shown below expression of FSH in this vector makes use of the SV40 late promoter and the FSH splicing signals (Figure 5).

## Propagation of the Vectors in CY-1 Cells

The vectors, cloned as BamH I fragments in pBR322, were digested with BamH I and ligated at low concentration of DNA to form self-ligated circles. This process eliminates the pBR322 portion of DNA because it cannot be propagated in CV-1 cells since it lacks a mammalian origin of replication. Similarly, ptsA58 DNA (SV40 viral DNA containing a temperature-sensitive mutation in the coding region of Large T) cloned into the BamH I site of pBR322 was digested with BamH I and self-ligated.

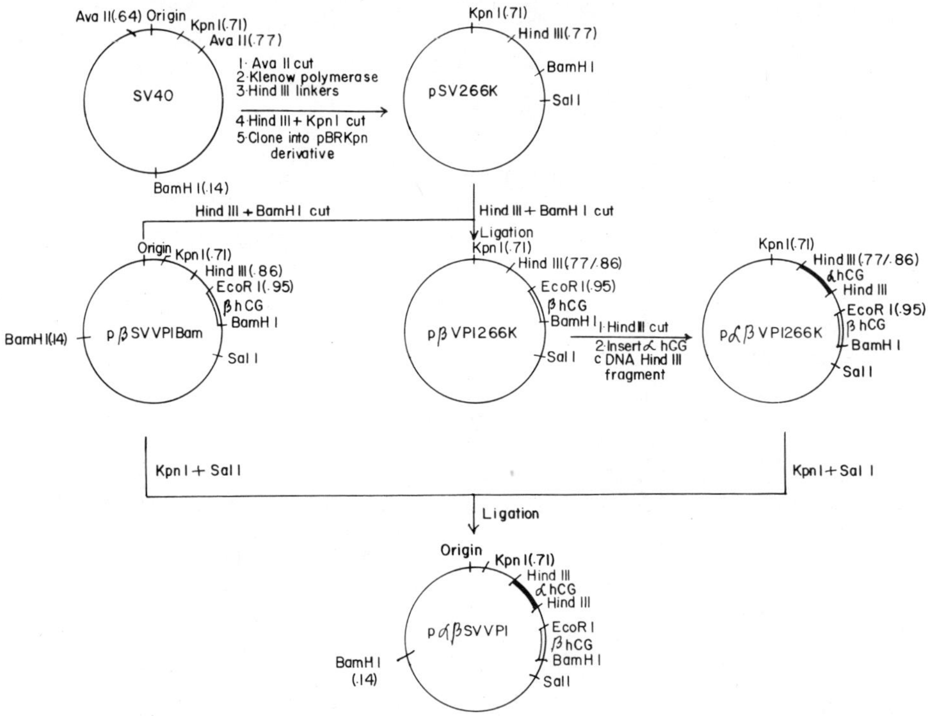


Figure 4: Constructions of double replacement vector, pαβSVVP1, which after transfection into CV-1 cells, express dimeric hCG. Similar vectors were constructed for the expression of dimeric hLH and hFSH by replacing the βhCG cDNA with βhLH and βhFSH cDNAs.

In the first case, 5ug of pα SVVP1 Bam, 5ug of pβ SVVP1 Bam and 1ug of tsA58 were mixed and used for transfection. In the second case, 10ug of pαβ SVVP1 and 1ug tsA58 were used for transfection.

Transfection was carried out by using DEAE-dextran method (15). The DNAs were precipitated with ethanol and dissolved in 10ul of sterile water. They were mixed with 2ml of TBS buffer and 1ml of DEAE-dextran (2mg/ml) solution and added to a monolayer of CV-1 cells (in a T-75 flask, approximately $10^6$ cells) which had been washed twice in 10ml of TBS buffer (16). After incubation at 37°C for 1-2 hours with occasional shaking, the cells were washed twice with TBS buffer, fed with 10ml of DMEM containing 5% fetal calf serum, and left at 40°C for 10-15 days. After complete cell lysis, the medium along with cell debris was transferred into a test tube, frozen and thawed four times and used to infect fresh CV-1 cells at 40°C.

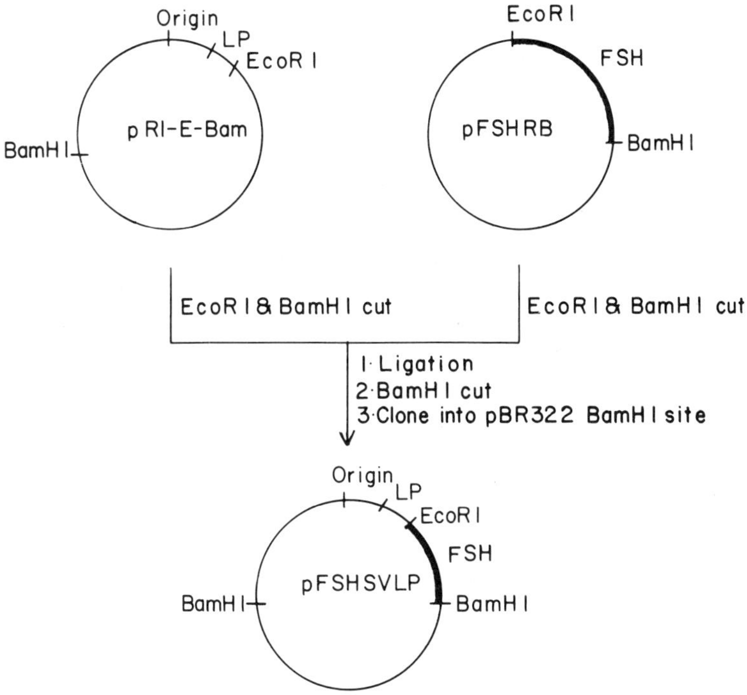


Figure 5: Construction of late replacement vector, pFSHSVLP. βFSH genomic DNA (2kb long) is linked to the SV40 late promoter and the FSH mRNA production is dependent on the removal of the 1600 nucleotide long intron.

## Expression and Detection of Dimers and Subunits in CV-1 Cells

The hCG produced by infected CV-1 cells was detected immunochemically by using two commercially available assays. The first was the subunit-specific BetaIII hCG radioimmunoassay produced by Serono Laboratories, the second was a dimer-specific enzyme-linked immunoassay (Tandem E hCG) supplied by Hybritech.

There is no method currently available to determine the dimer content of the hLH and hFSH. Therefore, hLH and hFSH production was determined by β subunit-specific RIA which reflected both free subunits and dimers. However, the dimer content was estimated by the mouse uterine weight assay (17). Two milliliters of tissue culture supernantants were injected intra-peritonially into a series of C57BL/6J female mice, between 19 and 22 days old, over a 60 hour period. Control and experimental animals were sacrificed 72 hours after the initial injection, and the uteri were dissected out, blotted dry and weighed. Commercially available hormones were also assayed as positive controls. As shown in Table 1, the recombinant hCG, for example, increased the weight of the uteri by two or three fold compared with the uteri of the control animals. Similar results were obtained with recombinant hLH and hFSH. The following figure depicts the increase in mass of the mouse uteri (Figure 6).

Table 1: C57BL/6J females, 19 to 21 days old, were injected with commercially obtained hCG (Profasi: Serono Laboratories) and tissue culture supernatants, or their dilutions. In each case, a total of 2ml was used for inoculating each animal. Weights of freshly dissected blotted uteri were determined on an analytical balance. IU, international units.

| Sample | N | Uterine Weight (mg) |
|---|---|---|
| Control | 3 | 9.9 |
| Profasi (0.2 IU) | 3 | 13.8 |
| Profasi (0.4 IU) | 4 | 28.1 |
| Recombinant hCG (diluted, 1:1) | 3 | 15.4 |
| Recombinant hCG (undiluted) | 3 | 30.1 |

Left Right

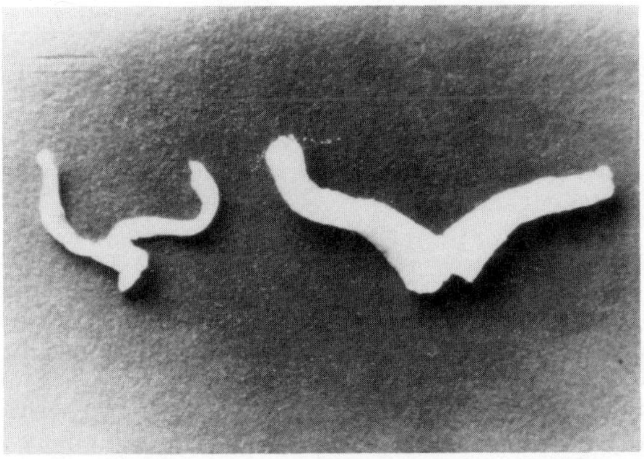

Figure 6: Photograph of the uteri of a control mouse (left) and a mouse treated with recombinant hCG (right). The mice were injected with 2ml of tissue culture supernatants.

hCG, hLH and hFSH were identified in the supernatants of CV-1 cells infected with the recombinant viruses by the assays described above. The presence of the dimers as well as subunits in the tissue culture medium suggests that they were processed correctly in CV-1 cells. Maximum expression (greater than 20mg/L/24 hr.) in CV-1 cells was observed only for the $\alpha$ hCG subunit, when CV-1 cells were infected with $\alpha$ SVVP1Bam. Only low levels of $\beta$ subunit were found in the medium when CV-1 cells were infected with $\beta$ SVVP1Bam alone. This may be due to the instability of the free $\beta$ subunit. As shown in the following table (Table 2), considerable expression levels were observed when CV-1 cells were infected with $\alpha\beta$ SVVP1 or with two recombinant viruses containing $\alpha$ and $\beta$ subunits separately. In the case of $\alpha\beta$ SVVP1 infected CV-1 cells, the $\beta$ subunit is expressed at higher levels than the $\alpha$ subunit because the former is associated with the more efficient 16S splice of SV40. Consequently, the production of dimers is dependent on the expression levels of $\alpha$ subunit.

Table 2: Expression levels of monomeric and dimeric godadotropins

| Recombinant | Productions (mg/L/24 hr.) |
|---|---|
| $\alpha$ SVVP1 Bam | 20 |
| $\beta$ SVVP1 Bam | 0.08 |
| $\alpha$ SVVP1 Bam + $\beta$ SVVP1 Bam | 2.0 |
| $\alpha\beta$ SVVP1 | 2.3 |
| $\alpha\beta$ hLHSVVP1 | 1.6 |
| $\alpha\beta$ hFSHSVVP1 | 1.5 |
| $\alpha$ SVVP1 Bam + $\beta$ hFSHSVLP | 3.2 |

We have analyzed the subunit proteins secreted by the CV-1 cells by labelling the cells with $^{35}S$ cysteine, immuno-precipitations using anti-sera raised against the dimers or subunits and SDS gels (18). Analysis of immunoprecipitations from cells infected with $\alpha\beta$ SVVP1 showed protein bands of apparent molecular weights of 22,000 and 35,000 daltons. Identical bands were observed, as shown below (Figure 7), from BeWo cells (19), which are known to produce hCG dimers. Cultures of CV-1 cells infected with $\alpha\beta$ hLHSVVP1, after immunoprecipitation, showed protein bands of apparent molecular weights of 16,000 and 22,000 daltons. Immunoprecipitation of culture supernatants with anti-$\beta$ hFSH gave a protein band with an apparent molecular weight of 18,000 daltons.

## RNA Analysis

CV-1 cells were grown to confluence in roller bottles and infected with the recombinant virus stock ($\alpha\beta$ SVVP1). Five days

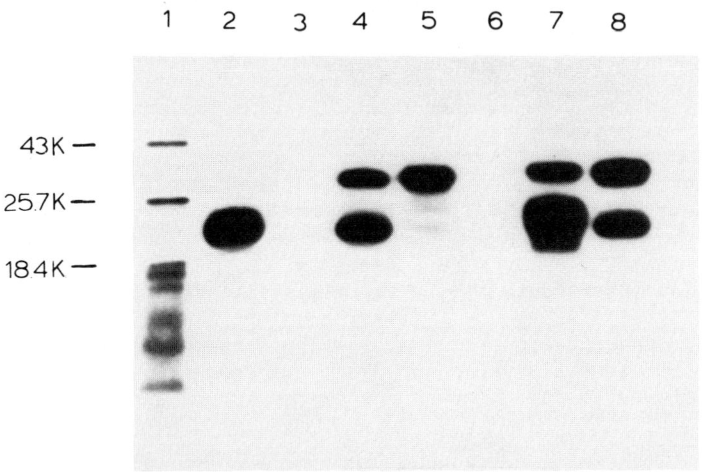


Figure 7: Autoradiogram of the $^{35}$S-labeled α and β hCG subunits. CV-1 cells were infected with either αSVVP1 Bam alone (Lane 2) or αβSVVP1 (Lanes 4, 5) and labeled with $^{35}$S-cysteine. BeWo cells, known to produce hCG dimer, were also labeled with $^{35}$S-cysteine (Lanes 7, 8). The supernatants were immunoprecipitated with α hCG antiserum (Lanes 2, 4 and 7) and β hCG antiserum (Lanes 5 and 8). Lane 1 is markers and Lanes 3 and 6 are immunoprecipitations of the supernatants of uninfected CV-1 cells with α and β hCG antisera. Only a faint band in the place of α hCG was observed in Lane 5 and the reason for this is not known.

after infection, the cells were trypsinized and collected by centrifugation. Cytoplasmic RNA was extracted by Penman's procedure (20) and poly A RNA was selected by oligo-dT cellulose chromatography. The RNA was electrophoresced on formaldehyde/agarose gels (21), transferred to nitrocellulose and hybridized with $^{32}$P labeled α and β hCG cDNAs. As shown in Figure 8, 2.1Kb and 1.1Kb long poly $A^+$ RNA species hybridized to α and β hCG cDNAs, respectively. The α hCG cDNA hybridized only to the larger species, whereas the β hCG cDNA probe hybridized to both the large and small RNAs. This result is in accord with the published analysis of the RNA transcripts of SV40 (22), and indicates that the 2.1Kb mRNA is processed as if it were SV40 19S RNA species and that the 1.1Kb mRNA is processed like the SV40 16S species. It should be pointed out that the 2.1Kb RNA of αβSVVP1 contains both α and β hCG coding sequences and that it hybridizes to both cDNA probes. The Figure 9 depicts the generation of mRNAs from the recombinant late region of αβSVVP1. It is interesting to note that the 1.1Kb RNA is produced in greater quantities (5-10 fold) than the 2.1Kb RNA. This is expected because the former uses the more efficient SV40 16S splicing signals.

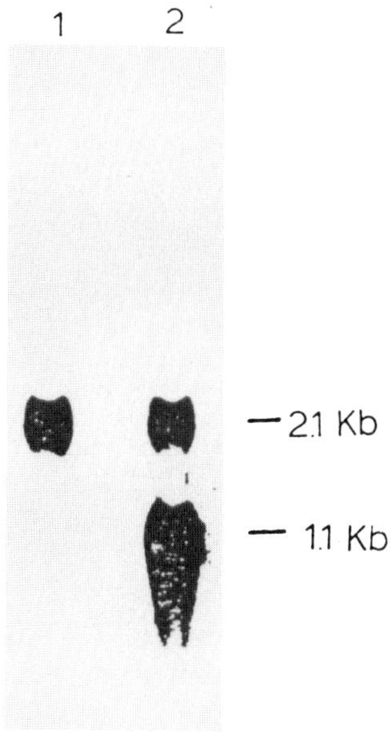


Figure 8: RNA blot analysis of poly A RNA from CV-1 cells infected with $\alpha\beta$SVVP1. RNA was immobilized on nitrocellulose paper and hybridized to $^{32}$p-labeled $\alpha$ hCG cDNA (Lane 1) or $\beta$ hCG cDNA (Lane 2). Size determinations were based on the unlabeled and denatured DNA markers.

## CONCLUSION

We reported here that the SV40 late region is suitable to express one or two distinct cDNAs under the control of the late promoter and the 19S and 16S splicing signals (24). It is interesting to note that $\alpha$ hCG subunit was the only one which was expressed in large amounts (greater than 20mg/L/24 hr.). This may be due to the intrinsic stability of the $\alpha$ subunit compared to $\beta$ subunit and may be attributed to factors other than glycosylation. The yield of the dimers can be improved by two to five fold by increasing the availability of the $\alpha$ subunit inside the cells. This was accomplished by co-infecting the cells, for example, with $\alpha$ SVVP1Bam and $\beta$ SVVP1Bam. An alternative is constructing two kinds of double replacement vectors, for example, $\alpha\beta$SVVP1 and $\beta\alpha$SVVP1, and infecting the CV-1 cells with both vectors at 1:1 ratio.

Although the lytic nature of the SV40 recombinant system is a clear disadvantage for large scale production, the ease with which the vectors can be constructed and the relatively simple growth requirements make this an attractive system to isolate small quantities of material for research purposes. For instance, mutant subunits with altered glycosylation sites can be made rapidly using this system. Assembly of the glycoprotein hormones and structural features that are essential for their activity can also be studied by means of expression vectors as reported here. It is tempting to speculate that hybrid glycoprotein subunits can be made using SV40 expression vectors in order to assess their biological activity and their antigenicity in humans.

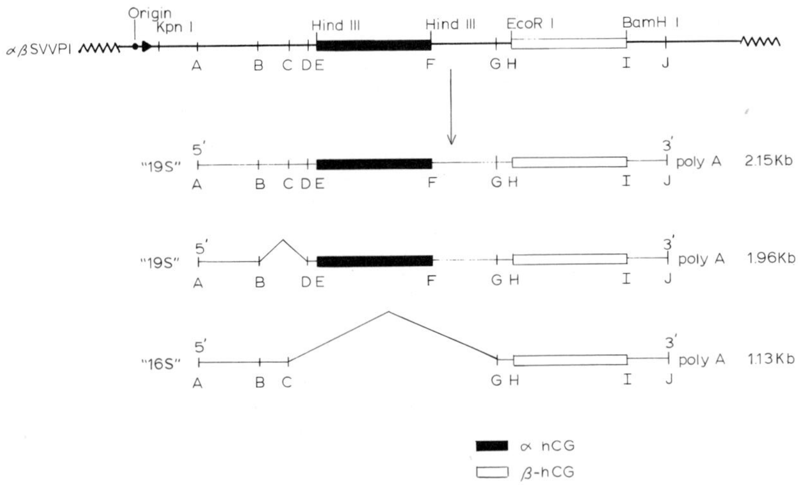


Figure 9: Schematic representation of the biogenesis of late mRNAs from αβSVVP1. Relevant positions on the SV40 genome (23) are: A, transcriptional initiation point at residue 243; B, 5' end of major 19S splice junction at residue 291; C, 5' end of major 16S splice at 444; D, 3' end of the 19S splice at nucleotide 476; E, Ava II site converted to a Hind III site; F, Hind III site at position 968; G, 3' end of the 16S splice at position 1381; H, Hind III site at 1411 converted into an EcoR I site; I, BamH I site at residue 2455; and J, 3' termini of late mRNAs at 2592.

## References


1. Canfield, R.E., Birkens, S., Morse, J.H. and Morgan, F.J. (1976) in Peptide Hormones, ed. Parsons, J.A. (Univ. Park Press, Baltimore), pp. 299-315.

2. Pierce, J.G. and Parsons, T.F.A. (1981) Annu. Rev. Biochem. 50, 465-495.

3. Kessler, M., Reddy, M.S., Shah, R.H. and Bahl, O.P. (1979) J. Biol. Chem. 254, 7901-7908.

4. Kessler, M.J., Mise, T., Ghai, R.D. and Bahl, O.P. (1979) J. Biol. Chem. 254, 7909-7914.

5. McKerns, K.W. (1978) Structure and Function of the Gonadotropins (Plenum Press, New York and London).

6. Hamer, D.H. and Leder, P. (1979) Nature (London) 281, 35-40.

7. Gething, M.J. and Sambrook, J. (1981) Nature (London) 293, 620-625.

8. Gluzman, Y. (1982) Eukaryotic Vectors (Cold Spring Harbor Laboratory, Cold Spring Harbor, N.Y.).

9. Gluzman, Y. (1981) Cell, 23, 175-182.

10. Maxam, A. and Gilbert, W. (1980) Methods Enzymol. 65, 499-599.

11. Fiddes, J.C. and Goodman, H.M. (1979) Nature (London) 281, 351-356.

12. Fiddes, J.C. and Goodman, H.M. (1980) Nature (London) 286, 684-687.

13. Talmadge, K., Vamvakopoulos, N.C. and Fiddes, J.C. (1984) Nature (London) 307, 37-40.

14. Maniatis, T., Hardison, R.C., Lacy, E., Laurer, J., O'Connell, C., Quon, D., Sim, G.K. and Efstrantiadis, A. (1978) Cell, 15, 687-701.

15. Sompayrac, L.M. and Danna, K.J. (1981) Proc. Natl. Acad. Sci., USA 78, 7575-7578.

16. Kimura, G. and Dulbecco, R. (1972) Virology 49, 79-81.

17. Loraine, J.A. and Brown, J.B. (1959) J. Endocrinol. 18, 77-84.

18. Laemmli, U.K. (1970) Nature (London) 227, 680-685.

19. Patillo, R.A. and Grey, G.O. (1968) Cancer Res. 28, 1231-1236.

20. Penman, S. (1966) J. Mol. Biol. 17, 117-130.

21. Maniatis, T. Fritsch, E.F. and Sambrook, J. (1982) Molecular cloning: A Laboratory Manual (Cold Spring Harbor Laboratory, Cold Spring Harbor, N.Y.).

22. Bhaskara Reddy, V., Ghosh, P.K., Lebowitz, P. and Weissman, S.M. (1978) Nucleic Acids Res. 5, 4195-4213.

23. Reddy, V.B., Thimmappaya, B., Dhar, R., Subramanian, K.N., Zain, B.S., Pam, J., Ghosh, P.K., Celma, M.L. and Weissman, S. (1978) Science 200, 494-502.

24. Reddy, V.B., Beck, A.K., Garramone, A.J., Vellucci, V., Lustbader, J. and Bernstine, E.G. (1985) Proc. Natl. Acad. Sci., U.S.A. 82, 3644-3648.

# CLONING AND EXPRESSION OF LUTROPIN GENES

William W. Chin and Soheyla D. Gharib

Department of Medicine, Brigham and Women's Hospital; Howard Hughes Medical Institute Laboratories; and Section on Molecular Genetics, Joslin Diabetes Center, One Joslin Place, Boston, MA

## INTRODUCTION

In man, lutropin (LH) and chorionic gonadotropin (CG) belong to a group of hormones known collectively as the glycoprotein hormones. LH along with follicle-stimulating hormone (follitropin, FSH) and thyroid-stimulating hormone (TSH) is produced and secreted by the anterior pituitary gland and CG by the placenta. LH and FSH, the pituitary gonadotropins, stimulate the production of the sex steroid hormones and gametogenesis. As such, they are important for sexual development and function, and reproduction. CG, whose maximal levels appear in early pregnancy, is essential for the function of the corpus luteum (1, 2).

The production of the glycoprotein hormones is tissue-specific. LH is produced by gonadotropes in the anterior pituitary gland and CG is synthesized by the syncytiotrophoblasts of the placenta. However, on rare occasions, CG, and/or one of its subunits may be produced eutopically by trophoblastic tissue in the non-pregnant individual, and ectopically by non-trophoblastic tissues such as cancers of the lung, breast, and gastrointestinal tract.

The pituitary glycoprotein hormones, LH, FSH and TSH, and, to a lesser extent, CG are synthesized and released under complex hormonal control. LH stimulates the gonadal tissues to produce sex steroid hormones such as testosterone and estrogen which, in turn, act at the pituitary gland directly or indirectly to diminish the gonadotropin output of the gonadotrope.

LH, like other members of the glycoprotein hormone family, contains two different units named α and β in a non-covalent dimer. These subunits are products of separate genes; there is apparently a single α-subunit gene in most mammalian species, and separate β subunit genes. The apoproteins of the α and β subunits are small and contain 89 to 96 and 112 to 121 amino acid residues, respectively. Each subunit contains multiple disulfide linkages that are essential during the biosynthesis of the subunits to allow the subunits to obtain the appropriate conformation for subunit-subunit interaction in order to form biologically active dimers. In addition each subunit contains one or more N- or O-linked carbohydrate moieties (1).

In view of the critical roles that LH and CG play in the reproductive life of mammals, we have recently embarked on a research program to study the genes encoding the subunits of these hormones and to determine the hormonal regulation of the synthesis of these hormones at the pre-translational level. Recent advances in molecular biology and recombinant DNA biology have allowed the isolation and characterization of cDNAs and the natural genes that encode the subunits. The availability of such DNAs allows us not only to better understand the structure and organization of the genes within the genome but also to explore the precise molecular mechanisms involved in the hormonal regulation of expression of these genes. In this regard, the ability to introduce foreign DNAs into heterologous cells will allow careful dissection of the structure-function relations involved in this hormonal regulation.

## BIOSYNTHESIS OF GLYCOPROTEIN HORMONES--GENERAL VIEW

The pathway for the biosynthesis of any protein in a mammalian cell is now well characterized (2, 3). Hence, a glycoprotein hormone-subunit is encoded by a gene which contains coding regions or exons, and non-coding regions or introns or intervening sequences. The first step in the expression of such a gene is the transcription of the gene in its entirety to yield immature mRNA which contains both coding and non-coding sequences. Rapidly, the nucleus processes this mRNA precursor to its mature form by removing introns, capping the 5'-end and polyadenylation of 3'-end. The mature RNA procedes to the cytoplasm where it interacts with the protein translational machinery. At this point newly synthesized protein precursors are found. During translation several important steps occur. These include (1) cleavage of a leader peptide (hydrophobic 20 to 30 amino acid region found at the $NH_2$-termini of the precursors of most secretory and membrane proteins) and (2) addition of core carbohydrate chains. These nascent proteins then are further processed as they traverse the endoplasmic reticulum and Golgi apparatus. These post-translational modifications include glycosylation, and possibly phosphorylation, acetylation, methylation and sulfation. As a result, the subunits obtain the appropriate secondary and tertiary conformations to enable them to form dimers and hence biologically active hormones. They are then stored in secretory granules and are released when signalled by the appropriate effectors (2). This paper evaluates the synthesis of LH at the pre-translational level as regulated by gonadal sex steroid hormones. Hence, we will focus on the

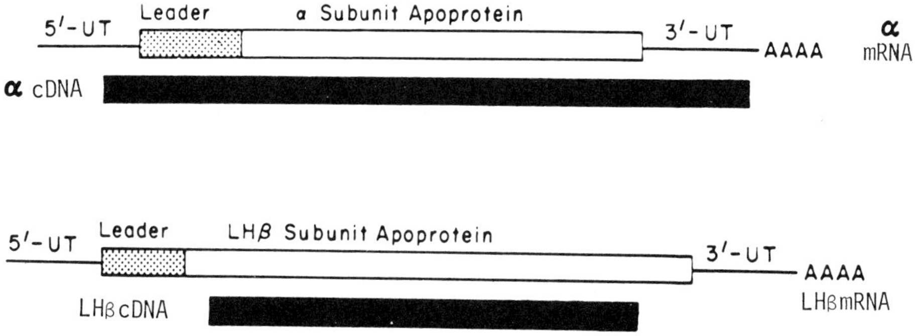


Figure 1. Schematic diagram of mRNAs and cloned cDNAs encoding the α and β subunits of rat LH. The top section in each group depicts a schematic diagram of either α or LH β mRNA. The open box areas denote the regions of the mRNA that encode the subunit precursors; the stippled areas indicate the leader peptide and the remainder represent the apoproteins. The solid boxes indicate the extent of mRNA representation for the α (pαl, [4]) and LH β (pLHβ-2, [5]) cDNAs. UT = untranslated region.

effects of these hormones on the levels of mRNAs which encode the subunits of LH.

**MOLECULAR CLONING**

We have recently isolated and characterized cDNAs and natural genes encoding the rat α and LHβ subunits (4-6). A cDNA library was prepared from pituitary gland poly A+ RNA of ovariectomized Sprague-Dawley rats using the P t I site of pBR322 and G:C homopolymers. The rat α and LHβ subunit cDNAs were selected by colony hybridization using labeled mouse α and human CGβ cDNAs, respectively. The two cDNAs are shown schematically in Figure 1. The nucleotide and deduced amino acid sequences of the cDNAs encoding rat α and LH β subunits are shown in Figures 2 and 3, respectively. The rat α subunit precursor contains 120 amino acid residues (24 amino-acid residue leader peptide and 96 amino-acid residue apoprotein) and is encoded by a mRNA that is 800 bases in size. The rat LH β subunit precursor contains 141 amino-acid residues (20 amino-acid residue leader peptide and 121 amino-acid residue apoprotein) and is encoded by a mRNA that is approximately 700 bases in extent.

```
                                                          -24
5'...CTGCCCACAACACATCCTTCCAAGATCCAGAGTTTGCAGGAGAGCT   Met Asp Cys
                                                       ATG GAT TGC

    -20                 -15                 -10                 -5          -1  +1              +5
Tyr Arg Arg Tyr Ala Ala Val Ile Leu Val Met Leu Ser Met Val Leu His Ile Leu His Ser Leu Pro Asp Gly Asp
TAC AGA AGA TAT GCG GCT GTC ATT CTG GTC ATG CTG TCC ATG GTC CTG CAT ATT CTT CAT TCT CTT CCT GAT GGA GAC

                +10                                     +20                                     +30
Leu Ile Ile Gln Gly Cys Pro Glu Cys Lys Leu Lys Glu Asn Lys Tyr Phe Ser Lys Leu Gly Ala Pro Ile Tyr Gln
CTT ATT ATT CAG GGT TGT CCA GAA TGT AAA CTA AAG GAA AAC AAA TAC TTC TCC AAG CTG GGT GCC CCC ATC TAT CAG

                                +40                                     +50
Cys Met Gly Cys Cys Phe Ser Arg Ala Tyr Pro Thr Pro Ala Arg Ser Lys Lys Thr Met Leu Val Pro Lys Asn Ile
TGT ATG GGC TGT TGC TTC TCC AGG GCA TAC CCG ACT CCC GCA AGG TCC AAG AAG ACA ATG TTG GTT CCA AAG AAT ATT

        +60                                     +70                                     +80
Thr Ser Glu Ala Thr Cys Cys Val Ala Lys Ser Phe Thr Lys Ala Thr Val Met Gly Asn Ala Arg Val Glu Asn His
ACC TCG GAG GCC ACG TGC TGT GTG GCC AAA TCA TTT ACT AAG GCC ACA GTG ATG GGA AAC GCC AGA GTG GAG AAC CAC

                        +90                     +96 Stop
Thr Asp Cys His Cys Ser Thr Cys Tyr Tyr His Lys Ser
ACG GAC TGC CAC TGT AGC ACT TGT TAC TAC CAC AAG TCG TAG  CTTCCATGTGTGCCAAGGGCTGCGCTGACGACTGCTGACCCGTGCG

ATGGCACTGAGTGTCGCCACCTCCTCCTTACCAGACTTCTGACACGCTTCAGTCATACACTGCTGCTTTCCTGTCACATCCCTTATACTTCAGTACCATCGAC

AGTCTCTTCTCATTAGGGGAAAATGTGTATCTACCATGGTCCCATCAGAAAT...3'
```

Figure 2. Nucleotide and deduced amino acid sequences of cDNAs encoding the rat α subunit (4). The composite nucleotide sequence of rat α mRNA is shown. The deduced amino acid sequence of this cDNA reveals that there is an open reading frame of 120 amino acids representing the rat α subunit precursor. The sequence reads from 5' to 3' and the numbers above the sequences indicate the amino acid residues in the precursor (-24 to -1 = leader peptide, and +1 to +96 = α apoprotein). Modified from Figure 2 of reference 4.

## SUBUNIT GENE ORGANIZATION

Each glycoprotein subunit is encoded by a separate gene (2). We and others have recently determined the chromosomal localization of these genes in mouse and man using blot hybridization analyses of DNA derived from somatic cell hybrids whose chromosome constitutions have been well-characterized by karyotype and enzyme analyses (7, 10, 11). Table 1 indicates that the α and LHβ genes in mouse and man are located on separate chromosomes. In addition, in man, it appears that there are at least seven CGβ genes and a single LHβ gene located on the same chromosome (7, 10, 11). In contrast, in the rat, there is a single LHβ gene but no CGβ or CGβ-like gene (6, 12, 13). These data and others involving the analysis of the gene structures indicate that the CGβ gene evolved from LHβ late in the mammalian radiation.

TABLE 1. Chromosomal localization of the glycoprotein hormone subunit genes in mouse and man (7-9).

| SPECIES | SUBUNIT GENE | CHROMOSOME # |
|---|---|---|
| mouse | α | 4 |
| | LH β | 7 |
| | TSH β | 3 |
| man | α | 6 |
| | LH/CG β | 19 |

```
      -20                                     -10                                     -1  +1
      Met Glu Arg Leu Gln Gly Leu Leu Leu Trp Leu Leu Leu Ser Pro Ser Val Val Trp Ala Ser Arg Gly Pro Leu
5' ..GA ATG GAG AGG CTC CAG GGG CTG CTG CTG TGG CTG CTG CTG AGC CCA AGT GTG GTG TGG GCC TCC AGG GGC CCC CTT

                  +10                                     +20                                     +30
      Arg Pro Leu Cys Arg Pro Val Asn Ala Thr Leu Ala Ala Glu Asn Glu Phe Cys Pro Val Cys Ile Thr Phe Thr
      CGG CCA CTG TGC CGG CCT GTC AAC GCA ACC CTG GCT GCA GCG AAT GAG TTC TGC CCA GTC TGC ATC ACC TTC ACC

                                      +40                                     +50
      Thr Ser Ile Cys Ala Gly Tyr Cys Pro Ser Met Val Arg Val Leu Pro Ala Ala Leu Pro Pro Val Pro Gln Pro
      ACC AGC ATC TGT GCC GGC TAC TGT CCT AGC ATG GTT CGA GTA CTG CCA GCT GCC TTG CCT CCC GTG CCT CAG CCA

                  +60                                     +70                                     +80
      Val Cys Thr Tyr Arg Glu Leu Arg Phe Ala Ser Val Arg Leu Pro Gly Cys Pro Pro Gly Val Asp Pro Ile Val
      GTG TGC ACC TAC CGT GAG CTG CGC TTC GCC TCT GTC CGC CTC CCT GGC TGC CCA CCT GGT GTA GAC CCC ATA GTC

                                      +90                                 +100
      Ser Phe Pro Val Ala Leu Ser Cys Arg Cys Gly Pro Cys Arg Leu Ser Ser Ser Asp Cys Gly Gly Pro Arg Thr
      TCC TTT CCT GTG GCC CTC AGC TGC CGC TGT GGG CCC TGC CGT CTC AGT AGC TCT GAC TGT GGG GGT CCC AGG ACT

                 +110                                     +120+121
      Gln Pro Met Thr Cys Asp Leu Pro His Leu Pro Gly Leu Leu Leu Phe  ***
      CAA CCA ATG ACC TGT GAC CTT CCC CAC CTC CCC GGC CTT CTC CTC TTC  TGA  TGCCCACCCACTAACTCCCCATTCTTCTG

      GAGCCAGCAGGTGTTCTAACCATCCCTCCCAATAAAGGCTTTACAACTGC poly A ..3'
```

Figure 3. Nucleotide and deduced amino acid sequences of cDNAs encoding rat LHβ subunit (5). The composite nucleotide sequence of the rat LHβ mRNA is shown. The cDNAs encode a precursor of rat LHβ that contains 141 amino acid residues. The numbers above the sequences indicate the amino acid residues in the precursor (-20 to -1 = leader peptide, and +1 to +121 = LHβ apoprotein). The *** indicates the proposed <u>stop</u> codon for the LHβ subunit.

## HORMONAL REGULATION OF LH SUBUNIT GENE EXPRESSION

In order to evaluate the effect of gonadal sex steroid hormones on the steady-state levels of LH subunit mRNAs, we utilized the following in vivo model systems: (1) ovariectomized (OVX) female Sprague-Dawley rats, and (2) steroid-hormone-replaced OVX rats. We determined the time course of the changes of the subunit mRNAs in the pituitary gland of these animals in relation to the changes in the plasma LH levels. The results are shown in Fig. 4 and 5. Briefly, there is a gradual increase with time in the steady-state levels of both α and LHβ mRNAs, measured by blot hybridization analysis, in the pituitary glands of OVX animals tht mimic the gradual increase in the LH levels (Fig. 4). Replacement with 17β-estradiol benzoate (2 μg/100g bw/d ip) of OVX (three to four weeks) rats results in rapid decreases of both subunit mRNAs in parallel with an abrupt decline in the plasma LH levels (Fig. 5). We have obtained similar results using castrate and testosterone-treated castrate rats (Gharib and Chin, unpublished data). These data along with those in sheep and rat (14-16) using blot hybridization and cell-free translation techniques provide strong evidence that gonadal sex steroid hormones regulate the levels of LH subunit mRNAs. Whether this regulation is effected at the transcriptional or mRNA stability levels is not yet clear. However, recent data by Shupnik et al. (17) suggest that thyroid hormone suppression of TSH biosynthesis, a parallel regulation system, occurs in large part at the level of transcription. The effects of gonadal sex steroid hormones on the rate of LH subunit gene transcription is under active investigation in our laboratory.

## SUMMARY

We have recently cloned and characterized cDNAs and genes encoding the subunits of rat LH. These cDNAs have served as molecular probes to determine the levels of LH subunit mRNAs in the pituitary glands of hormonally-manipulated animals using a blot hybridization assay. Removal of estrogen by ovariectomy results in increases of the subunit mRNAs whereas replacement of estrogen to these animals results in the rapid decline of the subunit mRNAs. Work is in progress to determine whether these changes occur at transcriptional and/or mRNA stability levels.

The availability of the genes encoding the LH subunits and techniques of in vitro mutagenesis of DNA and gene transfer in heterologous cells provide hope that we may someday understand the mechanism of action of these hormones at the molecular level.

## ACKNOWLEDGEMENTS

We wish to thank Nancy Patterson for her expert assistance in typing this manuscript. This work was supported, in part, by NIH HD 19938.

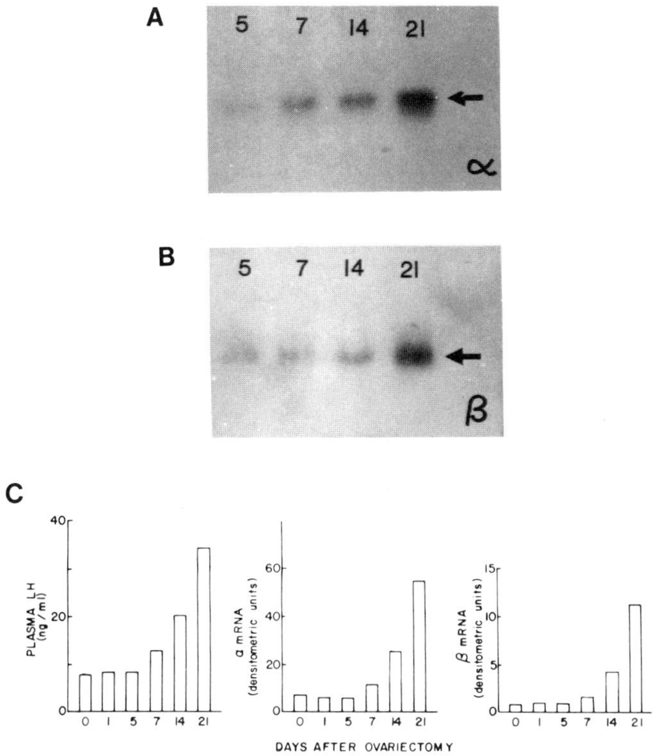


Figure 4. Effect of ovariectomy on the steady-state levels of α and LHβ subunit mRNAs in the anterior pituitary gland in the rat. Female Sprague-Dawley rats (200-225g) were surgically oophorectomized and animals sacrificed by decapitation at various times after the operation. Steady-state levels of the subunit mRNAs were determined by blot-hybridization techniques using cloned cDNAs encoding the rat α and LHβ subunits. Plasma LH in trunk blood was determined by radio-immunoassay. **A:** autoradiogram of a blot-hybridization analysis using RNA from pituitaries at 5, 7, 14, and 21 d post-ovariectomy, and probed with labeled rat α subunit cDNA. **B:** autoradiogram of the blot used in panel A but probed with labeled rat LHβ subunit cDNA. **C:** summary of the hybridization studies using data obtained by semiquantitative densitometric analyses of autoradiograms in A and B, compared with plasma LH levels. Messenger RNA levels are expressed in terms of arbitrary densitometric units, and plasma LH is expressed in ng/ml post-ovariectomy. Reprinted from Chin, W.W. in The Pituitary Gland (1985) edited by H. Imura, Raven Press, New York; pp. 103-125.

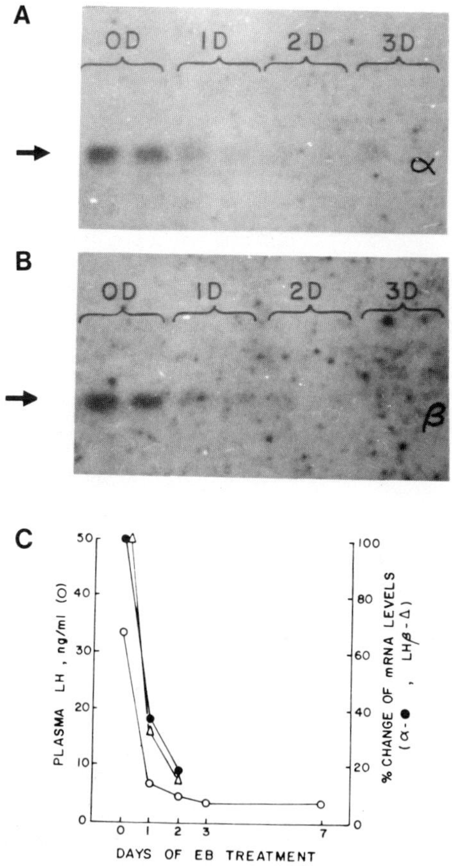


Figure 5. Effect of 17-β estradiol on the steady-state levels of α and LHβ subunit mRNAs in the anterior pituitary gland of the ovariectomized rat. Experiments were begun 3 to 4 weeks after the ovariectomy of 200-225g rats. Animals were then treated with 17-β estradiol benzoate (EB) (2 μg/100g bw/day) by intraperitoneal injection. Animals were sacrificed at 0, 1, 2, 3, and 7 days after initiation of hormone treatment. Steady-state levels of rat α and LHβ subunit mRNAs and plasma rat LH were determined as described in Fig. 4. **A:** autoradiogram of a blot-hybridization described for Fig. 4, panel A using the rat α subunit cDNA probe. **B:** autoradiogram of a blot-hybridization analysis described for Fig. 4 panel A using the rat LHβ subunit cDNA probe. **C:** summary of the mRNA and plasma LH data as described in Fig. 4. Messenger RNA levels are expressed as the percent change of the levels from the untreated state. Plasma rat LH is expressed as nanograms per milliliter. Reprinted from Chin, W.W. in The Pituitary Gland (1985) edited by H. Imura, Raven Press, New York; pp. 103-125.

## REFERENCES


1. J.G. Pierce and T. F. Parsons, Glycoprotein hormones: structure and function. Ann. Rev. Biochem. 50:465-495 (1981)
2. W. W. Chin, Organization and expression of glycoprotein hormones gene. In: "The Pituitary Gland," Imura, H (ed)., Raven Press, New York, (1985).
3. J. Darnell, Variety in the level of gene control in eucaryotic cells. Nature 297:365-371 (1982).
4. J. E. Godine, W. W. Chin, J. F. Habener, α subunit of rat pituitary glycoprotein hormones: primary structure of the precursor determined from the nucleotide sequence of cloned cDNAs. J. Biol. Chem. 257:365-371 (1982).
5. W. W. Chin, J.E. Godine, D. R. Klein, A. S. Chang, L. K. Tan and J. F. Habener, Nucleotide sequence of the cDNA encoding the precursor of the β subunit of rat lutropin. Proc. Natl. Acad. Sci. USA 80:4649-4653 (1983).
6. J. L. Jameson, W. W. Chin, A. N. Hollenberg, A. S. Chang and J. F. Habener, The gene encoding the β subunit of rat luteinizing hormone: analysis of gene structure and evolution of nucleotide sequence. J. Biol. Chem. 259:15474-15480 (1984).
7. S. L. Naylor, W. W. Chin, H. M. Goodman, P. A. Lalley, K. H. Grzeschik and A. Y. Sakaguchi, Chromosomal assignment of genes encoding the α and β subunits of glycoprotein hormones in man and mouse. Somat. Cell Genet. 9:757-770 (1983).
8. C. Julier, D. Weil, P. Couillin, J. C. Cote, V. C. Nguyen, C. Foubert, A. Boue and C. Junien, The beta chorionic gonadotropin-beta luteinizing hormone gene cluster maps to human chromosome 19. Hum. Genet. 67:174-177 (1984).
9. I. A. Kourides, P. E. Baker, J. A. Gurr, D. D. Pravtcheva and F. H. Ruddle, Assignment of the genes for the α and β subunits of thyrotropin to different mouse chromosomes. Proc. Natl. Acad. Sci. USA 81:517-519 (1984).
10. K. Talmadge, N. C. Vamvakopoulos, and J. C. Fiddes, Evolution of the genes for the β subunits of human chorionic gonadotropin and luteinizing hormone. Nature 307:37-40 (1984).
11. W. R. Boorstein, N. C. Vamvakopoulos and J. C. Fiddes, Human chorionic gonadotropin β-subunit is encoded by at least eight genes arranged in tandem and inverted pairs. Nature 300:419-422 (1982).
12. M. A. Tepper and J. L. Roberts, Evidence for only one β-luteinizing and no β-chorionic gonadotropin gene in the rat. Endocrinol. 115:385-391 (1984)
13. F. E. Carr and W. W. Chin, Absence of detectable chorionic gonadotropin mRNAs in rat placenta during gestation. Endocrinol. 116:1151-1157 (1985).
14. T. Landefeld and J. Kepa, Regulation of LH beta subunit mRNA in the sheep pituitary gland during different feedback states of estradiol. Biochem. Biophys. Res. Commun. 122:1307-1313 (1984).

15. J. H. Nilson, M. T. Nejedlik, J. B. Virgin, M. E. Crowder and T. M. Nett, Expression of α subunit and luteinizing hormone β genes in the ovine anterior pituitary. J. Biol. Chem. 258:12087-12090 (1983).
16. M. Corbani, R. Counis, A. Starzec and M. Jutisz, Effect of gonadectomy on pituitary levels of mRNA encoding gonadotropin subunits and secretion of luteinizing hormone. Molec. Cell Endocrinol. 35:83-87 (1984).
17. M. A. Shupnik, W. W. Chin, J. F. Habener and E. C. Ridgway, Transcriptional regulation of the thyrotopin subunit genes by thyroid hormone. J. Biol. Chem. 260:2900-2903 (1985).

# DEVELOPMENT OF oFSH AS A VACCINE FOR THE MALE - A STATUS REPORT ON THE RECENT REASEARCHES CARRIED OUT USING THE BONNET MONKEY (M.RADIATA)

N.R. Moudgal[1], G.S. Murthy[1], A.J. Rao[1]
N. Ravindranath[1], M.R. Sairam[2]
S.G. Kotagi[1] and F. Martin[1]

[1]Center for Advanced Research in Reproductive Biology
Laboratory of Endocrine Biochemistry
Indian Institute of Science, Bangalore 560012, India
[2] Reproduction Research laboratory
Clinical Research Institute of Montreal, Montreal
Quebec H2W 1R7, Canada

## INTRODUCTION

It is currently accepted that immunocontraception is a feasible procedure for the female. The possibility of using such an approach in the male is still under experimental manipulation. Among the different immunogens suggested three antigens - one tissue specific and two hormonally based appear promising and as such are currently being tested. Development of any contraceptive for the male has to contend with the effect it may have on testosterone production and consequently libido. Most hormonally based contraceptives under development for the male therefore advocate supplementation with an androgen. The one exception to this appears to be FSH. The observation that FSH is involved in regulating sperm production and fertility of the adult male primate in itself is of recent origin. It was shown in 1979 that continuous neutralization of endogenous FSH of proven fertile adult male bonnet monkeys over a period of 90-230 days with characterized FSH antibody effects testicular funcion, the monkeys becoming infertile as a consequence of it[1-4]. Such neutralization, however, did not effect testosterone production or libido. This basic observation particularly with respect to the effect passive immunization with FSH antiserum produces on the quality and quantity of sperm production was soon confirmed using the rhesus[5] and cynomolgous[6] monkeys. Yet another evidence for the involvement of FSH in regulating testicular function of the adult male primate was obtained recently by chronically dosing adult proven fertile male bonnet monkeys with an ovine testicular inhibin preparation. This led, as in the case of FSH antibody to testicular dysfuction, exemplified here by acute oligospermia and infertility[7].

The above studies encouraged us to propose oFSH as an effective contraceptive vaccine for the male. A recent report from Neischlag's laboratory[8] indicating that rhesus monkeys actively immunized with oFSH over a 4 1/2 year period show recovery of sperm production despite exhibiting high FSH antibody titers, however, puzzled us and led to close examination of the bonnet monkeys actively immunized with oFSH over a period of 7-13 years. It may be pertinent to point out here that the male bonnet unlike the rhesus does not exhibit seasonal testicular recrudescence; instead like in man, the sperm and testosterone production of the bonnet monkey remain unchanged throughout the year[2]. Consequently the bonnet and the cynomolgous[7] as well, appear more suitable than the rhesus for testing male contraceptive agents.

## EXPERIMENTAL

### 1. Effect of long-term active immunization of adult male bonnet monkeys with oFSH

A group of 4 adult proven fertile male bonnet monkeys actively immunized with oFSH over a 7-13 year period were examined with respect to a antibody titers and cross-reactivity with primate FSH; b testicular histology and c sperm production.

These monkeys were initially immunized at the start of our passive immunization study and as such the protocol of immunization has been described earlier[2]. The antibody titer in these monkeys, however, was kept up by periodic boosting. In Table 1 are provided details of the immunization record of these monkeys. Excepting for monkey # 603 which received a booster in November 1984, the other 3 monkeys received a booster injection of oFSH (250 μg oFSH given in saline) almost 2-3 years ago. Freunds complete adjuvant was used during primary immunization. The oFSH used for immunization was a highly purified preparation passed through an oLH antibody immunoaffinity column to remove any contaminating LH present in the FSH preparation.

Table 1. Details of longterm active immunization of bonnet monkeys with oFSH

| Monkey Number | Present age (approx)yrs | Start of immu-nization date | Adjuvant used | Last booster given |
|---|---|---|---|---|
| 308 | 15 | Dec 1977 | FCA* | May 1983 |
| 322 | 15 | Nov 1977 | FCA | May 1983 |
| 320 | 16 | Oct 1978 | FCA | Aug 1982 |
| 603 | 20 | Dec 1972 | FCA | Nov 1984 |

*FCA = Freund's Complete Adjuvant

The antibody titer of sera, obtained at two recent bleedings, towards oFSH (the homologous antigen) and hFSH (used here as a representative of primate FSH) are provided in Table 2. Since a large portion of the cross-reacting antibody must be used up in neutralizing endogenous mFSH, that binding to hFSH represents only the 'excess' free antibody. It is perhaps for this reason that the antibody titers towards hFSH (compared to that exhibited for oFSH) is relatively low. Despite this low titer its ability to neutralize the biopotency of hFSH as tested in an *in vitro* bioassay was quite high (Table 3). The antisera of these monkeys have also been successfully used to block endogenous FSH of cycling female bonnet monkeys, as little as 25 µl per monkey being needed to block follicular maturation[10].

Table 2. Current antibody titer in the longterm actively immunized monkeys

| Monkey number | A/s dilution required to provide 50% binding of | | |
|---|---|---|---|
| | $^{125}$I oFSH | $^{125}$I hFSH | |
| | Apr'85 | Apr'85 | May'85 |
| 308 | 1:625 | 1:203 | 1:156 |
| 322 | 1:3906 | 1:125 | 1:227 |
| 320 | 1:178 | 1:13 | 1:20 |
| 603 | 1:3125 | 1:50 | 1:125 |

Table 3. Bioneutralizing potency of antisera (a/s) obtained from actively immunized bonnets (tested in an in vitro system using granulosa cells)

| Treatment | | ng progesterone/0.5x10$^6$ cells/4h (mean ± S.D.) | Neutralizing capacity µg hFSH/ml a/s |
|---|---|---|---|
| Hormone 50 ng hFSH | Serum 5µl | | |
| - | NMS* | 0.75 ± 0.02 | - |
| + | NMS* | 4.00 ± 0.01 | - |
| + | a/s 308 | 2.25 ± 0.02 | 5.4 |
| + | a/s 322 | 2.40 ± 0.01 | 4.9 |
| + | a/s 320 | 2.80 ± 0.02 | 3.7 |
| + | a/s 603 | 2.50 ± 0.01 | 4.6 |

*NMS = Normal Monkey Serum

The serum testosterone levels of the actively immunized monkeys were comparable to that seen in a group of 4 control monkeys of the same age group (Table 4). The actively immunized monkeys, however, exhibited a state of acute oligospermia to azoospermia as tested following 3 electroejaculations conducted 1 week apart. The controls during the same period showed on an average a total sperm count 273 millions/ejaculate (Table 4).

Histological examination of testicular biopsy samples revealed that there was arrest in spermatogenesis in most of the tubules at the primary spermatocyte stage but in some tubules there were foci of spermatogenic activity and fully formed spermatids could be clearly seen. The basement membrane of the tubule appeared thickened. In contrast, the biopsy samples of control monkeys revealed normal spermatogenesis with normal tubular organization.

Table 4. Testosterone and sperm counts in a set of control and actively immunized monkeys

| Group | Monkey number | Age approx. | Testosterone ng/ml 10 a.m./10 p.m. | Total sperm count million/ejaculate |
|---|---|---|---|---|
| CONTROL | 310 | 15 | 2.8/7.2 | 140 |
| | 309 | 15 | 2.8/5.2 | 444 |
| | 314 | 16 | 4.2/7.5 | 150 |
| | 345 | 18 | 7.0/21.0 | 360 |
| EXPERIMENTAL | 308 | 15 | 4.8/8.5 | 0/0/1 |
| | 322 | 15 | 5.0/7.5 | 0/5/25 |
| | 320 | 16 | 3.1/5.0 | 5/6/0 |
| | 603 | 20 | 6.3/16.0 | 0/0/3 |

* refer to sperm counts obtained at three ejaculations done a week apart

## 2. The choice of the immunogen

It has been suggested, considering that the $\alpha$-subunit of FSH and LH are common, that it may be advisible to use the FSH $\beta$-subunit instead of the whole hormone as an immunogen to obtain antibodies capable of specifically neutralizing only FSH bioactivity. This fear, however, appears unfounded as immunization with intact FSH has not resulted, as tested in the bonnet[2], rhesus[5] and cynomolgous[6] monkeys in any reduction in endogenous testosterone levels, a classic event that occurs if antibodies capable of cross-reacting with primate LH were to be present. Although oFSH $\beta$-subunit has been successfully used by Raj and coworkers[6] as an immunogen in the cynomolgous monkey, it does not appear to offer any special advantage over intact oFSH. Following a suggestion of Dr. Robbins of NIH, Bethesda, it was felt worthwhile to determine if derivatization of oFSH-like desialation, deglycosylation or conjugation to tetanus toxoid - would lead to increased immunogenicity. The desialated and deglycosylated oFSH was prepared by Dr. M.R. Sairam at the Clinical Research Institute, Montreal, Canada while the oFSH-tetanus toxoid conjugate was made by Dr. Talwar's group at the National Institute of Immunology, New Delhi, India. Immunization was carried out in groups of adult male rats (n per group=6), the immunogen being given in each case adsorbed on aluminium hydroxide. Each rat received a total dose of 50 ug of oFSH spread over a period of 6 weeks. The antisera obtained at autopsy following a booster dose of oFSH or its derivative was analysed for antibody titer as well as bioneutralizing activity. The results described in this paper (Fig.1 and Table 5) considered together with our ealier observation would indicate that intact unaltered oFSH is unmatched in its ability to produce high titer antibodies capable of neutralizing ovine as well as primate FSH.

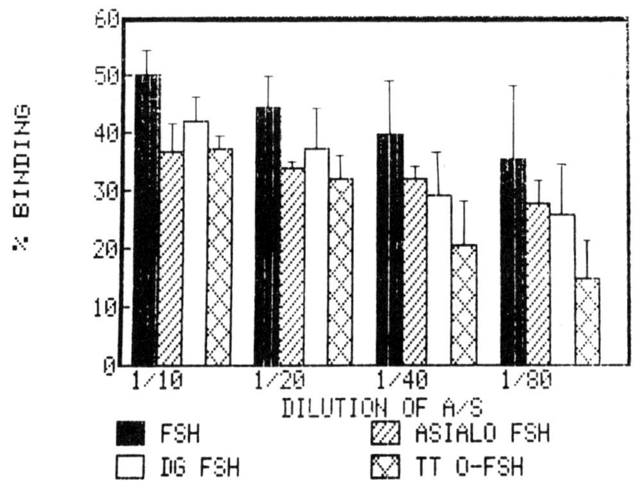


Fig. 1. Relative immunogenicity of oFSH and its derivatives- A study in rats

Table 5. Bioneutralizing activity of antisera (a/s) raised in rats to derivatives of oFSH in the rat granulosa cell bioassay

| Treatment NRS(5µl | A/s(5µl) | ng prog/0.5x10$^{6}$ cells/4h mean ± S.D. | % inhibition |
|---|---|---|---|
| + * | - | 0.61 ± 0.04 | - |
| + | - | 1.60 ± 0.27 | - |
| - | oFSH | 0.81 ± 0.02 | 80 |
| - | Asialo FSH | 0.81 ± 0.08 | 80 |
| - | dg FSH | 0.93 ± 0.15 | 68 |
| - | TT FSH | 1.00 ± 0.14 | 61 |

* All tubes excepting that marked with * received 100 µg oFSH

## CONCLUSION

Two primary conclusions can be arrived at from the present study. Firstly it suggests that long-term active immunization of non-seasonal nonhuman primates like the bonnet monkey with oFSH results in continued maintenance of testicular dysfunction leading to acute oligospermia or azoospermia. Eventhough the period of immunization in the current study was long (7-13 years), the animals appear in good health, have normal testosterone levels, exhibit normal libido and can be electroejaculated with ease. Histological examination of testicular biopsy samples revealed spermatogenic process to be effected. These results are in contrast to that reported for the rhesus monkey. While we are unable to offer a specific explanation for this, it is possible that seasonal testicular recrudescence the rhesus exhibit could be effecting the ability of the FSH antibody to neutralize the increased level (?) of FSH that may be outpouring at the beginning of every season when testis becomes active. Recently using a fresh group of 4 bonnet monkeys, we have been able to induce within 200 days acute oligo/azoospermia by immunizing them with a highly purified oFSH preparation given adsorbed on Aluminium hydroxide, an adjuvant cleared for human usage. The current series of experiments thus demonstrate that the observed effect is highly reproducible, everyone of the monkeys thus far immunized showing an effect on sperm production. Interestingly, long term immunization of rhesus moneys with oFSH has been reported [8] not to prouce any immunopathologic lesions.

Intact oFSH in itself appears to be the most suitable immunogen as derivatization of this did not in our hands lead to an increase in immunogenicity. oFSH being heterologous in nature it is not necessary to conjugate it to tetanus toxoid like in the case of hCG to increase its immunogenicity. The antisera produced to oFSH has been shown both in the present study and elsewhere as being capable of effectively neutralizing both monkey and hFSH. As immunization with oFSH does only seem to effect only sperm production and not testosterone levels and libido, the advantage of using this protein as a vaccine becomes all the more significant. Presently it is unclear how FSH lack brings about infertility. Our earlier study showed that such of those bonnet monkeys which were rendered only oligospermic by passive immunization with FSH antiserum were all the same unable to impregnate proven fertile females.

The likelihood of spermatozoa produced under a state of 'FSH deficiency' being qualitatively deficient to bring about fertilization has been mooted and experiments are currently underway to test this hypothesis.

Although FSH has been shown to be essential for initiating spermatogenesis in the human[11], the recent results of Matsumoto et al[12] using testosterone to suppress both endogenous FSH and LH in adult human male suggests that supplementation with exogenous LH/hCG alone is able to maintain spermatogenesis atleast qualitatively. This is currently puzzling and it is not clear if excess testosterone (that given to block gonadotropin secretion plus that produced following LH injection) in the presence of LH can override an FSH requirement. It appears that the simplest way of determining the physiologic need for FSH in maintaining testicular function of normal fertile human males is to immunize human volunteers or chimpanzees with either oFSH or preformed characterized FSH antibody for a period of 90-120 days. Such an experiment would set at rest the continuing debate on this subject and determine the validity of using oFSH as a contraceptive vaccine in man.

## ACKNOWLEDGEMENT

The authors wish to thank Dr. H.G.M. Raj for the gift of the antisera raised by him in cynomolgous monkeys and Prof. M.R.N. Prasad for his expert opinion on the histology preparations. The financial assistance provided by the ICMR, New Delhi and the WHO, Geneva during the various phases of this programme is also gratefully acknowledged.

## REFERENCES

1. C.S. Sheela Rani, G.S.R.C. Murty, and N.R. Moudgal, Effect of chronic neutralization of endogenous FSH on testicular function in the adult male bonnet monkey - assessment using biochemical parameters, Intl. J. Andrology 1:32 (1978).

2. G.S.R.C. Murty, C.S. Sheela Rani, N.R. Moudgal, and M.R.N. Prasad, Effect of passive immunization with specific antiserum to FSH on the spermatogenic process and fertility of adult male bonnet monkeys (Macaca radiata), J. Reprod. Fert., Suppl. 26:147 (1979).

3. G.S.R.C. Murty, C.S. Sheela Rani, and N.R. Moudgal, The role of FSH in regulating testicular function - a study involving the use of specific FSH antibodies, Proc. VI Intl. Cong. Endocrinol., Melbourne Australia (1980).

4. N.R. Moudgal, A need for FSH in maintaining Fertility of adult male subhuman primates, Arch. Andrology 7:117 (1981).

5. E.J. Wickings, K.H. Usadel, G. Dathe, and E. Nieschlag, The role of FSH in testicular function of the mature rhesus monkey, Acta Endocrinol. 95:117 (1980).

6. H.G.M. Raj, M.R. Sairam, M. Dym, N. Kotite, F.S. French, C. Sloan, and R. Chendy, Effect of immunization against follicle stimulating hormone on spermatogenesis in the rat and the monkey, in : "Nonhuman primate models for study of human reproduction", T.C. Anand Kumar, ed., Karger (Basel), (1980).

7. N.R. Moudgal, H.M. Shashidhara Murthy, G.S. Murthy, and A.J. Rao, A role for inhibin in regulating FSH levels in the adult male bonnet monkey, Proc. of Satellite Symposium on Gonadal Protein and Quebec, Canada, World Scientific Publishers, Singapore, p21 (1984).

8. B.R. Srinath, E.J. Wickings , C. Witting, and E. Nieshlag, Active immunization with follicle stimulating hormone for fertility control: a 4 1/2 year study in male rhesus monkeys, Fertil. Steril. 40:110 (1983).

9. H.G.M. Raj, Effefct of active immunization with FSH on spermtogenesis in the adult crab eating monkey - evaluation for male contraception, See chapter in this book.

10. C.S. Sheela Rani, N. Ravindranath, and N.R. Moudgal, Role of FSH in follicular development in the bonnet monkey: studies using an antiserum to FSH, Proc. 7th Intl. Cong. Endocrinol. (1984).

11. A.M. Matsumoto, A.E. Karpas, C.A. Paulsen, and W.J. Bremer, Reinitiation of sperm production in gonadotropin suppressed normal men by administration of FSH, J. Clin. Invest. 72:1005 (1983).

12. A.M. Matsumoto, A.C. Paulsen, and W.J. Bremer, Stimulation of sperm production by human luteinizing hormone in gonadotropin suppressed normal men, J. Clin. End. Metab. 59:882 (1984).

# IMMUNIZATION AGAINST FSH AS A METHOD OF MALE CONTRACEPTION

Jeffrey Spieler

Research Division
Office of Population
Agency for International Development
Washington, DC 20523

In May 1985 I had the opportunity of participating in an International Workshop on Male Contraception in Geneva, Switzerland sponsored by the Program for Applied Research on Fertility Regulation (PARFR), Northwestern University. PARFR invited Professor Eberhard Nieschlag of the Max Planck Clinical Research Unit for Reproductive Medicine, Munster, Federal Republic of Germany, to present a paper on immunization against FSH as a male method of fertility regulation. Professor Nieschlag informed PARFR that the results of his work in this area were discouraging and that his group had abandoned the approach. Not dissuaded by negative results, PARFR reinvited Professor Nieschlag to present a paper on the reasons for abandoning immunization against FSH as an approach to male fertility regulation.(1) Because Professor Nieschlag was unable to attend the Fogerty Symposium I would like to summarize some of his findings for you.

The preclinical primate studies conducted by Nieschlag's group between 1977 and 1983 began under the classical concept that LH controlled Leydig cell function and that FSH was responsible for the control of spermatogenesis. If this concept were true then the suppression, or inactivation, of FSH alone should lead to azoospermia without affecting androgen levels and libido. However, if the findings in rats that testosterone alone could maintain spermatogenesis held true for humans, than selective inhibition of FSH may not be an effective method for men.

In an attempt to elucidate the role of FSH in human spermatogenesis, non-human primates were studied. Since sufficient quantities of monkey gonadotrophins were not available to perform the necessary replacement studies in hypophysectomized animals, the experimental protocol chosen called for the neutralization of FSH bioactivity with antibodies to FSH.

The results of passive immunization studies with ovine FSH in adult rhesus monkeys showed a clear suppression of spermatogenesis and testicular volume without affecting Leydig cell function and ejaculatory behavior. Although azoospermia was not reached, the role of FSH in maintaining spermatogensis in primates was established.(2)

The next study conducted was aimed at assessing the long term (4 1/2 years) effects of active immunization against FSH.[3] Four adult male rhesus monkeys were immunized with purified ovine FSH. The animals developed high titers of antibodies to FSH that did not cross react with rhesus LH. Serum testosterone remained in the normal range throughout the experiment. Testicular volumes decreased to an extent similar to that of hypophysectomized animals, with lowest volumes reached six months after immunization. Sperm counts during the first two years were severly reduced and azoospermia was observed intermittently. After two years, however, sperm counts returned to the low normal range, with normal motility and morphology. Mating studies were not performed at any time, but in vitro studies during the third year of the project indicated that the sperm were capable of penetrating zona-free hamster eggs. Testicular biopsies after 4 1/2 years showed that the initial impairment of spermatogenesis (reduction of tubular diameter) reversed spontaneously for the most part, but cell numbers (spermatids) were still reduced. Immunization with FSH did not render the animals infertile; azoospermia had not been consistently achieved. However, no circulating nor precipitated immune complexes were detected in a wide variety of tissues examined.

Additional studies were conducted in monkeys to help to clarify the relative importance of FSH, LH and testosterone for spermatogenesis in primates. Testosterone alone, administered in physiological doses to intact mature rhesus monkeys, was capable of slowing down testicular atrophy and preventing azoospermia which accompanies high-dose treatment with LHRH agonists. Testosterone alone was shown to be capable of maintaining some degree of spermatogenesis in hypophysectomized adult rhesus monkeys, and an increase in testes volume (the seminal epithelium begins to develop) and spermotogenesis in immature intact or hypophysectomized cynomolgus monkeys. Also, the administration of 250 ug per week of testosterone enanthate to pituitary stalk sectioned adult rhesus monkeys resulted in an increase in testes volume with sperm observed in the ejaculate. Pulsatile GNRH administered to these animals further improved testes volume and spermatogenesis.

Nieschlag concluded from these experiments that testesterone alone could initiate, maintain and reinitiate spermatogenesis qualitatively, but not quantitatively when compared to normal animals. However, the combination of FSH and testosterone is required to observe normal spermatogenesis in primates. In Nieschlag's clinical opinion, the neutralization of FSH alone in normal men would not be sufficiently effective to be used as a male contraceptive. Data from Raj (4) in cynomolgus monkeys immunized with ovine FSH or the B-subunit of oFSH support Nieschlag's conclusions. However, studies conducted in bonnet monkeys immunized with FSH raise questions about this position. Moudgal (5,6) found that a reduction in sperm count without azoospermia was accompanied by a loss of fertility in immunized animals. In Nieschlag's opinion these findings are difficult to explain and may be a result of studying too few animals. However, because Nieschlag's group had not conducted mating experiments, data on the actual fertility of oligospermic monkeys in his study are not available.

Nieschlag's premise is that unless azoospermia is obtained, an acceptably effective level of male contraception will not be reached. This issue has been debated for years and forms the basis of the WHO's Task Force on Male Methods of Fertility Regulation efforts to develop safe, acceptable and effective contraceptives for men. It is time to conduct clinical trials in oligospermic, but otherwise normal, men to see, if in fact, azoospermia is a prerequisite for effective fertility regulation in men.

REFERENCES


1. E., Nieschlag, Reasons for abandoning immunization against FSH as an approach to male fertility regulation, in: "Male Contraception: Advances and Future Prospects," G. I. Zatuchni, A. Goldsmith, J. J. Sciarra and J. M. Spieler, eds., Harper and Row, Philadelphia (1986, in preparation).

2. E. J., Wickings, Usadel, K. H. Dathe, G. and Nieschlag, E., The role of follicle stimulating hormone in testicular function of the mature rhesus Monkey, Acta Endocr. 95:117 (1980).

3. B. R., Srinath, Wickings E.J., Witting, C. and Nieschlag, E., Active immunization with follicle stimulating hormone for fertility control: A 4 1/2-year study in male rhesus monkeys, Fertil. Steril. 40:110 (1983).

4. H.G.M., Raj, Murty, G.S.R.C., Sairam, M.R. and Talbert, L.M., Control of spermatogenesis in primates: Effects of active immunization against FSH in the monkey, Int. J. Androl., Suppl. 5:27 (1982).

5. G.S.R.C., Murty, Rani, C.S.S., Moudgal, N.R. and Prasad, M.R.N., Effect of passive immunization with specific antiserum to FSH on the spermatogenesis process and fertility of adult male bonnet monkeys (Macaca radiata), J. Reprod. Fertil., Suppl. 26:147 (1979)

6. N.R. Moudgal, - This Symposium

# EFFECTS OF ACTIVE IMMUNIZATION WITH FOLLICLE STIMULATING HORMONE (FSH) ON SPERMATOGENESIS IN THE ADULT CRAB EATING MONKEY- EVALUATION FOR MALE CONTRACEPTION

H.G. Madhwa Raj

Reproduction Research Laboratories
Section of Reproductive Endocrinology
Departments of Obstetrics, Gynecology
and Biochemistry

## INTRODUCTION

It is well known that both follicle stimulating hormone (FSH) and luteinizing hormone (LH) are required for normal testicular function. The role of FSH in spermatogenesis has been the subject of intense investigation in the last few years. In the rat, FSH is required during the first wave of spermatogenesis, but not in the adult (Madhwa Raj and Dym, 1976; Dym et al., 1977; Madhwa Raj et al., 1980). However, in the adult bonnet (Sheela Rani et al., 1978; Murty et al., 1979, 1980) and the rhesus (Wickings and Nieschlag, 1980) monkeys, FSH has been shown to play an important role in spermatogenesis. In the studies mentioned above, both passive and active immunization procedures have been employed. We first reported the effects of active immunization with FSH and FSH-$\beta$ subunit in the crab eating monkey (Madhwa Raj et al., 1980). Considerable interest has been evinced in evaluatig methods that might selectively suppress spermatogenesis leaving androgen production and androgen dependent parameters intact, for purpose of achieving male contraception. Thus it is important to examine the role of FSH in spermatogenesis and effects of selective withdrawal of this hormone on fertility and sexual behaviour in the primate model. We report here the chronic effects of neutralizing FSH (by active immunization with ovine FSH or ovine FSH-$\beta$ subunit) in the male crab eating monkey,Macaca fasicularis.

## MATERIALS AND METHODS

### Animals

Adult male crab eating monkeys purchased from Primate Imports, New Jersey, were used in the present study. The animals were quarantined for a period of 40 days, after which they were housed individually in temperature and humidity controlled rooms with 12 hours of light and 12 hours of dark periods. They were fed with monkey chow (Purina Lab Chows, St. Louis, Mo.) supplemented with fruits and vegetables, and water was given, ad libitum. The monkeys were weighed regularly and subjected to tuberculin tests at 3-month intervals.

## Hormones and immunization

Highly purified ovine FSH and FSH-$\beta$ subunit preparations were used for immunizing the monkeys at regular intervals. The biological potency of FSH was 770 IU/mg. The preparation of FSH and FSH-$\beta$ subunit has been described previously in detail (Sairam, 1979).

Five monkeys were immunized with FSH and four with FSH-$\beta$ subunit using a slight modification of the multiple-site intradermal immunization technique as described by Vaituikitis et al. (1979). Initially, 500 ug of hormone was injected at 15-day intervals for immunization. Later, it was found that 100 ug could be injected at monthly intervals without loss of titres, and this regimen was adopted for immunization. The hormone was dissolved in 0.2 ml of distilled water and emulsified with an equal volume of Fruends incomplete adjuvant (Difco Laboratories, Detroit, Michigan) and administered intradermally at 6-8 sites. This procedure was repeated at monthly intervals. The animals were bled from the femoral vein at bimonthly intervals. The serum was separated and stored for further characterization. Five additional monkeys served as controls.

## Antibody titres

Serial dilutions of serum from immunized monkeys were incubated with a trace (1 ng) of $^{125}$I labeled ovine FSH for 24 hours at 37 C. Protein A (0.1 ml of 5% solution, Enzyme Center, Boston, Massachusettes) was used to separate the antibody-bound hormone from free hormone. After an additional incubation of 1 hour at 37 C, the antibody-bound hormone was separated by centrifugation and the pellet counted in a Packard gamma spectrometer. The antibody titre is defined as the dilution of the serum that binds 50% of the labeled radioactive hormone.

## Neutralization of biological activity

The neutralizing ability of the sera from immunized monkeys was tested using the immature rat testis tubule assay for FSH as described by Rao and Ramachandran (1975). Tubule preparations from 21-day-old rat testis were incubated either with 100 ng ovine FSH or 50 ug of monkey pituitary extract (representing monkey FSH) in the presence of normal monkey serum or serum from immunized monkeys. FSH stimulated increase in cyclic AMP was used as the end point. Cyclic AMP was measured by the protein kinase binding method of Gillman et al. (1970).

## Collection and analysis of semen

Semen from normal and immunized monkeys were obtained by electro-ejaculation using a rectal probe. The monkeys were lightly anesthesized with Ketamine hydrochloride (Ketalar, Parke-Davis Co., Detroit, Michigan) and the rectum was douched with normal saline prior to the insertion of the probe. Sperm motility was evaluated in the liquified part of the semen. Motility was rated on a subjective scale of 0-100%. The semen samples were incubated for 1 hour at 37 C, in the presence of 2% trypsin to dissolve the clot and to facilitate total sperm count measurements. The sperm counts are expressed as concentration per milliliter of ejaculate. A small part of the liquid semen was diluted and stained with 0.05% eosin to analyze the live and the dead sperm by standard techniques.

Testosterone measurement

Testosterone levels were measured in ether extract of serum samples using a radioimmunoassay as described by Bartke et al. (1973), with slight modifications. Sephadex-LH-20 column chromatography was omitted and a specific antiserum was used for the assay.

RESULTS

All immunized animals maintained generally good health throughout the period of immunization, and showed no weight loss.

Antibody titres

Circulating antibodies could be detected 4-6 weeks after the initiation of immunization. From there on, the antibody titres rose steadily and reached peak levels of 1:10,000 to 1:50,000 by 4-5 months. Such titres were maintained throughout the rest of the immunization period. Recently we have also examined the binding of labeled human FSH to the sera of immunized monkeys. Sera from all the monkeys bound human FSH; however the antibody titres, when expressed in terms of human FSH binding ability, were slightly lower than ovine FSH. Nevertheless, the potency of the antibody to combine with this heterologous FSH was considered extremely good.

Biological neutralization

In the in vitro testis tubule assay (Table 1) 100 ng of ovine FSH was able to stimulate cyclic AMP production by about 6-fold over controls. Inclusion of either FSH antiserum or FSH-$\beta$ antiserum (100 $\mu$l) consistently inhibited this response, bringing it to control levels. Similarly, 50 $\mu$g of monkey pituitary extract caused a 2-3 fold stimulation of cAMP levels and this was inhibited by antibody to either FSH or FSH-$\beta$.

Table 1. Inhibition of FSH stimulated cAMP response by serum from monkeys immunized with ovine FSH or ovine FSH

| Gr. | Treatment | cAMP, pM/mg* |
|---|---|---|
| None | NMS | 6.7 |
| oFSH, 100 ng | NMS | 38.2 |
| oFSH, 100 ng | FSH A/S | 7.9 |
| oFSH, 100 ng | FSH B A/S | 8.2 |
| MPE, 50 $\mu$g | NMS | 21.5 |
| MPE, 50 $\mu$g | FSH A/S | 4.9 |
| MPE, 50 $\mu$g | FSH B A/S | 6.1 |

Immature rat testis tubule preparation was used according to Rao and Ramachandran (1975).
NMS=Normal monkey serum
MPE=Monkey pituitary extract: representing monkey FSH.
*Mean of duplicate determinations.

### Semen analysis

Ejaculates can be obtained throughout the year in this species of monkeys, and we observed no seasonal fluctuations (Figure 1). However, a wide variation in sperm counts was seen in the individual monkeys, the concentrations ranging from 200 million to 1200 million/ml of semen. In all the immunized monkeys, sperm concentrations began to decline by day 70-140 of immunization (Figures 2 & 3). This decline became pronounced by about day 200 after immunization. However, consistent azoospermia was not observed in these monkeys. Though a reduction in motility was observed in a few monkeys, there were no consistent changes in motility or abnormality in the immunized groups taken as a whole (data not shown).

### Testosterone levels

Serum testosterone levels were measured in representative blood samples throughout the immunization period. It can be seen from Table 2 that the mean serum levels of this hormone are similar in immunized monkeys and controls, indicating that LH was not neutralized during active immunization.

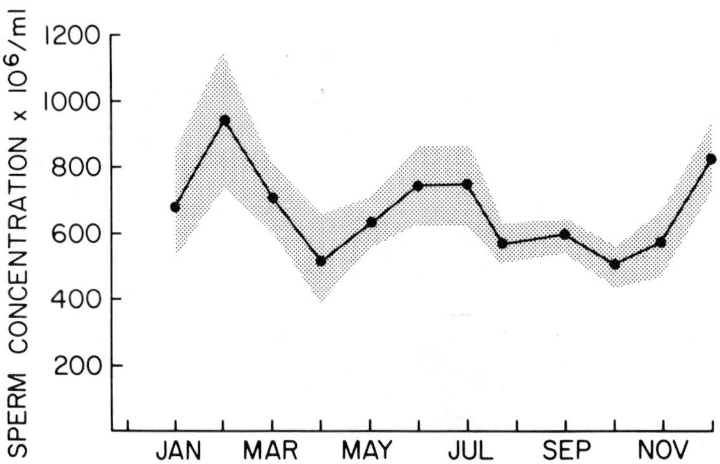


Fig. 1. Sperm concentration of normal monkeys throughout the year.

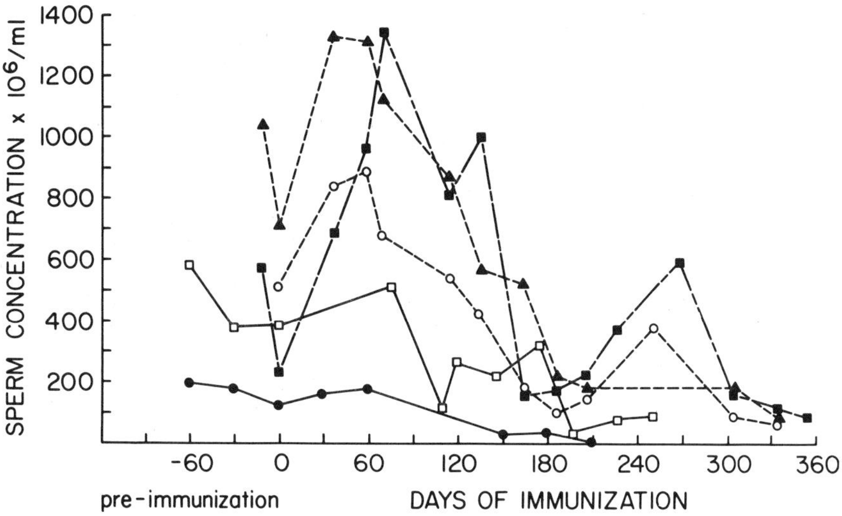


Fig. 2. Effect of active immunization with FSH on sperm counts in 5 monkeys

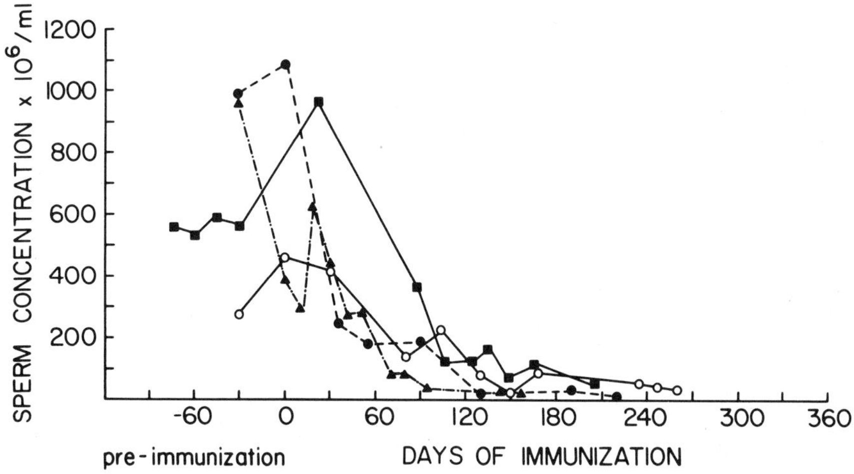


Fig. 3. Effect of active immunization with FSH B-subunit on sperm counts in 4 monkeys

Table 2. Serum testosterone level in monkeys

| | N | ng/ml, mean + SD |
|---|---|---|
| Controls* | 42 | 9.14 ± 4.7 ← |
| Postimuunization+ | 40 | 8.97 ± 3.96@ ← |

N = number of samples
* = includes preimmunization levels from immunized monkeys
\+ = values from throughout the immunization period
@ = not significantly different (p=0.1)

DISCUSSION

The present study demonstrates that FSH is necessary for optimal spermatogenic response in the adult male crab eating monkey, M.fasicularis. Suppression of FSH action was achieved by active immunization with either FSH or FSH-$\beta$ subunit. The antibodies generated were capable of binding to ovine and human FSH. Further, such binding resulted in loss of biologic activity as evidenced by the in vitro rat testis tubule assay which is specific to FSH. In this assay, the activity of FSH present in monkey pituitary extracts was also abolished. This indicates that the antibodies to ovine FSH or its $\beta$-subunit could neutralize endogenous FSH activity of immunized monkeys. LH dependent testosterone levels were not altered in these monkeys, thus indicating that LH activity was not neutralized.

Active immunization with FSH resulted in lowering of sperm counts in all the monkeys; however, consistent azoospermia was not achieved. This is consistent with the observations in the bonnet (Murty et al., 1979, 1980) and rhesus monkeys (Wickings and Nieschlag, 1980). In addition, loss of fertility has been demonstrated in bonnet monkeys passively immunized with FSH antibody (Murty et al., 1979, 1980). No seasonal fluctuations were observed in sperm concentration of this species of monkeys in our colony. This is borne out by the data on control monkeys, and is in agreement with the observations of Mahone and Dukelow (1979) in this species of monkey.

In the adult monkey, pituitary support is essential for spermatogenic function of the tesis. Thus, Smith (1942, 1944) demonstrated that following hypophysectomy, there is a cessation of mitosis and total disappearence of spermatids and fully formed spermatozoa in the seminiferous tubules. Daily injections of 25-50 mg. testosterone propionate caused an increase in diameter of tubules and brought about a clearcut restoration of sperm production in many tubules. However, he observed that size of the testis, and of tubules as well as restoration of spermatogenesis in the tubules did not reach normal levels (Smith, 1944). He concluded that some other factors may be necessary for normal maintenance of the testis. Recent investigations of Marshell et al. (1982) corroborate these findings. In this study, testicular regression was brought about by pituitary stalk section of adult rhesus monkeys. Weekly administration of 250 mg. testosterone enenthate could restore sermatogenesis as assessed by analysis of ejaculated semen. This restoration appears to be partial (17 to 60 x $10^6$/ml sperms in testosteroe enenthate treated vs. 110 to 1100 x $10^6$/ml sperms in normal adult rhesus monkeys, Wickings and Nieschlag, 1980). From these, it is evident that in the absence of pituitary support testosterone alone can restore sermatogenesis, but not to the full extent. Thus, other factors (FSH?) may be required for normal spermatogenic function as assessed by size of testis, tubules and normal sperm count in ejaculates. This is supported by our current observations that sperm counts are lowered upon neutralizing FSH activity, despite normal serum testosterone levels. Similarly, Karpas et al. (1982) demonstrated that in man, selective FSH difficiency brought about by chronic hCG administration results in reduction of sperm counts. They suggested that FSH is important in maintaining quantitatively normal spermatogenesis, though it may not be absolutely required for qualitative maintenance of sperm production. The mode of action of FSH in supporting quantitative spermatogenesis has been investigated. FSH administration drastically reduces spermatogonial degeneration occuring during spermaogenesis in the immature rat (Huckins et al., 1973). Recent investigations of Matsumoto et al. (1982) demonstrated that FSH alone could reinitiate sperm production in man during gonadotropin suppression induced by exogenous testosterone enenthate administration. They hypothesize that FSH could be responsible for increasing intratesticular testosterone (necessary for sprmatogenesis) through sitmulation of androgen binding protein in the tubular compartment.

It is now well accepted that FSH receptors exist on the Sertoli cell and this is the specific target cell type for FSH in the testis. It is also well known that Sertoli cell plays a central role in spermatogenesis, performing several important functions. Thus we have catalogued at least 7 functions of the Sertoli cell, relevent to spermatogenesis (Dym, Madhwa Raj and Chemes, 1977). Recent observations from the group of Clermont have shown that during late phase of spermatogenesis, a Sertoli cell cytoplasmic organelle is 'donated' to the developing spermatid. The importance of this event in determining sperm motility, fertilizability and viability is not completely understood and needs to be investigated. Also whether FSH directly or indirectly regulates such a process and therefore determines the quality of the sperm, also needs to be evaluated. In this context, it is important to discuss the prerequisites for any drug acting at the level of spermatogenesis, to qualify as a male contraceptive. It is currently held that any such drug should bring about consistent azoospermia. None of the agents tried so far, including LHRH agonists, antagonists and steroid formulations have qualified under this definition. Similarly FSH immunization also will not qualify if this definition is used. However, the preliminary results from Moudgal's group (Murthy et al., 1979) indicate that the immunized monkeys became totally infertile, despite not achieving azoospermia. These results indicate that a 'biochemical lesion' has been induced in these sperms, rendering them unsuitable. The exact nature of this lesion(s) if any, needs to be defined. We are currently investigating the penetrability, fertilizability of sperms from FSH immunized monkeys and post fertilization development, using monkey eggs as well as the zona free hamster egg system. In addition, a number of biochemical parameters as sperm hyaluronidase ad cyclic AMP are also under investigation under the sponsorship of US-India technology initiative program. These will help us in better understanding the role of FSH and its mechanism of action in regulating spermatogenesis and in evaluatig its potential for use in achieving male contraception. If it is borne out that immunization with FSH affects fertility by bringing about qualitative changes in the sperm, this will be an ideal male contraceptive, from the point of acceptability. Such a contraceptive effect will not be accompanied by a drastic ( >50% ) reduction in the size of the testis, which occurs wih total inhibition of spermatogenesis (eg. with hypophysecomy or LH antiserum treatment, Madhwa Raj and Dym, 1976). Our preliminary observations indicate that upon immunization with FSH, viability of spermatozoa in ejaculated semen is impaired. Further ability of such sperms to attach to monkey eggs is also severely reduced in *in vitro* fertilization studies.

Another aspect of the investigations on active immunization with FSH that needs to be clarified is the duration of inhibition. Recent investigation from Nieschlag's group (Srinath et al.,1983) in the rhesus monkey showed return of normal sperm counts after a prolonged immunization of 4 years. This occured despite high antibody titres. A careful examination of their study by this investigator showed that the recovery was not complete. Further, the last injection of FSH had been given several months earlier. Also data on fertility of these monkeys or any data on penetrability and fertilizing capacity of sperms from these monkeys in in vitro egg penetration tests, and any biochemical changes in the sperms are not available in this study. These need to be evaluated before concluding the suitability of this method for male contraception and extended to othr species of non human primates. Such information will be of vital imporatance to not only for contraceptive development, but also to fully evaluate the role of FSH in spermatogenesis which could help treatment of male infertility.

ACKNOWLEDGEMENT

Supported by NIH-HD 20072 & NSF under the US-India technology initiative program. The author wishes to thank Mrs. Mala M. Murthy for excellent secretarial assistance.

REFERENCES

Bartke, A., Steel, R.E., Musto, N., and Caldwell, B.V., 1973, Fluctuations in plasma testosterone levels in adult male rats and mice, Endocrinology, 92:1223.

Dym, M., Madhwa Raj, H.G., and Chemes, H.E., 1977, Response of the testis to selective withdrawal of LH or FSH using antigonadotropic sera, in: "New Concepts of the testis in normal and infertile men: Morphology, Physiology and Pathology," H. Nankin and P. Teoen, ed., Raven Press, NY.

Gliman, A.G., 1970, A protein binding assay for adenosine 3':5'-Cyclic monophosphate, Proc. Natl. Acad. Sci. (USA), 67:305.

Huckins, C., Mills, N., Besch, P., and Means, A.R., 1973, Spermatogonial differentiation in immature testis: regulation by FSH, Endocrinol. Suppl., 92:A-94.

Karpas, A.E., Matsumoto, A.M., Paulsen, C.A., and Bremner, W.J., 1982, Effect of selective FSH deficienty induced by chronic hCG administration on spermatogenesis in normal men, Proceedings of the Endocrine Society, 64th Annual Meeting, June 1982, Abstract #473, pg. 198.

Madhwa Raj, H.G., and Dym, M., 1976, The effects of selective withdrawal of FSH or LH on spermatogenesis in the immature rat, Biol. of Reprod., 14:489.

Madhwa Raj, H.G., Sairam, M.R., Dym, M., Kotite, N., French, F.S., Sloan, C.and Dy, Ruth Chen, 1980, Effect of immunization against follicle stimulating hormone on spermatogenesis in the rat and the monkey, in: "Non-human primate models for study of human reproduction," Satellite Symp. 7th Congr. Int. Primatol. Soc. Bangalore, T.C. Anand Kumar, ed., Karger, Basel.

Mahone, J.P., Dukelow, W.R., 1979, Seasonal variation of reproductive parameters in the laboratory-housed male cyomologus macaque (Macaca fasicularis), J. Med. Primatol., 8:179.

Marshall, G.R., Wickings, E.J., Ludecke, D.K., and Nieschlag, E., 1982, Restoration of spermatogenesis in primates by testosterone alone, Proc. of the Endocrine Society, 64dth Annual Meeting, June 1982, Abstract #471.

Matsumoto, A.M., Paulsen, C.A., and Bremner, W.J., 1982, Follicle stimulating hormone reinitiates sperm production in gonadotropin-suppressed normal men, Proc. of the Endocrine Society, 64th Annual Meeting, June 1982, Abstract #472.

Murty, G.S.R.C., Sheela Rani, C.S., Moudgal, N.R., and Prasad, M.R.N., 1979, Effect of passive immunization with specific antiserum to FSH on spermatogenic process and fertility of adult male bonnet monkeys (Macaca radiata), J. Reprod. Fert. Suppl, 26:1.

Murty, G.S.R.C., Sheela Rani, C.S., and Moudgal, N.R., 1980, The role of FSH in regulating testicular function - A study involving the use of specific FSH antibodies, in: "Endocrinology 1980," I.A. Cumming, J.W. Funder, F.A.O. Mendelsohn, eds, Elsevier/North Holland Biomedical Press, Amsterdam, New York, Oxford.

Rao, A.J., and Ramachandran, J., 1975, cAMP production in isolated rat seminiferous tubule cell preparations: A potential in vitro assay for FSH, Life Sci., 17:411.

Srinath, B.R., Wickings, E.J., Witting, C., and Nieschlag, E., 1983, Active immunization with follicle stimulating hormone for fertility control: a 4 year study in male rhesus monkeys, Fertil. Steril., 40:110.

Wikings, E.J., Nieschlag, E., 1980, Suppression of spermatogenesis over two years in rhesus monkeys actively immunized with follicle stimulating hormone, Fertil. Steril., 34:269.

# LHRH IMMUNONEUTRALIZATION: BASIC STUDIES AND PROSPECTS FOR PRACTICAL APPLICATION

Hamish M. Fraser

MRC Reproductive Biology Unit
37 Chalmers Street
Edinburgh EH3 9EW

## INTRODUCTION

The hypothalamic decepeptide, pGlu-His-Trp-Ser-Tyr-Gly-Leu-Arg-Pro-Gly-$NH_2$, luteinizing hormone releasing hormone (LHRH) or gonadotrophin releasing hormone, plays a central role in reproduction in all mammalian species. Our understanding of its physiological role has been guided on one hand by effects of administering LHRH at different doses and frequencies to humans or experimental animals who lack the hormone, and on the other by studying the consequences of desensitizing the pituitary by repeated exposure to agonist analogues, by blocking the LHRH receptors by chemical antagonists or by the neutralizing endogenous LHRH by antibodies (Fig. 1). These studies have shown that for continued stimulation, the pituitary gonadotroph must be exposed to small pulses of LHRH at a frequency of one per 60-120 min (1-3) which appear to the pattern of normal hypothalamic activity as reflected by the frequency of luteinizing hormone (LH) pulses from the pituitary gland and from what is known from measuring LHRH in the hypophysial portal blood (4).

The first experiments on neutralization of LHRH by antibodies established this central role by the observation that passive immunization blocked ovulation in rats (5,6) while active immunization caused testicular involution and arrest of spermatogenesis in rabbits (5,7). Later work helped establish the intimate relationship between LHRH and secretion of LH pulses from the pituitary (8,9) and the more distant relationship with follicle stimulating hormone (FSH) (8). More recently, LHRH antibodies have become the ideal tool by which to study the role of LHRH in controlling its receptor numbers on the pituitary gonadotroph.

Although the methodology for using LHRH immunization has been available for over a decade it has not been developed for clinical or contraceptive use. Instead, the most significant applications of LHRH manipulation have been developed from the phenomenon of pituitary densitisation or down regulation which occurs when agonist analogues of LHRH are administered chronically on a daily basis, or by constant release from a long acting slow release depot. This ability of low doses of agonist to suppress reproductive function is being evaluated in humans for control of fertility and in the treatment of hormone dependent tumours (2,3).

The more logical alternative approach of occupying the LHRH receptor by a chemical antagonist with no LH-releasing activity has been extensively investigated during the last decade, but the fact that it has taken the synthesis of over 1,000 modifications of LHRH to obtain compounds sufficiently potent to block the action of LHRH in monkeys and in humans is an indication of the difficulties in taking this concept to reality. The antagonists are invaluable experimental tools, but it will take the devleopment of even more potent modifications before these expensive analogues can be used in practical doses in large animals and man. In comparison, suppression of pituitary gonadotrophin secretion by LHRH neutralization has proven cheaper and more versatile as active immunization has permitted long-term suppression in monkeys, sheep, dogs, deer and cattle as well as the common laboratory species.

LHRH immunization has not been seen in terms of a contraceptive in the human because of its markedly suppressive effects on gonadal steroids, problems with predicting the strength and duration of the antibody response and the need for an immunological adjuvant. LHRH immunization was proposed over a decade ago as a method of treatment of hormone dependent tumours (10) and as a non-surgical, reversible approach of castrating domestic species (11). While the impact of the chemist in overcoming the structural problems of low potency of LHRH analogues has been considerable, the imput of the immunologist in overcoming the immunological problems of LHRH immunization has been disappointing so neither of these aims have yet been achieved, although some important recent developments in producing an 'LHRH vaccine' will be described during this symposium.

The original methods of conjugation and immunization against LHRH have been reviewed in detail previously (12) as have the effects of active (12,13) and passive immunization (14). In this chapter I will summarize the effects of LHRH immunoneutralization in a variety of species and highlight some recent developments.

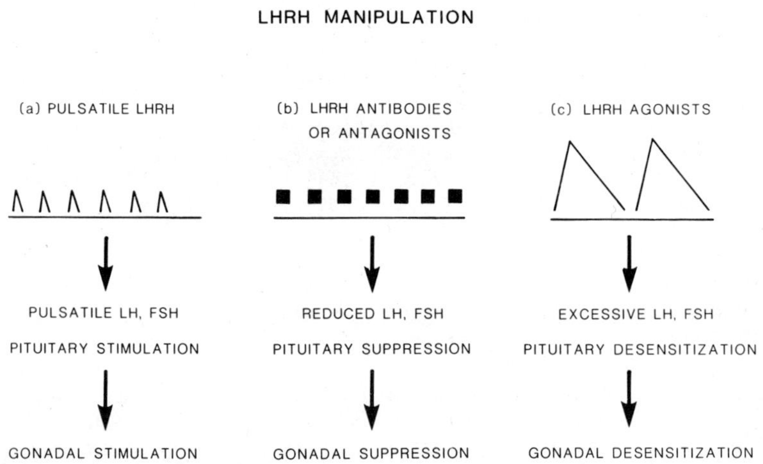


Fig. 1 Diagram to illustrate how (a) physiological pulses of LHRH stimulate the pituitary gonadotroph while this can be prevented by (b) neutralization by antibodies or receptor occupancy by LHRH antagonists to reduce LH and FSH release; and (c) chronic overstimulation to cause target-organ desensitisation.

In adult male rats (13) and in the ram (8), passive immunization by an LHRH antiserum results in a rapid suppression of serum concentrations of LH and testosterone, establishing the dependence between these 3 hormones (e.g. Fig. 2). Suppression is maximal during the first few days then is followed by a slow recovery. Suppression of FSH is much less and is slower showing that unlike LH its secretion is not governed closely in the short term by LHRH. Perhaps FSH release is maintained by low levels of LHRH remaining after antibody administration and partially controlled by a negative feedback effect of testicular products specifically upon FSH secretion at the pituitary level. There is no doubt, however, that the chronic effects of repeated passive immunization (15) or active immunization against LHRH suppress both LH and FSH in blood (13,16) and in the anterior pituitary gland (16,17) (Fig. 3) and this argues against the alternative possibility of a separate FSHRH. This likely suppression of synthesis of gonadotrophin is reflected in small size and inactive appearance of the pituitary gonadotrophs in actively immunized animals (13,18).

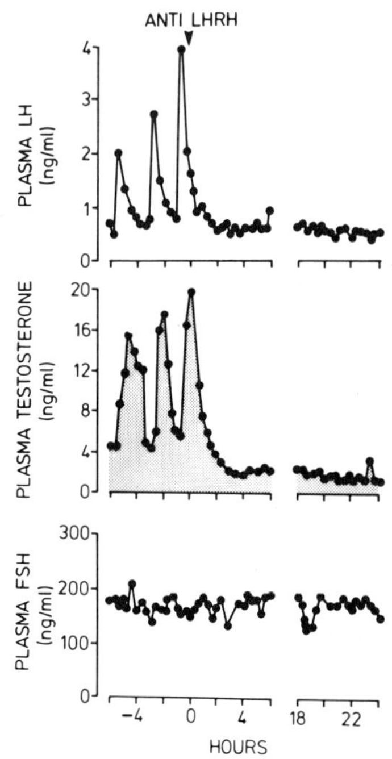


Fig. 2 Effect of an i.v. injection of an ovine antiserum to LHRH on the plasma concentrations of LH, testosterone and FSH in a Soay ram. The time of injection is indicated by the arrow. From Lincoln & Fraser (8).

Pituitary LHRH receptor numbers in the intact rat fall to about 70 per cent of control values 24h after injection of LHRH antibodies (13,19) while active immunization reduced receptors to 30 per cent of normal (17). Castration results in a doubling of LHRH receptor numbers. Injection of antibodies at time of castration in rats abolishes the rise in LHRH receptors, while antibody administration to chronically castrate rats causes a marked suppression of the elevated LHRH receptor numbers (19). Since testosterone is virtually non-detectable in both castrates and in rats actively immunized against LHRH the low number of receptors in the latter group support the idea of a primary role for LHRH in regulating its own receptors (Fig.3) (20).

Active immunization against LHRH has been shown to induce testicular involution in the rat (16) rabbit (5,7) dog (21) deer stag (22,23) ram (24) bull (25,26) marmoset monkey (27) and rhesus monkey (28). Provided antibody titres are sufficiently high, by 3 or more months after immunization an arrest of spermatogenesis is observed with a failure to produce cells beyond the spermatocyte stage. The ability of the Leydig cells _in vivo_ to release testosterone in response to LH is markedly reduced (22) and binding of hCG to rat Leydig cells and their response to hCG stimulation _in vitro_ is minimal (29).

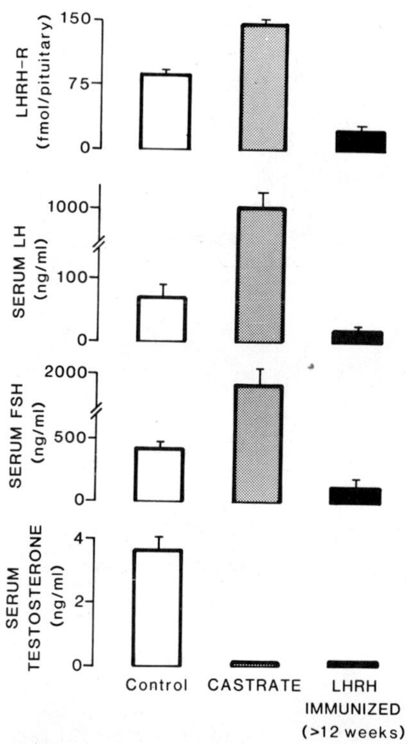


Fig. 3 Effect of castration or immunization against LHRH on pituitary LHRH receptors and serum concentrations of LH and FSH in adult male rats. Five rats per group, values are means ± SEM. All values for treated animals significantly different ($P < 0.001$) by Student's t-test.

## LHRH IMMUNONEUTRALIZATION IN THE FEMALE

As in the male, passive immunization against LHRH causes an immediate cessation of LH pulses in the intact and castrate animal (6,30,32) while suppression of FSH concentrations in blood is minimal. This was shown most prominently when ewes were injected with antiserum during the late follicular phase and a rise in serum FSH was observed during the following 24h (Fig.4)(30) and by the observation that antibodies to LHRH failed to prevent the rise in serum FSH concentrations which occurs during the first few hours after ovariectomy in the rat (33). Antibodies to LHRH also fail to block the rise in FSH which occurs after the pre-ovulatory LH/FSH surge in the rat (37,38) and ewe (39). The most likely explanation for these results is that products from the active ovarian follicle act to selectively suppress FSH by acting upon the pituitary gonadotroph. If these products are removed by blocking LH stimulation of the follicle or by ovariectomy then there is a temporary rise in FSH as a result of removal of this negative influence. In chronically ovariectomized rats (6) ferrets (34) rhesus monkeys (35) and stumptailed monkeys (36) administration of antibodies to LHRH results in suppression of FSH, but the effect takes longer than for LH. These results suggests differences within the gonadotroph between synthesis and release of LH and FSH, giving FSH secretion a degree of autonomy for a few days after LHRH deprivation or it may be that the effect is due to low levels of biologically active LHRH.

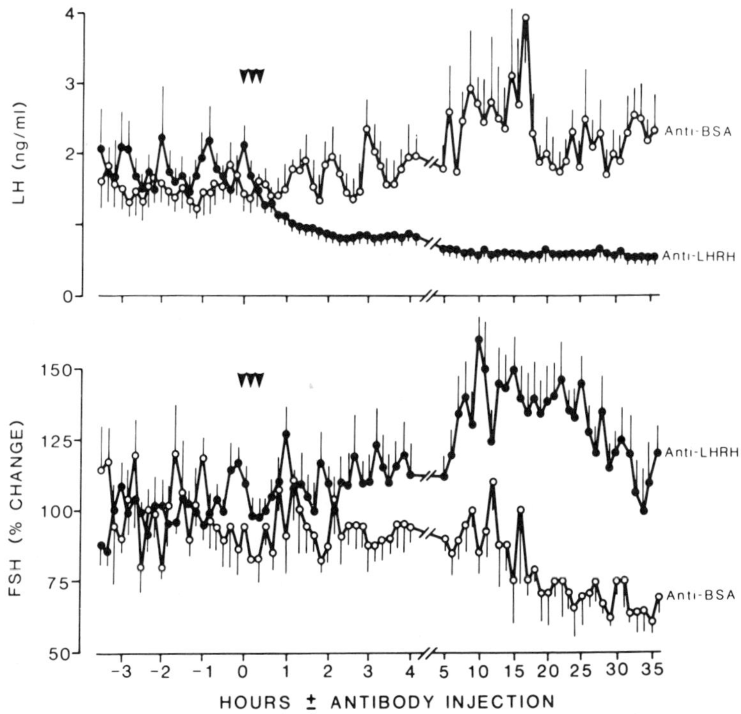


Fig. 4 Effect of an i.v. injection of antiserum to bovine serum albumin (control) or antiserum to LHRH on the mean plasma concentrations of LH and FSH during the follicular phase of the oestrous cycle in the ewe. Values are means $\pm$ SEM for 5 control ewes and 6 LHRH antiserum treated ewes. Times of injection shown by arrows. From Fraser & McNeilly (30).

It should be emphasised that any rise in FSH after LHRH antibodies is only transitory and is not observed in all stages of the follicular phase. For example, Fig. 5 shows how in the stumptailed macaque, injection of antibodies to LHRH during the mid-follicular phase suppressed further rises in FSH and LH for 8 days and prevented further follicular development during this period as shown by the fall in oestradiol secretion.

Active immunization against LHRH will suppress FSH as well as LH in the female rat (40,41,43) and stumptailed macaque (42) and block follicular development and ovulation (Figs.6 & 7). Although a significant decline in FSH was not observed in an early study in the ewe (44) recent more detailed studies have demonstrated a clear suppression in FSH secretion (46).

Antibodies to LHRH have proved useful in elucidating the changes in pituitary LHRH receptor numbers observed during the rat oestrous cycle. We have examined the role of the various components in the hypothalamic-pituitary-ovarian axis by either immunoneutralization of LHRH, to remove both stimulation of gonadotrophin and ovarian function, or immunoneutralization of LH to remove the stimulus for ovarian steroid production leaving the hypothalamic system intact. Active

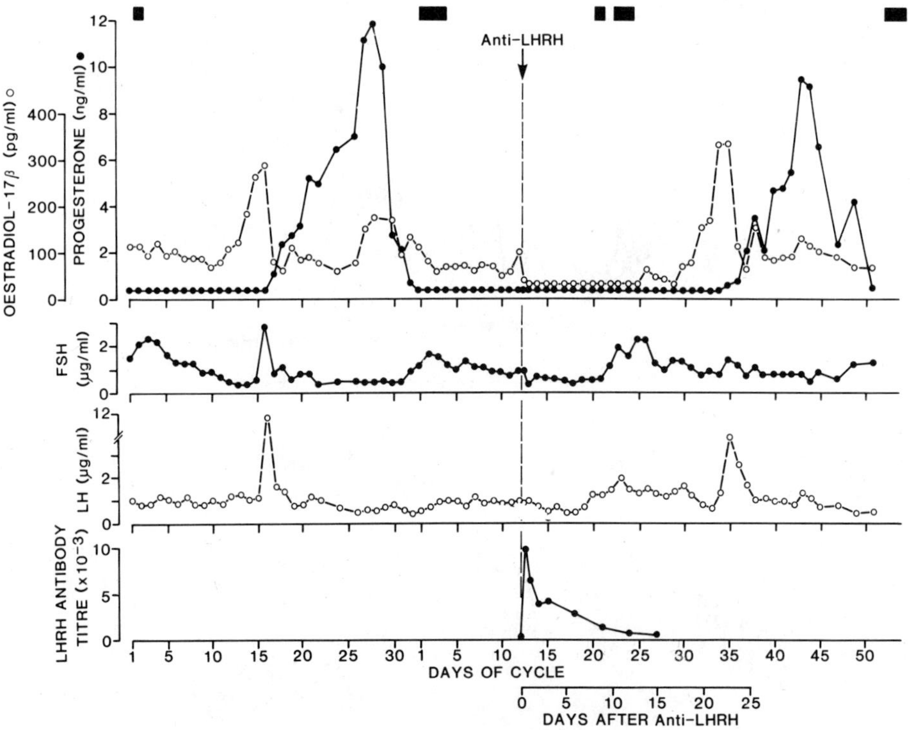


Fig. 5 Serum concentrations of LH, FSH, oestradiol and progesterone during a pre-treatment control cycle and during the following cycle after an i.v. injection of LHRH gamma globulin during the mid-follicular phase of the stumptailed macaque. Bottom panel shows titre of LHRH antibodies in the circulation. Bars show menstrual bleeding. From Fraser et al (36)

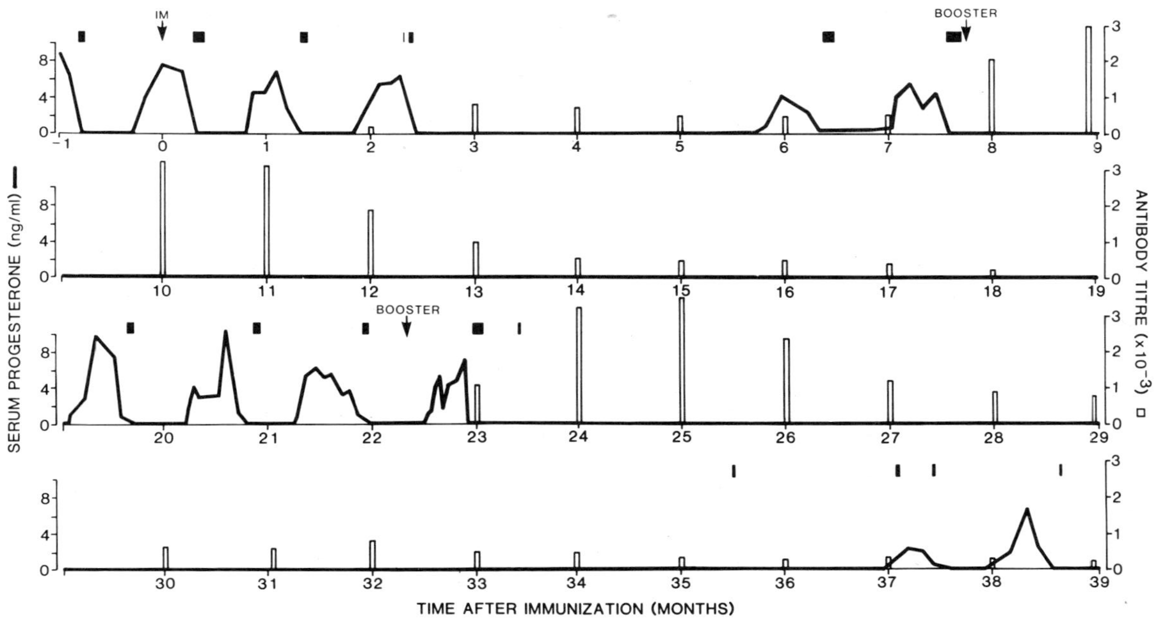


Fig. 6 Effect of active immunization against LHRH (arrow, rime 0) on serum concentrations of progesterone (▬▬), menstrual bleeding ( ■ ) and LHRH antibody titre ( □ ) in a stumptailed monkey (No. 51). LHRH was conjugated to tetanus toxoid as carrier, and administered, emulsified with Freunds complete adjuvant, at 10 s.c. sites. From Fraser (42).

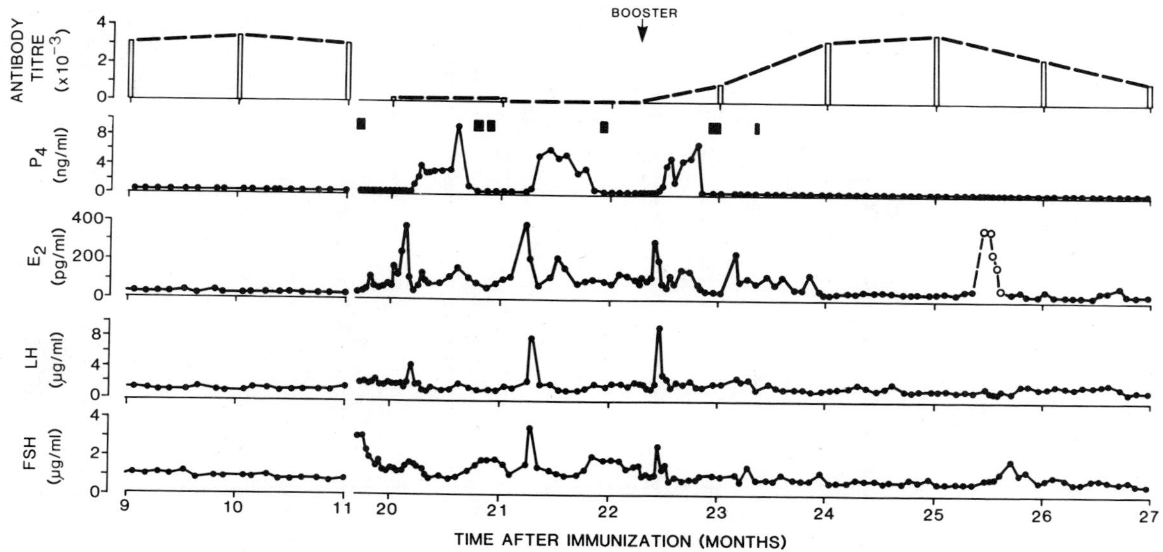


Fig. 7 Effect of active immunization against LHRH on serum concentrations of progesterone ($P_4$), oestradiol ($E_2$), LH and FSH, and menstrual bleeding in monkey No. 51. The periods shown demonstrate changes during a period when LHRH antibody titres (top panel) are high (months 9-11 after primary immunization, low antibody levels (months 20-23) and after booster immunization (arrow) to restore antibody titres. Injection of oestradiol benzoate (open circles) failed to induce an LH surge. From Fraser (42).

immunization against LHRH or LH has a similar suppressive effect on oestrous cycles but markedly different effects on pituitary LHRH receptors. LH immunization increases receptor numbers as after ovariectomy (47), while there is a marked decrease in receptors after LHRH immunization (Fig.8) supporting the positive autoregulatory role of LHRH (20).

In the normal cycling rat, pituitary LHRH receptors begin to rise on dioestrus day one, reaching maximal levels during the morning of pro-oestrus, after which numbers fall to a nadir at oestrus (48,49). This increase in receptors has been suggested to be due to ovarian steroids or the autoregulatory action of LHRH (48,49). Injection of antibodies to LH on the first day of dioestrus prevented oestrogen secretion as evidenced by the absence of a rise in uterine weight, but failed to block the rise in LHRH receptors (Fig.9). However, treatment with an LHRH antiserum over the same time period completely abolished the rise (50). Since the essential difference between the treatments was the removal of LHRH by the LHRH antiserum, these results suggest that the primary driving force for the rise in pituitary LHRH receptors at pro-oestrus in the rat is LHRH itself. There is a decline in LHRH receptors between noon on pro-oestrus and the morning of oestrus which seems to be independent of LHRH since administration of antibodies to LH or LHRH at noon on pro-oestrus to neutralize the respective hormones and to block ovulation failed to alter the changes in LHRH receptors (Fig. 10) (50).

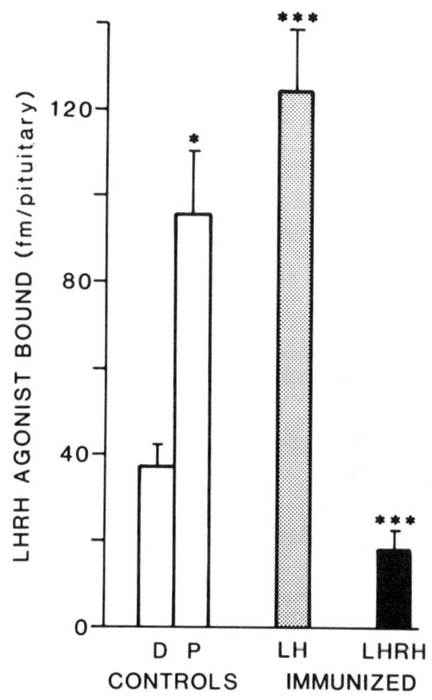


Fig.8 Effect of active immunization of adult female rats against LH (shaded bars) or LHRH (closed bars) on pituitary LHRH receptors. Values for control rats (open bars) are shown at 10.00h on the first day of dioestrus and at 12.00h on the day of pro-oestrus. Values are means ± SEM (5 rats in each of control groups, 10 LHRH-immunized and 6 LH-immunized groups). *** $P < 0.001$ for immunized compared to dioestrus control value. From Popkin & Fraser (47).

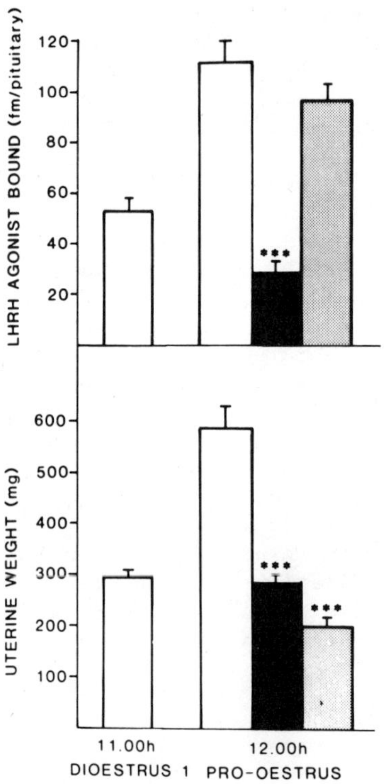


Fig. 9 Effect of administration of antiserum to LHRH (closed bars) or LH (shaded bar) at 11.00h on the first day of dioestrus on pituitary LHRH receptors at 12.00h pro-oestrus and on uterine weight. Values are means ± SEM (5 rats per group) ***$P < 0.001$ than controls at pro-oestrus. From Popkin & Fraser (50).

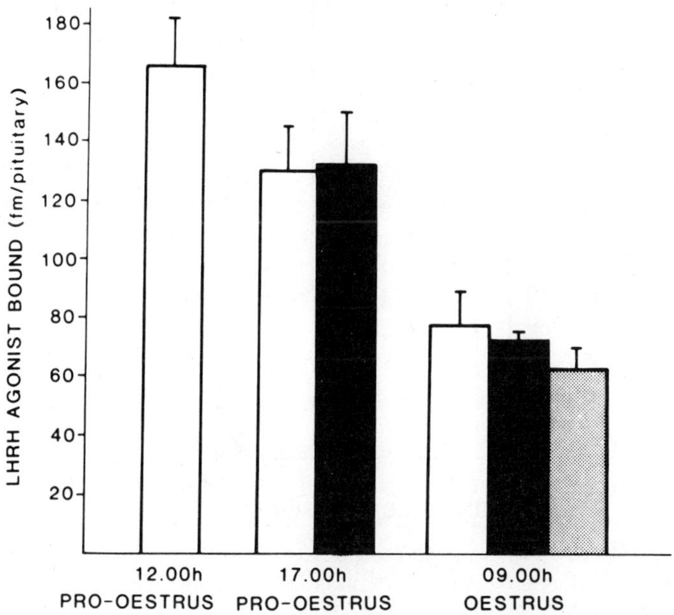


Fig.10 Absence of effect of administration of antiserum to LHRH (closed bars) or LH (shaded bar) at 12.00h pro-oestrus on the fall in pituitary LHRH receptors at 17.00h pro-oestrus and 09.00h oestrus. Both treatments blocked ovulation. Values are means ± SEM (5 rats per group). From Popkin & Fraser (50).

Passive immunization against LHRH blocks the pre-ovulatory LH/FSH surge in the rat (6) when given as late as a few hours prior to its expected onset. This is also observed in the hamster (51) and in the ewe (Fig. 11) showing that these species LHRH is essential during the period of the LH surge (52). In the rhesus monkey (35) and stumptailed macaque monkey (36) it has not been possible to block the LH surge by administration of antibodies during the late follicular phase of the normal cycle (Fig. 12) or when a surge is induced by exogenous oestradiol. In our studies in the stumptailed macaque the same antiserum could suppress the cycle if given during the mid-follicular phase (Fig. 5) and block the LH surge and ovulation in the rat at a lower circulating antibody titre. As expected, chronic deprivation of LHRH by active immunization of the stumptailed macaque does prevent the surge induced by exogenous oestrogen (42). These results suggest that in the primate, oestrogen has a powerful action directly on the pituitary to release LH provided the gonadotrophs have been suitably primed by LHRH pulses previously as suggested by the studies of Knobil and co-workers (1).

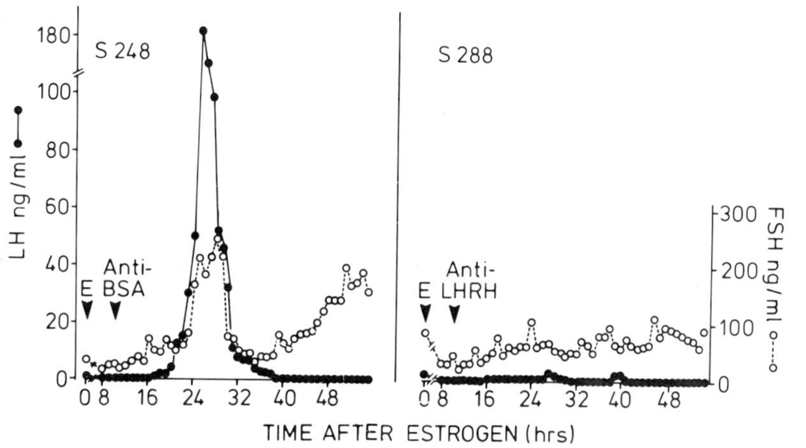


Fig. 11 Effect of an i.v. injection of antiserum to bovine serum albumin (control) or antiserum to LHRH on the surges of LH and FSH induced by oestradol benzoate (E) injection (50 µg in arachis oil) in the ewe. Times of injection shown by arrows. From Fraser & McNeilly (52).

Follicular development is blocked by passive LHRH immunoneutralization as shown by suppression of oestradiol secretion in the hamster (51) the ewe (30,31) and in the stumptailed macaque if given in the early but not the late follicular phase (Figs. 5 & 12)(36). These findings are primarily related to the absence of the LH pulses. The continued rise in oestradiol in the macaque may be due to an increased sensitivity and prolonged responsiveness of the mature follicle to the gonadotrophin stimulation prior to LHRH antibody administration or to low levels of gonadotrophins produced after injection. Active immunization also suppresses follicular development as shown by low serum levels of oestradiol and by the predominance of small or atretic follicles in immunized rats (40,41) and ewes (46). In rats producing low titre

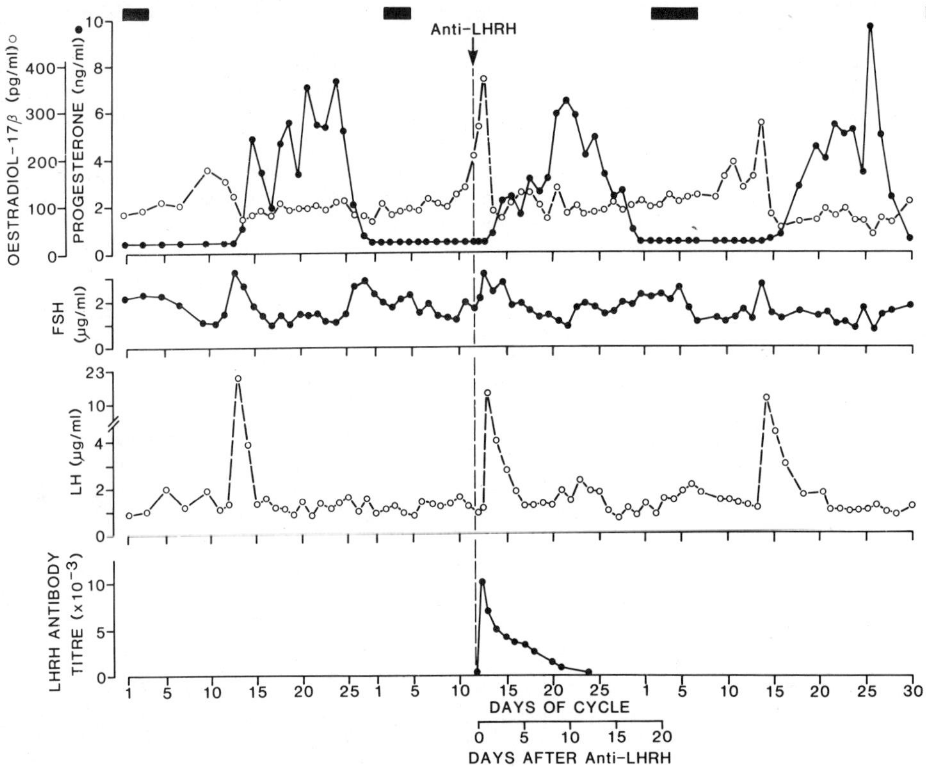


Fig. 12 Serum concentrations of LH, FSH, oestradiol and progesterone during a pre-treatment control cycle and during the following cycle after an i.v. injection of LHRH gamma globulin during the late follicular phase of a stumptailed macaque. Other details as in Fig. 5 From Fraser (36).

antibodies to LHRH, cystic follicles are also observed, presumably stimulated by low basal gonadotrophin secretion occurring with an absence of a pre-ovulatory surge (40).

There have been few investigations using LHRH antibodies to elucidate the role of LHRH in luteal function and in early pregnancy. Prelimary observations in the stumptailed macaque (36) supported by more detailed work with antagonists (53) suggest that the corpus luteum of the monkeys is dependent on LH secretion stimulated by LHRH. The question of whether LHRH antibodies can block early pregnancy in the primate once chorionic gonadotrophin is being produced has only recently been investigated (54) and it is anticipated that these studies, together with similar work with LHRH antagonists, will help solve the question of the control of luteal function. Although early pregnancy in the rat can be blocked by LHRH antibodies (55) the species difference in dependence for LH and oestradiol secretion for implantation and maintainance of pregnancy make it essential to repeat these studies in other mammals.

## PRACTICAL APPLICATIONS OF LHRH IMMUNONEUTRALIZATION

Passive immunization against LHRH using both antiserum and monoclonal antibodies (54,56) should continue to prove an extremely useful tool to investigate the physiological role of LHRH in controlling pituitary and gonadal function but is unlikely to be used for practical application. Active immunization against LHRH has the potential to inactivate the pituitary-gonadal axis for long periods of time without the need for repeated applications of drugs and at much less cost than with LHRH analogues. However, the use of the technique for contraception in humans seems remote because in men the suppression in LH and FSH which would cause an arrest of spermatogenesis would also be associated with an unacceptable suppression of testosterone. Also, suppression of follicular development as well as ovulation in women leading to low oestradiol secretion would cause menopausal symptoms. Similar dilemmas are being faced with use of LHRH analogues for contraception (2,3) although with this approach more control is possible. Although the proposal that LHRH immunization could be used to treat sex hormone dependent cancer was valid a decade ago (10) this use also has been superseded by the development of LHRH analogues.

In addition to these endocrine side effects, active immunization against LHRH shares the problems of immunization against several other antigens in the reproductive system in that the strength and duration of the antibody response will vary between individuals and improved adjuvants are needed for practical application. For example, by three months after immunization, most animals will have produced antibodies of high titre which are sustained for several more months, while others have produced only a low titre for a shorter period. Animals with high LHRH antibody titres will demonstrate the changes described in this chapter while the poor responders have incomplete suppression of pituitary and gonadal function (18,25,26,28,40,41). Although, booster immunizations help reduce these differences there are often some individuals, particularly of certain species which tend to respond poorly to immunization such as the dog (18) and cattle (25,26), in whom the treatment cannot be considered as successful.

The best prospects for practical application seem to be in veterinary practice where an inexpensive method of reversibly controlling gonadal function using a small number of vaccine applications would be more suitable than use of expensive LHRH analogues. The most useful application seems to be in meat production where short-term manipulation of sex hormones can have considerable effects on the body composition of an animal being kept for 1-2 years before slaughter. Thus in pre-pubertal bulls active immunization against LHRH has been demonstrated as a more profitable alternative to surgical castration, suppressing aggressive behaviour of the animals while producing higher quality meat that bulls or surgically castrated animals (25,26).

Acknowledgements It is my pleasure to acknowledge the collaboration of Drs. A.S. McNeilly, R.M. Sharpe, R. Popkin, G.A. Lincoln and J. Sandow in these studies and the excellent technical assistance of Miss M. Abbott, Miss. N. Anderson and Mr. N. Laird.

## REFERENCES


1. E. Knobil, The neuroendocrine control of the menstrual cycle. Rec. Prog. Horm. Res. 36:53 (1980).
2. J. Sandow, Clinical applications of LHRH and its analogues. Clin Endocrinol. 18:571 (1983).
3. H.M. Fraser, New prospects for luteinising hormone releasing hormone as a contraceptive and therapeutic agent. Br. Med. J. 285:990 (1982).
4. I.J. Clarke and J.T. Cummins, The temporal relationship between gonadotropin releasing hormone (GnRH) and luteinizing hormone (LH) secretion in ovariectomized ewes. Endocrinology 111:1737 (1982).
5. H.M. Fraser and A. Gunn, Effects of antibodies to luteinizing hormone releasing hormone in the male rabbit and on the rat oestrous cycle. Nature 244:160 (1973).
6. Y. Koch, P. Chobsieng, U. Zor, M. Fridkin and H.R. Lindner, Suppression of gonadotrophin secretion and prevention of ovulation in the rat by antiserum to synthetic gonadotrophin-releasing hormone. Biochem biophys Res Commun 55:623 (1973).
7. A. Arimura, H. Sato, T. Kumasaka, R.B. Worobec, L. Deleljuk, J. Dunn and A.V. Schally, Production of antiserum to LH-releasing hormone (LH-RH) associated with gonadal atrophy in rabbits: development of radioimmunoassays for LH-RH. Endocrinology 93:1092 (1973).
8. G.A. Lincoln and H.M. Fraser, Blockade of episodic secretion of luteinizing hormone in the ram by the administration of antibodies to luteinizing hormone releasing hormone. Biol. Reprod 21:1239 (1979).
9. G.B. Ellis, C. Desjardins and H.M. Fraser, Control of pulsatile LH release in male rats. Neuroendocrinology 37:177 (1983).
10. H.M. Fraser, 'Effects of antibodies to luteinizing hormone releasing hormone on reproductive functions in rodents'. in: "Immunization with Hormones in Reproduction Research" E. Nieschlag, ed., North-Holland Publishing Company, Amsterdam (1975)
11. H.M. Fraser, A. Gunn, R. Borthwick and A.F. Fraser, Sterilising by immunization. Vet. Rec. 96:323 (1975).
12. H.M. Fraser, Inhibition of reproductive function by antibodies to luteinizing hormone-releasing hormone, in: "Immunological aspects of reproduction and fertility control" J.P. Hearn, ed., MTP Press, Lancaster, U.K. (1980).
13. H.M. Fraser, R.M. Sharpe, G.A. Lincoln and A.J. Harmer, LHRH antibodies: Their use in the study of hypothalamic LHRH and testicular LHRH-like material, and possible contraceptive applications in: "Progress Towards a Male Contraceptive" S.L. Jeffcoate and M. Sandler eds., John Wiley & Sons Ltd. (1982).
14. H.M. Fraser, A.S. McNeilly and R.M. Popkin, Passive immunization against LHRH: elucidation of the role of LHRH in controlling LH and FSH secretion and LHRH receptors in: "Immunological Aspects of Reproduction in Mammals" B. Crighton ed., Butterworths (1984).
15. I.T. Huhtaniemi, J.M. Stewart, K. Channabasavaiah, H.M. Fraser and R.N. Clayton, Effect of treatment with GnRH antagonist, GnRH antiserum and bromocriptine on pituitary - testicular function of adult rats. Mol. Cell. Endocrinol 34:127 (1984).
16. H.M. Fraser, A. Gunn, S.L. Jeffcoate and D.T. Holland, Effect of active immunization to luteinizing hormone releasing hormone on serum and pituitary gonadotrophins, testes and accessory sex organs in the male rat. J. Endocrinol 63:399 (1974).

17. H.M. Fraser, R.M. Popkin, A.S. McNeilly and R.M. Sharpe, Changes in pituitary LHRH receptor levels in situations of increased or decreased gonadotrophin secretion in the male rat. Mol Cell Endocrinol 28:321 (1982).
18. B.D. Schanbacher, H.F. English, D. Gross, R.J. Santen, M.F. Walker and R.E. Falvo, Animal model of isolated gonadotropin deficiency I. Hormonal responses to LHRH immunoneutralization. J. Androl 4:233 (1983).
19. R.N. Clayton, R.M. Popkin and H.M. Fraser, Hypothalamic regulation of pituitary GnRH receptors: effects of gonadotrophin-releasing hormone immunoneutralisation. Endocrinology 110:1116 (1982).
20. R.N. Clayton and K.J. Catt, Gonadotropin-releasing hormone receptors: characterization, physiological regulation, and relationship to reproductive function. Endocrine Reviews 2:198 (1981).
21. H.F. English, B.D. Schanbacher, D. Gross, M.F. Walker, R.E. Falvo and R.J. Santen, Animal model of isolated gonadotropin deficiency II. Morphologic responses to LHRH immunoneutralization. J. Androl. 4:240 (1983).
22. G.A. Lincoln, H.M. Fraser and T.J. Fletcher, Antler growth in male red deer Cervus elaphus following active immunization against luteinizing hormone releasing hormone. J. Reprod. Fert. 66:703 (1982).
23. G.A. Lincoln, H.M. Fraser and T.J. Fletcher, Induction of early rutting in male red deer Cervus elaphus by melatonin and its dependence on LH-RH. J. Reprod Fert. 72:339 (1985).
24. B.J. Keeling and D.B. Crighton, Reversibility of the effects of active immunization against LH-RH in: "Immunological Aspects of Reproduction in mammals" D.B. Crighton ed., Butterworths, London (1984).
25. I.S. Robertson, J.C. Wilson, A.C. Rowland and H.M. Fraser, Further studies on immunological castration in male cattle. Vet. Rec 108:381 (1981).
26. I.S. Robertson, H.M. Fraser, G.M. Innes and A.S. Jones, The effect of immunological castration on sexual and production characteristics in male cattle. Vet Rec 111:529 (1982).
27. J.K. Hodges and J.P. Hearn, Effects of immunisation against luteinizing hormone releasing hormone on reproduction of the marmoset monkey Callithrix jacchus Nature 265:746 (1977).
28. S.C. Chappel, W.E. Ellinwood, C. Huckins, D.C. Herbert and H.G. Spies, Active immunization of male rhesus monkeys against luteinizing hormone releasing hormone. Biol. Reprod 22:333 (1980).
29. R.M. Sharpe and H.M. Fraser, Leydig cell function in rats chronically deprived of normal gonadotrophic stimulation: the effect of treatment with hCG. Int. J. Androl 2:395 (1979).
30. H.M. Fraser and A.S. McNeilly, Differential effects of LH-RH immunoneutralization on LH and FSH secretion in the ewe. J. Reprod Fert 69:569 (1983).
31. A.S. McNeilly, H.M. Fraser and D.T. Baird, Effect of immunoneutralization of LH releasing hormone on LH, FSH and ovarian steroid secretion in the preovulatory phase of the oestrous cycle in the ewe. J. Endocr 101:213 (1984).
32. M.C. Snabes and R.P. Kelch, Acute inhibitory effects of antiserum to gonadotropin-releasing hormone in ovariectomized rats. Neuroendocrinology 29:34 (1979).

33. M. Kawakami and T. Higuchi, Effects of active and passive immunization with LH-RH on gonadotrophin secretion and reproductive function in female rats. Acta endocr 91:616 (1979).
34. B. Gledhill, H.M. Fraser and B.T. Donovan, Effect of passive immunization against LH-RH gonadotrophin secretion in the ferret. J. Reprod. Fert 64:19 (1982).
35. J.T. McCormack, T.M. Plant, D.L. Hess and E. Knobil, The effect of luteinizing hormone releasing hormone (LHRH) antiserum administration on gonadotrophin secretion in the rhesus monkey. Endocrinology 100:663 (1977).
36. H.M. Fraser, A.S. McNeilly, M. Abbott, W.R.A. Brown and R.A. Steiner, The effect of LHRH immunoneutralization on fillicular development, the LH surge and luteal function in the stumptailed macaque. J. Reprod. Fert (1985).
37. C.A. Blake and R.P. Kelch, Administration of antiluteinizing hormone-releasing hormone serum to rats: effects on periovulatory secretion of luteinizing hormone and follicle-stimulating hormone. Endocrinology 109:2175 (1981).
38. Y. Hasegawa, K. Miyamoto, C. Yazaki and M. Igarashi, Regulation of the second surge of follicle-stimulating hormone; effects of antiluteinizing hormone-releasing hormone serum and pentobarbital. Endocrinology 109:130 (1981).
39. K. Narayana and H. Dobson, Effect of administration of antibody against GnRH on preovulatory LH and FSH surges in the ewe. J. Reprod Fert. 57:65 (1979).
40. H.M. Fraser and T.G. Baker, Changes in the ovaries of rats after immunization against luteinizing hormone releasing hormone. J. Endocr 77:85 (1978).
41. M. Takahashi, J.J. Ford, K. Yoshinaga and R.O. Greep, Active immunization of female rats with luteinizing hormone releasing hormone (LHRH) Biol. Reprod. 17:754.
42. H.M. Fraser, Active immunization of stumptailed macaque monkeys against luteinizing hormone releasing hormone, and its effects on menstrual cycles, ovarian steroids and positive feedback. J. Reprod Immunol. 5:173 (1983).
43. H.M. Fraser, S.L. Jeffcoate, A. Gunn and D.T. Holland, Effect of active immunization to luteinizing hormone-releasing hormone on gonadotrophin levels in ovariectomized rats. J. Endocr 64:191 (1975).
44. I.J. Clarke, H.M. Fraser and A.S. McNeilly, Active immunization of ewes against luteinizing hormone releasing hormone and its effects on ovulation and gonadotrophin, prolactin and ovarian steroid secretion. J. Endocr 78:39 (1978).
45. H.M. Fraser, I.J. Clarke and A.S. McNeilly, Effect of oestrogen and an LH-RH agonist on the release of gonadotrophins in ovariectomized ewes deprived of LH-RH. J. Reprod Fert 62:131 (1981).
46. A.S. McNeilly, J.A. Jonassen and H.M. Fraser, Suppression of follicular development after long-term immunoneutralization of LHRH in the ewe. J. Reprod. Fert (submitted) (1985).
47. R.M. Popkin and H.M. Fraser, Changes in pituitary and ovarian LHRH receptors after active immunization of female rats against LH or LHRH. J. Reprod Fert. 73:491 (1985).
48. R.T. Savoy-Moore, N.B. Schwartz, J.A. Duncan and J.C. Marshall, Pituitary gonadotropin-releasing hormone receptors during the rat oestrous cycle. Science 209:942 (1980).

49. R.N. Clayton, A.R. Solano, A. Garcia-Vela, M. Dufau and K.J. Catt, Regulation of pituitary receptors for gonadotropin- releasing hormone during the rat estrous cycle. Endocrinology 107:699 (1980).
50. R.M. Popkin and H.M. Fraser, The effects of immunoneutralization of LHRH or LH on pituitary LHRH receptors during the rat oestrous cycle. Mol Cell Endocr 33:305 (1983).
51. A. de la Cruz, A. Arimura, K.G. de la Cruz and A.V. Schally, Effect of administration of anti-serum to luteinizing hormone-releasing hormone on gonadal function during the oestrous cycle in the hamster. Endocrinology 98:490 (1976).
52. H.M. Fraser and A.S. McNeilly Effect of immunoneutralization of LHRH on the estrogen-induced LH and FSH surge in the ewe. Biol Reprod 27:548 (1982).
53. H.M. Fraser, D.T. Baird, G.I. McRai, J.J. Nestor and B.H. Vickery Suppression of luteal progesterone secretion in the stumptailed macaque by an antagonist analogue of luteinizing hormone releasing hormone. J. Endocr 104:R1-R4 (1985).
54. C. Das. Anti-GnRH monoclonals: pituitary and extrapituitary actions in control of fertility. This symposium.
55. N. Nishi, A. Arimura, K.G. de la Cruz and A.V. Schally, Termination of pregnancy by sheep anti-LH-RH gamma globulin in rats. Endocrinology 98:1024 (1976).
56. D.W. Silversides, B.D. Murphy, V. Misra and R.J. Mapletoft, Monoclonal antibodies against LHRH: development and immunoactivity in vivo and in vitro. J Reprod Immunol 7:171 (1985).

# IMMUNIZATION AGAINST LHRH WITHOUT THE USE OF FREUND'S COMPLETE ADJUVANT

C. Shaha, S. Kaul, M. Kini, M. Chowdhury, R. Anand,
C. Das and G.P. Talwar

National Institute of Immunology, Post Box No.4922
New Delhi-110 029, India

## INTRODUCTION

Neutralization of endogenous LHRH by active immunization has been reported in several species including rodents (Fraser et al, 1974) and monkeys (Chappel et al, 1980). Antibodies to LHRH inhibit LHRH presumably at the level of portal blood vessels before the hormone reaches the pituitary. Due to interception of LHRH, no LH or FSH is released thereby disrupting the production of testicular steroids and subsequently spermatogenesis in the male.

LHRH by itself is not expected to be immunogenic. Two approaches have been used to make it immunogenic. One of them is linkage with a carrier. The most commonly employed carrier has been the bovine serum albumin (Arimura et al, 1973, Koch et al, 1973) but several other proteins have also been used such as the human serum albumin (Arimura et al, 1975), thyroglobulin (Copeland et al, 1979), horseradish peroxidase(Sternberger et al, 1978) guineapig $\gamma$-globulin (Kerdeltue et al, 1976) human lactoferrin (Tennissen et al, 1976) and key hole Limpet Haemocyanin (Shastri et al, 1981). Comparative studies have shown that tetanus toxoid is a better carrier than bovine serum albumin if alum is used as adjuvant (Shastri et al, 1981).

## SYNTHETIC VACCINES

Recently an alternate approach has been suggested to render LHRH immunogenic. This was by linkage of the decapeptide to an adjuvant. We tested LHRH linked through lysine with muramyl dipeptide (MDP) in both male and female rats but have failed to get antibody response. Immunological castration of rats was reported on treatment with synthetic peptide in which LHRH has been linked in a similar way through lysine to MDP (Carelli et al, 1985). The reason we did not get a response may be due to possible differences in the compounds synthesized by the two laboratories.

Two other synthetic compounds were made. One of these is a 16-amino acid peptide (LHRH-ala-ala-Tuftsin) in which a tetrapeptide adjuvant tuftsin was attached to the decapeptide LHRH through a bridge of two alanines (Fig. 1). This compound has been tested in both male and female rats for immunogenicity and has been found to be a poor immunogen . Another compound synthesized was a 30 amino-acid peptide in which a 16 amino acid immuno-determinant of Hepatitis-B surface protein was linked on one

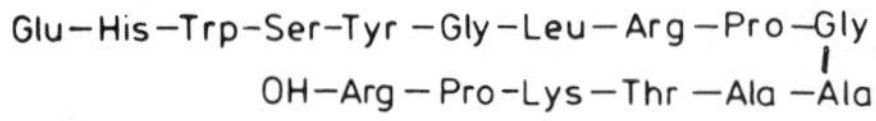

LHRH-Ala-Ala-Tuftsin

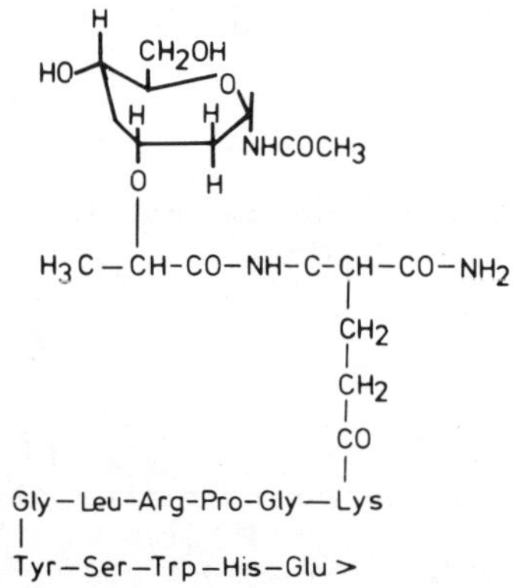

LHRH-lys-MDP

Fig. 1. Figure showing the structures of LHRH-ala-ala tuftsin and LHRH lysine MDP.

side to LHRH and on the other to the tetrapeptide Tuftsin (Fig. 2). This peptide is currently under evaluation.

## INDUCTION OF ANTIBODY RESPONSE WITH LHRH PROTEIN CARRIER CONJUGATES

Tested by us in rodents and monkeys was LHRH linked to tetanus toxoid through tyrosine. It is possible to produce antibodies against LHRH using tetanus toxoid as a carrier, without using Freund's complete adjuvant (FCA). Depicted in Fig. 3 is antibody titres obtained in a female bonnet monkey immunized initially with three injections of LHRH-TT (tetanus toxoid). The conjugate was adsorbed on alum. A derivative of MDP 1[2-(2-hexamido-2-deoxy-D-glucose-3-oxyl)-D-propionyl-L-alanyl-D-isoglutaminel] was also included in the formulation. A booster injection of LHRH-TT with an innocuous preparation, a lipidic metabolizable emulsion LBA (Leiras Basic adjuvant, available from Leiras Pharmaceutical Plant, Huhtamaki Oy, Turku, Finland) was given which produced high enough antibody titres to interfere with normal cyclicity of the animal. The duration of the response was fairly long for example for 140 weeks. We have similar data in a baboon whose fertility and cyclicity was blocked for 160 weeks by immunization with LHRH-TT given on alum with SPLPS (sodium pthalyl derivative of lipo-polysaccharide) was included instead of MDP in the first injection. Primary

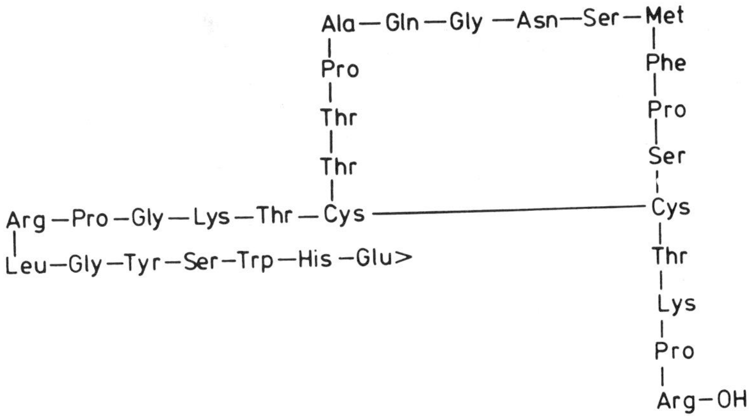


LHRH-Hepatitis B-Tuftsin

Fig. 2. The structure of LHRH-Hepatitis-B Tuftsin.

injection was followed by a booster with LBA. The sex steroid levels measured in these animals at various time points were very low. The antibody titres produced by this approach were sustained for a sufficient length of time and were bioeffective.

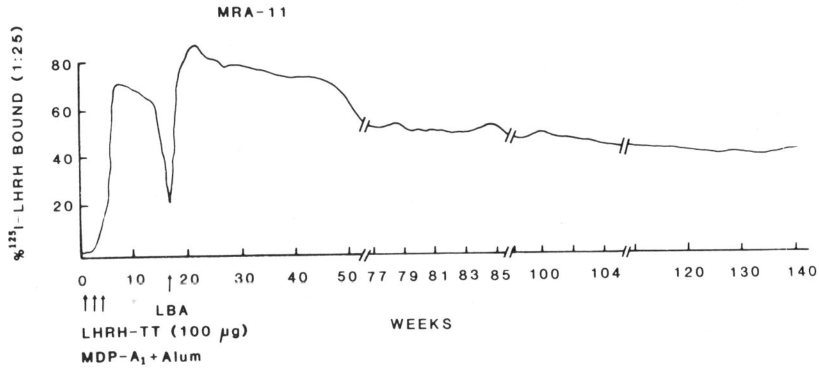


Fig. 3. Antibody titres to LHRH in a monkey immunized with LHRH-TT followed by boosters of LHRH-TT with LBA.

Different groups of male rats were treated with this compound after adsorption on alum and also after emulsification with CFA. Comparable antibody titres were obtained with both the groups whether adsorbed on alum or administered with CFA (Fig. 4). A drop in serum testosterone was observed in both the groups but the values did not decline below biological levels (Fig. 5). On autopsy, accessory reproductive organs were weighed, the weight of organs in the group treated with LHRH-TT with CFA was significantly lower as compared to controls but the same was not the case in the LHRH-TT on alum group (Fig. 6).

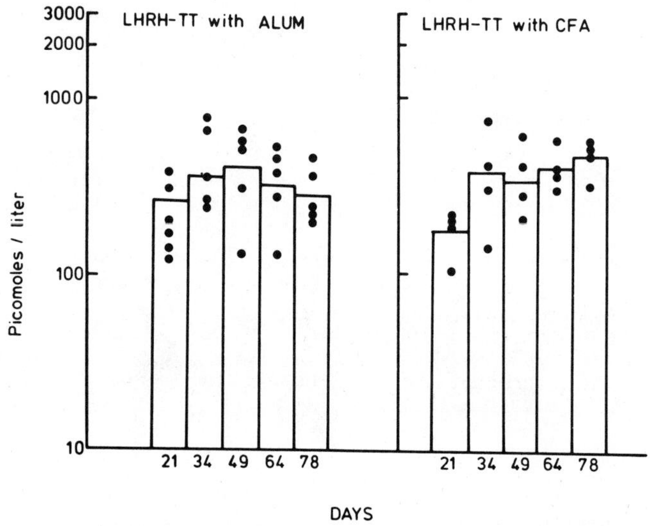


Fig. 4. LHRH antibody titres in male rats immunized with LHRH-TT on alum and with Complete Freund's adjuvant.

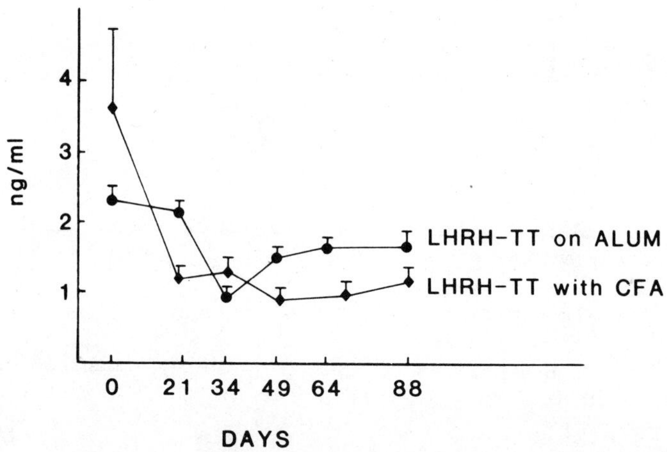


Fig. 5. Serum testosterone levels of male rats immunized with LHRH-TT on alum and with Complete Freund's adjuvant.

Histological observations on testes showed extensive defoliation of cells in the lumen of the seminiferous tubules and degeneration of about 75% of seminiferous tubules per cross sectional area in the group treated with LHRH-TT on alum as compared to controls (Fig 7 a,b & c). Groups treated with LHRH-TT with Complete Freund's adjuvant had drastic atrophy of the testes. Spermatogenesis was arrested at the spermatogonial stage (Fig.7c). There was a marked reduction in the diameter of the tubules also (Fig. 8).

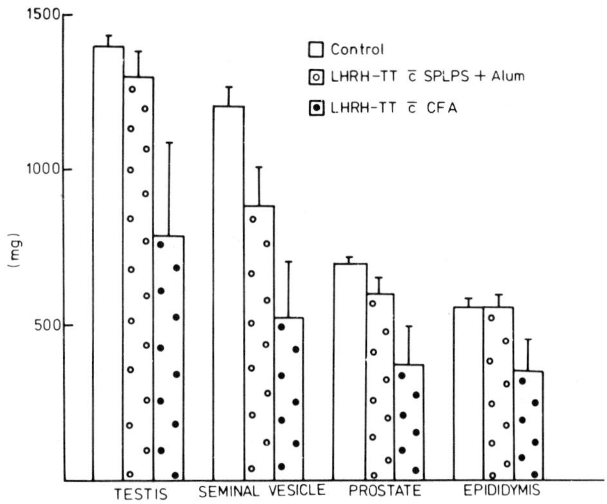


Fig. 6. Weights of accessory sex organs of male rats immunized against LHRH-TT.

Examination of pituitary from control and treated animals where pituitary sections were immunohistochemically stained for LH secreting cells revealed a difference between the control and experimental groups. Control groups had 45.9 $\pm$ 2.9 immunostainable cells per cross sectional area whereas treated groups had 9.9 $\pm$ 2.1 and 21.68 $\pm$ 7.7 (A&C) cells per cross sectional area. The cells in the treated groups also appeared to be smaller in size as compared to control animals (A-Alum, C-CFA).

LHRH-TT administered to female rats also produced sufficient antibody titres (Fig. 9). There was a direct correlation between the cycle length and extent of antibody response.

BINDING CHARACTERISTICS OF ANTIBODIES

Antibodies from both the monkey and baboon that elicited a long term antibody response on immunization with LHRH-TT were similar in some respects. Antibodies in both cases were of high affinity, the Ka was of the order of $10^{10}$-$10^{11}$ Liters/Mol. The antibodies reacted maximally with the native LHRH ($NH_2$) but did not react at all with the LHRH free acid. A minor change at the C-terminus e.g. replacement of glycine amide by acid group (-COOH) abolished totally the recognition (Singh et al, 1985). These antibodies did not bind the synthetic fragments of LHRH, the tripeptide (amino acid 4-6), the tetrapeptide (amino acid 4-10), in contrast to the binding characteristics of a bioeffective monoclonal (Talwar et al, 1985).

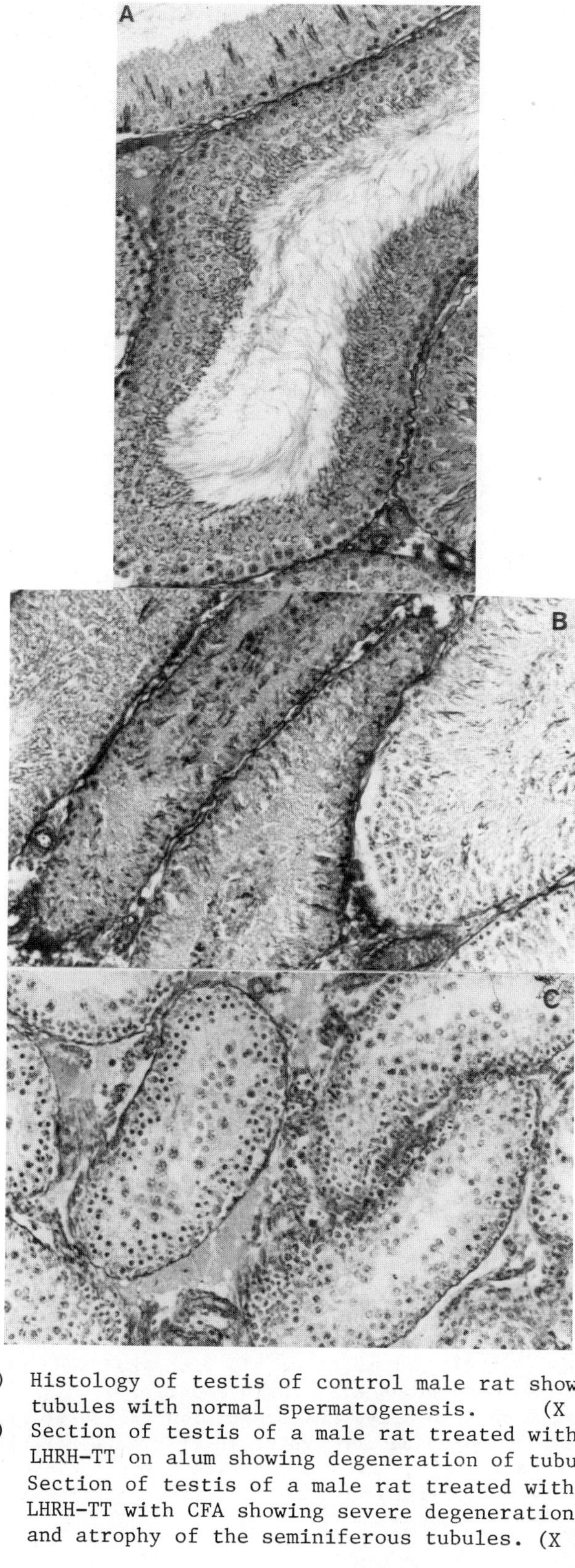


Fig. 7. (a) Histology of testis of control male rat showing tubules with normal spermatogenesis. (X 100)
(b) Section of testis of a male rat treated with LHRH-TT on alum showing degeneration of tubules. (X 100)
(c) Section of testis of a male rat treated with LHRH-TT with CFA showing severe degeneration and atrophy of the seminiferous tubules. (X 100)

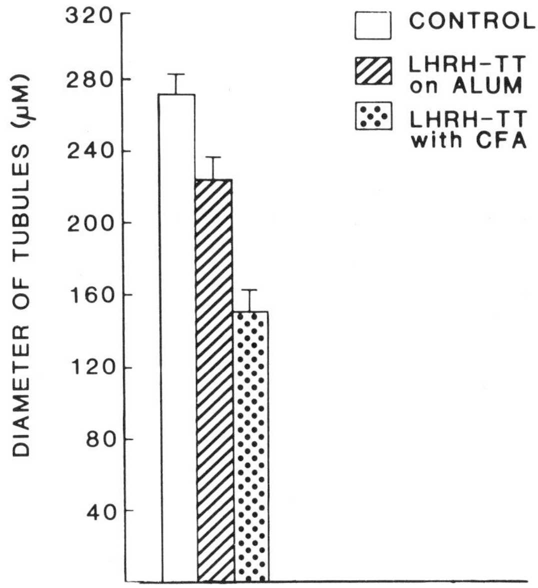


Fig. 8. Effect of immunization with LHRH-TT on diameter of seminiferous tubules.

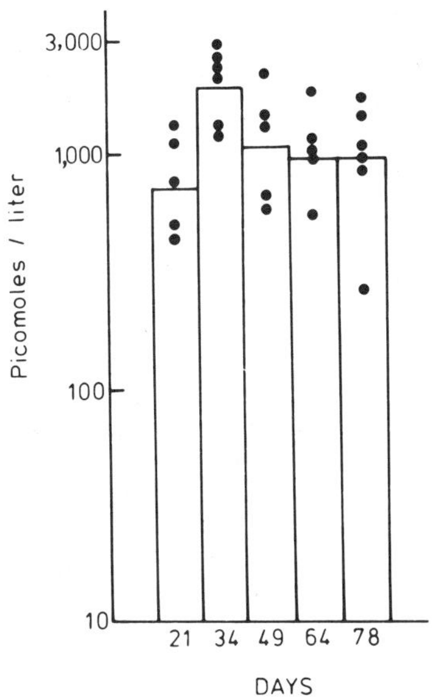


Fig. 9. LHRH antibody titres produced in female rats after immunization with LHRH-TT on alum.

These observations clearly indicate that biologically effective antibody titres can be produced by administration of LHRH linked to a suitable proteinic carrier and given with a suitable adjuvant. It is evident from the studies in monkeys and baboons that for a long term sustainance of antibody titres, and therefore a pronounced biological effect, a booster injection is required to be given at the time of falling antibody titres. With the male rats in our study a more drastic effect could have been achieved if a booster was given and titres maintained for a longer time.

## REFERENCES


Arimura, A., Sato, H., Loy, D.H. Worobec, R.B., Schally, A.V., Yanaihara, N., Hashimoto, Y., Yanihara, C. and Sukura, H., 1975, The determinant of the LH-releasing hormone for the 3 different anti-sera. Acta Endocrinol (Copenhagen). 78:222.

Arimura, A., Sato, H., Kumasaka, T., Worobec, R.B., Dunn, L., Debljuk, L.& Schally, A.V., 1973, Production of antiserum to LH-releasing hormone (LH-RH) associated with gonadal atrophy in rabbits. Development of radioimmunoassay for LHRH. Endocrinology. 93 : 1092.

Carelli, C., Amdibert, F., Gaillard, D.T.& Chedid, L., 1985, Immunological Castration of male mice by a totally synthetic vaccine administered in Saline. Proc. Natl. Acad. Sci. USA. 79 : 5392

Chappel, S.C., Evin Wood, B.W.E., Huckings, C., Herbert, D.C., Spies, and Spies, H.C., 1980, Active Immunization of male rhesus monkeys against luteinizing hormone releasing hormone. Biol. Reprod. 22 : 333.

Copeland, K.C., Anbert, M.L., Rivier, J.& Sizonenko, P.C., 1979, Luteinizing hormone releasing hormone, releasing hormone, sequential versus conformational specificity of anti-luteinizing hormone releasing hormone sera. Endocrinology, 104 : 1504.

Fraser, H.M., Gunn, A., Jeffcoate, S.L.& Holland, D.T., (1974) Effect of active immunization to luteinizing hormone releasing hormone on serum and pituitary gonadotropins, testes and accessory sex organs in the male rat. J. Endocrinology. 63 : 339.

Kerdeltue, B., Catin, S. Kordon, C. & Jutisy, M., 1976, Delayed effects of in vivo LH-RH immuno neutralization of gonadotropins and prolactin secretion in the female rats. Endocrinology. 98 : 1539.

Koch, Y., Wilchek, M., Fridkin, M., Chobsung, P. Zor, V. & Lindner, H. R., 1973, Production and characterization of an antiserum to synthetic gonadotropin releasing hormone. Biochem. Biophy. Res. Commun. 616.

Shastri, N., Manhar, S.K.& Talwar, G.P., 1981, Important role of the carrier in the induction of antibody response without Freund's complete adjuvant against a "self" peptide luteinizing hormone releasing hormone (LHRH). Am. J. Reprod. Immunol. 1 : 262.

Singh, V., Singh, O., Kaul, S. & Talwar, G.P., 1985, The dominant role of amide group at C-terminus for recognition by antibody in primates against gonadotropin releasing hormone. J. Steroid. Biochem. In Press

Sternberger, L.A., Petrali, J.P., Joseph, S.A., Meyer, H.G. & Mills, K.R., 1978 specificity of the immunocytochemical luteinizing hormone releasing hormone receptor reaction. Endocrinology 102 : 63.

Talwar, G.P., Gupta, S.K., Singh, V., Sahal, D., Iyer, K.S.N. and Singh O., 1985, Bioeffective monoclonal antibody against the decapeptide gonadotropin-releasing hormone : Reacting determinant and action on ovulation and estrus suppression. Proc. Natl. Acad. U.S.A. 82 : 1228.

Tennissen, B., Thomas, K. & Ferin, J., Coupling of carboxyme thylated (Itis)$^2$., 1976, luteinizing hormone releasing hormone to poly-DL-alanine chains (tracer groups) polymerised on human lactroferrin FEBS Le 72 : 341.

# SPERM ANTIGENS, IMMUNOLOGIC INFERTILITY AND CONTRACEPTION

A. C. Menge

Department of Obstetrics and Gynecology
University of Michigan
L1221 Women's Hospital
Ann Arbor, Michigan 48109

The demonstration at the turn of the century that sperm cells are antigenic and capable of eliciting autoantibodies initiated an era of experimentation which continues to expand. As early as the 1920's speculation arose concerning the possible role of immunologic reactions involving sperm in human infertility.[1] Indeed, early studies in experimental animals suggested infertility could be induced in females by immunization with semen.[2] These reports surely stimulated the attempts that followed to immunized women by multiple injections of human semen. Whereas, the report on subcutaneous injections of semen in three women suggested a failure to induce serum antibodies to sperm,[3] a more extensive study in 20 women injected by the intramuscular route reported induction of both antibody and infertility.[4] The antibody detected was cytotoxic to sperm and appeared in the sera of all but one woman and in the cervical secretions of half the cases. No pregnancies were reported in the presence of serum antibody but, unfortunately, the short followup period did not permit adequate evaluation. However, this study definitely showed the iso-antigenicity of human sperm in women and that the concept of an immunologic contraceptive based on sperm antigens is plausible. During the same time frame the hypothesis was advanced suggesting that the occurrence of spontaneous antisperm antibodies in women could induce infertility. It was not until the 50's and 60's however, when several different groups of clinical investigators working with men and women of infertile couples reported that the evidence supported an association between human infertility and antibodies to sperm.[5,6,7] A survey of retrospective and prospective studies overall suggests significant negative association between serum titers of antisperm antibodies of either partner and capacity to produce viable offspring.[8] Likewise, the presence and titer of local antibodies to sperm in the cervical secretion of infertile women or on the sperm of infertile men is negatively associated with subsequent fertility.[9,10] Therapy with corticosteroids, especially in men, has resulted in decreased antibody titer and subsequent ability to achieve fertility in 30 to 40% of the treated individuals.[11,12]

Animal studies have proven the potential of immunization with sperm or sperm and testis fractions in females to induce infertility that wanes with time. Immunization in males, however, where effective in decreasing fertility has done so by induction of immune orchitis resulting in aspermatogenesis and azoospermia.[13] This appears in contrast to results in men experiencing natural occurrence of sperm autoantibodies from unknown causes, infection or vasectomy in which there appears to be little or no testicular involvement but the antifertility effect is exerted through antibody binding to sperm cells in the ejaculate. The presence and role of the secretory immune system is well established in the female reproductive tract but less well defined for the male tract. The components of secretory IgA antibodies as well as IgG antibodies are found in the cervical secretions of women and uterine secretions of experimental animals.[14] Specific antisperm antibodies of both IgA and IgG classes have been identified in secretion of the lower female reproductive tract as well as in the semen of men. The exact source or point of entry of the antibodies in the male reproductive tract has yet to be carefully evaluated. Though evidence from vasovasostomy men suggest entry on the testicular side of the former occlusion or lesion since in the majority of cases antisperm antibodies appear in the ejaculate after the reconnection of the vas deferens.[15] Whatever the source it appears that antibodies against sperm of either IgA or IgG class are effective in interrupting normal fertility. In addition, serum antibodies especially of the IgG class probably enter the lumen of the reproductive tract of either sex at different points and in different quantities. The ovarian Graffian follicle has levels of IgG and IgA quite similar to that of the serum so the egg-cumulus mass complex may be literally saturated with antibodies.[16]

In summary, animal and human studies have suggested that antisperm antibodies produce infertility be direct effects on the following events of the fertility process:

1. Sperm passage to the site of fertilization;[1,6,8,9,10]

    a. Antibody originating from either the male or female reproductive tracts can inhibit sperm from freely swimming through the cervical canal in women.
    b. Cervical secretions of women may also contain antibody that immobilize sperm cells.
    c. In experimental animals antibody reduces significantly the number of sperm entering the oviducts and reaching the infundibular area.

2. Capacitation and acrosome reactions of sperm cells have been suggested as possible processes interfered with by antibodies.

3. Sperm interactions with the ovum.[8,17,18]

    a. Binding to zona pellucida
    b. Penetration of zona pellucida
    c. Fusion with vitelline membrane

4. Postfertilization cleavage and development of the embryo.[1,8,9,21]

    a. Consequences of antibody treatment of sperm reflected through effects on cleavage of fertilized eggs.
    b. Direct effects of antisperm antibodies on cleaving and developing embryos or fetuses.

These various effects of antisperm antibodies that have been observed and elucidation of antigens by different techniques suggest the presence of numerous sperm antigens that could be targets for immunologic contraception. The identification and purification of specific antigens have been achieved by Goldberg and colleagues[19] for LDH-C4 and by O'Rand[20] for RSA using the more classical methods, whereas utilizing hybridoma technology additional antigens have been identified and partially characterized.[21,22] The most suitable targets of immunologic contraception appear to be intrinsic antigens or unremovable bound peripheral antigens of the plasma membrane of sperm. The epitopes must be specific to sperm and readily accessible to binding by antibodies of the IgA and IgG classes. That the antigens have functional roles which are blocked by bound antibody may be desirable but perhaps not exclusively necessary. Some of the normal events in fertilization require receptor-like interactions and whether or not the receptor molecule itself is bound or the adjacent molecules are antibody bound as to cause steric hindrance of function may yield the same result. A contraceptive vaccine should possibly contain a mixture of immunogenic components representing different antigens of the sperm membrane to ensure a greater effectiveness. These antigenic components need to be complementary and noncompetitive in terms of immune response, antibody binding and inhibition of fertility.

While elucidation of the antigens of sperm should receive high priority, studies also need to proceed on the stimulation and maintenance of the local immune response in the reproductive tract as well as systemic immunity and the further elaboration of the mechanisms by which antisperm antibodies and cellular immunity to sperm inhibit fertility. Knowledge of these factors would be of value also for development of therapy for cases of clinical infertility due to spontaneous immunity against sperm cells.

## REFERENCES


1. W.R. Jones, Immunological aspects of infertility, in: Immunology of Human Reproduction, J.S. Scott & W.R. Jones, eds, Academic Press, London, 375 (1976).
2. S. Katsh, Immunology, fertility and infertility: A historical survey, Am J Obstet & Gynecol 77:946 (1959).
3. S.S. Rosenfield, Semen injections with serologic studies, Am J Obstet Gynec., 37:385 (1926).
4. M.J. Baskin, Temporary sterilization by the injection of human spermatozoa - a preliminary report, Amer J Obstet Gynec, 24:892 (1932).
5. P. Rumke, and G. Helleuga, Autoantibodies against spermatozoa in sterile men, Am J Clin Path, 32:357 (1959).
6. B. Fjallbrant, Sperm antibodies and sterility in men, Acta Obstet Gynecol Scand, 47:1 (1968).
7. R. Franklin and C.D. Dukes, Studies on sperm-agglutinating antibody and unexplained infertility, J Am Med Assoc, 190:682 (1964).
8. A.C. Menge, Clinical immunologic infertility: diagnostic measures, incidence of antisperm antibodies, fertility and mechanisms, in: Immunological Aspects of Infertility and Fertility Regulation, D.S. Dhindsa & G.F.B. Schumacher, eds, Elsevier/North-Holland, New York, 205 (1980).
9. A.C. Menge, N.E. Medley, C.M. Mangione, and J.W. Dietrich, The incidence and influence of antisperm antibodies in infertile human couples on sperm-cervical mucus interactions and subsequent fertility, Fertil Steril, 38:439 (1982).
10. J.M. Paslow, T.A. Poulton, G.M. Besser and W.F. Hendry, The clinical relevance of classes of immunoglobulins on spermatozoa from infertile and vasovasostomized men. Fertil Steril 43:621 (1985).
11. T.B. Hargreave and Elton, Treatment with intermittent high dose methylprednisolone or intermittent betamethasone for antisperm antibodies: preliminary communication, Fertil Steril 38:587 (1982).
12. J.F. Shulman and S. Shulman, Methylprednisolone treatment of immunologenic infertility in the male, Fertil Steril 38:591 (1981).
13. K.S.K. Tung, and A.C. Menge, Sperm and testicular autoimmunity,in; The Autoimmune Diseases, editors N.R. Rose and I.R. Mackay, Academic Press, New York In Press.

14. G.F.B. Schumacher, Humoral immune factors in the female reproductive tract and their changes during the cycle, in: Immunology Aspects of Infertility and Fertility Regulation, D.S. Dhindsa & G.F.B Schumacher, eds. Elsevier/North-Holland, New York, 93 (1980).
15. J. Linnet, T. Hjort, and P. Fogh-Anderson, Association between failure to impregnate after vasovasostomy and sperm agglutinins in semen, Lancet 1:117 (1981).
16. D.J. Kay, B. Boettcher, J.L. Yovich and J.D. Stanger, Antisperm antibodies in human follicular fluid, Amer J Reprod Immunol Microbiol 7:113 (1985).
17. R.A. Bronson, G.W. Cooper, D.L. Rosenfeld, Sperm specific isoantibodies and autoantibodies inhibit the binding of human sperm to the human zona pellucida, Fertil Steril 38:724 (1984).
18. A.C. Menge, C.S. Black, Effect of antisera on human sperm penetration of zona-free hamster ova, Fertil Steril 32:214 (1979).
19. E. Goldberg, T.E. Wheat, J.A. Shelton, Sperm-specific LDH and development of a synthetic contraceptive vaccine, In Reproductive Immunology, ed S. Isojima and W.D. Billington, Elsevier Science Publishers, New York 215 (1983).
20. M.G. O'Rand, J.P. Porter, Purification of rabbit sperm autoantigens by preparative SDS gel electrophoresis: Amino acid and carbohydrate content of RSA, Biol Reprod 27:713 (1982).
21. R.K. Naz, B.B. Rosenblum and A.C. Menge, Characterization of a membrane antigen from rabbit testis and sperm isolated by using Monoclonal antibodies and effect of its antiserum on fertility, Proc Natl Acad Sci (USA) 81:857 (1984).
22. R.K. Naz, J.J. Alexander and M. Isahakia, Monoclonal antibody against a human germ cell membrane glycoprotein that inhibits fertilization, Science 225:342 (1984).

# TRANSFORMATION OF THE NUCLEUS DURING MAMMALIAN SPERMATOGENESIS AND FERTILIZATION: IMPLICATIONS FOR CONTRACEPTIVE DEVELOPMENT

Anthony R. Bellvé, Stuart B. Moss,
Michael J. Donovan and Marion C. Usselman

Department of Physiology and Biophysics and Laboratory
of Human Reproduction and Reproductive Biology
Harvard Medical School
Boston, MA

## INTRODUCTION

Formation of the mammalian spermatozoon requires the precise temporal synthesis and assembly of many unique polypeptide and glycoprotein constituents. These processes occur primarily, if not exclusively, during meiosis and spermiogenesis[65,66], while the differentiating germ cells are located within the central compartment of the seminiferous epithelium, behind the Sertoli cell junctions[8]. The advanced spermatocytes and spermatids, therefore, are excluded from immune surveillance and so many constituents involved in sperm biogenesis are auto-antigenic. These germ cell-specific components provide potential targets for immunological probes designed to act as contraceptive vaccines. The principal questions then reside in: 1) identifying suitable antigens with known functions, hence allowing for predictable actions and consequences of the immune vaccination, 2) selecting a mode of delivery and effect that ensures optimal specificity and efficacy, and 3) designing a procedure that allows "normal" expression of physiological and behavioral sex. In the case of male contraceptive vaccines directed against sperm antigens, some level of finesse will be required to abrogate the potential induction and deleterious effects of allergic orchitis. The choice of physiological mechanisms and pathways necessitates an understanding of the structural and functional organization of the mature spermatozoon. This article will focus on outlining some of the more provocative insights into the molecular organization of the mammalian sperm nucleus and their implications for post-fertilization events. These paradigms will be considered in the context of possible mechanisms for the biological targeting of "vaccines" to "neutralize" the function of components vital to the sperm cell.

## MOLECULAR ORGANIZATION OF THE SPERMATOZOON NUCLEUS

Sperm nuclei occur in condensed and elongated shapes, each form being characteristic of a mammalian species. The nucleus generally is uniform in density[29], although in some species freeze-fracture studies

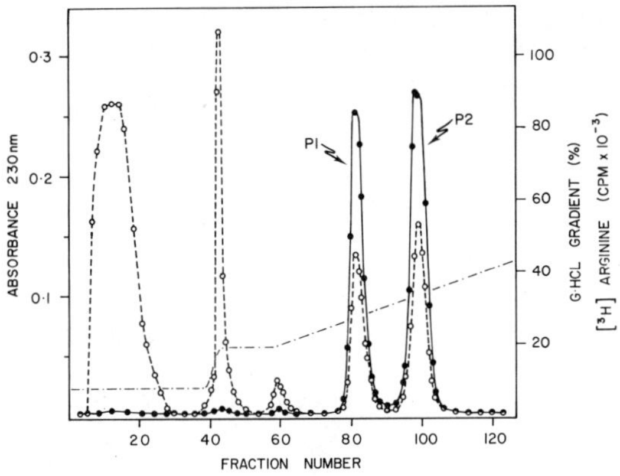


Fig. 1. Separation of the nonprotamine "chromosomal" proteins (NPCPs) and the two mouse protamines, P1 and P2, by ion exchange chromatography on Bio Rex 70. Sperm nuclei were dissociated in 6M G•HCl and 50 mM DTT; alkylated and subjected to ultracentrifugation. Soluble proteins were applied to Bio Rex 70 in 8% G•HCl and 0.1 M $PO_4$ buffer (pH 6.8). Acidic NPCPs were eluted with 8% G•HCl, moderately-basic proteins with 18% G•HCl, and the two protamines, P1 and P2, were resolved with a linear gradient of 20-50% G•HCl. The two protamines were prelabeled <u>in vivo</u> with [$^3$H]arginine (●). Absorbance, 230 nm (o), G•HCl (•-•).

have revealed chromatin fibers arranged in stacked lamellar patterns[31,45,46]. Two known exceptions, human and mouse sperm, contain nucleoprotein in a fibrogranular organization[7,44]. The difficulties encountered in studying the dense, native chromatin have led some investigators to utilize sulfhydryl reducing agents, proteases and/or chemical denaturants to partially disperse the chromatin for observation. Chromatin of human and bull sperm, on exposure to alkaline thioglycolate and critical point drying, exhibits an irregular network of branching fibers with diameters ranging from 14-24 nm[52,53]. These fibers may be dispersed further by treatment with dithiothreitol (DTT) and the ionic detergent Sarkosyl to yield a mesh of 2-3 nm fibrils interconnecting larger spherical and cord-like bodies. The 2-3 nm fibrils may represent naked DNA strands[28].

The extreme condensation and distinctive shape of the sperm nucleus has been attributed to the presence of unique chromosomal basic proteins[29], which replace the somatic histones during spermatogenesis[8]. The protamines now have been isolated from sperm of several mammals[6,14,21,25,42,47,60]. By comparison to the somatic histones, the mammalian protamines are smaller, contain a higher molar content of arginine and cysteine, and have distinct primary sequences[8]. Although not highly conserved phylogenetically, the known protamines do have a relatively invariant N-terminal region and central arginyl domains. These conclusions are based on comparisons of the primary sequences of bull[25] and boar[86] protamines, partial sequences of those from stallion, ram[60], rat[41] and human[33,47], and the protein sequence predicted from the cDNA for mouse protamine 1 mRNA[43]. Most mammalian sperm appear to have only a single protamine species, but those of mouse[6,13,14] and human[47] contain at least two distinct arginine-rich polypeptides: a typical type 1 protamine and a more prominent type 2 protamine having a high histidine content [8,12,13,47] (Fig. 1). Thus, any model of protamine-DNA interactions in these two species must allow for the unique primary structure of the more abundant type 2 protamines.

Protamine interactions with DNA have been examined using physical, biochemical and morphological techniques[5,19]. Studies of nonmammalian sperm chromatin and reconstituted DNA-protamine complexes suggest these polypeptides stabilize DNA in a β* conformation[30,78,90]. One model depicts the protamine molecule lying along the minor groove of the DNA double helix, with the successive arginyl moieties interacting alternately with the phosphate groups of the two DNA strands[30]. The conserved N-terminal extension of each protamine molecule is predicted to fold back and interact with an inner domain of the peptide. The more variable C-terminal region, having cysteinyl and tyrosinyl groups[60], are thought to interact with another protamine molecule overlapping in the same minor groove. Alternatively, the C-terminus, which usually contains some arginyl groups[60], could interact with an adjacent DNA double helix to insure close, parallel packing of the chromatin strands. In either case, the alignment of the cysteinyl groups probably facilitates formation of the intermolecular disulfide bonds that are prevalent in mammalian sperm chromatin. Those disulfide bonds occurring between protamine molecules located on apposed DNA helices would render the chromatin resistant to dispersion by high salt, urea and guanidine hydrochloride. The general concepts of nucleoprotamine conformation are not compatible with the existence of nucleosomes in sperm chromatin, a

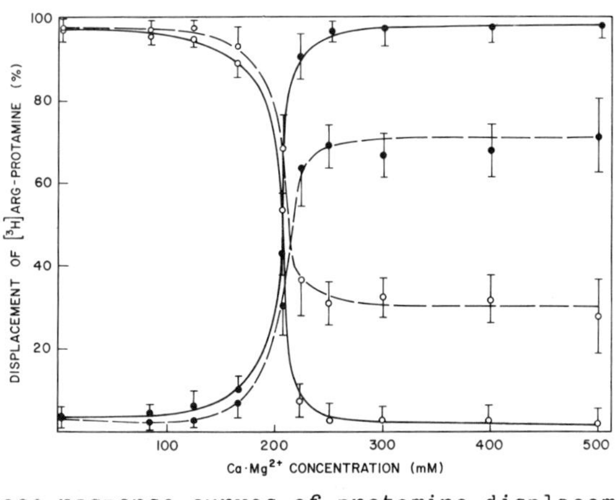


Fig. 2. Dose response curves of protamine displacement from sperm nuclei by the divalent cations, $Ca^{2+} \cdot Mg^{2+}$. Sperm were cleaved into head and tail components by brief homogenization in 1% SDS. Nuclei were isolated to 99% purity by sucrose gradient centrifugation, incubated in 50 mM DTT, 1 mM PMSF, 20 mM Tris•HCl (pH 8.3) for 30 min, and exposed to $Ca^{2+} \cdot Mg^{2+}$ (3:2; mol:mol) either directly (---), or in progressive increments (—), at the total concentrations designated. All samples were subjected to sucrose gradient centrifugation for 13 hr at 100,000 g. The resulting supernatants and pellets were quantified for soluble (●) and DNA-bound [$^3$H]protamine (o).

conclusion confirmed by nuclease digestion studies[95]. Yet, a few morphological studies report observing nucleosome-like structures (12-15 nm) in the sperm of dogfish, bull, ram[87] and man[35]. Also, timed proteolysis of mammalian sperm chromatin produces limit digests of protamine[56,96], reminiscent of the histone fragments remaining after controlled proteolysis of somatic nucleosomes[91]. Such studies raise interesting questions. and so more detailed studies are required to resolve the specific mechanisms and mode of protamine-DNA interactions.

The role of protamines in promoting chromatin condensation is established, but the functions of virtually all other sperm nuclear proteins have yet to be defined[7,8,65,66]. These proteins (Fig. 1) may include structural components, such as residual histones[47,65,71,73] and constituents of the perinuclear theca[7,65], and several enzymes, including the DNA[67,93] and RNA polymerases[36] and a possible chromatin-bound protease[56]. Presumably, a limited number of proteins polymerize to form the discrete regional domains of the enveloping perinuclear theca. Others may have regulatory roles in sperm function, or may be activated only after fertilization, either to facilitate pronucleus formation or to initiate hypothetical enzyme cascades essential to early development. However, despite their potential significance, few studies have focused on the nonprotamine "chromosomal" proteins (NPCPs), and so their various roles in chromatin organization and nuclear structure have yet to be defined.

## DETERMINANTS OF SPERM NUCLEAR SHAPE

The sperm nucleus acquires its polar architecture during the terminal stages of spermiogenesis[7,8]. Some reports based on nonmammalian species, suggest an array of microtubules acts as an extrinsic determinant by molding the nucleus into shape[59]. In mammalian spermatids, this complex array of microtubules, the manchette, appears in the cytoplasm at the onset of chromatin condensation, in close apposition to the lateroposterior margin of the nucleus. Because of this association, the manchette has been implicated in imposing the truncated pyrimidal shape upon the posterior pole of the nucleus. Support for this concept is not substantial. In fact, the manchette detaches from the caudal pole and angles obliquely away from the nucleus during the early phases of nuclear condensation[29]. In the Wooly opossum nuclear condensation occurs in a transverse plane relative to the manchette and the longitudinal axis of the cell[68]. Moreover, in some species the spermatids lack microtubular arrays[69]. These and other observations suggest the manchette may act as an external scaffold to guide nuclear events rather than provide a direct mechanical force[63,64]. Thus, nuclear shape may be determined primarily by factors intrinsic to the nucleus[8]; including the 1) elimination of most NPCPs; 2) transformation to a nucleoprotamine complex; and 3) assembly of a nuclear skeleton, the perinuclear theca.

The perinuclear theca may act as a determinant of nuclear shape. Constituents of the perinuclear theca, the NPCPs, are synthesized primarily during spermiogenesis coincident with nuclear transformation[66]. Also, by analogy, somatic cells contain an extensive nuclear matrix that is contiguous with the pore-lamina complex, a structural element of the nuclear envelope[1,2,16,17]. This pore-lamina-matrix complex, in addition to its direct involvement in nuclear events, is thought to define nuclear shape in somatic cells[32].

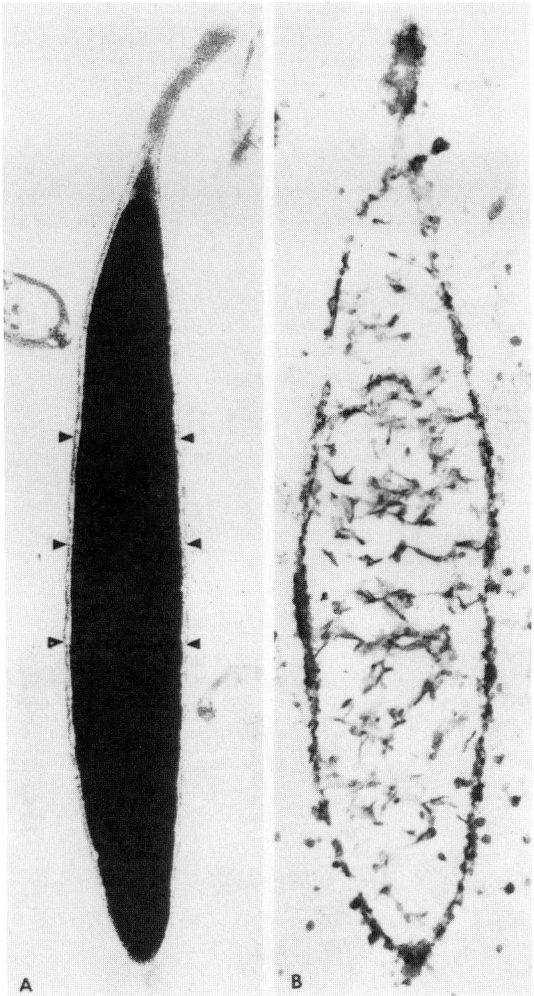


Fig. 3. Electron micrograph of a mouse sperm nucleus (A) and an isolated perinuclear theca-matrix (B). (A) Sperm nuclei were isolated and fixed as described[13]. The SDS protocol decapitates the sperm, and removes the acrosome and nuclear envelope from the nucleus. The perinuclear theca (arrow heads) remains associated closely with the dense nucleus. (B) Sperm perinuclear theca-matrix prepared by exposing nuclei to a total final concentration of ~250 mM $Ca^{2+} \cdot Mg^{2+}$ (3:2; mol:mol), 50 mM DTT, and 100 µg DNase/ml. Whereas both protamines and DNA are displaced, the perinuclear theca with an internal network of coarse transverse fibers remains relatively intact and approximates the shape and size of the original nucleus.

It is significant, therefore, that a skeletal matrix conforming to the original size and shape of the sperm nucleus can be isolated by selectively removing protamines and DNA[7]. The basic protocol involves 1) reduction of protamine disulfide bonds with dithiothreitol (DTT), 2) displacement of protamine(s) with $Ca^{2+} \cdot Mg^{2+}$ (3:2; mol:mol), and

3) digestion of the DNA with DNase I. Direct exposure to a total concentration of 250-500 mM $Ca_2^{+} \cdot Mg^{2+}$ (3:2; mol:mol), followed by 100 μg DNase I/ml displaces only the histidine-rich type 2 protamine, whereas stepwise increments in $Ca^{2+} \cdot Mg^{2+}$, from 125 to 150, 175, 200 and then to 250 mM, in the continued presence of DNase I, causes displacement of both protamine species (Fig. 2). The former procedure appears to lead to a nonspecific aggregation of protamine 1 with residual DNA and NPCPs. Both treatments remove protamine(s) and bulk DNA without influencing the original conformation and size of the sperm nucleus.

Nuclei exposed to 125-250 mM $Ca^{2+} \cdot Mg^{2+}$ (3:2; mol:mol) and digested simultaneously with DNase I reveal a relatively intact nuclear exoskeleton that is derived primarily from the perinuclear theca (Fig. 3). Interwoven proteinaceous fibers course across the nuclear interior and terminate on the perinuclear lamina. These transverse fibers appear to provide some degree of structural stability. By scanning microscopy, the sperm nuclear matrices retain the general configuration of the original nucleus (Fig. 4). Each has a clearly defined perforatorium and implantation fossa, and appears to be comprised of a coarse fibrous reticulum. The denser reticular network of the posterior pole, is delimited by a well-defined line of demarcation angling obliquely across the equatorial zone. This

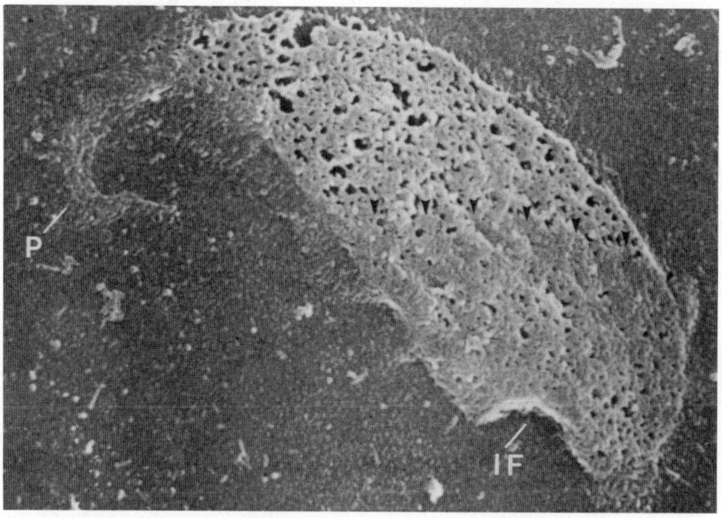


Fig. 4. Mouse sperm perinuclear theca-matrix, as viewed by scanning electron microscopy. Isolated sperm nuclei were exposed to progressive increments of $Ca^{2+} \cdot Mg^{2+}$ (125-250 mM), in the presence of 50 mM DTT and 100 μg DNase I/ml, to remove both protamines and DNA. These nuclear matrices, each consisting primarily of the perinuclear theca, have a well-defined apical perforatorium and caudal implantation fossa. Comprised of a coarse, dense reticulum, the matrix has discernible anterior and posterior domains demarcated by a margin of the oblique equatorial zone (arrows).

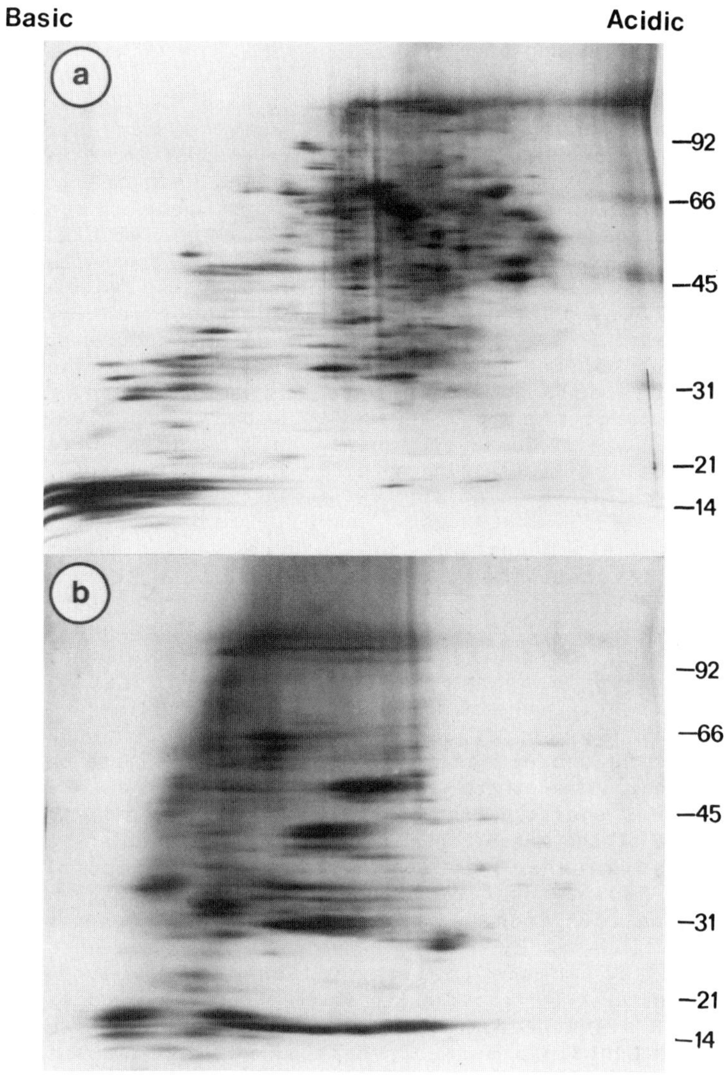


Fig. 5. Two-dimensional, electrophoretic analysis of nuclear matrix proteins prepared from purified populations of mouse spermatids (steps 1-8) and mature sperm. The respective nuclear matrix preparations were solubilized and resolved initially by non-equilibrium, isoelectric focusing, gel electrophoresis (NEFGE). These gels were equilibrated in SDS-sample buffer and further resolved by SDS-PAGE using a linear, 7-18% polyacrylamide gradient. Substantial differences are evident in the polypeptide composition of spermatid and sperm nuclear matrices. Fewer and more basic proteins exist in the sperm nuclear matrix. Samples include nuclear matrix proteins of (a) spermatids (steps 1-8) and (b) mature sperm. $M_r$ standards ($x\ 10^{-3}$) are denoted.

perinuclear structure is comprised primarily of NPCPs, ranging in $M_r$s from ~80,000 to 8,000 and with pIs of 4.5 to 7.8. Surprisingly, a high proportion of the constituent polypeptides appear to be relatively basic in character (Fig. 5).

This novel perinuclear theca-matrix is assembled during the final stages of spermiogenesis[50], concomitant with the marked changes in nuclear matrix morphology and polypeptide composition (Fig. 5). The period of nuclear transformation also coincides with the major phase of NPCP synthesis[65,66], which occurs both concurrent with or immediately following the deposition of protamines within the sperm nucleus[66]. The substantial change in polypeptide constituents during late spermiogenesis is most evident on comparing two-dimensional NEFGE-SDS PAGE patterns of polypeptides recovered from nuclear matrices isolated from spermatids (steps 1-8) and mature sperm (Fig. 5). Thus, the polypeptide complexity reduces substantially during late spermiogenesis, with an apparent loss of many high-$M_r$ polypeptides and the appearance of prominent, low-$M_r$, basic constituents. Some of these components have been identified by SDS PAGE-immunoblot analyses using specific antisera, both polyclonal and monoclonal in origin (Moss et al., in preparation).

Finally, the perinuclear theca can be removed selectively from sperm nuclei by incubating the latter in DTT and cetyltrimethylammonium bromide (CTAB). This treatment removes two prominent polypeptides of $M_r$s 16,000 and 18,000 daltons, together with a few minor components. Subsequent treatment with 175-200 mM $Ca^{2+} \cdot Mg^{2+}$ now causes all nuclear elements to disperse considerably (~10- to 15-fold), reflecting the removal of essentially all major structural constraints. Subsequent digestion with DNase I yields a collapsed aggregate of the proteinaceous nuclear material. These observations suggest the perinuclear theca contributes to nuclear shape by acting as a structural scaffold that envelops, and perhaps also protects the haploid genome of the mature spermatozoon. This structure may contain actin and myosin which could provide the mechanistic force for transforming nuclear conformation (Moss et al., in preparation). Actin has been localized to the sperm nucleus of several mammalian species[23,24,85], primarily within the perinuclear theca at either the anterior[4,22,88] or the posterior pole[23,24]. Interestingly, NBD-phalloidin, a probe specific for filamentous actin, does not bind to the mature sperm head. Therefore, regardless of where actin is localized, the protein presumably exists in a nonfilamentous form. Two other structural proteins also have been found in the human sperm; vimentin in the equatorial region and myosin in a narrow band at the neck region[88].

Collectively, these studies suggest distinct skeletal domains exist in the mature sperm head, with their presence inferring functional roles during spermiogenesis. One feasible explanation may be that filamentous actin assembles around the spermatid nucleus, and, guided by the microtubular manchette, molds the nucleus into its predetermined shape. Continual assembly of the perinuclear theca could provide the alloplastic properties required for this structure to assume new conformations with changing nuclear shape[50]. At late spermiogenesis, non-contractile theca constituents may stabilize nuclear morphology by forming intra- and inter-molecular disulfide bonds, thereby allowing the F-actin to depolymerize.

The lamin proteins may act as intrinsic structural elements of the sperm nucleus. In somatic nuclei lamins A, B, and C having $M_r$s of ~70,000, 68,000 and 63,000, respectively, form the peripheral

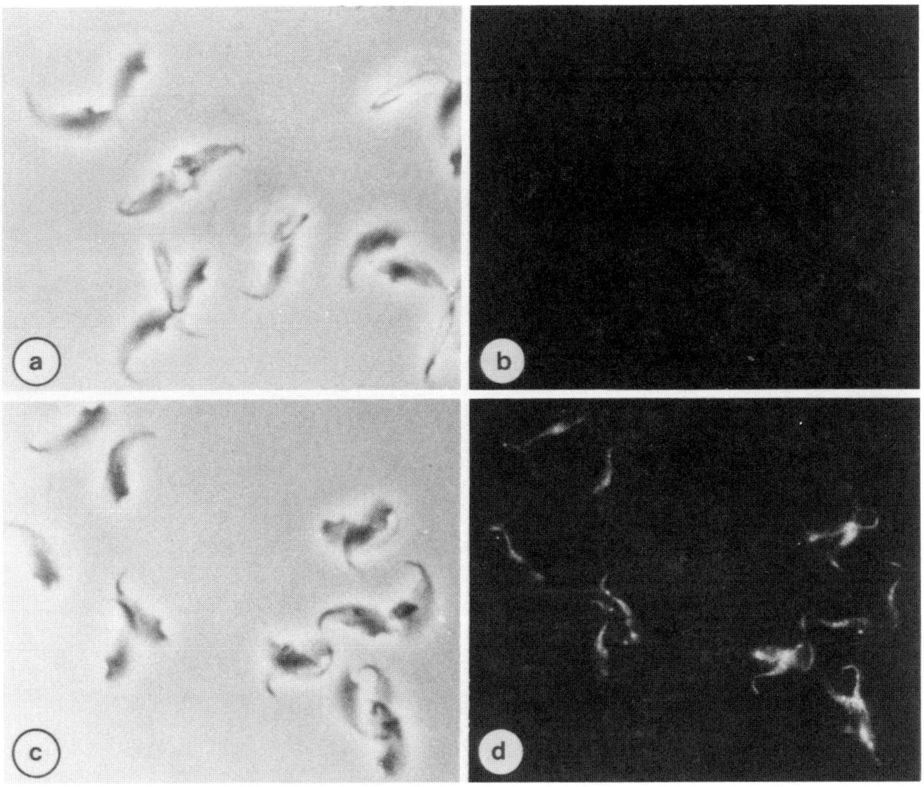


Fig. 6. Distribution of lamins AC and lamin B in sperm nuclei as observed by indirect immunofluorescence. Sperm nuclei were attached to poly-L-lysine-coated coverslips, and incubated with a monospecific, anti-lamin AC or an anti-lamin B, guinea pig IgG. The nuclei were washed extensively with PBS and then incubated with a fluorescein-conjugated, anti-guinea pig, goat IgG. Note that anti-lamin AC binding is negative, whereas anti-lamin B binds to a narrow domain extending along the anterio-ventral edge of the nucleus and obliquely across the equatorial region. Figures depict nuclei following incubation with anti-lamin AC (a,b) and anti-lamin B (c,d) antibodies by phase contrast (a,c) and epifluorescence microscopy (b,d).

pore-lamina complex, a non-membranous, meshwork juxtaposed to the inner nuclear membrane. This fibrous lamina is known to depolymerize and reassemble at distinct points in the cell cycle[34]. Based on these and other observations it has been suggested that the fibrous lamina may aid in organizing interphase chromatin[51], mediate nuclear envelope disassembly and reassembly during mitosis[34], and facilitate chromosome condensation during meiosis[82,83]. It is important, therefore, to determine whether these particular proteins exist in the sperm nucleus.

Significantly, the lamin proteins appear to be expressed differentially in the mouse sperm nucleus. Thus, an antibody specific for somatic lamins A and C does not bind to either sperm nuclei or matrices (Fig. 6). The apparent lack of lamins A and C is not due to

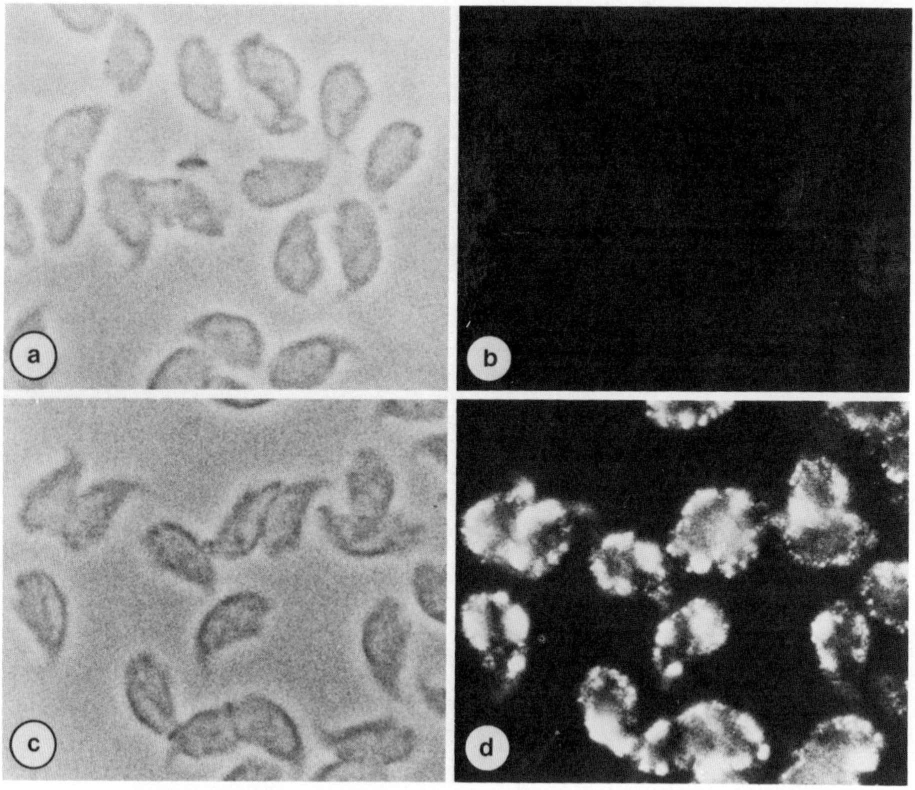

Fig. 7. Distribution of lamins AC and lamin B in sperm nuclei depleted of the enveloping perinuclear theca. Sperm nuclei were exposed briefly to a 1% cetyltrimethylammonium bromide (CTAB) to remove the peripheral theca, and then incubated with the anti-lamin AC or anti-lamin B antibodies, followed by a biotinylated, secondary antibody and then streptavidin-fluorescein. Note that anti-lamin AC binding still remains negative, whereas anti-lamin B now binds to the entire nuclear periphery in a punctate pattern. Photomicographs include theca-depleted nuclei by phase contrast (a,c) and by epifluorescence (b,d) microscopy after exposure to anti-lamin AC (a,b) and anti-lamin B (c,d).

the masking of antigenic determinants by the enveloping perinuclear theca, since the selective removal of the theca with DTT-CTAB does not expose reactive sites (Fig. 7). Furthermore, no proteins from sperm nuclear matrices bind anti-lamin AC on SDS-PAGE immunoblots, again eliminating the possibility of masked antigenic sites (Fig. 8). By contrast, the 68,000-$M_r$ lamin B polypeptide is present in both sperm nuclei and isolated nuclear matrices, as detected by using an antibody specific for somatic lamin B. However, unlike the perinuclear staining observed with the differentiating spermatogenic cells, the lamin B antigenic determinants in sperm nuclei are restricted to a narrow domain along the anterio-ventral edge of the nucleus, and obliquely across the equatorial region (Fig. 6). After removing the perinuclear theca with CTAB-DTT, the anti-lamin B antibody then localizes to the nuclear periphery in a punctate pattern (Fig. 7). This difference in immunoreactivity presumably represents an

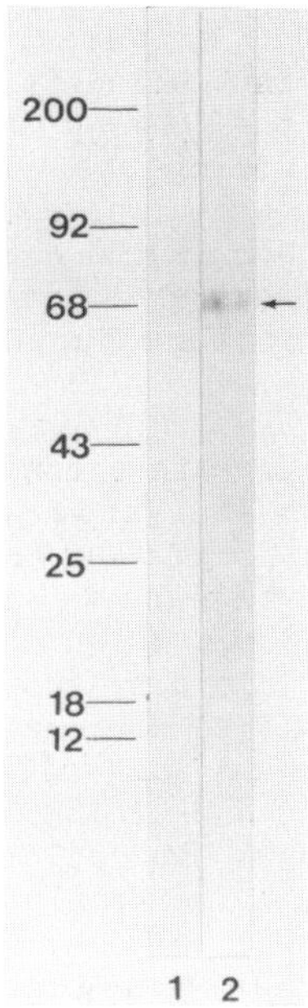


Fig. 8. Immunoblots of antigenic determinants in sperm nuclear matrices recognized by anti-lamins AC and anti-lamin B. Polypeptides of isolated nuclear matrices were subjected to SDS-PAGE, electrophoretically transferred to nitrocellulose paper, and then incubated with either antibody, followed by a biotinylated, goat anti-guinea pig IgG and then streptavidin. Note that neither lamins A nor C are detectable, whereas lamin B gives a positive reaction at 68,000 $M_r$. Sample lanes, (1) anti-lamin AC and (2) anti-lamin B. $M_r$ standard proteins (x $10^{-3}$).

unmasking of determinants underlying the peripheral theca. Finally, on immunoblots anti-lamin B reacts with a 68,000-$M_r$ polypeptide of sperm nuclear matrices, corresponding in $M_r$ to lamin B of somatic nuclear matrices (Fig. 8). The presence of a lamin B-like protein in mature sperm implies that the polypeptide has a conserved function, possibly in maintaining the spatial organization of chromatin around the periphery of the nucleus. Whether this lamin-B-like polypeptide is a germ cell-specific variant has yet to be determined.

## FATE AND ROLE OF SPERM NUCLEAR PROTEINS AFTER FERTILIZATION

Condensation and shaping of the germ cell nucleus protects the haploid genome and facilitates the processes leading to fertilization. These events include sperm penetration, dissolution of the nuclear envelope, dispersion of chromatin, appearance of nucleoli, and formation of the pronucleus[3,79,93,94]. The diverse roles of the sperm nuclear proteins in these complex events are unknown. Protamine molecules may persist for only a brief period after fertilization[27,48,49,76]; their removal possibly being facilitated by proteolysis[55,95,96], phosphorylation[92] and/or local changes in their ionic interactions with DNA[75]. Presumably, these polypeptides are replaced by histones stored in the oocyte cytoplasm, thereby allowing reformation of nucleosomes in the forming male pronucleus[76]. Whether other nuclear proteins, including the complement of RNA[36] and DNA polymerases[68,74], later serve special roles during early embryogenesis has not been investigated. Nor is there any information in regard to the many other sperm nuclear proteins[8,65] that could have structural, enzymatic, or regulatory functions during fertilization and early embryogenesis.

Accumulating evidence suggests sperm contribute an extra-genomic factor that is essential for embryonic development. Mouse sperm subjected to paternal hyperthermia during epididymal maturation are able to fertilize and activate early embryogenesis but mortality ensues at the blastocyst to early somite stages[9,10,11]. Parthenogenetic embryos made diploid by suppressing second polar body formation with cytochalasin D also die during early development, never surviving beyond the early somite stages[39]. Blastomeres from these parthenogenones can be rescued and ultimately contribute to a chimeric adult when aggregated with normal embryos[80,81] or injected into normal blastocysts[62]. One such chimeric female has produced offspring that are derived from germ cells of parthenogenetic origin[80]. Developmental failure of parthenogenones could be due to the expression of recessive lethal genes that are exposed by the high degree of homozygosity. However, evidence has been reported of "uniparental mice" being obtained from fertilized mouse oocytes after one pronucleus has been removed and the other diploidized[38]. Moreover, fertilized mouse eggs, after being enucleated and then microinjected with diploidized nuclei taken from parthenogenetic inner cell mass can develop and form offspring of the same genotype as the parthenogenetic parent[37]. In another novel approach to this question, Surani et al.[84] have reported obtaining different results with normally fertilized embryos after suppressing formation of the second polar body and then restoring the diploid state by surgically removing one of the three pronuclei. Normal development ensues when either of the two maternal pronuclei are removed. But when the paternal pronucleus is removed each embryo soon degenerates, suggesting that only those having both male and female genetic complements can develop normally. Likewise, when artificially-activated eggs are given a male pronucleus the embryos develop to term, but those receiving a second female pronucleus suffer from retarded development and preimplantation death[84]. Thus, it appears that parthenogenetic lethality may be due not to the lack of some cytoplasmic factor(s), but rather to an inherent defect in the parthenogenetic pronuclei. The inference being that the male pronucleus, X or Y chromosome-bearing, contains some imprinted genomic signal or a nuclear factor that plays a critical role in ensuring normal embryonic development.

## DYNAMICS OF LAMIN PROTEINS DURING MEIOTIC MATURATION AND FERTILIZATION

The rapid dispersal of the sperm head to form the male pronucleus after fertilization suggests substantial changes may occur in the complement of structural and regulatory proteins. In addition, the apparent lack of lamins A and C in the sperm nucleus raises questions concerning the temporal reappearance of these particular proteins, or their variants, during pronucleus formation and the early cleavage divisions. Based on current studies, lamins A, B and C undergo

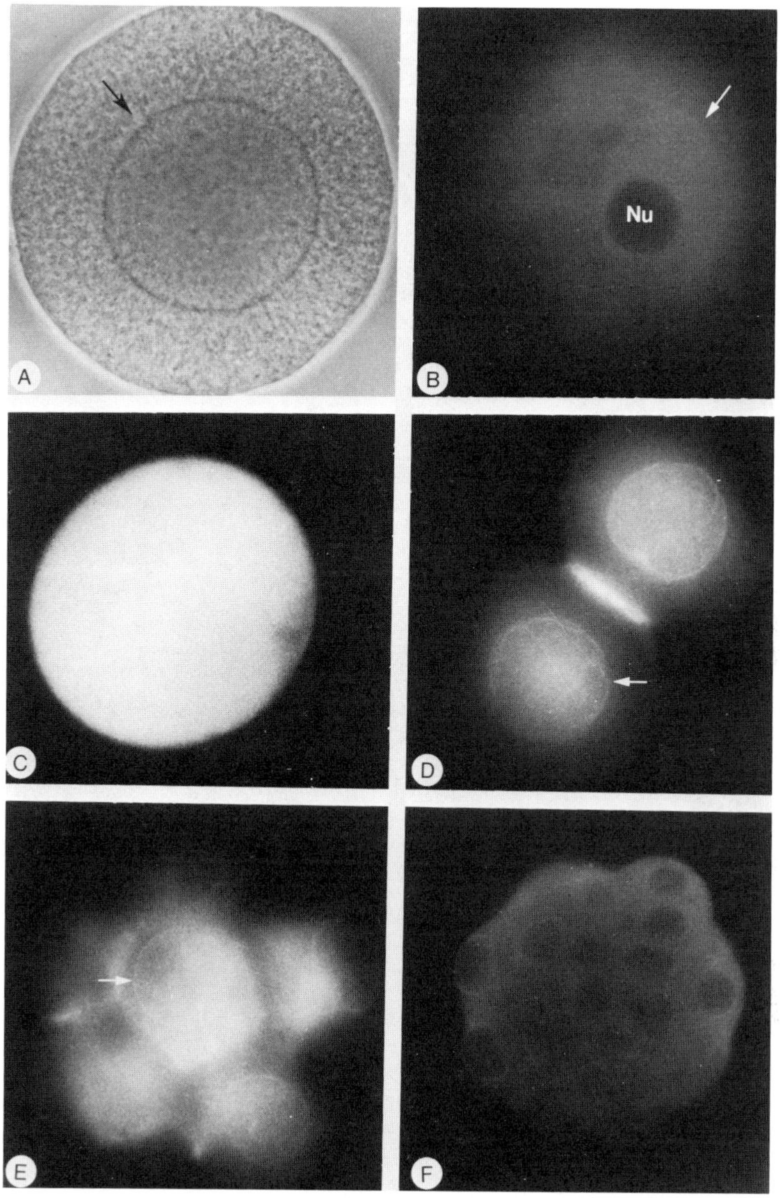


Fig. 9. Micrographs of mouse oocytes, zygotes and early embryos after binding anti-lamin B, using procedures described previously. (A) Phase contrast image of a diplotene oocyte, with germinal vesicle (arrow), after being recovered from an ovarian follicle. (B) Corresponding epifluorescent micrograph showing staining of germinal vesicle and surrounding nuclear envelope (arrow); but not the central nucleolus (Nu). (C) Zygote recovered at 14 hr post-hCG depicting intense cytoplasmic staining. (D) Two-cell embryo with strong labeling of the nuclear envelopes (arrow) and a low level of cytoplasmic fluorescence. (E) Eight-cell embryo with staining of the nuclear envelope (arrow) and increased cytoplasmic labeling. (F) Morula-stage embryo with diminished staining of the nuclear envelope, and low levels of cytoplasmic staining.

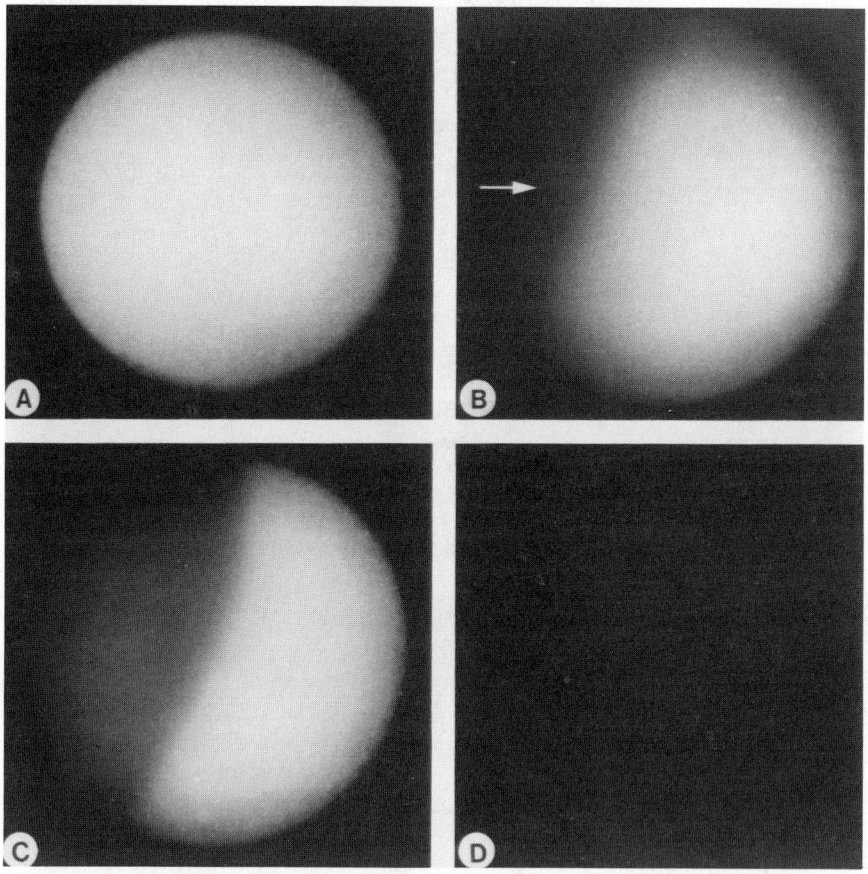

Fig. 10. Immunofluorescent images obtained on reacting with anti-lamins AC during _in vitro_ fertilization of mouse eggs. The patterns reflect a wave-like "loss" of antigenic determinants progressing across the zygote cytoplasm. (A) Secondary oocyte recovered at 14 hr post-hCG showing an intense level of cytoplasmic staining. (B) Zygote recovered at 3 min post-fertilization exhibiting a polar "loss" of cytoplasmic reactivity. (C) Zygote recovered at ~3 min with half-polar "loss" of antigenic determinants. (D) Zygote recovered at 4 to 6 min post-fertilization depicting a complete lack of reactivity.

marked changes in distribution during meiotic maturation, fertilization, and the early cleavage divisions of mouse embryogenesis. Immunofluorescence and immunoblot analyses demonstrate "stores" of lamins A and B in the oocyte's cytoplasm, and the discrete localization of these polypeptides to the forming pronuclear envelopes and to the nuclear envelopes of cleavage-stage blastomeres (Fig. 9). However, in early zygotes _no immunoreactive sites_ are detected by anti-lamin AC, even though binding of anti-lamin B remains strongly positive by immunofluorescence (Fig. 10). This apparent disappearance of antigenic determinants occurs soon after _in vivo_ fertilization. In fact, during _in vitro_ fertilization, the immunoreactive determinants are "lost" within 2-5 min in a "wave-like" pattern originating from the site of initial sperm contact (Fig. 11). After induction of polyspermy, supernumerary sperm attached to the zygote's plasma membrane do not promote a similar response. Later, during pronucleus formation immunoreactivity for lamin A gradually returns, initially in a central zone, and then expanding centripetally throughout the zygote's cytoplasm. This process does not appear to involve rapid proteolysis, since lamin A continues to be detectable by immunoblot analyses throughout the zygote's early phase of development (Donovan et al., submitted). Also, in the presence of the ionophore A23187 the

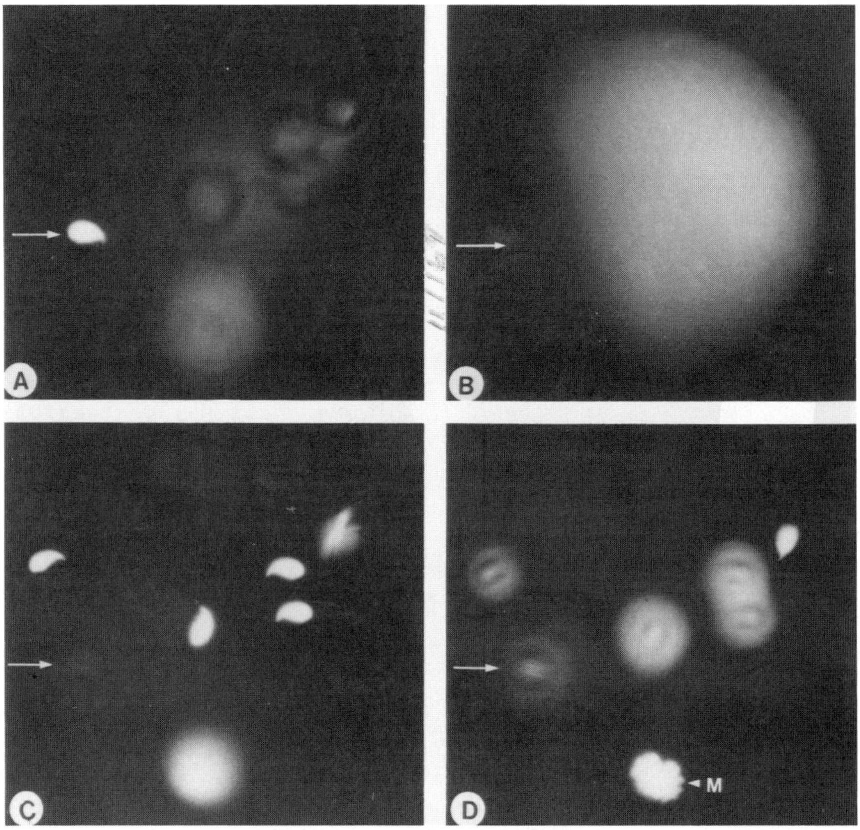


Fig. 11. Single activated zygote, with attached supernumerary sperm, showing a polar loss of immunoreactivity to anti-lamins AC in a region corresponding to the "fertilizing spermatozoon (arrows). (A) Sperm nucleus within the zygote depicted by staining with the DNA-specific fluorochrome, Hoechst 33258. (B) Corresponding immunofluorescent pattern of zygote showing the polar "loss" of determinants to anti-lamins AC in the area of the fertilizing spermatozoon. (C) Supernumerary sperm attached to the zygote at another focal plane, but with no corresponding loss of fluorescence (cf. Fig. 11B). (D) Third focal plane of the same zygote showing another attached sperm and maternal metaphase chromosomes (M).

immunoreactivity for lamin A and probably lamin C is lost within 2 to 3 min. By contrast, binding of anti-lamin B is not sensitive to the $Ca^{2+}$-specific ionophore. Finally, this apparent "loss" of determinants for anti-lamin AC is not prevented by prior incubation of oocytes with protease inhibitors. The process, therefore, appears to involve a $Ca^{2+}$-dependent masking or conformational change of the antigenic sites specifically on lamins A and C.

## NOVEL BIOLOGICAL PROCESS FOR ACCESSING ANTIBODIES TO THE DIFFERENTIATING SPERM CELL

The processes of nuclear transformation during spermatogenesis, fertilization and early embryogenesis involve unusual polypeptide constituents. Many of those assembled into the spermatozoon are synthesized during the terminal phases of meiotic prophase and spermiogenesis[66], while the germ cells are located within the central compartment of the seminiferous epithelium, a site normally excluded from the surveillance of the immune system. Thus, those constituents unique to the spermatozoon generally are autoantigenic on immunization, readily eliciting immune responses, followed by allergic orchitis. This biological phenomenon makes sperm constituents, particularly those having vital regulatory functions, before or after fertilization, suitable candidates for targeted vaccines. Selection of the most appropriate target(s), single or multiple, will require more research. The principal question is whether such components extra- or intra-cellular, will be accessible _in vivo_ to lytic or neutralizing immunological probes. In this regard it may be feasible to take advantage of a known and novel biological process.

Sertoli cells play both structural and sustentacular roles in promoting mammalian spermatogenesis. Aside from hormonal interactions, these epithelial cells have been demonstrated to secrete lactate and to facilitate the transfer of transferrin from serum to the central compartment. Both substances appear to be essential for sustaining spermatogenesis. Another novel process for transferring vital macromolecules into germ cells involves the exocytotic-endocytotic transfer of Sertoli cell hyaloplasm into the cytoplasm of spermatids during the latter half of spermiogenesis[61,89]. In this process, the Sertoli cell forms multiple finger-like, cytoplasmic protuberances that project into evaginations of the spermatid cytoplasm (Fig. 12). These complex structures become surrounded by elongated cisternae of endoplasmic reticulum in the form of a fenestrated sleeve with connections to other regions of reticulum throughout the spermatid cytoplasm. After formation, constrictions appear along the length of the Sertoli cell processes, yielding a series of spherical, double-walled vesicles. These "fenestrated spherules" remain interconnected by bridging cisternae (Fig. 12). Flattened membranous structures appear in the Sertoli cell cytoplasm adjacent to the membrane delimiting each spherule. Then, as the Sertoli cell membrane undergoes a lytic process, single-walled vesicles are released into the spermatid cytoplasm. This complex process is presumed to serve as a mechanism for transferring macromolecules to the spermatid during the crucial period of flagella formation and nuclear transformation. In this context the process is comparable to a multiple microinjection system.

It may be feasible, given this novel exocytotic-endocytotic process and recent developments in immunology, to target monoclonal antibodies to the appropriate antigenic determinants and thereby effectively "neutralize" sperm function. This approach may use either

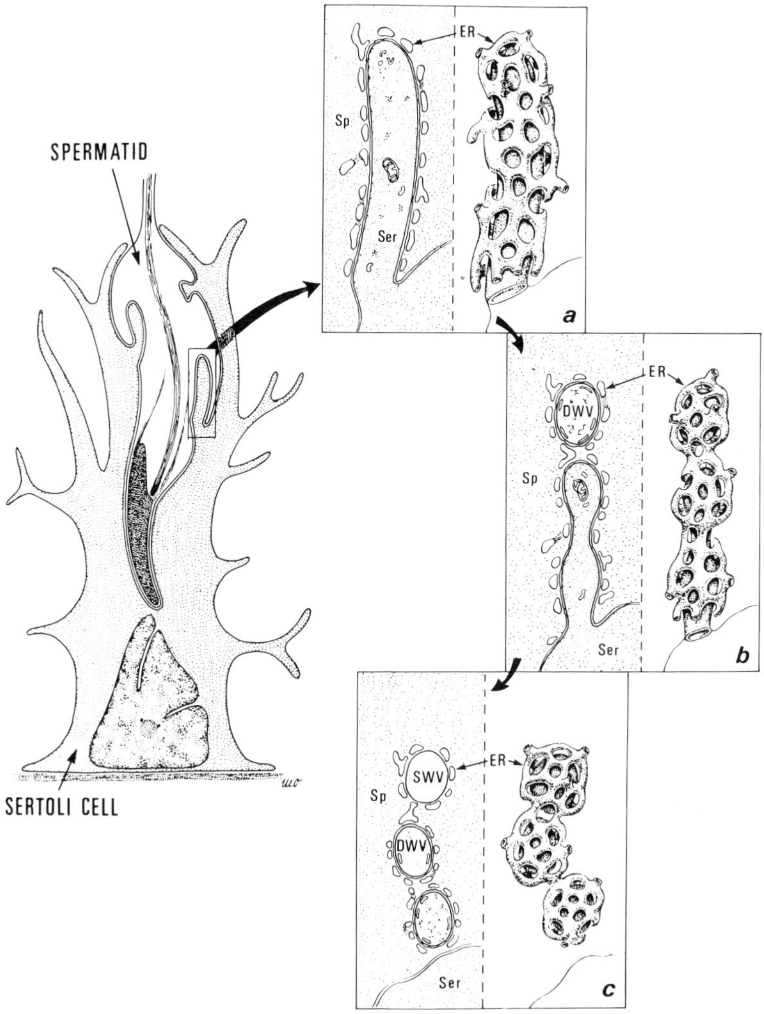


Fig. 12. Schematic diagram depicting the evolution of Sertoli cell cytoplasmic processes penetrating and forming spherical vesicles within the cytoplasm of rat spermatids (steps 8-19). The finger-like protuberance (Ser) of the Sertoli cell (left) on invading the spermatid cytoplasm (Sp): (a) becomes surrounded by elongated cisternae of endoplasmic reticulum of germ cell origin, (b) buds off to form double-membraned, vesicular bodies (DWV), and finally (c) yields single-walled vesicles (SWV) or "fenestrated spherules" after lysis of the Sertoli cell membrane. (From Clermont et al., 1982; by permission of the Editor, Anatomical Record).

human bivalent monoclonal antibodies or their Fab and $F(ab')_2$ fragments[15]. It may be possible even to construct bispecific antibodies from the $F(ab')_2$ fragments of two different monoclonal antibodies having the appropriate specificities[20]. With one recognition site directed against the target antigen, the other could be anti-idiotypic for a specific peptide hormone cell surface receptor, and thereby facilitate entry into the Sertoli cell cytoplasm. Alternatively, translocation across the plasma membrane may be accomplished by coupling the antibody (or $F(ab')_2$ fragments) directly to the hormone binding subunit. Conjugation of the antibody and hormone through the use of a heterobifunctional cross-linking agent, one that yields an acid-labile linker[18] would allow separation of the two macromolecules within the acidic environment of the Sertoli cell lysosomes. The released IgG (or $F(ab')_2$) then may be transferred from the Sertoli cell to the spermatid via the novel "exocytotic-endocytotic" process, and thereby gain access to the target antigen. Thus, by allowing imagination to prevail, these or other similar mechanisms may yield contraceptive methods having an appropriate level of simplicity and specificity.

ACKNOWLEDGMENTS

The authors express appreciation for the excellent technical assistance of Ms. Brenda L. Burnham and Patricia Mayhew, for the photography skills of Steven Borack, and for the manuscript preparation by Barbara Lewis. The preparation of this article was supported in part by NICHHD grants HD 08270 and HD 17633.

REFERENCES

1. Aaronson RP and Blobel G. Proc Natl Acad Sci U.S.A. 1975; 72:1008-1011.
2. Aaronson RP and Blobel G. J Cell Biol. 1974; 62:746-754.
3. Anderson E, Hoppe PC, Whitten WK and Lee GS. J Ultrastruct Res. 1975; 50:231-252.
4. Baccetti B, Bigliardi E and Burrini AG. J Ultrastruct Res. 1980; 72:232-287.
5. Balhorn R. J Cell Biol. 1982; 93:298-305.
6. Balhorn R, Gledhill BL and Wyrobek AJ. Biochemistry 1977; 16:4074-4080.
7. Bellve AR. In: "Prospects for Sexing Mammalian Sperm" (RP Amann and GE Seidel, Jr., eds.). Boulder, Colorado: Colorado Associated University Press, 1982, pp. 69-102.
8. Bellve AR. In: Oxford Reviews of Reproductive Biology (CA Finn, ed.). Oxford: Oxford University Clarendon Press, 1979; 1:159-261.
9. Bellvé AR. Biol Reprod. 1976; 15:632-646.
10. Bellvé AR. J Reprod Fert. 1973; 35:393-403.
11. Bellvé AR. J Reprod Fert. 1972; 30:71-81.
12. Bellvé AR and Carraway R. J Cell Biol. 1978; 79:177a.
13. Bellvé AR, Anderson, E and Hanley-Bowdoin, L. Develop Biol. 1975; 47:349-365.
14. Bellvé AR and O'Brien DA. In: Mechanisms and Control of Fertilization (JF Hartmann, ed.). New York: Academic Press, 1983; 55-137.
15. Bellvé AR and Moss SB. Biol Reprod. 1983; 28:1-26.
16. Berezney R. In: The cell nucleus (H Busch, ed.). Vol. VII. 1979; 413-456.
17. Berezney R and Coffey DS. Biochem Biophys Res Commun. 1974; 60:1410-1417.
18. Blattler WA, Kuenzi BS, Lambert JM and Senter P. Biochemistry 1985; 24:1517-1524

19. Bode J and Lesemann D. Hoppe-Seyler's Z Physiol Chem. 1977; 358:1505-1512.
20. Brennan M., Davison PF and Paulus H. 1985; 229:81-83.
21. Calvin HI. Biochim Biophys Acta. 1976; 434:377-399.
22. Campanella G, Gabbiani G, Baccetti B, Burrini AG and Pallini V. J Submicro Cytol. 1979; 11:53-71.
23. Clarke GN, Clarke FM and Wilson S. Biol. Reprod. 1982; 26:319-327.
24. Clarke GN and Yanagimachi R. J Exp Zool. 1978; 203:125-132.
25. Coelingh JP, Monfoort CH, Rozijn TH, Leuven JAG, Schiphof R, Styn-Parve CP, Braunitzer G, Schrank B and Rahfus A. Biochim Biophys Acta 1972; 285:1-14.
26. Ducibella T and Anderson E. Devel Biol. 1975; 47:45-58.
27. Ecklund PS and Levine L. J Cell Biol. 1975; 66:251-262.
28. Evenson DP, Witkin SS, deHarven E and Bendich A. J Ultrastruct Res. 1978; 63:178-187.
29. Fawcett DW, Anderson WA and Phillips DM. Develop Biol. 1971; 26:220-251.
30. Feughelmann M, Landgridge R, Seeds WE, Stokes AR, Wilson HR, Hooper HR, Wilkins MHG, Barclay LK and Hamilton LD. Nature (Lond). 1955; 275:834-838.
31. Flechon JE. J Microsc. 1974; 19:59-64.
32. Franke WW, Scheer U, Krohne G and Jarasch TD. J Cell Biol. 1981; 91:39s-50s.
33. Gaastra W, Lukkes-Hofstra J and Kilk AHJ. Biochem Genet. 1978; 16:525-529.
34. Gerace L, and Blobel G. Cell 1980; 19:277-287.
35. Gusse M and Chevaillier P. J Cell Biol. 1980; 87:280-284.
36. Hecht NB and Williams JL. Biol Reprod. 1978; 19:573-579.
37. Hoppe PC and Illmensee K. Proc Natl Acad Sci. 1982; 79:1912-1916.
38. Hoppe PC and Illmensee K. Proc Natl Acad Sci. 1977; 74:56.
39. Kaufman MH, Barton SC and Surani MAH. Nature 1977; 265:53-55.
40. Kierszenbaum AL and Tres LL. Fed Proc. 1978; 37:2512-2516.
41. Kistler WS, Keirn PS and Heinrikson RL. Biochim Biophys Acta. 1976; 427:752-757.
42. Kistler WS, Geroch ME and Williams-Ashman HG. J Biol Chem. 1973; 248:4532-4543.
43. Kleene KC, Distel RJ and Hecht NB. Biochemistry 1985; 24:719-722.
44. Koehler JK. J Ultrastruct Res. 1972; 34:529-539.
45. Koehler JK. J Ultrastruct Res. 1970; 33:598-614.
46. Koehler JK. J Ultrastruct Res. 1966; 31; 359-375.
47. Kolk A and Samuel T. Biochim Biophys Acta. 1975; 393:307-319.
48. Kopecny V. Z Zellforsch Mikrosk Anat. 1970; 109:414-419.
49. Kopecny V and Pavlok A. J Exptl Zool. 1975; 191:85-96
50. Lalli M and Clermont Y. Amer J Anat. 1981; 160:419-434.
51. Lewis CD and Laemmli UK. Cell 1982; 29:171-181.
52. Lung B. Ultrastruct Res. 1968; 22:485-493.
53. Lung B. J Cell Biol. 1972; 52:179-186.
54. Marks JL Science 1985; 229:455-456.
55. Marushige Y and Marushige K. Biochim Biophys Acta. 1978; 518:440-449.
56. Marushige Y and Marushige K. Biochim Biophys Acta. 1974; 340:498-508.
57. Mayer JF, Chang TSK and Zirkin BR. Biol Reprod. 1981; 25:1041-1051.
58. Mayer JF and Zirkin BR. J Cell Biol. 1979; 81:403-410.
59. McIntosh JR and Porter KR. J Cell Biol. 1967; 35:153-173.
60. Monfoort CH, Schiphof R, Rozijn TH and Steyn-Parve DP. Biochim Biophys Acta. 1973; 322:133-177.
61. Morales C and Clermont Y. Anat Rec. 1982; 203:233-244.

62. Moustafa LA. Genetics. 1978; 88:70-71.
63. Myles DG and Hepler PK. J Cell Sci. 1977; 23:57-83.
64. Myles DG and Hepler PK. Develop Biol. 1982; 90:238-252.
65. O'Brien DA and Bellvé AR. Develop Biol. 1980; 75:386-404.
66. O'Brien DA and Bellvé AR. Develop Biol. 1980; 75:405-418.
67. Philippe M and Chevaillier P. Biochem J. 1978; 77:27-34.
68. Phillips DH. J Ultrastruct Res. 1970; 33:369-380.
69. Phillips DM. J Cell Biol. 1974; 62:911-917.
70. Platz RD, Grimes SR, Meistrich ML and Hnilica L. J Biol Chem. 1975; 250:5791-5800.
71. Pongswasdi P and Svasti Z. Biochim Biophys Acta. 1976; 474:462-473.
72. Pruslin FH and Rodman TC. Exptl Cell Res. 1983; 144:115-126.
73. Puwaravutipanich T and Panyim S. Exp Cell Res. 1975; 90:153-158.
74. Richards JM and Witkins SS. J Reprod Fertil. 1978; 54:43-47.
75. Rodman TC, Pruslin FG and Allfrey VG. J. Cell Sci. 1982; 53:227-244.
76. Rodman TC, Pruslin FG, Hoffman HP and Allfrey VG. J Cell Biol. 1981; 90:351-361.
77. Sapsford CS and Rae CA. Aust J Zool. 1969; 17:415-445.
78. Suau P and Subirana JA. J Mol Biol. 1977; 117:909-926.
79. Stefanini M, Oura C and Zamboni L. J Submicrosc Cytol. 1969; 1:1-23.
80. Stevens LC. Nature 1978; 276:266-267.
81. Stevens LC, Varnum DS and Ekler EM. Nature 1977; 269:515-517.
82. Stick R and Schwarz H. Cell Differentiation 1982; 11:235-243.
83. Stick R and Schwarz H. Cell 1982; 33:949-958.
84. Surani MAH, Barton SC and Norris ML. Nature 1984; 308:548-550.
85. Tamblyn TM. Biol Reprod. 1980; 22:727-734.
86. Tobita T, Tsutsumi H, Kato A, Suzuki N, Nomoto M, Nakano M and Ando T. Biochim Biophys Acta 1983; 744:141-146.
87. Tsanev R and Avramova Z. Eur J Cell Biol. 1981; 24:139-145.
88. Virtanen I, Badley RA, Paasivo R and Lehto V-P. J Cell Biol. 1985; 99:1-83-1091.
89. Vogl AW, Soucy LJ and Foo V. Amer J Anat. 1985; 172:75-86.
90. Warrant RW and Kim SH. Nature 1978; 217:130-135.
91. Weintraub H. Proc Natl Acad Sci U.S.A. 1975; 72:1212-1216.
92. Wiesel S and Schultz GA. Gamete Res. 1981; 4:25-34.
93. Witkin SS, Evenson DP and Bendich A. In: The Molecular Biology of the Mammalian Genetic Apparatus (P Ts'o, ed.) New York: Elsevier/North-Holland Biomedical Press. 1977; 345-351.
94. Yanagimachi R and Noda YD. Am J Anat. 1970; 128:429-462.
95. Young RJ and Sweeney R. Genetic Res. 1979; 19:265-282.
96. Zirkin BR, Chang TSK and Heaps J. J Cell Biol. 1980; 85:116-121.

# SPERM ANTIGENS RELATED TO INFERTILITY

Nancy J. Alexander and Mohamed Isahakia

[1]Reproductive Biology and Behavior, Oregon
Regional Primate Research Center, Beaverton, Oregon
[2]Institute of Primate Research, P.O. Box 34505
Nairobi, Kenya

## ANTIBODIES AND INFERTILITY

How antibodies to sperm interfere with fertility has been argued at many scientific meetings. No clear-cut answer is available from either epidemiological or experimental studies. We know that animals immunized with whole sperm or sperm extracts have high antibody levels and become infertile. When the antibody titers fall, fertility returns. Men and women with antisperm antibodies are less likely to be fertile than those lacking such antibodies. Further evidence comes from the finding that the levels of antibodies that develop in men after vasectomy can be used to predict fertility after vasovasostomy. When we measured sperm-agglutinating and sperm-immobilizing antibodies in a prospective study of 160 men, we found agglutinating antibodies in 63%, immobilizing antibodies in 37%, and antibodies in the seminal plasma in 3% (Fuchs and Alexander, 1983). In a postoperative evaluation most men had no significant change in agglutinating or immobilizing antibody levels. The incidence of men with antibodies in their seminal plasma rose after vasovasostomy to 16%. This rise most likely occurred because of the contribution of the epididymal segment to the seminal plasma. Pregnancy rates were inversely correlated with antibody levels. No man in our study caused a pregnancy if he had a titer of greater than 1:160. Sutherland and associates (1984) observed similar findings in men who underwent a vasectomy reversal and Rümke (1959) obtained similar results from men who were infertile and had antibodies but had not had a vasectomy.

## CORTICOSTEROID TREATMENT

If antibodies to sperm can affect fertility, one might expect people with such antibodies to have their levels reduced by corticosteroids; such treatment should enhance pregnancy rates. We tested this hypothesis (Alexander et al., 1983) by administering prednisone to 24 patients; 26 patients with similar antibody levels were not treated and served as controls. Both men and women with antisperm antibodies were studied. In men, the drug did not change sperm count, motility, or the percentage of sperm with normal forms. It did cause significant reductions in levels of circulating sperm-immobilizing antibodies in both sexes. Fourteen pregnancies occurred in the four-month evaluation period. We thought that pregnancies in response to the therapy should occur within that time period. Significantly more pregnancies occurred in the treatment group than in the control group (45% vs 16%, $p < 0.025$). Prednisone treatment did not always eliminate circulating antisperm antibodies (we measured the levels 2 months after treatment). We do not know if doses other than 60 mg or longer treatment periods (we used 7 days) would be more effective. A study by Hendry and associates (in press) suggests that lower levels may be effective in some patients.

## HOW DO ANTIBODIES REDUCE FERTILITY?

In order to better understand how antisperm antibodies could affect fertility, we added serum samples from patients with antisperm antibodies to sperm. Would sperm coated with antibodies be able to penetrate hamster eggs? Six serum samples totally blocked and another 10 substantially reduced penetration. Only two samples yielded data comparable to that of the controls. To determine whether sperm-egg penetration was reduced owing to the antibodies, we purified the serum samples and used the IgG fraction. This fraction caused a reduction similar to that found with whole serum, an indication that the observed effect was present in the immunoglobulin fraction of serum (Alexander, 1984).

No one antisperm antibody type was particularly associated with infertility. Agglutinating antibodies, immobilizing antibodies and those revealed by immunofluorescence were found in specimens affecting egg penetration.

We tested whether exposure of sperm to antisperm antibodies would reduce the ability of sperm to penetrate cervical mucus as well. We observed that 21% of the serum samples did reduce cervical mucus penetration. So antisperm antibodies affect cervical mucus penetration as well as oocyte fusion (Alexander, 1984).

The precise mechanism of antisperm-antibody-mediated infertility in humans and animals is unknown. Sperm antibodies influence gametes during and after fertilization, as well as during preimplantation development (Tung and Goldberg, 1979; Naz et al., 1983). Although the antibodies have been extensively studied in humans, less has been published about the characterization of the corresponding spermatozoal antigens.

Analysis of mammalian cell membrane ontogeny during spermatogenesis has indicated that distinctive macromolecules specific to the sperm appear during spermatogenesis and are subsequently polarized into discrete structural and functional domains (Friend and Fawcett, 1974; Elias et al., 1979; Koehler, 1978). Sperm maturation within the epididymis further modifies these antigenic domains on the sperm surface and thus the fertilizing capacity is acquired (Bedford, 1975). The exact mechanism of maturation is unclear, but antigenic moieties are believed to be transferred from the apical surface of epithelial principal cells to the sperm plasmalemma in the proximal and corpus epididymidis (Moore, 1980, 1981). The secretion of specific sperm binding or coating proteins or glycoproteins by various regions of the epididymis has been demonstrated by Feuchter et al. (1981) and Moore et al. (1980) in mice and hamsters.

## MONOCLONAL ANTIBODIES TO HUMAN SPERMATOZOA

A detailed study of the consequences of immune reactions to sperm autoantigens is essential to the rational development of immunologic contraception. Characterization of sperm target antigens is important; such studies involve not only determination of cell specificity, but also whether or not the antigens are membrane-bound or subsurface antigens since only the former are accessible to immunologic attack. The biological functions of sperm antigens and particularly their roles in sperm capacition and fertilization are equally important to an understanding of how immunologic infertility is induced. In recent years the two basic features of fertilization discussed by Lille in 1919, namely, sperm capacitation and sperm-egg interaction have become amenable to study through the use of monoclonal antibody (MCA) probes.

We recently developed a library of MCAs to human sperm surface antigens (Isahakia and Alexander, 1984). These are mainly specific for the acrosomal region of the sperm, even though a few recognize the midpiece, equator- and tail regions. Thus, the mammalian sperm surface, as visualized in our studies, is a dramatic example of cell surface differentiation. The human sperm surface contains distinctive molecules having a striking level of topographic organization (Figs. 1-3). An understanding of the locations of antigens on human sperm and their molecular composition sugggests that the sperm surface is a complex mosaic in which one domain has several distinctive molecules (84K, 220K, 53K, 34K, 21K, 26-40K antigens occupy the acrosome as recognized by MA1, MA2, MA3, MA8, MA11 and MA13). Specific sperm functions, e.g., the acrosome reaction and subsequent sperm-egg interaction have been localized to particular regions of the sperm acrosome that correlate with the domains defined by our MCAs. This phenomenon has also been reported by Primakoff and Myles (1984), who found a multiplicity of antigenic determinants occupying one domain on guinea-pig sperm. The data on both the human and guinea-pig sperm raise questions concerning the functional roles of the many groups of antigens occupying one region. Are they part of a multistep process that occurs specifically in that region? Or do they function independently in several distinct region-specific surface roles? The different effects some of our MCAs with similar regional sperm specificities have in the sperm penetration assay (SPA) point to the latter hypothesis. Several MCAs (MA12, MA24) tested in the SPA blocked sperm penetration, presumeably through different mechanisms (Table 1). Nevertheless, our findings suggest that the respective sperm antigens are directly involved in a process essential to fertilization.

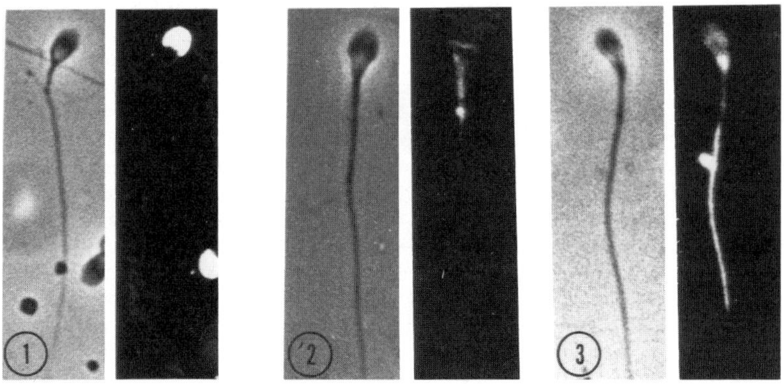


Fig. 1 Indirect immunofluorescence reveals that monoclonal antibodies as directed against specific antigenic domains on methanol-fixed human spermatozoa. Each figure represents a phase contrast and a fluorescence photomicrograph of the same spermatozoon. Figure 1 depicts an antibody reaction to the acrosome; Figure 2, to the midpiece; and Figure 3, to the postacrosomal region and tail.

Table 1. Effect of Monoclonal antibodies on the human sperm-hamster egg penetration assay.

| Clone | Immunofluorescence pattern | No. of oocytes penetrated/No. recovered | %Fertilization |
|---|---|---|---|
| MA12 | Neck | 0/34 | 0% |
| MA24 | Tail/Neck | 0/33 | 0 % |
| MA5 | Equatorial | 30/34 | 89% |
| NS-1 myeloma ascites | None | 34/34 | 100% |

*MA12 - Inhibits sperm penetration but not sperm attachment on to the eggs.

MA24 -Inhibits both sperm penetration and attachment to eggs.

We have been able to further characterize one such antigen recognized by MA24 (Naz et al. 1984). This 23-K antigen has been purified by affinity chromatography and has been shown to be involved in both iso- and autoimmune-mediated infertility in humans. Thus it could be a candidate for a sperm-based contraceptive vaccine. Lakoshi and Saling (1984) described a MCA against the acrosome of mouse sperm that could inhibit in vitro fertilization of zona-intact mouse oocytes in a manner similar to that shown by MA24 (Naz et al. 1984). However, whether these two antibodies (generated by different procedures) recognize common determinants in humans and mice is unclear. Both antibodies display cross-specificity for the acrosome. Many of our MCAs appear to be specific for the acrosome of several species (Table 2). This presence of identical antigenic determinants on mammalian sperm raises the question of whether or not common mammalian sperm antigenic determinants with specific functions have been phylogenetically conserved through evolution (for review, Ohno, 1970). Investigation of antigenic determinants having phylogenetically diverse and limited distributions may therefore provide important clues for understanding the fundamental steps in fertilization. This idea is supported by the observation that MA24 inhibits human and mouse sperm-egg interaction. It has enormous practical implications for efforts to develop a contaceptive vaccine. There is a need to establish appropriate animal models, e.g., the mouse, for in vivo and in vitro fertility studies. These animals can also serve as an abundant source of antigen.

A better understanding of sperm capacitation may allow the development of methods to interfere with this process in spermatozoa. We have found that intrinsic changes on the human sperm surface might be contolled by intracellular metabolic changes that lead to capacitation.

Table 2. Interspecies cross-reactivity of sperm antigens defined by monoclonal antibodies.

| Clone | Human | Monkey | Dog | Rabbit | Mouse | Rat |
|---|---|---|---|---|---|---|
| MA7 | A | A | A | A | A | A |
| MA10 | A | - | - | - | - | - |
| MA14 | T/M | - | E | - | - | - |
| MA16 | PA | - | PA/A | - | M | - |
| MA19 | A | A | A | A | A | A |
| MA22 | A | A | A | A | T | - |
| MA27 | T | - | - | - | - | - |

Abbreviations: A-Acrosome; T-Tail; M-Midpiece; PA-Postacrosome; E-Equatorial.

The position of MA5 on the equatorial region changes during incubation in a capacitating medium and subsequently there is staining of parts of the tail (Fig. 4-5). This indicates that some sperm antigens are most probably mobile in the lateral plane of the membrane during capacitation. Whether such a change would be a prerequisite for the final acrosome reaction is not yet known. Thus, MA5 antibody might be a marker for capacitation.

The use of MCAs to bind specific, single antigenic determinants will be critical to the development of a sperm-based contraceptive vaccine. We

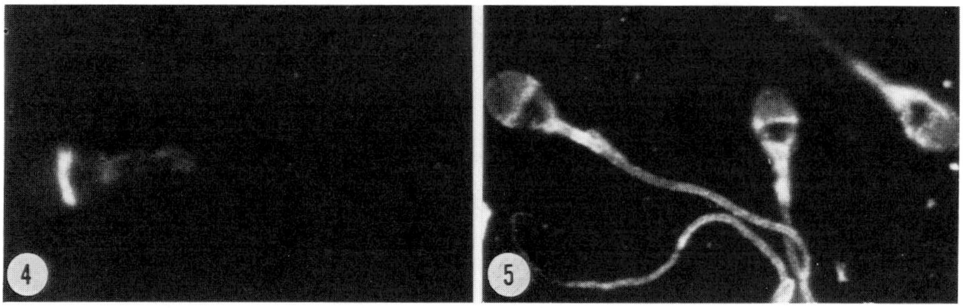


Fig. 2 Figures 4 and 5 are of the reaction of monoclonal antibodies to freshly washed and capacitated spermatozoa. Capacitation results in increased binding to the postacrosomal and tail regions.

have been able to identify several MCAs having the ability to cause: (a) total loss of sperm mobility through agglutination or immobilization or (b) sperm failure to penetrate and fuse with hamster eggs in vitro. Given the unique specificities of these antibodies, we are currently isolating specific antigens through affinity chromatography for fertility trials in animal models.

## ACKNOWLEDGMENT

The work described in this chapter, Publication No. 1405 of the Oregon Regional Primate Research Center, was supported by National Institutes of Health Grants RR-00163 and HD-14572.

## REFERENCES

Alexander, N.J. (1984) Antibodies to human spermatozoa impede sperm penetration of cervical mucus or hamster eggs. Fertil. Steril. 41:433-439.

Alexander, N.J., Sampson, J.H., and Fulgham, D.L. (1983) Pregnancy rates in patients treated for antisperm antibodies with prednisone. Int. J. Fertil. 28:63-67.

Bedford, J.M. (1975) Maturation, transport and fate of spermatozoa on the epididymis. In: Hamilton, Greene. Handbook of Physiology, Section 7: Endocrinlogy, Vol. V: Male Reproductive System, p. 303 (American Physiological Society, Washington).

Elias, P.M., Friend, D.S., and Goerke, J. (1979) Membrane sterol heterogenity: freeze fracture detection with saponins and filipin. J. Histochem. Cytochem. 27:1247-1249.

Feuchter, F.A., Vernon, R.B. and Eddy, E.M. (1981) Analysis of the sperm surface with monoclonal antibodies. Topographically restricted antigens appearing in the epididymis. Biol. Reprod. 24:1099-1110.

Friend, D.S., and Fawcett, D.W. (1974) Membrane differentiation in freeze-fractured mammalian sperm. J. Cell Biol. 63:641-645.

Fuchs, E.F., and Alexander, N.J. (1983) Immunological considerations before and after vasovasostomy. Fertil. Steril. 40:497-499.

Hendry, W.F., Treehuka, K., Hughes, L., Stedronska, J., Parslow, J.H., Wass, J.A.H., and Besser, G.M. (In press). Cyclical prednisolone therapy for male infertility associated with autoantibodies to spermatozoa. Fertil. Steril.

Isahakia, M., and Alexander, N.J. (1984) Interspecies cross-reactivity of monoclonal antibodies directed against human sperm antigens. Biol. Reprod. 30:1015-1026.

Kohler, J.K. (1978) The mammalian sperm surface: Studies with specific labeling techniques. Int. J. Devel. Cytol. 54:73.

Lakoski, K.A., and Saling, P.M. (1984) Development of the acrosome: Sperm antigens involved in fertilization probed with monoclonal antibodies. (Abstract) Biol. Reprod. (Suppl.) 30:134.

Lillie, F.R. (1919) Problems of Fertilization. Univ. of Chicago Press, Chicago, Il.

Moore, H.D.M. (1980) Localisation of specific glycoproteins secreted by the rabbit and hamster epididymis. Biol. Reprod. 22:705-718.

Moore, H.D.M. (1981) Glycoprotein secretion of the epididymis in the rabbit and hamster: localisation on epididymal spermatozoa and the effect of specific antibodies on fertilization in vivo. J. Exp. Zool. 215:77-85.

Moore, H.D.M., and Hartman, T.D. (1984) Localisation by monoclonal antibodies of various surface antigens of hamster spermatozoa and the effect of antibody on fertilization in vitro. J. Reprod. Fertil. 70:175-183.

Naz, R.K., Saxe, J.M., and Menge, A.C. (1983) Inhibition of fertility in rabbits by monoclonal antibodies against sperm. Biol. Reprod. 28:249-254.

Naz, R.K., Alexander, M.J., Isahakia, M., and Hamilton, M.S. (1984) Monoclonal antibody to a human germ cell membrane glycoprotein that inhibits fertilization. Science 225:342-344.

Ohno, S. (1970) Evolution by Gene Duplication. Springer-Verlag, Berlin, Heidelberg, New York.

Primakoff, P., and Myles, D.G. (1983) A map of the guinea-pig sperm surface constructed with monoclonal antibodies. Dev. Biol. 98:417-428.

Rümke, P., and Hellinga, G. (1959) Autoantibodies against spermatozoa in sterile men. Am. J. Clin. Pathol. 32:357-363.

Tung, K.S.K., and Goldberg, F.H. (1979) Immunobiological consequence of immunization of female mice with homologous spermatozoa: Induction of fertility. J. Reprod. Immunol. 1:145-151.

# TOWARD THE DEVELOPMENT OF AN ANTI-SPERM CONTRACEPTIVE VACCINE

Rajesh K. Naz

Department of OB/GYN
The George Washington University Medical Center
2150 Pennsylvania Ave. NW
Washington, DC 20037

Development of a vaccine based on sperm antigens represents a promising approach to contraception. The feasibility of this approach is based upon two evidences. The first type of evidence comes from the studies of involuntary immunoinfertility in humans. Presence of antisperm antibodies have been reported to be one of the major causes of immunoinfertility in both men and women.[1] Second type of evidence is provided by the experimental immunization studies. Immunization of male and female animals of various species with extracts of sperm or mature testis results in a significant reduction in fertility by causing either fertilization failure or preimplantation embryo mortality or both.[2-5] The whole sperm cannot be used as an immunogen for the development of an antisperm vaccine due to the presence of numerous antigens on germ cells which could be shared with other somatic tissues. The utility of an antigen as an immunocontraceptive vaccine is contingent upon its tissue-specificity, its homogeneity, strong immunogenicity and its involvement in fertilization and fertility.

A few sperm-specific antigens have been isolated in homogeneous form and characterized, and some of these are relevant to fertility. The known antigens of sperm include acrosin, hyaluronidase, rabbit sperm autoantigen (RSA-1) and lactate dehydrogenase-X (LDH-$C_4$). Acrosin and hyaluronidase are enzymes present in spermatozoa and are required for a successful fertilization process. Though these are required for the penetration of spermatozoa into the oocytes, active immunization with these enzymes did not inhibit fertility in female rabbits[6] and sheep.[7] Antiserum to another antigen purified from rabbit sperm[8] (RSA-1) resulted in decreased fertility on artificial insemination of female rabbits with treated-sperm. Immunization with testis-specific LDH-$C_4$ resulted in a significant reduction of fertility in mice, rabbits and baboons.[9-10] However immunization with LDH-$C_4$ caused a reduction rather than a complete block in fertility even when strong adjuvants like Freund's complete adjuvant (FCA), which are potentially toxic and nonpermissible for humans, were employed for immunization. LDH-$C_4$ is rarely if at all involved in involuntary immunoinfertility in humans. So there is an obvious need to isolate more sperm-specific antigens which are relevant to fertility.

With the advent of hybridoma technology it has been possible to identify and isolate such antigens in homogeneous form. Some of these antigens which are relevant to the fertilization process and subsequent embryonic development are described below.

a) THE GERM-CELL ANTIGEN (GA-1) INVOLVED IN POST-FERTILIZATION EMBRYONIC DEVELOPMENT

Monoclonal antibodies (MCA's) were prepared against rabbit sperm antigens by the standard technique.[11] Five of these subclones secreting antisperm antibodies as checked by enzyme-linked immonosorbent assay (ELISA) and indirect immunofluorescence technique (IFT), were tested for their effect on fertility in female rabbits.

Two of the hybridomas (8C4.1 and 8C10.5) demonstrated a significant reduction in fertility based on the percentage of 9 days-viable implants to corpora lutea ratio. [12] These two MCA's were negative in sperm immobilization technique (SIT) and tray agglutination technique (TAT), methods usually employed for the detection of antisperm antibodies.[13,14] These MCA's in a localized manner reacted with the plasma membrane on acrosomal region of the sperm.

Both MCA's recognized an antigen of 63KDa on the Western blot with rabbit whole testis membrane extract. This germ-cell antigen (GA-1) was not recognized by the antiserum raised against the whole testis extract. The GA-1 has been isolated using monoclonal antibody (8C10.5) by immunoaffinity chromatography.[16] This testicular glycoprotein has been partially characterized and its immunological and biochemical properties are summarized in Table 1.

Recently we actively immunized female rabbits (n=6) and female mice (n=29) with GA-1 purified from rabbit testis. There was a significant reduction of fertility after immunization.[17] In immunized rabbits percentage of implants were 36% as compared to controls in which they were 86% (Table 3). In mice there was a reduction in fertility as seen by mean implants per mated mouse actively immunized with GA-1 (GA-1, 1.2-3.8; control 8.0-10.1)(Naz and Menge, unpublished data).

The mechanism by which antibodies (monoclonal or polyclonal) to GA-1 inhibit fertility seem to be at the postfertilization preimplantation embryonic development stage. The incidence of fertilization with anti-GA-1 antibodies-treated sperm were not significantly different from controls. The antibodies did not have anti-blastocyst activity. The normally fertilized zygotes cleaved and developed into normal embryos when cultured in a medium containing antibodies to GA-1. The effect is not due to polyspermy or parthenogenetic activation of eggs. The antibodies may affect some extranuclear signal(s) on the sperm plasma membrane which is necessary for viable embryo formation.

b) THE FERTILIZATION ANTIGEN (FA-1) INVOLVED IN FERTILIZATION PROCESS

Of 40 putative clones secreting antibodies to human sperm,

Table 1. CHARACTERISTICS OF THE GERM-CELL ANTIGEN (GA-1) ISOLATED BY SODIUM DEOXYCHOLATE SOLUBILIZATION

| | | |
|---|---|---|
| 1. | Apparent molecular weight | 63 kDa on 10% gel<br>on reduction form two subunits composed of numerous spots in 50-70kDa range in 2D-gel |
| 2. | Amino acid analysis | High percentage of glycine |
| 3. | Carbohydrate analysis | 21% carbohydrate |
| 4. | Topographic localization | Plasma membrane antigen localized on the acrosomal region of the sperm<br>also present in the intrastructure of tail |
| 5. | Ontogenesis | Synthesized in testis<br>first develop on spermatocytes |
| 6. | Phylogenetic relationship | Cross reacting antigen on mouse, rabbit, bull, monkey and human |
| 7. | Immunogenicity | Immunogenic in mice and rabbits<br>Tissue specific polyclonal antiserum inhibits fertility |

one (MA-24) was of special interest. The MA-24 clone belonging to IgG2a subclass was germ-cell specific but cross-reacted with sperm from other species namely mouse, rabbit, bull, rhesus monkey and human. The MA-24 clone bound to the postacrosome, midpiece and tail of human spermatozoa. The tissue-specific but not species-specific MA-24 antibody completely blocked (0%) binding and penetration of zona-free hamster ova by human sperm. MA-24 also significantly inhibited fertilization in vitro of mouse eggs (up to 0%) by murine sperm.[18] MA-24 antibody was negative in the agglutination and immobilization assays.

MA-24 recognized a single protein band of 23kDa or its dimer of 47kDa when a detergent-solubilized membrane preparation of testis or sperm was used in a Western blot enzyme immunobinding assay. MA-24 did not react with seminal plasma from vasectomized men.

Using immunoaffinity chromatography with MA-24 immunoglobulins, we isolated the fertilization antigen (FA-1) from human testes. As the availability of human germ cells is limited for use in the isolation of FA-1 required for large scale practical use, we recently isolated the homologous antigen from murine testes. The antigen isolated in DOC, may have limited biological utility and may change its immunogenicity. We also isolated it from lithium diiodosalicylate (LIS) - solubilized testes. The FA-1 isolated from murine testes is very homogeneous and has been well characterized.[19] Some of the properties of FA-1 are summarized in Table 2.

Table 2. CHARACTERISTICS OF THE FERTILIZATION ANTIGEN (FA-1) ISOLATED FROM MURINE TESTES

| | | Method | Result |
|---|---|---|---|
| a) | Apparent molecular weight | 1D-SDS-PAGE<br>Sucrose and Cesium cloride gradient<br>High performance chromatography size exclusion | Monomer of 23-kDa and/or dimer of 46-kDa<br>Forces involved in dimerisation are ionic and not disulfide linkage |
| | | 2D-PAGE | 4-5 polypeptide spots of same molecular weight |
| b) | Amino acid analysis | | High percentage of aspartic acid and glutamic acid<br>Serine and aspartic acid are N-terminal amino acids |
| c) | Carbohydrate analysis | | 18.8% of the total mass |
| d) | Topographic localization | | Plasma membrane localized on the post acrosome, mid piece and tail of sperm |
| e) | Ontogenesis | | Testicular antigen |
| f) | Phylogenetic relationship | | Cross reacts with mouse, rabbit, bull, monkey and human |
| g) | Immunogenicity | | Mice, rabbits and humans |

A single intraperitoneal injection of MA-24 ascites significantly inhibited fertilization *in vivo* in mice. Recently six female rabbits were actively immunized with FA-1. All rabbits responded to FA-1 by showing a drastic reduction in fertility as seen by percentage of 9 days-viable implants to corpora lutea ratio. Many rabbits had a total block of fertility with zero(%) implants (Table 3).

The antisera collected from these rabbits showed binding only with the specific protein band in the Western blot procedure. The antisera did not agglutinate or immobilize sperm.

The purified FA-1 gave a strong cross reaction with sera from involuntary immunoinfertile patients in the enzyme linked immunosorbent assay (ELISA) or dot blot enzyme linked immunosorbent assay. In our successful human *in vitro* fertilization - embryo transfer (IVF-ET) program[20] sometimes we observed failure of fertilization. The sera of infertile couples

Table 3. EFFECT OF ACTIVE IMMUNIZATION WITH PURIFIED ANTIGENS ON FERTILITY OF DOES

| Treatment | Rabbit No. | Percent implants* | Mechanisms |
|---|---|---|---|
| 1. GA-1 | 6 | 36.3[a] | Post fertilization pre-implantation embryonic mortality |
| 1a. Controls | 3 | 85.7[b] | |
| 2. FA-1 | 6 | 24.4[c] | Fertilization inhibition |
| 2a. Controls | 3 | 93.9[d] | |

Significance based upon chi-squared analysis, a vs b, $P < 0.05$; c vsd, $P < .001$.

*based upon the ratio of viable implants to corpora lutea ratio.

showing a failure in IVF demonstrated a strong binding with FA-1. In many cases sera from both husband and wife demonstrated antibodies to FA-1 These preliminary results are encouraging and indicate strong immunogenicity (both auto- and iso-) of the FA-1 in humans. These results also indicate that once the sufficient antibodies are available, these can cause a total block of fertilization and fertility in humans.

The mechanism(s) by which antibodies to FA-1 inhibits fertilization and fertility is under study. Since both binding and penetration are inhibited in fertilization systems _in vitro_, these antibodies may hinder interactions between sperm and ovum or receptor recognition; the block is not due to agglutination or immobilization of sperm. MA-24 did not bind to ova, which shows the sperm specificity of the antibody. In the murine fertilization assay performed _in vitro_, MA-24 inhibited fertilization only in ova with intact zonae and not when zonae were removed, indicating that the inhibition occurs at the level of interaction between sperm and zona pellucida. However, in the heterogametic assay, MA-24 completely blocked binding and penetration of human sperm in the zona-free hamster ova, an assay that has been reported to measure capacitation indirectly.[21] These antibodies may be directed to a sperm component (enzymatic or nonenzymatic) that is vital for capacitation.

FA-1 appears to be incorporated into zygote during normal fertilization. So antibodies to FA-1 may have dual action: these will block fertilization; and if a spermatozoon escapes and the fertilization does occur, these may be able to inhibit embryonic development.

FA-1 constitutes a very promising cnadidate for the development of an anti-sperm immunocontraceptive vaccine and also for the diagnosis and treatment of involuntary immunoinfertility in humans.

c) THE CLEAVAGE SIGNAL (CS-1), THE ANTIGEN INVOLVED IN FIRST CLEAVAGE

Besides the GA-1 and FA-1, we are engaged in identifying, isolating and characterizing other sperm-specific membrane antigens which are involved in the fertilization process, subsequent cleavage and embryonic development. We have developed antisperm antibodies which when injected into female mice cause inhibition of the first cleavage. Fertilization is normal, but the zygotes do not divide into 2-cell *in vitro* or *in vivo*. We are presently engaged in characterizing the CS-1. The CS-1 does not seem to cross react with GA-1, which is involved at the later stages of embryonic development. These results indirectly indicate that sperm plasma membrane antigen(s) constitute extra nuclear signal(s) for the oocyte to cleave, develop and blastulate.

The use of sperm specific antigens appears to be a promising approach to contraception. Two considerations are important in using sperm-specific antigens for the development of an immunocontraceptive vaccine. First is efficacy and second is reversibility. The general consensus is that a vaccine which has less than 90% effectiveness would not be acceptable.[22] For sperm antigens it is generally argued that no one has as yet reported a total block of fertility even after immunizing with crude extracts that presumably contain most of the sperm and/or testis antigens. Immunization with intact sperm may not result in antibodies against surface proteins that are weakly immunogenic, but involved in fertilization and fertility e.g., immunization of mice with intact isologous epididymal sperm leads to the fomation of antisperm antibodies against various antigens but not against weak immunogens like LDH-$C_4$,[23] and immunization of animals with heterologous or isologous intact zona pellucida results in antizona antibodies that are not directed against immunogenically weak sperm receptors on the zona pellucida.[24,25]

Antibodies to the right type of antigen(s) can cause a total block of fertility. Many immunoinfertile patients have a complete block of fertility which can be attributed to antisperm antibodies.

The contraceptive approach using sperm specific antigens will probably be reversible either naturally by allowing the immune response to simply wear off or through standard infertility treatments such as abstinence and steroids or even *in vitro* fertilization. Besides, these purified antigens will also help in diagnosis and treatment of involuntary immunoinfertility by specifically neutralizing antisperm antibodies and leaving sperm free for fertilization.

In conclusion, anti-sperm approach constitutes very promising line for development of an immunocontraceptive vaccine. Besides LDH-$C_4$, RSA-1, GA-1, CS-1, the FA-1 constitutes the most promising candidate at the present time. Its homogenity, strong immunogenicity, involvement in involuntary immunoinfertility in humans, and a drastic reduction in fertilization and fertility by antibodies against it are some of the strong points in favor of its candidature.

ACKNOWLEDGEMENTS

The work on GA-1 was done in collaboration with Dr. Alan Menge. We thank Drs. T.M. Phillips, B.B. Rosenblum, Nancy Alexander for useful suggestions. The work on GA-1 was supported in part by grants from the National Institutes of Health Grant HD05200 and on FA-1 by the Program for Applied Research on Fertility Regulation, Northwestern University, under a Cooperative Agreement with the U.S. Agency for International Development (DPE-0546-A-00-1003-00).

REFERENCES

1. A.C. Menge, Clinical immunologic infertility: Diagnostic measures, incidence of antisperm antibodies, fertility mechanisms, in: "Immunological Aspects of Infertility and Fertility Regulation," D.S. Dhindsa and G.F.B. Schumacher, eds., Elsevier-North Holland, New York (1980).

2. S. Katsh, Infertility in female guinea pigs induced by injection of homologous sperm, Am. J. Obstet. Gynecol. 78:276 (1959).

3. R.G. Edwards, Immunological control of fertility in male mice, Nature (London) 203,50 (1964).

4. C.A. Kiddy, and R.M. Rollins, Infertility in female guinea pigs injected with testis, Biol. Reprod. 8,545 (1973).

5. A.C. Menge, Immune reaction and infertility, J. Reprod. Fertil. Suppl. 10,171 (1970).

6. F.N. Syner, B.S. Kuros, and K.S. Moghissi, Active immunization of female rabbits with purified rabbit acrosin and effect on fertility, Fertil Steril. 32,468 (1979).

7. D.B. Morton, and P.A. McAnulty, The effect on fertility of immunizing female sheep with ram sperm acrosin and hyaluronidase, J. Reprod. Immunol. 1.61 (1979).

8. M.G. O'Rand, Inhibition of fertility and sperm-zona binding of antiserum to the rabbit sperm membrane autoantigen RSA-1, Biol. Reprod. 25,621 (1981).

9. E. Goldberg, Effects of immunization with LDH-X on fertility, in: "Immunologic Approaches to Fertility Control," E. Diczfalusy, ed., Karolinska Institute, Stockholm (1974).

10. E. Goldberg, T.E. Wheat, J.E. Powell, and V.C. Stevens Reduction of fertility in female baboons immunized with lactate dehydrogenase-C-4, Fertil. Steril. 35,214 (1981).

11. G. Kohler, and C. Milstein, Derivation of specific antibody-producing tissue culture and tumor lines by cell fusion, Eur. J. Immunol. 6,511 (1976).

12. R.K. Naz, J.M. Saxe, and A.C. Menge, Inhibition of fertility in rabbits by monoclonal antibodies against sperm, Biol. Reprod. 28,249 (1983).

13. J. Friberg, A simple and sensitive micro method for demonstration of sperm - agglutinating activity in serum from infertile men and women, Acta Obstet. Gynecol. Scand. 74,21 (1974).

14. S. Isojima, T.S. Li, and Y. Ashitaka, Immunological analysis of sperm - immobilizing factor found in sera of women with unexplained infertility, Am. J. Obstet. Gynecol. 101,677 (1968).

15. R.K. Naz, C.R. Bradford, and A.C. Menge, Isoantigenicity of rabbit sperm, testis and their extracts as demonstrated by Western blot enzyme immunobinding procedure, Arch. Androl. 13,279 (1985).

16. R.K. Naz, B.B. Rosenblum, and A.C. Menge, Characterization of a membrane antigen from rabbit testis and sperm isolated by using monoclonal antibodies and effect of its antiserum on fertility, Proc. Natl. Acad. Sci., U.S.A. 81,857 (1984).

17. R.K. Naz, R.J. Poffenberger, and A.C. Menge, Reduction of fertility in female rabbits and mice actively immunized with a germ-cell antigen (GA-1) from the rabbit, Biol. Reprod. Submitted.

18. R.K. Naz, N.J. Alexander, M. Isahakia, and M.S. Hamilton, Monoclonal antibody against a human germ cell membrane glycoprotein that inhibits fertilization, Science 225, 342 (1984).

19. R.K. Naz, T.M. Phillips, and B.B. Rosenblum, Characterization of the fertilization antigen (FA-1) isolated from murine testis plasma membrane for the development of an immunocontraceptive vaccine, Proc. Natl. Acad. Sci. U.S.A. Submitted.

20. R.K. Naz, B.A. Littman, and R.J. Stillman, Successful human pregnancy following in vitro fertilization using frozen semen, J. IVF, in press.

21. J.E. Gould, J.W. Overstreet, H. Yanagimachi, R. Yanagimachi, D.F. Katz, and F.W. Hanson, What functions of the sperm cell are measured by in vitro fertilization of zona-free hamster eggs? Fertil. Steril. 40,344 (1983).

22. In: "Research Frontiers in Fertility Regulation," G.I. Zatuchni, ed., PARFR, Chicago (1985).

23. K.S.K. Tung, E.H. Goldberg, E. Goldberg, Immunobiological consequence of immunization of female mice with homologous spermatozoa: Induction of infertility, J. Reprod. Immunol. 1, 14 (1979).

24. K.K. Ahuja, and S.J. Tzartos, Investigation of sperm receptors in the hamster zona pellucida by using univalent (Fab) antibodies to hamster ovary, J. Reprod. Fertil. 61,257 (1981).

25. R.J. Aitken, E. Rudak, D.W. Richardson, J. Dor, O. Djahanbakch, and A.A. Templeton, the influcence of anti-zona and anti-sperm antibodies on sperm-egg interactions, J. Reprod. Fertil. 62,597 (1981).

# CONTRACEPTIVE EFFECT OF TWO ANTI-SPERM MONOCLONAL ANTIBODIES, ADMINISTERED SINGLY AND IN COMBINATION, IN THE MOUSE

Patricia M. Saling, Paula C. Morton, and Robert Waibel

Department of Obstetrics and Gynecology
Duke University Medical Center
Durham, North Carolina 27710

## INTRODUCTION

Although many reports in the literature suggest an association between infertility and anti-sperm antibodies, the particular sperm antigen(s) that may be responsible is unknown. In an effort to sort out this dilemma, as well as to identify sperm components involved specifically at discrete steps of the gamete interaction process, we have generated anti-mouse sperm monoclonal antibodies (mAbs).

Using these mAbs, we have identified two sperm compomemts that are candidates for participation in two different events of the gamete interaction process. One of the mAbs, M29, localizes to the equatorial segment of the sperm head and appears to interfere with fusion between the sperm and egg plasma membranes when examined using *in vitro* fertilization conditions (Saling et al., 1983, 1985a). In contrast, a different anti-sperm mAb, M42, which localizes to the acrosomal crescent, a restricted region of plasma membrane overlying the acrosome, blocks mouse fertilization *in vitro* by preventing sperm penetration through the zona pellucida (Saling and Lakoski, 1985).

Here, we describe the passive effect of these mAbs on mouse fertilization *in vivo* when these reagents are administered either individually or together by intraperitoneal injection.

## MONOCLONAL ANTIBODIES - PRODUCTION, PURIFICATION AND LABELLING

The mAbs used in this study were generated by syngeneic immunization of Balb/c male mice with Balb/c testis homogenized in phosphate buffered saline (PBS), as described previously (Saling et al., 1983, 1985a). The hybridoma cell lines which resulted following the fusion of spleen cells from the immunized male mouse with mouse myeloma cells (X63/Ag8) were screened using indirect immunofluorescence on formaldehyde-fixed cauda epididymal mouse sperm. This procedure selected for the presence of anti-sperm antibodies directed toward antigens that arose in the testis and persisted on the sperm throughout spermatogenesis and epididymal maturation. It also facilitated the detection of mAbs that localize to very restricted domains on the sperm cell. After cloning the appropriate hybridoma lines twice in semi-solid agarose, ascites fluids containing the mAbs in high concentration were produced in Pristane-primed Balb/c mice. These ascites fluids could be diluted greater than 1:20,000 to produce an intense immunofluorescent signal, and were the source of purified mAb used in the experiments described below.

Use of indirect immunofluorescence as a screening technique permitted detection of the localization patterns of the different mAbs from the outset. In the studies presented here, two different pairs of mAbs were used: the first pair, M42 and M41, share the same localization pattern, both being confined to the acrosomal crescent, whereas the second pair, M29 and M2, are both restricted to the equatorial segment. These mAbs were chosen as pairs because of the high degree of similarity that was found between the two mAbs in each pair. For instance, both M42 and M41 display the same tissue and species cross reactivity, antigen solubility characteristics, and immunoglobulin class (although their subclasses differ, i.e., M42 = $IgG_1$ and M41 = $IgG_{2a}$) (Saling and Lakoski, 1985; Saling et al., 1985b). However, the mAbs in each pair differ in two significant aspects: functional capacity and antigen recognition. M42 blocks sperm penetration of the zona pellucida, while M41 has no effect on fertilization; M29 blocks fusion between the sperm and egg plasma membranes, while M2 displays no effect at any level of the fertilization process. Thus, the non-inhibitory mAb in each pair can serve as a control for possible non-specific effects caused by its partner.

Both M2 and M29 belong to the immunoglobulin M class and were purified from ascites fluid by gel filtration on Sephacryl S-300 (Pharmacia) equilibrated with PBS made up to 0.5 M NaCl. Material eluting in the void volume was pooled, concentrated, and washed using a filter with a molecular weight cut-off of 500,000. Both M41 and M42 were purified from ascites fluid chromatographically on Protein A using the MAPS buffer system, as described by Bio-Rad (Richmond, CA). For all purified mAbs, protein concentrations were determined according to the method of Lowry et al. (1951). The purity of the resulting preparations, as assessed electrophoretically on 12% SDS-polyacrylamide gels, was approximately 90%.

To determine the mAb concentration within the mouse oviduct following passive administration of mAb, both M29 and M42 were labelled with $^{125}I$ using Chloramine T as described by Hunter and Greenwood (1962). Iodination was terminated by the addition of metabisulfite. In the case of M29 IgM, labelled material was separated from free iodine by dialysis at 4°C against 3 x 4 liters PBS. For M42 IgG, labelled antibody was separated from free iodine on Sephadex G-10. Both the $^{125}I$-M29 IgM and the $^{125}I$-M42 IgG were used within 4 days of preparation.

## PASSIVE IMMUNIZATION PROTOCOL

For all of the fertilization <u>in vivo</u> studies, CD-1 mice (Charles River Breeding Co.) were used. Superovulation was achieved by injecting female mice (5 - 8 wks) intraperitoneally with 5 I.U. of pregnant mare's serum gonadotropin (PMSG) followed 56 hrs later with 5 I.U. of human chorionic gonadotropin (hCG). The females were housed with males of proven fertility immediately after the hCG injection (2 females/male/cage). The following morning (12-15 hrs later), females were examined for the presence of vaginal copulation plugs; only those females with obvious plugs were included in the study. The females were sacrificed at 40-44 hrs post-hCG injection and the number of eggs/embryos flushed from the excised oviducts was determined. Fertilization was considered to have occurred normally if a 2-cell embryo, or later developmental stage, was observed at that time.

Female mice immunized passively with purified mAb received intraperitoneal injections of antibody (0.5, 1.0, 2.0, or 4.0 mg) in PBS at the time of both the PMSG and the hCG injections; thus, each immunized animal received 2 mAb doses. Regardless of the antibody dose delivered, a constant volume (0.5 ml) was injected into each animal.

## MONOCLONAL ANTIBODY INHIBITION OF FERTILIZATION *IN VIVO*

To determine whether inhibition of a single epitope on sperm is sufficient to generate a significant contraceptive effect, the mAbs, M29 IgM and M42 IgG, were administered individually to female mice. The results of a previous study demonstrated that M29 IgM is capable of producing a significant contraceptive effect following passive immunization (Saling & Waibel, 1985). As shown in Figure 1, it appears that passive administration of M42 IgG effectively reduces fertilization *in vivo* as well. M41 IgG, which displays no effect upon fertilization *in vitro*

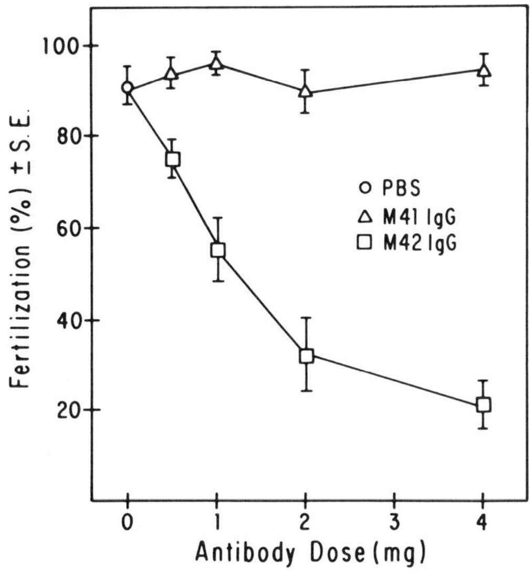


Figure 1: Effect of passive administration of either M41 IgG or M42 IgG upon mouse fertilization *in vivo*. Eggs/embryos were recovered 40-44 hrs post-hCG. The fertilization percentage was determined by dividing the number of embryos observed by the total number of eggs/embryos recovered.

(Saling and Lakoski, 1985), similarly shows no effect upon fertilization *in vivo*. In contrast, increasing doses of M42 IgG led to a significant reduction in the fertilization level. At the maximal M42 IgG dose (4 mg), 21% of 172 ovulated eggs were fertilized, as compared with 95% of 106 eggs in mice immunized with a similar dose of M41. In Figure 2, the effect of passive immunization with both M42 + M29 is shown. In this case, greater inhibition of fertilization is observed at each dosage; for ease of comparison, the fertilization levels achieved with M42 individually and with M29 individually are also shown in Figure 2. At the maximal dose of M42 + M29 (4 mg), 3% of 171 ovulated eggs were fertilized. These 5 fertilized eggs were found in two of the animals in this group; the remaining animals' oviducts contained no fertilized eggs.

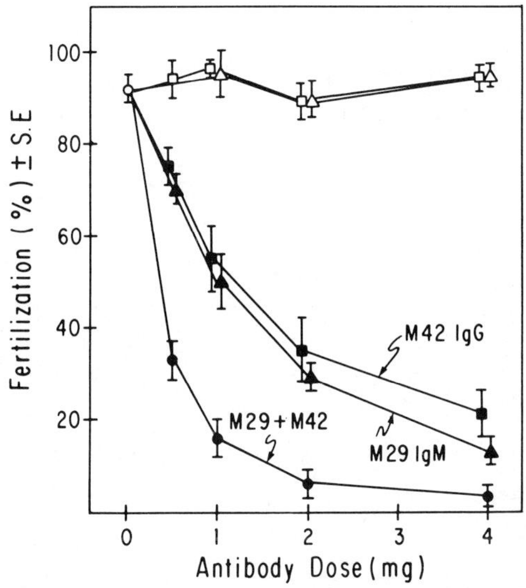


Figure 2: Comparison of the effect of individual administration or combined administration of the monoclonal antibodies M42 IgG and M29 IgM upon mouse fertilization *in vivo*. Eggs/embryos were recovered 40-44 hrs post-hCG. The fertilization percentage was determined by dividing the number of embryos observed by the total number of eggs/embryos recovered.

The possibility exists that the mAbs could exert their anti-fertility effect indirectly by reducing superovulation levels or causing egg degeneration. When the total number of eggs and embryos recovered from the immunized animals was analyzed (Table 1), no specific effect of passive immunization upon superovulation levels could be discerned. However, when the proportion of degenerate eggs in each treatment group was tabulated similarly, there appeared to be a tendency toward egg degeneration with high levels of M42 IgG, either when administered singly, or in combination with M29 IgM (Table 1). At present, we have no insight into this possible trend, particularly since M42 mAb was not found to display cross

TABLE 1

EFFECT OF ANTIBODY INJECTION UPON SUPEROVULATION AND OOCYTE DEGENERATION

| Treatment | Total Number of Eggs Examined | Mean Number of Tubal Eggs per Mouse | Degenerate Oocytes (%) |
|---|---|---|---|
| NONE | 267 | 33.4 | 14 |
| PBS | 281 | 31.2 | 6 |
| M29 IgM | | | |
| 0.5 mg | 257 | 42.8 | 4 |
| 1.0 mg | 247 | 24.7 | 7 |
| 2.0 mg | 251 | 25.1 | 9 |
| 4.0 mg | 304 | 30.4 | 9 |
| M42 IgG | | | |
| 0.5 mg | 181 | 30.1 | 13 |
| 1.0 mg | 248 | 31.0 | 13 |
| 2.0 mg | 243 | 30.4 | 10 |
| 4.0 mg | 172 | 28.6 | 28 |
| M29 IgM + M42 IgG | | | |
| 0.5 mg | 168 | 28.0 | 20 |
| 1.0 mg | 173 | 28.8 | 18 |
| 2.0 mg | 118 | 29.5 | 12 |
| 4.0 mg | 171 | 28.5 | 23 |

Eggs/embryos were flushed from excised oviducts 40-44 hrs post-hCG.

reactivity with ovarian tissue containing mouse eggs. Greater numbers of eggs/embryos need to be examined to examine this possible effect in detail.

## ACCESS OF Ig TO THE OVIDUCTAL LUMEN FOLLOWING INTRAPERITONEAL ADMINISTRATION

To determine the mAb concentration within the tubal lumen following intraperitoneal administration of antibody, female mice were injected according to the immunization schedule described above with a known ratio of unlabelled M29 IgM + $^{125}$I-M29 IgM or with unlabelled M42 IgG + $^{125}$I-M42 IgG. These animals were sacrificed approximately 14-16 hrs post-hCG, a time point close to that of fertilization under the conditions employed. The excised oviducts from these animals were bathed (x2) with 1 ml of Ham's F-10 medium each, blotted dry, cannulated with a blunted 30-gauge needle and then flushed with 0.5 ml of the same medium. The $^{125}$I present in the first and second external oviduct bath, the oviductal tissue itself, and the luminal flush was determined with a Beckman Gamma 5500 counter.

When material flushed from the tubal lumen was assayed, the results shown in Figure 3 were observed: the recovered luminal M42 IgG is close

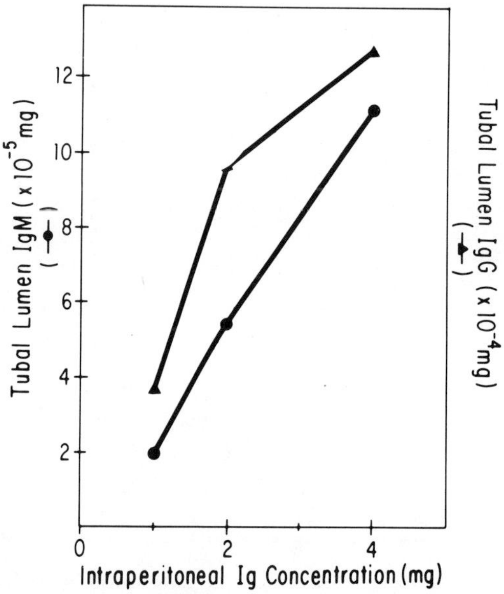


Figure 3: Amount of IgG vs. IgM in the lumen of the oviduct as a function of the Ig dose administered intraperitoneally. Oviducts were flushed 14-16 hrs post-hCG.

to a linear function of the intraperitoneally administered M42 IgG, such that an increase in the intraperitoneal M42 IgG dose increases the luminal M42 IgG amount. Since 95% of the $^{125}$I recovered in the luminal flush samples precipitated with TCA, it is most likely that we are measuring $^{125}$-I coupled to immunoglobulin.

The results of a previous study employing $^{125}$-I-M29 IgM alone are also shown in Figure 3. It is of interest to note that the intraluminal IgG content is consistently one order of magnitude greater than the IgM content at any designated intraperitoneal dose. At present, we do not have an explanation for this difference since it is not yet known by what route(s) the Ig enters the tubal lumen following intraperitoneal administration. Two factors which may influence the amount of IgG vs. IgM found within the tube under these circumstances may be: 1)the difference in half-life for members of these two immunoglobulin classes (Goding, 1983); or 2)the size and aggregation characteristics of the Ig molecules.

## DISCUSSION

Spermatogenesis occurs normally in a physiological compartment separated from the remainder of the organism by the blood-testis barrier. As such, it is a process that is protected from the immune system. One consequence of this arrangement is that the mature, highly differentiated spermatozoon contains antigens that are not recognized as "self". Until hybridoma technology appeared, few techniques were available to generate probes specific for individual autoantigenic sperm components. Currently, ten years after the advent of monoclonal antibodies, numerous reports have now appeared describing anti-sperm mAbs. This ability to examine specific sperm antigens individually is permitting useful investigation into the molecular basis of gamete interaction. Furthermore, this type of inquiry provides a rational basis for the construction of an anti-fertility vaccine.

In our own work with anti-sperm mAbs, we have identified two sperm antigens that appear to participate in separate events in the gamete interaction process. The mAb M29 recognizes a sperm component with subunit $M_r$ of 40,000; this antigen, localized to the equatorial segment of the sperm head, appears to be involved selectively with fusion between the sperm and egg plasma membranes (Saling et al., 1983, 1985a,b). In contrast, the mAb M42 interacts with a doublet or cluster of high molecular weight (220-240,000) sperm components; these antigens, located in a restricted region of the plasma membrane overlying the acrosome, appear to participate in sperm penetration through the zona pellucida (Saling and Lakoski, 1985; Saling et al., 1985b).

The potential utility of employing either or both of these mAbs (or their respective antigens) in the construction of an anti-fertilization vaccine has now been demonstrated: both M29 IgM and M42 IgG produce a significant contraceptive effect, by preventing fertilization, following passive immunization. Moreover, when M29 IgM + M42 IgG are administered together, the effect of their individual inhibitory capability is multiplicative. Prof. J. D. Biggers (1969, 1976) has developed a thoerem to describe the overall effect produced by the inhibition of multiple independent events. A multiplicative effect is predicted by use of this theorem. In the data presented concerning the effect of passive immunization with M29 IgM + M42 IgG, the observed values fall very closely to the predicted values based upon data generated using M29 IgM and M42 IgG individually (see Biggers, J. D., this volume). Because this effect is a multiplicative one, as the number of individual events that are inhibited increases, it can be predicted that much lower doses of each individual component would result in a highly efficacious agent.

We intend to proceed with work toward the eventual development of an immunocontraceptive vaccine by following two related approaches. The first approach will continue our work with anti-sperm mAbs in an attempt to more fully dissect the process of gamete interaction at a molecular level. In this way, we hope to identify the sperm components that participate in other, independent events of the fertilization process. Since it is most likely that active, rather than passive, immunization will be the method of choice for an actual contraceptive vaccine, our second approach will be devoted to purifying the antigens recognized by the mAbs described here. Once sufficient quantities are available, we shall proceed with active immunization studies. Concurrently, we plan to pursue a strategy similar to that illustrated by the elegant work of Goldberg and colleagues (Goldberg, 1983, and this volume; Goldberg et al., 1983) in their work concerning the development of a contraceptive vaccine utilizing a synthetic peptide of LDH-$C_4$, rather than the entire molecule, as immunogen.

Our ultimate goal is the construction of an immunocontraceptive "cocktail", comprised of multiple synthetic components, each component being capable of generating an immune response that will selectively inhibit a specific event in the fertilization process. A considerable amount of work needs to be accomplished before this becomes a reality, but at present sufficient information exists to use this scenario as a rational basis for the design and testing of a contraceptive vaccine.

ACKNOWLEDGEMENTS

The authors are grateful for the constructive criticism and assistance offered by Dr. C. P. Carron and Ms. K. A. Lakoski. This work has been supported by grants from the N.I.H (HD 18201) and the Ford Foundation (820-1096).

REFERENCES

Biggers, J. D., 1969, Are there general principles of contraceptive technology? Proc. Pakistan International Family Planning Conference at Dacca, Jan. 28 - Feb. 4, 1969. pp.283-288.

Biggers, J. D., 1976, General principles of contraceptive technology. IN: "Regulation of Human Fertility." K. S. Moghissi and T. N. Evans, eds. Wayne State University Press: Detroit. pp. 28-56.

Goding, J. W., 1983, "Monoclonal Antibodies: Principles and Practice." Academic Press: New York.

Goldberg, E., 1983, Current status of research on sperm antigens: Potential application as contraceptive vaccines. IN: "Research Frontiers in Fertility Regulation." Zatuchni, G.I., ed. PARFR, Chicago, Ill. Vol. 2, No.6.

Goldberg, E., T. E. Wheat, and V. Gonzales-Prevatt, 1983, Development of a contraceptive vaccine based on synthetic antigenic determinants of lactate dehydrogenase-$C_4$. IN: "Immunology of Reproduction." T. G. Wegman and T. J. Gill, eds. Oxford University Press: New York, pp. 491-504.

Hunter, W. M. and F. C. Greenwood, 1962, Preparation of iodine-131 labelled growth hormone of high specific activity. Nature 194: 495-496.

Lowry, O. H., N. J. Rosebrough, A. L. Farr, and R. J. Randall, 1951, Protein measurement with the Folin Phenol reagent. J. Biol. Chem. 193: 265-275.

Saling, P. M. and K. A. Lakoski, 1985, Mouse sperm antigens that participate in fertilization. II. Inhibition of sperm penetration through the zona pellucida using monoclonal antibodies. Biol. Reprod., in press.

Saling, P. M. and R. Waibel, 1985, Mouse sperm antigens that participate in fertilization. III. Passive immunization with a single monoclonal anti-sperm antibody inhibits pregnancy and fertilization in vivo. Biol. Reprod., in press.

Saling, P. M., L. M. Raines, and M. G. O'Rand, 1983, Monoclonal antibody against mouse sperm blocks a specific event in the fertilization process. J. Exp. Zool. 227: 481-486.

Saling, P. M., G. P. Irons, and R. Waibel, 1985a, Mouse sperm antigens that participate in fertilization. I. Inhibition of sperm fusion with the egg plasma membrane using monoclonal antibodies. Biol. Reprod., in press.

Saling, P. M., R. Waibel, and K. A. Lakoski, 1985b, Immunological identification of sperm antigens that participate in fertilization. IN: "The Molecular and Cellular Biology of Fertilization." J. L. Hedrick, ed. Plenum Press: New York, NY, in press.

# MONOCLONAL ANTIBODIES AGAINST HUMAN SPERM

Gurpreet Singh

National Institute of Immunology
All India Institute of Medical Sciences
New Delhi, India

We have developed a number of monoclonal antibodies (MoAb) against human sperm. 4 of them have been characterized to some extent. In the indirect immunofluorescence, clone $C_1$ reacts with acrosome, Clone $F_{11}G_1$ reacts with the main tail piece, Clone $6SPB_6$ stains the whole sperm and Clone $A_3$ stains the equatorial segment as well as the entire tail. None of the 4 MoAbs give reaction with human peripheral blood lymphocytes, human erythrocytes or human serum proteins in the sandwich type enzyme immunoassay. MoAb $F_{11}G_1$ cross-reacts with monkey and baboon sperm but not with mice, rat or hamster epididymal sperm. MoAb $6SPB_6$ and $A_3$ react with human, monkey and baboon sperm strongly but weakly with rat sperm. However, MoAb $C_1$ was found to react only with human sperm. Their efficacy to prevent fertilization is being tested *in vitro* in zona-free hamster egg system and in baboons *in vivo*.

# THE POTENTIAL EFFECTIVENESS AND SAFETY OF SECOND GENERATION VACCINES

John D. Biggers

Laboratory of Human Reproduction and Reproductive Biology
and Department of Physiology and Biophysics
Harvard Medical School
45 Shattuck Street
Boston, Massachusetts 02115

Several times during this symposium on Immunological Approaches to Contraception and Promotion of Fertility, reference has been made to second generation vaccines (Talwar, 1985). A characteristic of these vaccines is that they simultaneously attack more than one vulnerable site. Intuitively it seems obvious that such a strategy should result in greater efficiency of the vaccine. The magnitude of the gain in efficiency to be expected is less obvious because it will be strongly influenced by the correlations between the effects of the different components.

Second generation contraceptive vaccines are a particular subset of multihit contraceptives defined by Biggers (1969) in which a number of vunerable sites are attacked simultaneously by the joint use of two or more contraceptive agents. Provided the separate agents act independently, a simple probability model can provide an initial framework for the discussion of the gains that can be expected from multihit contraceptive strategies (Biggers, 1973).

The way this model can be used to predict the efficiency of second generation contraceptive vaccines is outlined in this note, illustrated by data presented at this Symposium by Saling et al. (1985). The data concern the action of two passively administered monoclonal antibodies on the fertilization of mouse ova _in vivo_. Antibody M29 blocks mouse fertilization at the plasma membrane, while antibody M42 blocks fertilization at the zona pellucida. The results of the effects of these antibodies separately and jointly on _in vivo_ fertilization are shown in Table 1.

Table 1. The effect on the proportion of mouse ova fertilized in vivo of monoclonal antibodies M29 and M42, given separately and jointly. The observed data are expressed in parentheses as the number of ova unfertilized/number of ova exposed to spermatozoa. (Data of Saling et al., 1985)

| Dose (mg) | Antibody | | |
|---|---|---|---|
| | M29 ($p_1$) | M42 ($p_2$) | (M29+M42) ($J_2$) |
| 0.5 | 0.300 (77/257) | 0.249 (45/181) | 0.673 (113/168) |
| 1.0 | 0.498 (123/247) | 0.452 (112/248) | 0.838 (145/173) |
| 2.0 | 0.709 (178/251) | 0.679 (165/243) | 0.941 (111/118) |
| 4.0 | 0.868 (264/304) | 0.791 (136/172) | 0.971 (166/171) |

Let $p_1$ and $p_2$ be the probabilities of antibodies M29 and M42 blocking fertilization when used individually. If the two antibodies act independently, the probability of their blocking fertilization when administered simultaneously is given by:

$$\begin{aligned} J_2 &= p_1 + (1-p_1)\ _2. \\ &= p_2 + (1-p_2)p_1 \\ &= 1 - (1- p_1)(1-p_2). \qquad (1) \end{aligned}$$

Estimates of $p_1$, $p_2$ and $J_2$ (observed) have been calculated from the observations for the four doses of antibody shown in Table 1. The values of $p_1$ and $p_2$ have then been inserted in equation (1) to estimate $J_2$ (expected). The results are summarized in Table 2. As reported by Saling et al. (1985), the combination of two antibodies is much more effective in blocking fertilization than using them singly. However, the model defined by equation (1) only predicts the outcome of joint administration for the two higher doses of antibody used. At the two lower doses the probability of fertilization failure when both antibodies are used is very significantly underestimated, suggesting that at these doses the two antibodies are not acting independently. The reason for this dosage effect needs further study.

Table 2. Values of $J_2$ (observed) estimated from the data of Table 1, and the value of $J_2$ (expected) calculated using equation (1).

| Dose (mg) | $J_2$ (Observed) | $J_2$ (Expected) | $\chi^2_{[1]}$ |
|---|---|---|---|
| 0.5 | 0.673 | 0.474 | 26.63*** |
| 1.0 | 0.838 | 0.725 | 11.13*** |
| 2.0 | 0.941 | 0.907 | 1.60 |
| 4.0 | 0.971 | 0.972 | 0.01 |

***P<0.001

Equation (1) can be generalized for the case of $n$ simultaneously administered antibodies. Let each antibody be given in a dosage expected to render a proportion $p_i$ ( $i = 1,2,\ldots,n$) of a population infertile. If the antibodies produce their effect independently, then their joint effectiveness is given by:

$$J_2 = 1 - \prod_{i=1}^{n} (1-p_i). \qquad (2)$$

A special case of (2) is when all antibodies are equally effective. Here

$$J_n = 1 - (1-p)^n$$

By expressing $p$ as a function of $J_n$ and $n$, we obtain

$$p = 1 - (1- J_n)^{1/n}.$$

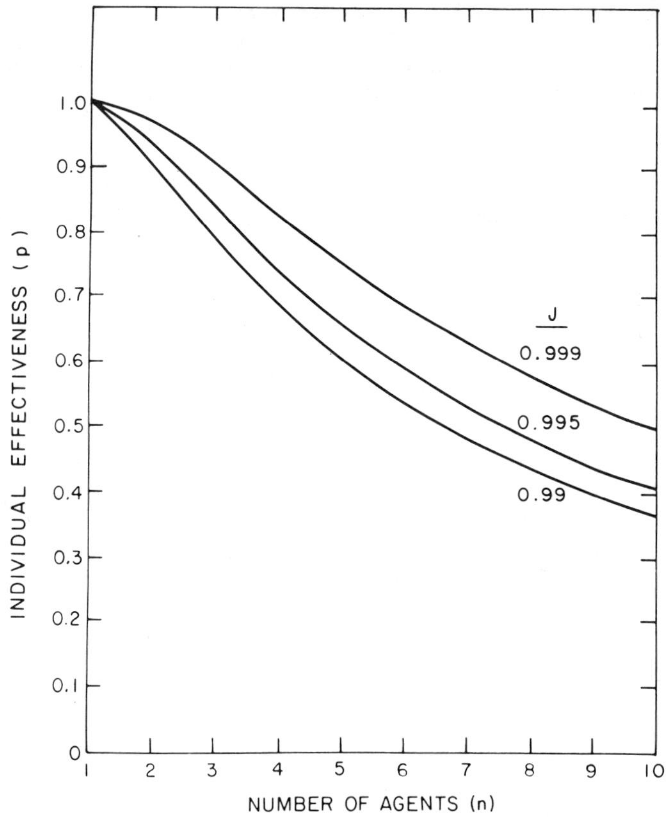


Figure 1. The relation between the number of agents ($n$) used simultaneously, and the required level of individual effectiveness of each agent ($p$), required to ensure a desired overall probability of infertility ($J$). It is assumed that the individual effectiveness ($p$) of all agents is equal. (From Biggers, 1976)

Figure 1 shows the dependency between $p$ and $n$ for several values of overall effectiveness ($J$). It is clear that very high levels of effectiveness can be achieved by the combination of a relatively low number of antibodies at levels which individually are relatively ineffective. Thus by combining three agents, each of 84 percent individual effectiveness, an overall effectiveness of 99.5 percent effectiveness can be expected.

The ability to use doses of antibodies in combination that are only partially effective may also have the additional, very significant advantage of reducing the incidence of undesirable side effects. A simulation analysis of a parametric model representing the distributions of the threshold doses resulting in infertility and undesirable effects, when several contraceptive agents are used simultaneously in sub-maximal doses, suggests that the incidence of undesirable effects may fall exponentially as the number of vulnerable sites blocked is increased (Biggers, 1976).

## ACKNOWLEDGMENT

I am indebted to Dr. Patricia M. Saling for the data shown in Table 1.

## REFERENCES

Biggers, J.D. (1969). Are there general principles of contraceptive technology? Proc. Pakistan Intern. Family Planning Conf., Dacca, 1969:283-288.

Biggers, J.D. (1973). Reproductive biology and human welfare. Perspectives Biol. Med. 16: 630-649.

Biggers, J.D. (1976). General principles of contraceptive technology. In: Moghissi, K.S. and Evans, T.N., eds. Regulation of Human Fertility. Detroit: Wayne State University Press, 1976:28-56.

Saling, P.M., Morton, P.C., and Waibel, R. (1985). Contraceptive effect of two antisperm monoclonal antibodies, administered singly and in combination, in the mouse. This volume.

Talwar, G.P. (1985). The Need, Basic Premise, and Over-view. This volume.

# FACTORS AFFECTING THE GENERATION AND CONTRACEPTIVE EFFECTIVENESS OF IMMUNE RESPONSES TO SPERM

Deborah J. Anderson

Fearing Research Laboratory
Department of Obstetrics and Gynecology
Harvard Medical School, Boston, MA 02115

## INTRODUCTION

In recent years it has been demonstrated that anti-sperm immunity is often associated with infertility in men and women, and a number of immunogenic sperm-specific antigens have been identified and characterized. It is now possible to mass produce these antigens by genetic engineering technology for use in contraceptive vaccine trials. However, knowledge of the complexities of the immune system and the manipulation of immune responses especially in the reproductive tissues lags considerably behind these more precise technological advances. Male and female reproductive tissues are naturally potential immunologic targets protected by immunologic barriers, immunosuppressive factors and possibly other immunoregulatory mechanisms. This area remains a largely unexplored research frontier and it is likely that considerable research on fundamental questions of reproductive immunology shall have to be performed before an effective contraceptive vaccine can be developed. In this chapter, I review certain classical immunologic considerations in the development of vaccines, focusing on immunological peculiarities of reproductive tissues and their antigens that require special consideration.

### Physical and Biochemical Immunological Barriers in Reproductive Tissues

The blood-testis barrier system of the male reproductive tract, comprised of tight junction-interlaced Sertoli cells in the testis, and interdigitated epithelial cells in the rete testis, epididymides and vas deferens (Dym, 1973; Hamilton, 1975), excludes high molecular weight molecules (ie: antibody and complement) and immunocompetent cells from the germ cell compartment. It is likely that the blood-testis barrier would protect the male reproductive tract form humoral and cellular immune responses generated by sperm antigen-based vaccines. This barrier system is most competent at the level of the testis; in some species the epididymis appears to be permeable at least to antibody (Weininger et al., 1982). The permeability of the human epididymis to immunologic cells and factors has not been systematically investigated. Potent immunosuppressive factors can also be bound in male reproductive tissues, and may serve as a backup mechanism to suppress immune responses directed against germ cell antigens. Different immunosuppressive factors are found in the epididymis, prostate and seminal vesicle (Anderson and Tarter, 1982; Tarter and Isahakia, 1982); these seminal plasma factors inhibit natural killer cell activity (Glater and Anderson,

1985; James and Ssymaniec, 1985), macrophage function (James et al., 1983), lymphocyte activation by mitogens and antigens (Anderson and Tarter, 1982; Stites and Erickson, 1975; Lord et al., 1972) and complement-dependent antibody cytotoxicity in vitro (Tarter and Alexander, 1982), and humoral immune responses to sperm and other antigens in vivo (Anderson and Tarter, 1982). It appears that such immunosuppressive factors not only would interfere with the generation and effect of immune responses directed against sperm in the male, but also with antisperm immune responses in the female reproductive tract.

The female reproductive tract does not contain tight junction physical barriers and therefore is more accessible to cells and soluble mediators of immunological responses; however, there is evidence that complement levels are insufficient to achieve complement-mediated cytolysis by antibody at midcycle in the cervix (Murdoch et al., 1982), and that uterine glands produce immunosuppressive factors that could block humoral as well as cellular immune responses (Bulmer and Johnson, in press). Therefore, although it appears that the female reproductive tract is accessible to immunologic factors which could affect fertility, mechanisms could exist to naturally block mediators of such responses and could interfere with vaccine effectiveness.

## Immunogenetic Influences on Antisperm Antibody Responses

Immune response (Ir) genes can regulate immune responses to foreign antigens. They were discovered through experiments which demonstrated that certain strains of inbred mice characteristically produced high antibody titers to a particular well-defined synthetic polypeptide antigen, while other strains made intermediate or undetectable responses. This effect was antigen dependent; strains developing high titers to one antigen were often low responders to other kinds of antigens that elicited high responses to other kinds of antigens that elicited high responses in other strains of mice. Genetic backcross studies mapped the Ir genes to a single autosomal dominant region mapping between H-2K and Ss loci of the Major Histocompatibility Complex on chromosome 17 of the mouse. A comparable genetic region, HLA-D, has been mapped to chromosome 6 in man. The gene products of the Ir regions of mice and men are involved in antigen presentation, and several theories have been proposed for mechanisms of immune response regulation by Ir gene products (recently reviewed by Anderson, in press).

Sperm immunization studies in genetically defined inbred strains of experimental animals have revealed high and low responder strains, providing evidence that humoral immune responses to sperm antigens are genetically controlled. In many of the studies, genetic backcross studies are difficult to interpret because complex antigen mixtures (ie: homogenized tissues) were used. Using a single sperm antigen as an immunogen, and highly inbred experimental animal strains, Tung et al. (1981) and Kille et al. (1978) found no MHC association in humoral immune responses to single testicular antigens, TSDA and LDH-C4 respectively, suggesting that non-MHC genetic loci may be involved in regulating anti-sperm immune responses. Teuscher et al. (in press) recently reported that experimental autoimmune orchitis induced in mice by administration of a combination of Bordetella pertussis and testicular antigens is controlled by at least 2 genes: a disease susceptibility gene mapping to the H-2 region, and a disease resistance gene controlled by a non-MHC associated region in orchitis-resistant strains. Studies by Taguchi and Nishizuka (1981) demonstrated that certain (not all) inbred strains of mice develop antisperm antibodies and autoimmune orchitis at puberty if they are given thymectomies shortly after birth, a procedure which reduces peripheral suppressor T cell levels. These results indicate that humoral immune responses to sperm and testicular antigens may be tightly regulated by suppressor cells, and that evaluation of the immunogenetic factors in antisperm immunity must separate genetic effects on this mechanism from genetic effects governing antibody production.

When dealing with complex antigen systems such as whole sperm immunization protocols, it is useful to use Western blots to analyze antibody responses directed against individual antigens in complex immunizing materials. Through such an approach we have shown striking interstrain heterogeneity in sperm antigens generating humoral immune responses in mice of different genetic backgrounds (Madrigal et al., in press; Fig. 1). Vasectomy has provided a model in which antisperm immunity in men can be studied, although it is based on a complex antigen system. Sperm continue to be produced after vasectomy, and often stimulate high titers of antisperm antibodies that persist for several years (Alexander and Anderson, 1979). However, only 40-60% of vasectomized men develop detectable antisperm antibodies (Alexander, 1977); men that fail to develop antibodies may represent a nonresponder population. One group has reported an association between antisperm antibodies in vasectomized men and the HLA phenotypes A-28 and B-22, providing evidence that human antisperm antibody responses may be regulated by MHC-associated genes. We detected highly heterogeneous antibody patterns in Western blot analyses of human antisperm antibodies from infertile women and vasectomized men (Fig.s 2a & 2b) indicating that natural sperm immunization is a complex model with qualitative as well as quantitative differences in response.

Do sperm antigens induce immunological tolerance?

This area has not been adequately explored, but several experimental findings indicate that sperm may induce immunological responses of a protective rather than harmful nature. Hertenbach et al. (1980) showed that autologous murine testicular germ cells induce tolerance in vitro, and also that sperm, when administered intravenously to mice, induce immune paralysis in vivo (Hertenbach and Shearer 1982). Ritchie et al. (1984) recently reported that interstitial tissues of the human epididymis are lined with $T8^+$ lymphocytes (suppressor T cell phenotype) indicating that suppressor T cells may be attracted to or activated by male reproductive tissues. We have found that supernatants of cultures of washed sperm suppress T cell and humoral immune responses (Pham and Anderson, unpublished). Taguchi et al., as mentioned in a previous section, demonstrated that neonatally thymectomized male mice of certain inbred strains will spontaneously develop autoimmune orchitis and epididymitis after puberty, and that this effect is abrogated by administration of syngeneic T cells (Taguchi and Nishizuka, 1981; Sakaguchi et al., 1985). Neonatal thymectomy, when performed between days 3 and 5 after birth, affects T cell development and results in a reduction in peripheral levels of suppressor T cells; thus, Taguchi's studies indicate that suppressor cells may be activated in normal males to suppress immune responses directed against testicular germ cells and sperm. This hypothesis is further supported by the research finding that male mice generally produce lower levels of antisperm antibodies than female mice after immunization with syngeneic sperm (Madrigal et al., in press; Marsh, 1981). That sperm antigens could elicit immunosuppressive rather than immunostimulation responses underscores the need for detailed studies of immune response kinetics in individuals immunized with sperm antigen vaccines.

Cell-mediated Antisperm Immunity

Most of the attention to immunologic mechanisms in infertility has been focused on antibody-mediated effects on fertility. However, cell-mediated immunological responses can be elicited by immunization using appropriate adjuvants, and the few reports that exist on the effects of anti-sperm cell-mediated immune responses on fertility indicate that such mechanisms could provide effective contraceptive protection. Cellular immune responses to

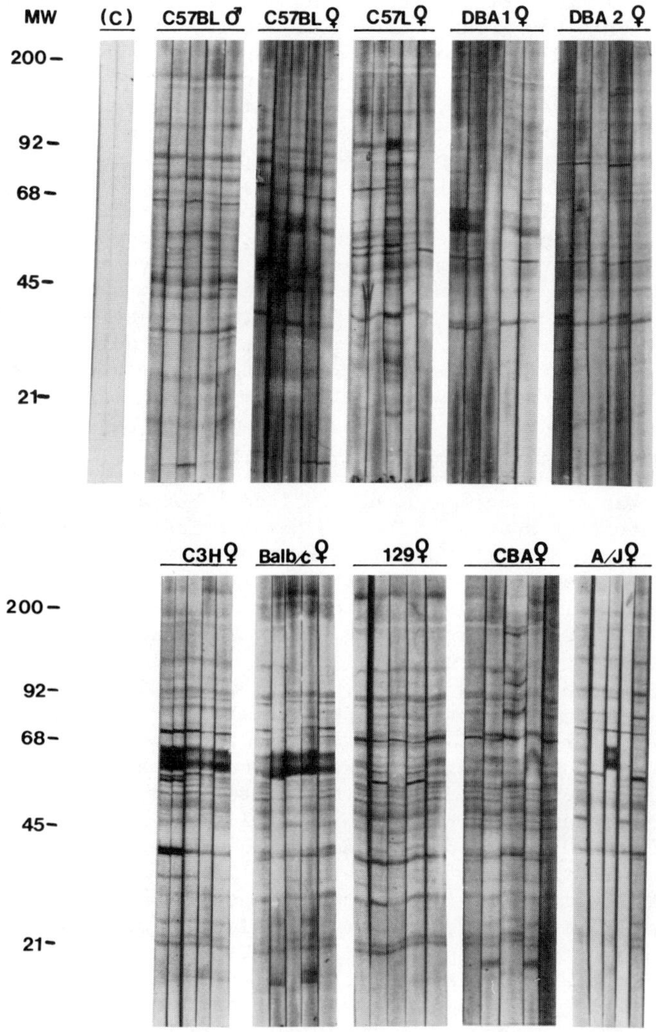


Fig. 1. Western blot profiles of individual sera from mice of several inbred strains that were immunized with syngeneic sperm in complete Freund's adjuvant. This technique reveals the complexity of the anti-sperm immune response and demonstrates striking inter- and intrastrain heterogeneity in response.

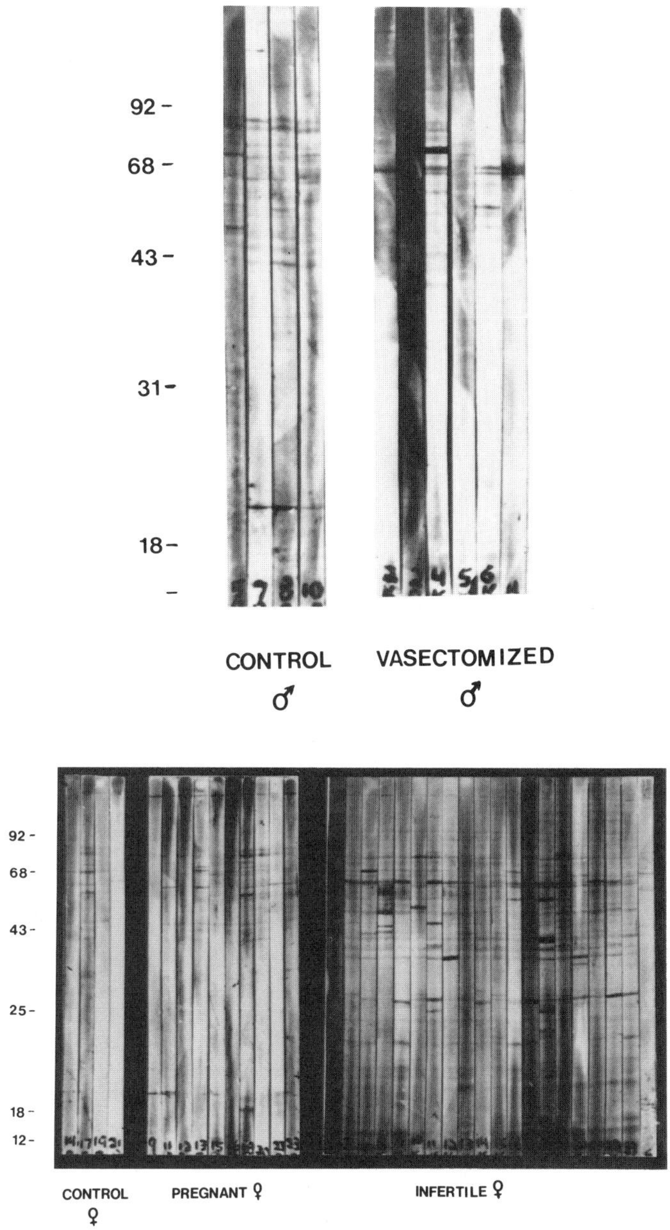


Fig. 2a. Western blot profiles of sperm-antibody-positive human vasectomy sera (6 out of 110 tested were positive) and sperm-antibody-negative nonvasectomized male control sera (4 most positive of 30).

2b. Western blot profiles of sperm-antibody-positive infertility sera (20/64), pregnancy sera and control sera (4/40) tested against sperm extracts (single donor). 25KD and 40 KD bands react with several infertililty sera. However, for the most part, reactivity patterns are extremely heterogeneous.

sperm antigens (measured by lymphokine release) have been detected in sperm-immunized experimental animals with impaired fertility (Dorsman et al., 1978), and in vasectomized men (Anderson et al., 1982; Nagarkatti and Rao, 1976) and infertile women (McShane et al., 1985). It is unlikely that activated cytotoxic lymphocytes directly kill spermatozoa since sperm do not express major histocompatibility Class I antigens which are required for cellular recognition by cytotoxic T cells (Anderson et al., 1982; Anderson et al., 1984), and because sperm migrate faster than lymphocytes. However, we have obtained preliminary data indicating that soluble mediators (lymphokines) produced by sperm-antigen-sensitized lymphocyte cultures from infertile women have adverse effects on sperm and embryo viability. It could turn out that cell-mediated antisperm immune responses are at least as effective as antibodies in achieving infertility effects.

## Environmental Factors that Influence Immune Responses to Reproductive Antigens

Prior exposure to an antigen (or a cross-reactive antigen) is an important parameter in predicting the effect of a vaccine. Prior exposure to sperm antigens could tolerize the host to subsequent antigen challenges (as may be the case in male mice immunized after puberty with sperm), or could sensitize the host so that a very vigorous secondary immune response is produced by the vaccine. It is critical to avoid IgE immune responses as these could lead to severe anaphylactic type reactions with reappearance of the antigen (ie: during intercourse). Recent advances in understanding the control of IgE immune responses was recently reviewed by Tung (in press). Patients with various types of immunodeficiencies as well as patients with parasitic infections are predisposed to isotype-specific IgE responses. It is therefore possible that a high incidence of IgE responses and anaphlactic type reactions may be seen in vaccinated populations suffering from malnutrition or parasites. Furthermore, some adjuvants such as alum preferentially elicit high IgE responses (Ishizaka, 1976) and must be avoided. Other factors that affect immune responses to vaccines include: the presence of bacterial infection at the injection site, the amount of antigen administered, route of administration and state of antigen (ie: degradation before immunization).

## Ways to optimize the antifertility efficacy and acceptability of a contraceptive vaccine based on sperm antigens

Variability in immune responses in an immunized population due to genetic or environmental influences can be minimized through a number of approaches:

1) Selection of appropriate adjuvant. Through use of different adjuvants (agents that act nonspecifically to increase specific immune responses to an antigen), different types of immune responses can be achieved. Adjuvants such as complete Freund's adjuvant enhance the antigen presenting capabilities of macrophages and other antigen-presenting cells and thus can overcome genetic (Ir) restrictions operating at that level. However, adjuvants that enhance antibody production and helper T cell function can depress the generation of cytotoxic T cell responses, possibly due to the stimulation of specific supppressor cells (Reinisch et al., 1976). Another class of adjuvants such as lipopolysaccharide (LPS) are polyclonal B cell activators that bypass the need for helper T cells, and may be useful in boosting already existing immunologic responses (Allison, 1979). Other adjuvants selectively activate mediators of cell-mediated immune responses (Allison, 1979).

2) Use of multiple epitope (antigenic determinant) vaccines would

improve the chance of achieving an immune response in a population heterogeneous in Ir gene status (see chapters by Saling and Biggers in this volume).

3) Lymphokines can be administered with the vaccine to boost immune responses. For example, $\gamma$-interferon enhances Ia expression on antigen presenting cells, and Il-2 partially bypasses the need for helper T cell activation in secondary immune responses (Janeway et al., 1984; Robb, 1984). It was recently demonstrated that administration of Il-2 at the site of antigen injection causes greatly enhanced antibody production in low-responder strains of animals (Kawamura et al., 1985).

4) Use of anti-idiotype antibodies in place of antigen. These antibodies can directly bind to specific antigen receptors on helper T cells and B cells, and bypass the need for antigen processing and presentation by macrophages (Roth et al., 1983; Cunningham, 1980).

5) Quality control of vaccine and standardization of immunization methods. Followup tests measuring IgE and cell-mediated immune responses to the antigen in addition to IgG and IgM responses.

## SUMMARY

It may be difficult to reproducibly achieve antifertility effects with reproductive-antigen based vaccines because of the numerous host defense mechanisms which have evolved to protect against such immune responses. Undoubtedly, however, a better understanding of immunological mechanisms of infertility will evolve from further studies on reproductive tissue:host interactions in experimental animals and man.

## ACKNOWLEDGEMENTS

Research described in this report was supported by NIH grants CA32132 and AICA 21141. I am grateful to Deirdre Meehan who assisted with the preparation of this manuscript.

## REFERENCES

Alexander, N.J., 1977, Summary of effects of vasectomy recorded in a number of species including man, in: "Immunological Influence on Human Fertility", p. 242, B. Boettcher, ed., Acad. Press, New York.

Alexander, N.J. and Anderson, D.J., 1979, Vasectomy: Consequences of autoimmunity to sperm antigens, Fertil. Steril., 32:253-260.

Allison, A.C., 1979, Mode of action of immunological adjuvants, J. Reticuloendothel. Soc., 26:619-630.

Anderson, D.J., Alexander, N.J., Fulgham, D.L., Vandenbark, A.A. and Berger, D.R., 1982, Immunity to tumor-associated antigens in vasectomized men, J. Natl. Cancer Inst., 69:551.

Anderson, D.J., Bach, D., Yunis, E.J. and DeWolf, W.C., 1982, Major Histocompatibility antigens are not expressed on human epididymal sperm, J. Immunol., 129:452.

Anderson, D.J. and Tarter, T.H., 1982, Immunosuppressive effects of mouse seminal plasma components *in vivo* and *in vitro*, J. Immunol., 128:535.

Anderson, D.J., Narayan, P. and DeWolf, W.C., 1984, Major Histocompatibility antigens are not detectable on post-meiotic human testicular germ cells, J. Immunol., 133:1962.

Anderson, D.J., in press, Immunogenetic considerations in the development of contraceptive vaccines based on testicular sperm anitgens, in: "Male Contraception: Advances and Future Prospects", G.I. Zatuchni, A. Goldsmith, J.M. Spieler and J.J. Sciarra, eds., Harper and Row Publishers, Philadelphia.

Bulmer, J. and Johnson, P.M., submitted.
Cunningham, A.J., 1980, Reliable vaccines using hybridoma products with defined idiotypes, in: "Strategies of Immune Regulation", p. 497, E. Sercarz, A.J. Cunningham, eds., Acad. Press, New York.
Dorsman, B.G., Tumbh-Oeri, A.G. and Roberts, T.K., 1978, Detection of cell-mediated immunity to spermatozoa in mice and man by the leukocyte adherance-inhibition test, J. Reprod. Fertil., 53:277.
Dym, M, 1973, The fine structure of the monkey (Macaca) Sertoli cell and its role in maintaining the blood-testis barrier, Anat. Rec., 175:639.
Glater, G.B. and Anderson, D.J., 1985, Human seminal plasma inhibits the cytotoxic effect of natural killer (NK) cells, J. Androl., 6:57.
Hamilton, D.W. 1975, Structure and function of the epithelium lining the ductuli efferentes, ductus epididymidis and ductus deferens in the rat, in: "Handbook of Physiology, Section 7, Endocrinology, Vol V, Male Reproductive System", P. 259, R.O. Greep, Amer. Physiol. Soc., Washington D.C..
Hertenbach, U., Morgenstern, F. and Bennett, D., 1980, Induction of tolerance in vitro by autologous murine testicular cells, J. Exp. Med., 151:1827.
Hertenbach, U. and Shearer, G.M., 1982, Germ cell-induced immune suppression in mice, effect of innoculation of syngeneic spermatozoa on cell-mediated immune responses, J. Exp. Med., 155:1719-1729.
Ishizaka, K., 1976, Cellular events in the IgE antibody response, Adv. Immunol., 23:1.
James, K., Harvey, J., Bradbury, A.W., Hargreave, T.B., Cullen, R.T. and Donaldson K., 1983, The effect of seminal plasma on macrophage function - a possible contributory role in sexually transmitted disease, AIDS Res., 1:45.
James, K. and Ssymaniec, S., 1985, Human seminal plasma is a potent inhibitor of natural killer cell activity _in vitro_, J. Reprod. Immunol., 8:61.
Janeway, C.A., Bottomly, K., Babich, J., Conrad, P., Conzen, S., Jones, B., Kaye, J., Katz, M., McVay, L., Murphy, D.B. and Tite, J., 1984, Quantitative variation in Ia antigen expression plays a central role in immune regulation, Immunol. Today, 5:99-105.
Kawamura, H., Rosenberg, S.A. and Berzofsky, J.A., 1985, Immunization with antigen and interleukin 2 in vivo overcomes Ir gene low responsiveness, J. Exp. Med., 162:381-386.
Kille, J.W., Wheat, T.E., Mitchell, G. and Goldberg, E., 1978, Strain differences in the immune response of mice to homologous sperm-specific lactate dehydrogenase (LDH-C4), Exp. Zool., 204:259-266.
Lord, E.M., Sensabaugh, G.P. and Stites, D.P., 1977, Immunosuppressive activity of human seminal plasma I. inhibition of _in vitro_ lymphocyte activation, J. Immunol., 118:1704.
Madrigal, J.A., Yunis, E.J. and Anderson, D.J., in press, Genetic effects on sperm immunity: Quantitative and qualitative differences in sperm antibody responses in mice of different inbred strains and sexes, J. Reprod. Immunol.
Marsh, J.A., O'Hern, P. and Goldberg, E., 1981, The role of an x-linked gene in the regulation of secondary humoral response kinetics to sperm specific LDH-C4 antigen, J. Immunol., 126:100.
McShane, P.M., Schiff, I. and Trentham, D., 1985, Cellular immunity to sperm in infertile women, J.A.M.A., 253:3555.
Murdoch, A.J.M., Buckley, C.H. and Fox, H., 1982, Hormonal control of the secretory immune system of the human uterine cervix, J. Reprod. Immunol., 4:23.
Nagarkatti, R.S. and Rao, S.S., 1976, Cell-mediated immunity to homologous spermatozoa following vasectomy in the human male, Clin. Exp. Immunol., 26:239.
Reinisch, C.L., Gleiner, N.A. and Schlossman, S.F., 1976, Adjuvant Regulation of T cell function, J. Immunol., 116:710-715.

Ritchie, A.W.S., Hargreave, T.B., James, K. and Chisholm, G.D., 1984, Intraepithelial lymphocytes in the normal epdidiymis. A mechanism for tolerance to sperm auto-antigens?, Brit. J. Urol., 56:79-83.

Robb, R.J., 1984, Interleukin 2: the molecule and its function, Immunol. Today, 5:203-209.

Roth, C., Somme, G. and Theze, J., 1983, Induction of an anti-GAT response in genetically responder and nonresponder mouse strains by monoclonal anti-idiotypic antibodies, Table Ronde Roussel U.C.L.A.F., 48:465.

Sakaguchi, S., Fukuma, K., Kuribayashi, K. and Masuda, T., 1985, Organ-specific autoimmune diseases induced in mice by elimination of T cell subset 1. Evidence for the active participation of T cell in natural self-tolerance, deficit of a T cell subset as a possible cause of autoimmune disease, J. Exp. Med., 161:72-87.

Stites, D.P. and Erickson, R.P., 1975, Suppressive effect of seminal plasma on lymphocyte activation, Nature, 253:727.

Taguchi, O. and Nishizuka, Y., 1981, Experimental autoimmune orchitis after neonatal thymectomy in the mouse, Clin. Exp. Immunol., 46:425.

Tarter, T.H. and Alexander, N.J., 1982, Complement-inhibiting activity of seminal plasma, Am. J. Reprod. Immunol., 6:28.

Tarter, T.H. and Isahakia, M., 1982, Inhibtion of complement-mediated hemolysis by aqueous extracts of monkey prostate and seminal vesicle, J. Androl., 3:10.

Teuscher, C., Smith, S.M., Goldberg, E.H., Shearer, G.M. and Tung, K.S.K, in press, Experimental autoimmune orchitis in mice: genetic control of susceptibility and resistance to induction of orchitis.

Tung, K.S.K., Teuscher, C., Goldgerg, E.H. and Wild, G., 1981, Genetic control of antisperm autoantibody response in vasectomized quinea pigs, J. Immunol., 127:835.

Tung, K.S.K., in press, Immunopathologic consideration of anti-fertility vaccine, in: "Male Contraception: Advances and Future Prospects", G.I. Zatuchni, A. Goldsmith, J.M. Spieler and J.J. Sciarra, eds.

Weininger, R.B., Fisher, S., Rifkin, J. and Bedford, J.M., 1982, Experimental studies on the passage of specific IgG to the lumen of the rabbit epididymis, J. Reprod. Fertil., 66:251-258.

# IMMUNOSUPPRESSION OF FERTILITY BY LDH-$C_4$

Erwin Goldberg and Joyce A. Shelton

Dept of Biochemistry, Molecular Biology & Cell Biology
Northwestern University
Evanston, Illinois 60201
U. S. A.

The natural response of the immune system to foreign proteins can be exploited in the development of a vaccine for control of fertility. Potential target antigens for such a vaccine include those that are found specifically on the surface of sperm and are absent from somatic tissues (reviewed by Aitken, 1982, Goldberg, 1983, Anderson and Alexander, 1983). Such antigens are uniquely suited to incorporation into a vaccine that may be applicable to both male and female use. They do not appear in the male until spermatogenesis begins, which is after the immune system has already become tolerant to "self-antigens". Even after they appear, they are isolated from the male immune system by the blood-testes barrier. They are not found at all in female tissues. Thus these antigens can provoke antibody formation in either males or females. Furthermore, a vaccine would have the advantage over currently available contraceptive methodologies of not interfering with hormonal and metabolic functions.

Although potential for a male-directed vaccine exists, emphasis has been placed on a vaccine suitable for use in the female. This is primarily due to difficulties in accessing the testicular compartment by circulating anti-sperm antibodies and possibilities of autoimmune inflammatory complications. Numerous studies document that infertility in females can be induced by immunization with sperm and sperm extracts (reviewed by Jones, 1982; Tung, 1983). In addition, there are many reports of antibodies to sperm being found in the sera of infertile men and women (reviewed by Beer and Neaves, 1979, Jones, 1980). These studies indicate the feasibility of using sperm antigens for immunological impairment of fertility; however, the development of a vaccine requires a pure antigen preparation. Therefore, more recent studies have emphasized the isolation and purification of sperm-specific proteins that may play a role in the fertilization process.

Both polyclonal and monoclonal antibodies have been used to identify and to isolate sperm antigens. These studies have been reviewed extensively by Goldberg (1983) and will only be highlighted here. Polyclonal antibodies have been used by O'Rand and his associates to isolate RSA-1, a 13kD protein found on rabbit sperm that appears to be involved in sperm penetration of the zona pellucida (O'Rand, 1981; O'Rand and Romrell, 1981; O'Rand and Porter, 1982). When antibody treated sperm are used to inseminate female rabbits, a 68% decrease in fertility results. *In vitro* fertilization is also inhibited (O'Rand, 1981). Monoclonal antibodies were raised against RSA-1 and two other sperm antigens RSA-2 and RSA-3. The monoclonals interfered with *in vitro* fertilization (O'Rand et al., 1984) and were reactive with human sperm (O'Rand and Irons, 1984).

Hybridoma technology, the production of monoclonal antibodies of high specificity, has been utilized extensively for antigen purification. Some examples of the use of monoclonal antibodies include isolation of FA-1 antigen from human sperm and testes by Naz et al. (1984; and this symposium). The monoclonal antibody to this antigen interferes with *in vitro* fertilization of mouse ova by mouse sperm and penetration of hamster ova by human sperm. Wolf et al. (1983) have found an antigen on the post-acrosomal region and midpiece of sperm with a monoclonal antibody. This antigen may be involved in capacitation. An 84 kD antigen shared by human, hamster and rabbit sperm has been detected by Saling et al. (1983). The antibody blocks egg penetration *in vitro*. These are only a few of the many sperm antigens to which monoclonal antibodies have been produced. However, while numerous antigens have been identified, few have been well-characterized. The major obstacle to progress in all of these investigations has been the inability to isolate enough pure antigen for further immunological and biochemical evaluation. Until this technical problem can be overcome, the limited availability of these antigens precludes an adequate assessment of their practical use in a contraceptive vaccine.

At present, the most completely characterized sperm antigen and the most promising candidate for an immunological contraceptive is the sperm-specific lactate dehydrogenase (LDH-$C_4$). This enzyme is readily isolated from the testes of mice and other animals and can be purified in relatively large quantities (Wheat and Goldberg, 1977). These factors have allowed extensive biochemical and immunological evaluation of this enzyme (Goldberg, 1977; Wheat and Goldberg, 1983; 1985).

Biochemical characterization has revealed that the LDH-$C_4$ molecule is composed of four identical subunits (Musick and Rossmann, 1979a). The three-dimensional structure of these subunits has been determined by X-ray crystallography (Musick and Rossmann, 1979b). Complete primary sequences are also available for both mouse and rat LDH-$C_4$ (Li et al., 1983a). The LDH-$C_4$ subunit is relatively homologous structurally to its LDH-A and LDH-B somatic isozymes (Li et al., 1983b) and they can form heterotetramers *in vitro* (Goldberg, 1977). However, there are major changes in the amino acid sequence of LDH-$C_4$ (Eventoff et al., 1977). Such primary sequence substitutions and ensuing modifications in its three dimensional structure account for the total lack of immunological cross-reactivity among LDH-$C_4$ and its somatic isozymes (Goldberg, 1971; Liang et al. in preparation). Thus, the immune response to LDH-$C_4$ is absolutely sperm-specific.

Previous studies designed to evaluate the immune response to LDH-$C_4$ have shown that parenteral immunization of males and females with mouse LDH-$C_4$ in combination with an adjuvant results in serum antibody production (Goldberg, 1971). These antibodies will react directly with LDH-$C_4$ on the surface of sperm (Beyler et al., 1985). Alvarez and Storey (1984) have determined biochemically that approximately 10% of LDH-$C_4$ activity is associated with the sperm plasma membrane and immunofluorescence has localized LDH-$C_4$ to the principle piece of the sperm tail (Beyler et al., 1985 ). Binding of anti-LDH-$C_4$ to sperm results in agglutination and cytotoxicity in the presence of complement

(Goldberg et al., 1981). Enzymatic activity is also inhibited by antibody binding (Goldberg, 1971), which suggests that sperm energy metabolism and, consequently, motility might also be immunologically impaired. Furthermore, antibodies to LDH-$C_4$ interfere with *in vitro* fertilization of mouse ova by mouse sperm and penetration of hamster ova by human sperm (Beyler and Goldberg, unpublished observations).

In addition to a humoral response, a cellular immune response is also elicited by systemic immunization. Mice immunized with LDH-$C_4$ exhibit delayed-type hypersensitivity (Kille and Goldberg, 1979). Cell-mediated cytotoxicity can be detected in LDH-$C_4$-immune mice by incubating their spleen cells with LDH-$C_4$-coated tumor cells containing $^{51}Cr$. A measure of the $^{51}Cr$ released by the tumor cells is indicative of specific cell lysis (Shelton and Goldberg, 1985).

Some or all of these immunological mechanisms may contribute to the suppressive effect that immunization with LDH-$C_4$ has on the fertility of females. This phenomenon has been well documented in a number of animal models. Following LDH-$C_4$ immunization, fertility is suppressed by 40-60% in mice (Lerum and Goldberg, 1974), while rabbits exhibit 70% fertility reduction (Goldberg and Wheat, 1976), and baboons 63% (Goldberg et al., 1981). The anti-fertility effect appears to be associated with high serum levels of antibody and is reversible as these levels decline after immunizations are discontinued (Goldberg et al., 1981).

The unique immunological and biochemical make-up of LDH-$C_4$ suggests that its incorporation into an anti-fertility vaccine is a viable approach to contraception. Two major obstacles, however, must be overcome before development of such a vaccine can proceed. These are the identification of a synthetic antigen that is a derivative of and can be substituted for the natural enzyme, and the enhancement of the immune response to LDH-$C_4$ in order to achieve complete fertility inhibition. Our present investigations, therefore, reflect this two-pronged attack.

We have approached the problem of developing a synthetic antigen by identifying the sites on the LDH-$C_4$ molecule where antibodies bind. Once these epitopes have been pinpointed, they can be chemically synthesized, attached to a macromolecular carrier and used for immunization. Antibodies made to these synthetic peptide fragments are then tested for their ability to bind native LDH-$C_4$. To date, eight such sites have been identified (Table I) (Wheat and Goldberg, in press). Two tryptic peptides comprising sequences 5-15 (region 1), 211-220 (region 3) and a third sequence 97-110 have been chemically synthesized, attached to either diphtheria toxoid (DT) or to bovine serum albumin (BSA) and inoculated into rabbits (Wheat et al., in press). The 97-110 peptide cannot be isolated from a tryptic digest of LDH-$C_4$, but was chosen as a possible antigenic determinant because it comprises the coenzyme binding site of LDH-$C_4$, would be accessible to antibody, and shows extensive sequence modification from the other isozymic forms. Figures 1, 2, and 3 show the individual immune profiles of rabbits following immunization with these three peptides. While there was considerable variability among individual rabbits, certain patterns were observed. Clearly, the rabbits immunized with peptide 5-15 responded best regardless of the carrier (Fig. 1). Peptide 97-110 was the poorest antigen (Fig. 2) and 211-220 (Fig. 3) elicited a median response among the three peptides, with some differences in response appearing to be due to the carrier. BSA seemed to be slightly more effective than DT with the 211-220 peptide.

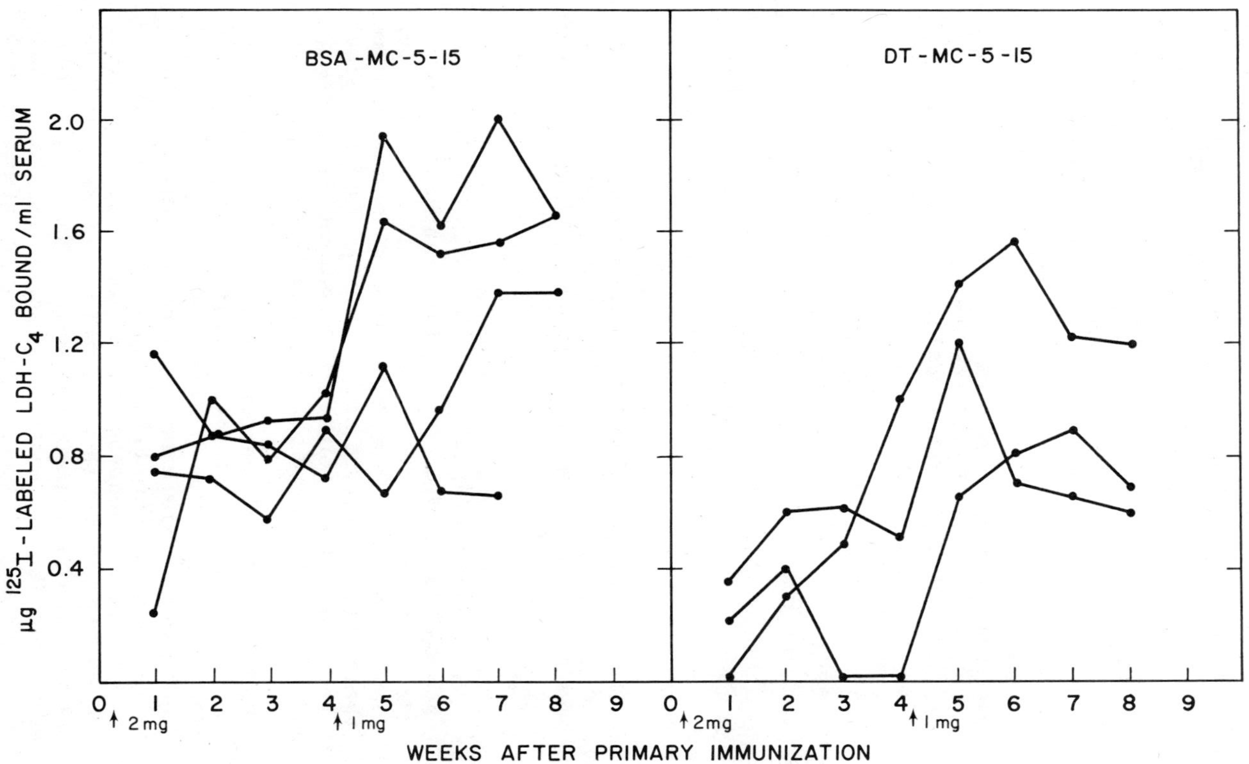


Figure 1. IMMUNE RESPONSE PROFILES OF INDIVIDUAL FEMALE RABBITS IMMUNIZED WITH BSA-MC5-15 AND DT-MC5-15. All rabbits received a 2mg primary immunization followed, in four weeks, by a 1mg secondary (designated by the arrows). These immunizations were administered in Freund's complete adjuvant at multiple subcutaneous sites. Results are expressed as μg of $^{125}I$-labeled LDH-$C_4$ bound/ml of serum as measured by a liquid phase radioimmunoassay.

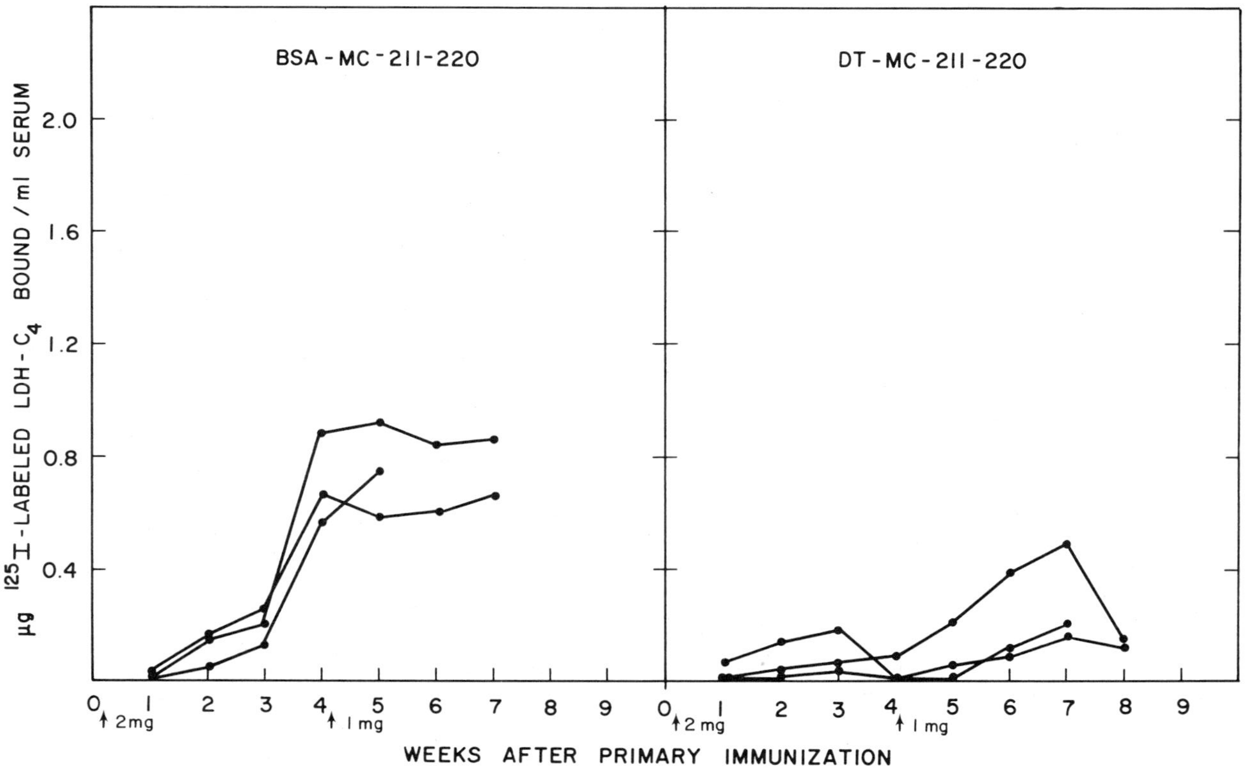


Figure 2. IMMUNE RESPONSE PROFILES OF INDIVIDUAL FEMALE RABBITS IMMUNIZED WITH BSA-MC211-220 AND DT-MC211-220. The immunizations were administered as described in Figure 1.

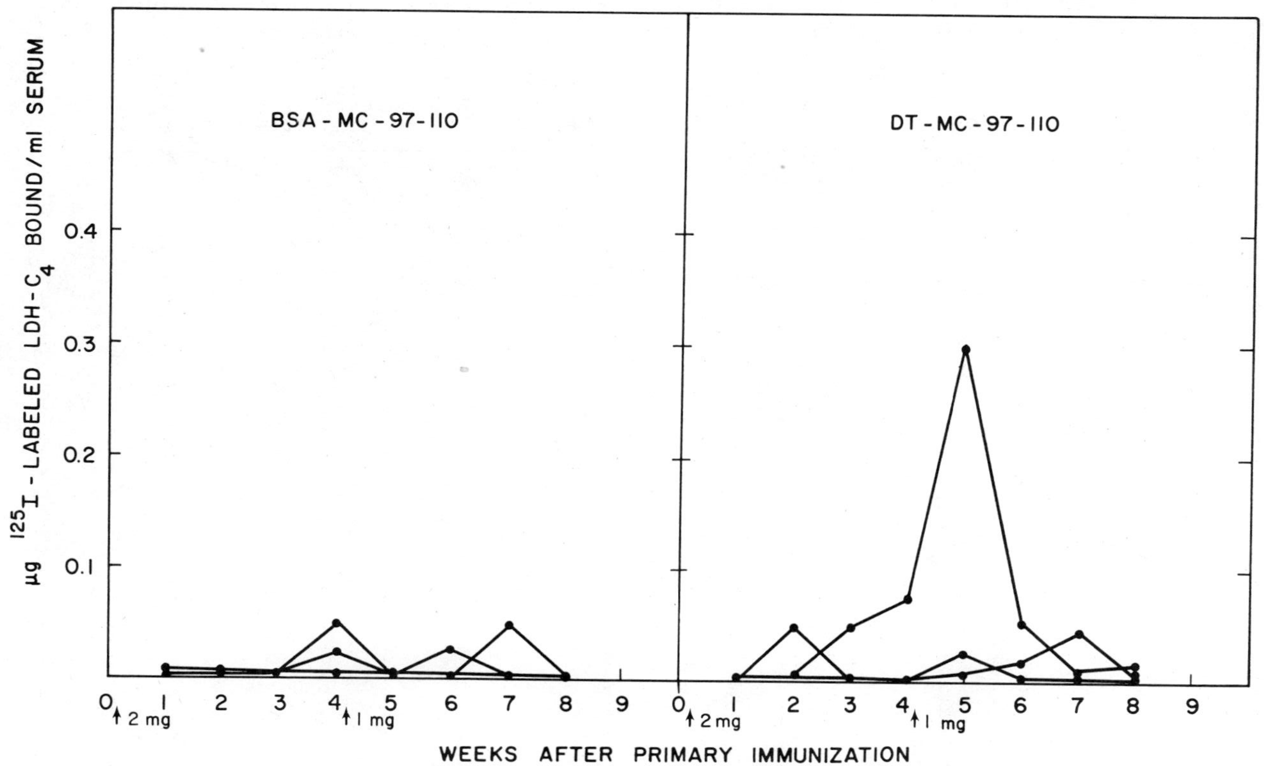


Figure 3. IMMUNE RESPONSE PROFILES FOR INDIVIDUAL FEMALE RABBITS IMMUNIZED WITH BSA-MC97-110 AND DT-MC97-110. The immunizations were given as described in Figure 1.

TABLE I

Antigenic Peptides of the LDH-C Subunit

| Region | Structure and Location |
|---|---|
| | 5 10 14a 14b |
| 1 | Glu-Gln-Leu-Ile-Gln-Asn-Leu-Val-Pro-Glu-Asp-Lys |
| | 41 50 55 |
| 2 | Gly-Leu-Ala-Asp-Glu-Leu-Ala-Leu-Val-Asp-Ala-Asp-Asp-Thr-Asp-Lys |
| | 211 220 |
| 3 | Ser-Leu-Asn-Pro-Ala-Ile-Gly-Thr-Asp-Lys |
| | 221 230 |
| 4 | Asn-Lys-Gln-His-Trp-Lys-Asn-Val-His-Lys |
| | 231 240 243 |
| 5 | Gln-Val-Val-Glu-Gly-Gly-Tyr-Glu-Val-Leu-Asp-Met-Lys |
| | 283 290 |
| 6 | Glu-Glu-Val-Phe-Leu-Ser-Ile-Pro-Cys-Val-Leu-Gly-Glu-Ser-Gly- |
| | 300 303 |
| | Ile-Thr-Asp-Phe-Val-Lys |
| | 304 310 316 |
| 7 | Val-Asn-Met-Thr-Ala-Glu-Glu-Glu-Gly-Leu-Leu-Lys-Lys |
| | 317 320 330 |
| 8 | Ser-Val-Asp-Thr-Leu-Trp-Asn-Met-Gln-Lys-Asn-Leu-Glu-Leu |

Based on these data, DT-MC5-15 was chosen for further immunization and fertility studies in the female baboon (Goldberg *et al.*, in preparation). Fourteen female baboons were immunized with DT-MC5-15 in squalene-arlacel A plus CGP 11,637, a muramyl dipeptide (MDP) adjuvant (generously provided by Ciba-Geigy Limited, Basel, Switzerland) (Stevens et al., 1981a). Fourteen control animals were immunized with the carrier plus adjuvant alone. All experimental animals produced antibodies to MC5-15 that also reacted with LDH-$C_4$. Figure 4 shows the typical immune response of an experimental animal. No antibodies to either MC 5-15 or to LDH-$C_4$ were detectable in control animals. Subsequently, fertility was tested by mating each animal at least four times following immunizations or until pregnant. The result was a 71% reduction in the fertility of the DT-MC 5-15 immunized baboons when compared to the control animals. Furthermore, when immunizations were discontinued, matings of experimental animals resulted in pregnancy . Thus, the immunological effect on fertility was reversible.

While these results demonstrate the promise that this approach holds, the percentage of fertility reduction must be increased to a level acceptable for human contraceptive practice. Certainly, one possibility is that, while MC5-15 immunization is effective in reducing fertility, another peptide or combination of peptides might be more immunogenic. This avenue is currently being explored. Our results also indicate that enhancement of the immune response to LDH-$C_4$ can be achieved by manipulation of several components of the immunization protocol. These include the choice of carrier, adjuvant, and

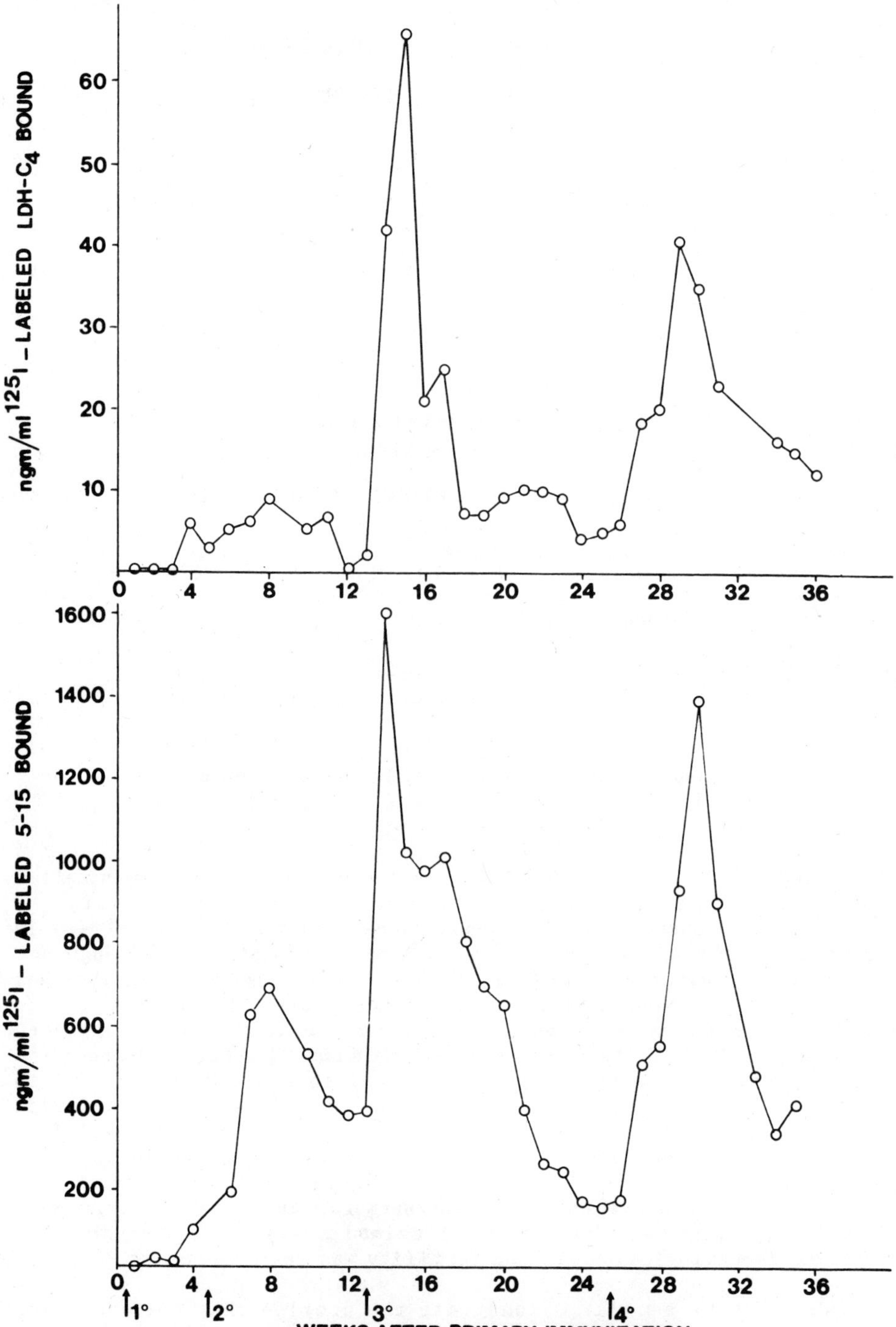


Figure 4. TYPICAL IMMUNE RESPONSE OF FEMALE BABOON FOLLOWING FOUR IMMUNIZATIONS WITH DT-MC5-15 IN SQUALENE-ARLACEL A PLUS CGP 11, 637 ADJUVANT (AT THE TIMES INDICATED BY THE ARROWS). Antibodies reacted with both 5-15 peptide and to the intact LDH-$C_4$. Results are expressed as ngm of $^{125}I$-labeled antigen bound/ml serum as measured by liquid phase radioimmunoassay.

immunization route. Design of the most effective immunization protocol, however, is restricted to parameters that will ultimately be acceptable for human application. In this regard, the choice of a carrier and an effective adjuvant is severely limited.

Two carriers that are considered safe for human use and have been used by ourselves and other investigators with some success are diphtheria toxoid and tetanus toxoid (Wheat et al., in press; Goldberg et al. in preparation; Stevens et al., 1981b). Since our results in rabbits immunized with the same peptide on two different carriers suggest that the carrier may indeed have differential effects on the response (Wheat et al. in press), it will be important to test various peptide antigens with more than one carrier. Another possibility is to design a synthetic carrier that will not cause harmful immune reactions, but will contain the appropriate side chain groups. Thus the most effective number of peptides can be attached and the environment of the attachment site will maintain the proper conformational stability of the peptide antigen.

Choice of a suitable adjuvant is also limited at the present time. Many adjuvants that have been effective in animal models, such as Freund's complete adjuvant and *Bordetella pertussis* cause painful inflammatory and allergic reactions. One new group of adjuvants that has been recently used is the synthetic muramyl dipeptides, which represent the active site of the bacterial cell wall component in Freund's complete adjuvant. They appear to be effective without producing strong inflammatory reactions. We have used such an adjuvant with MC5-15 in both female baboons (Goldberg et al., in preparation) and in rabbits (Shelton and Goldberg, unpublished observations). However, a number of preparations of these adjuvants exist and they are of varying potency and effectiveness. More testing needs to be done.

A third component that may be exploited to enhance the immune response is the route of immunization. While the systemic response consists primarily of IgG, which presumably enters the female reproductive tract as a transudate of serum (Kille and Goldberg, 1979), the major class of antibody bathing the reproductive tract is secretory IgA (sIgA), which is present locally in reproductive tract secretions (Tomasi, 1980). IgA is produced by plasma cells migrating from Peyers Patches to draining lymph nodes, and then to the mucosal lining of the reproductive tract. The secretory component is attached to dimeric IgA as it migrates through mucosal epithelium. Thus, an immunization designed to stimulate this mucosal immune response may ensure higher levels of antibody at the site of fertilization than those resulting from systemic immunization. We have immunized female mice with LDH-$C_4$ directly into the uterus. These animals produced secretory IgA specific for the enzyme in their uterine fluids. When mated, only 20% of the mice immunized with LDH-$C_4$ became pregnant as opposed to 70% of non-immune controls (Shelton et al., 1983; Shelton and Goldberg, in preparation). Local immunization is therefore an effective means of suppressing fertility. We are currently exploring the proper dose of immunogen and the possibilities of increasing the local response by indirect stimulation of the gut-associated lymphatic tissues (GALT) (Shelton et al., 1984), which would take advantage of the commonality of the mucosal immune system (Montgomery et al., 1980). The ability to administer a vaccine orally to stimulate the GALT and, indirectly, the mucosal lining of the reproductive tract, is an attractive one. In addition, the short duration of the memory response for sIgA should afford ready reversibility of the anti-fertility effects (Tomasi and Bienenstock, 1968).

Resolution of the problems of contraceptive vaccine technology seems much more likely with a biochemically and immunologically well-defined sperm antigen. Such an antigen is necessary for proper assessment and precise quantitation of immune responses, and it will allow for development of effective but safe synthetic analogues. Clearly, the sperm-specific LDH-$C_4$ fills such a role and, most importantly, it induces an immune response that effectively blocks pregnancy. These results provide encouragement that vaccine technology will offer an alternative form of contraception.

ACKNOWLEDGEMENTS

This work was supported by NIH grant HD-05863 and by the Program for Applied Research on Fertility Regulation, Northwestern University, under a cooperative agreement with the Agency for International Development (AID/DPE-0586-A-00-1003). The views of the authors do not necessarily reflect AID policy.

REFERENCES

Aitken, R. J., 1982, The contraceptive potential of antisperm antibodies, in: "Progress Towards a Male Contraceptive," S.J. Jeffcoate and M. Sandler, eds., John Wiley and Sons, Ltd., London, pp. 109-134.

Alvarez, J. G. and Storey, B. T., 1984, Assessment of cell damage caused by spontaneous lipid peroxidation in rabbit sperm, Biol. Reprod., 30:323-331.

Anderson, D.J. and Alexander, N. J., 1983, A new look at antifertility vaccines, Fertil. Steril., 40:557-571.

Beer, A. E. and Neaves, W. B., 1979, Antigenic status of semen from the viewpoints of the female and male, Fertil. Steril., 29:3-22.

Beyler, S. A., Wheat, T. E. and Goldberg, E., 1985, Binding of antibodies against antigenic domains of murine lactate dehydrogenase-$C_4$ to human and mouse spermatozoa, Biol. Reprod., 32:1201-1210.

Eventoff, W., Rossmann, M. G., Taylor, S. S., Torff, H. J., Meyer, H., Keil, W., and Kiltz, H. H., 1977, Structural adaptations of lactate dehydrogenase isozymes, Proc. Nat. Acad. Sci. U.S.A., 74:2677-2681.

Goldberg, E., 1971, Immunochemical specificity of lactate dehydrogenase-X, Proc. Nat. Acad. Sci. U.S.A., 68:349-352.

Goldberg, E., 1977, Isozymes in testes and spermatozoa, in: "Isozymes: Current Topics in Biological and Medical Research," M. S.Rattazzi, J.G. Scandelios, G. S. Whitt, eds., Alan R. Liss, Inc., New York, Vol. 1, pp. 79-124.

Goldberg, E., 1983, Current status of research on sperm antigens: potential applications as contraceptive vaccines, in: "Research Frontiers in Fertility Regulation," G. I. Zatuchni, ed., Program for Applied Research on Fertility Regulation, Chicago, Vol. 2, pp. 6-11.

Goldberg, E., Gonzales-Prevatt, V., and Wheat, T.E., 1981, Immunosuppression of fertility in females by injection of sperm-specific LDH-$C_4$ (LDH-X): prospects for development of a contraceptive vaccine, in: "Human Reproduction," Proceedings of the IIIrd World Congress, K. Semm and L. Mettler, eds., Excerpta Medica, Amsterdam, pp. 360-363.

Goldberg, E., Wheat, T.E., 1976, Induction of infertility in male rabbits by immunization with LDH-X, in: "Regulatory Mechanisms of Male Reproductive Physiology," C. H. Spilman, T. J. Lobl, K.

T. Kirton, eds., American Elsevier Publ. Co., New York, pp. 133-138.

Goldberg, E., Wheat, T. E., Powell, J. E., Stevens, V. C., 1981, Reduction of fertility in female baboons immunized with lactate dehydrogenase $C_4$, Fertil. Steril., 35:214-217.

Jones, W. R., 1980, Immunological factors in male and female infertility, in: "Immunological Aspects of Reproduction and Fertility Control," J. P. Hearn, ed., Univ. Park Press, Baltimore, pp. 105-140.

Jones, W.R., 1982, Immunization against spermatozoal antigens, in: "Immunological Aspects of Reproduction and Fertility Regulation," Blackwell Scientific Publications, Oxford, pp. 91-146.

Kille, J. W., Goldberg, E., 1979, Female reproductive tract immunoglobulin responses to a purified sperm-specific antigen (LDH-$C_4$), Biol. Reprod., 20:863-871.

Lerum, J. E., and Goldberg, E., 1974, Immunological impairment of pregnancy in mice by lactate dehydrogenase-X, Biol. Reprod., 11:108-115.

Li, S. S.-L., Feldman, R. J., Okabe, M., and Pan, Y.-C. E., 1983a, Molecular features and immunological properties of lactate dehydrogenase $C_4$ isozymes from mouse and rat testes, J. Biol. Chem., 258:7017-7032.

Li, S. S.-L., Fitch, W. M., Pan, Y.-C. E., and Sharief, F. S., 1983b, Evolutionaly relationships of vertebrate lactate dehydrogenase isozymes, $A_4$ (muscle), $B_4$ (heart), and $C_4$ (testis), J. Biol. Chem., 258:7029-7032.

Montgomery, P. C., Lemaitre-Coelho, I. M., and Vaer, J.-P., 1980, A common mucosal immune system. Antibody expression in secretions following gastro-intestinal stimulation, Immunol. Commun., 9:705-713.

Musick, W. D. L., and Rossmann, M. G., 1979a, The structure of mouse testicular lactate dehydrogenase isoenzyme $C_4$ at 2.9Å resolution, J. Biol. Chem., 254:7611-7620.

Musick, W. D. L., and Rossmann, M. G., 1979b, The tentative amino acid sequencing of lactate dehydrogenase $C_4$ by X-ray diffraction analysis, J. Biol. Chem., 254:7621-7623.

Naz, R., Alexander, N., Isahakia, M., 1984, Monoclonal antibody to a human germ cell membrane glycoprotein that inhibits fertilization, Science, 225:342-344.

O'Rand, M. G., 1981, Inhibition of fertility and sperm-zona binding by antiserum to the rabbit sperm membrane autoantigen RSA-1, Biol. Reprod., 25:621-628.

O'Rand, M. G., and Irons, G. P., 1984, Monoclonal antibodies to rabbit sperm autoantigens. II. Inhibition of human sperm penetration of zona-free hamster eggs, Biol. Reprod., 30:731-736.

O'Rand, M. G., Irons, G. P., and Porter, J. P., 1984, Monoclonal antibodies to rabbit sperm autoantigens. I. Inhibition of *in vitro* fertilization and localization on the egg, Biol. Reprod., 30:721-729.

O'Rand, M. G., and Porter, J. P., 1982, Purifications of rabbit sperm autoantigens by preparative SDS gel electrophoresis: amino acid and carbohydrate content of RSA-1, Biol. Reprod., 27:713-721.

O'Rand, M. G., and Romrell, L. J., 1981, Localization of a single sperm membrane autoantigen (RSA-1) on spermatogenic cells and spermatogonia, Dev. Biol., 84:322-331.

Saling, P. M., Raines, L. M., and O'Rand, M. G., 1983, Monoclonal antibody against mouse sperm blocks a specific event in the fertilization process, J. Exp. Zool., 227:481-486.

Shelton, J. A., Abe, M., and Goldberg, E., 1983, Cellular and local immunity to sperm-specific lactate dehydrogenase-$C_4$, J. Reprod. Immunol. (suppl. July), p. 26.

Shelton, J. A., Alexander, N. J., and Goldberg, E., 1984, Local secretory immunity to sperm-specific lactate dehydrogenase $C_4$ in the reproductive tract of the female rhesus macaque, Biol. Reprod., (suppl. #1), 30:74.

Shelton, J. A., and Goldberg, E., 1985, Induction of cell-mediated cytotoxic immunity to sperm-specific lactate dehydrogenase-$C_4$ in SJL/J female mice, Biol. Reprod., 32:556-560.

Stevens, V. C., Cinader, B., Powell, J. E., Lee, A. C., and Koh, S. W., 1981a, Preparation and formulation of a human chorionic gonadotropin anti-fertility vaccine: selection of adjuvant and vehicle, Amer. J. Reprod. Immunol., 1:315-321.

Stevens, V. C., Cinader, B., Powell, J. E., Lee, A. C., and Koh, S. W., 1981b, Preparation and formulation of a human chorionic gonadotropin anti-fertility vaccine: selection of a peptide immunogen, Amer. J. Reprod. Immunol., 1:307-314.

Tomasi, T. B., 1980, The secretory immune system, in: "Immunological Aspects of Infertility and Fertility Regulation", D. S. Dhindsa, and G. F. B. Schumacher, eds., Elsevier-N. Holland, Inc., New York, pp. 23-31.

Tomasi, T. B., and Bienenstock, J., 1968, Secretory immunoglobulins, in: "Advances in Immunology", F. J. Dixon, Jr. and H. G. Kunkel, eds., Academic Press, New York, Vol. 9, pp. 1-96.

Tung, K. S. K., 1983, Experimental models of autoimmunity and isoimmunity to sperm, in: "Immunology of Reproduction," T. G. Wegmann and T. J. Gall, eds., Oxford University Press, New York, pp. 404-423.

Wheat, T. E., and Goldberg, E., 1977, Isolation of the sperm-specific lactate dehydrogenase from mouse, rabbit and human testes and human spermatozoa, in: "Immunological Influences on Human Fertility", B. Boettcher, ed., Harcourt Brace Jovanovich, Australia, pp. 221-227.

Wheat, T. E., and Goldberg, E., 1983, Sperm-specific lactate dehydrogenase $C_4$: antigenic structure and immunosuppression of fertility, in: "Isozymes: Current Topics in Biological and Medical Research", M. C. Rattazzi, J. G. Scandelios, and G. S. Whitt, Alan R. Liss, Inc., New York, Vol. 7, pp. 113-130.

Wheat, T. E., and Goldberg, E., 1985, Antigenic domains of the sperm-specific lactate dehydrogenase, Molec. Immunol., in press.

Wheat, T. E., and Goldberg, E., 1985, Immunochemical dissection of the testes-specific isozyme, lactate dehydrogenase, Ann. NY Acad. Sci., 438:156-159.

Wheat, T. E., Shelton, J. A., Gonzales-Prevatt, V., and Goldberg, E., 1985, The antigenicity of synthetic peptide fragments of LDH-$C_4$, Molec. Immunol., in press.

Wolf, D. P., Tokoloski, J. E., Dandekar, P., and Bechtol, K. B., 1983, Characterization of human sperm surface antigens with monoclonal antibodies, Biol. Reprod., 29:713-723.

# CHARACTERIZATION OF AN ANTISPERM MONOCLONAL ANTIBODY INDUCING HUMAN SPERM AGGLUTINATION[1]

Yuan Chang Yan[2,*], Lin Fang Wang[3,*], Sumi M. Mitsudo,[+] and S. S. Koide[4,*]

*Center for Biomedical Research, The Population Council, 1230 York Avenue, New York, NY 10021 and [+]Department of Pathology, Montefiore Medical Center, Bronx, NY USA

## INTRODUCTION

Sera and cervical fluids of some infertile subjects of undetermined etiology contain antisperm antibodies inducing sperm agglutination and/or immobilization. These antibodies might be the underlying basis for the infertile condition (1-5). Non-agglutinating or non-immobilizing antisperm antibodies might also be involved in some cases of infertility by affecting in some unknown manner the fertilizing capacity of sperm or interfere with sperm-egg interaction. To identify the components constituting human sperm membrane that may act as antigens, we have raised monoclonal antibodies against human sperm membrane proteins. One of the cell lines produced antibodies that agglutinate human sperm (6). The interacting protein had an estimated mol. wt. of 84 kDa. In the present study, we have cultivated a second mouse fused spleen cell line raised against human sperm membrane proteins, producing antibodies that induce sperm agglutination. Localization of the antigen on the sperm surface and on colon carçinomatous cells was determined by an immunocytochemical method. Studies on the interaction of the antibodies with purified samples of carcinoembryonic antigen were carried out.

[1]This work was supported by a grant from the Mellon Foundation (S.S.K.) and from the Rockefeller Foundation (Y.C.Y. and L.F.W.).

[2]Present address: Shanghai Institute of Cell Biology, Academia Sinica, Shanghai, China.

[3]Present address: Institute of Basic Medical Sciences, Chinese Academy of Medical Sciences, Beijing, China.

[4]Correspondence to S.S. Koide, Center for Biomedical Research, The Population Council, 1230 York Avenue, New York, New York 10021.

## MATERIALS AND METHODS

Female mice of BALB/c strain were purchased from Jackson Laboratory (Maine). The myeloma cell line Sp2/0 was obtained from Dr. W. Prensky, Memorial Sloan-Kettering Cancer Center. Molecular weight calibration kit protein standards were purchased from Pharmacia Fine Chemicals. Dulbecco's phosphate buffered saline, RPMI-1640 medium, and fetal bovine serum were products of GIBCO Laboratory.

Fluorescein-conjugated IgG fraction of goat anti-mouse immunoglobulins was purchased from Cappel Laboratories (West Chester, PA); alkaline phosphatase-conjugated sheep F $(ab')_2$ anti-mouse immunoglobulins from New England Nuclear Corp. (Boston MA); Sigma 104 phosphate substrate, disodium p-nitrophenyl phosphate and Tween 20 (polyoxyethylene sorbitan monolaurate) from Sigma Chemical (St. Louis, MO).

Purified CEA was obtained from three sources: Dr. J. Krupey (Roche, Diagnostic Products, Pharmaceutical Operations (Belleville, NJ); standard reference CEA from the National Biological Standards Board, National Institute for Biological Standards and Control (Holly Hill, Hampstead, London) and Bioscan Continental (Pierrefonds, Quebec, Canada).

### Preparation of Human Sperm Membrane Proteins

Semen was obtained from healthy human donors. The spermatozoa were separated from seminal plasma by centrifugation at 1000g for 10 minutes. The sperm pellet was washed three times by suspension in 10 mM phosphate-buffered saline, pH 7.4. Spermatozoa were collected and resuspended in 10 mM Tris-HCl containing 0.5 M NaCl, pH 8.3. The suspension contained about $5 \times 10^9$ sperm per ml. Triton X-100 was added to the suspension of sperm to a final concentration of 1% (v/v). The homogenate was stirred at $4^{\circ}C$ for 12 hours and stored in the cold room overnight. Insoluble material was removed by centrifugation at 6000g for 30 min. The supernatant was dialyzed against deionized water overnight at $4^{\circ}C$, lyophilized, and store frozen at $-70^{\circ}C$.

### Monoclonal Antibody Production

The crude Triton X-100 extract of human sperm membrane protein (HSMP) was emulsified with complete Freund's adjuvant. A dose of 100 µg of HSMP was administered by subcutaneous injections to each BALB/c female mice at intervals of one week. Subsequent boosters were administered weekly for 3 weeks without adjuvant. Forty five-days after the initial injection a final booster injection of 100 µg of HSMP was administered intraperitoneally and cell fusion performed 3 days later. Sera were tested for sperm agglutinating antibodies and anti-CEA antibodies. A mouse producing significant titer of anti-CEA antibodies was selected. The spleen cells from the immunized mouse were fused with mouse myeloma cells (Sp 2/0) according to the method described by Goding (7) and Yan *et al*. (6).

## Cloning

Hybridoma cells secreting sperm agglutinating antibodies and anti-CEA antibodies were cloned in a 96-well tissue culture plate under condition of limiting dilution. A single hybridoma cell secreting sperm agglutinating antibodies and anti-CEA antibodies was plated into a well containing 2000 macrophages as feeder cells and designated as YWK-II cell line.

## Growth in Mice

Hybridoma cells ($2 \times 10^6$ to $6 \times 10^6$) were injected into the peritoneal cavity of BALB/c mouse, pretreated with 0.3 ml of pristane administered intraperitoneally 1 week prior to the inoculation. The ascitic fluid was collected 10-14 days after the inoculation with hybridoma cells.

## Microplate Enzyme-Linked Immunoassay: CEA Binding Test (ELISA)

Wells of microtiter plate were coated with 50 µl of antigen (5 µg of CEA per ml) dissolved in 0.04 M carbonate buffer, pH 9.6, and stored at 4°C overnight. Each well was filled with a solution of 1% BSA in 0.01 M Tris-HCl, 0.15 M NaCl buffer, pH 7.8, to block non-specific protein binding. After incubating for 3 hrs at 20-22°C, the antigen-coated plates were incubated with conditioned medium or diluted ascitic fluid of YWK-II cells. The plate was incubated at 37°C for 2 hrs. and washed with medium A, containing 0.1% BSA in a mixture of 0.01 M Tris-HCl, 0.15 M NaCl, pH 7.8, 0.05% Tween 20. Alkaline phosphatase-conjugated sheep $F(ab')_2$ anti-mouse immunoglobulins was then added as the second antibody. After washing with medium A, the colorimetric enzyme reaction was initiated by adding the substrate mixture (SIGMA 104, 6 tablets dissolved in 10 ml of 10% diethanolamine buffer containing 10 mM $MgCl_2$, pH 9.8). The plate was incubated at 20-22°C for 30 min and the reaction stopped with the addition of 50 µl of 2 N NaOH. Absorbance of each well was measured at 410 nm with a MR 600 microplate Reader (Dynatech Industries, Inc., Alexandria, VA).

## Immunofluorescence Localization of Sperm Antigen With Monoclonal Antibody

Fresh semen was obtained from human donors and incubated in glass tubes for 30 minutes at 37°C. Cellular debris in the liquified ejaculate was removed by centrifugation at low speed. Sperm were separated from the seminal plasma by centrifugation at 1000g; washed three times in Dulbecco's PBS buffer, and finally resuspended in this buffer. An aliquot of 30 µl of sperm suspension was placed in each well of a 10-well multispot slide. The sperm were allowed to settle and 1.8% formaldehyde added to fix the sperm. After 5 min of fixation, the slides were washed with distilled water, and subsequently with PBS buffer at least three times to remove the formaldehyde completely. To the fixed sperm of each slide 30 µl of the conditioned culture medium or ascitic fluid (diluted 1:100) of YWK-II cells were added separately. As negative controls, 30 μl of conditioned culture medium or ascitic fluid (diluted 1:100) of Sp 2/0 cells were used. As a second control 30 μl of a mixture composed of 1:1 volume of diluted ascitic fluid and 3% HSMP was used.

The slides were incubated at 4°C in a humidified plastic petri dish overnight and washed thoroughly with several changes of PBS over a 15-min period. A solution of second antibody consisting of 1:100 diluted fluorescein-conjugated IgG solution of goat anti-mouse immunoglobulins was added. After three hrs of incubation at 20-22°C, the slides were rinsed thoroughly three times with PBS as before and viewed under a Nikon fluorescence microscope.

Tissue Preparation for Immunocytochemistry

Surgically excised tissues were fixed in 10% buffered formaldehyde solution, dehydrated in ethanol and processed routinely into paraffin blocks. Sections were deparaffinized and washed with Dulbecco's phosphate-buffered saline (PHS), pH 7.3, (GIBCO Laboratory, Grand Island, NY), and incubated in 2% bovine serum albumin (BSA) in PBS at 20-22°C for 3 hrs. After rinsing with 0.1% BSA in PBS, the slides were incubated with monoclonal YWK-II ascitic fluid diluted 1:100 with 0.1% BSA in PBS at room temperature for 5 hrs, washed with 0.1% BSA in PBS containing 0.05% Tween-20 (Sigma Chemical, St. Louis, MO), and incubated with FITC fluorescein-conjugated IgG fraction of goat anti-mouse Ig (Cappel Lab, Cochranville, PA) diluted 1:100 at 20-22° for 4 hrs. The slides were washed with 0.1% BSA in PBS containing 0.05% Tween-20 three times, mounted while wet with 50% glycerol in PBS and examined under a fluorescence microscope.

As a negative control ascitic fluid obtained from mouse inoculated with Sp 2/0 cells diluted 1:100 with 0.1% BSA in PBS was used. As a second control, ascitic fluid was omitted from the incubation medium.

## RESULTS

ELISA for CEA

The binding of authentic CEA with monoclonal YWK-II antibodies was determined with the ELISA method. Positive reaction was obtained with the monoclonal YWK-II ascitic fluid diluted 1:2700 and CEA (5 μg/ml). Of the three reference samples of CEA tested, the absorbance of the reaction measured at 410 nm was highest with the sample obtained from Dr. Krupey (1.12 units), less with the authentic reference distributed by The National Biological Standard Board (0.29 units) and least with the sample from Bioscan (weak reaction).

To show that sperm membrane contain immunoreactive CEA-like material, the reaction between YWK-II antibodies and HSMP was determined with the ELISA method. Positive reaction was obtained on incubating YWK-II ascitic fluid diluted 1:900 with HSMP (100 μg/ml). The amount of immunoreactive-CEA in HSMP was estimated to be about 1%.

Sperm Agglutination

Agglutination of human sperm occurred on mixing with YWK-II ascitic fluid diluted at 1:30. The agglutination was of the mixed type.

Localization of Monoclonal YWK-II Antibody on Human Sperm and Colon Cancer Cells

The localization of the YWK-II antibodies on the surface of human sperm was determined by an indirect immunofluorescence method using ascitic fluid from BALB/c mouse inoculated with YWK-II fused spleen cells (Fig. 1). Moderate fluorescence staining occurred at the equatorial region of the head, midpiece and tail. No staining occurred when Sp 2/0 cell culture medium or ascitic fluid was used.

With sections of human colon adenocarcinoma intense staining occurred at the brush border or glycocalyx of the columnar epithelial cells and on the luminal boundary of tumor cells and lining and content of cystically dilated tumor glands (Fig. 2). Moreover, macrophages within the carcinomatous tissues stained intensely. No staining occurred, using ascitic fluid produced by Sp 2/0 cells.

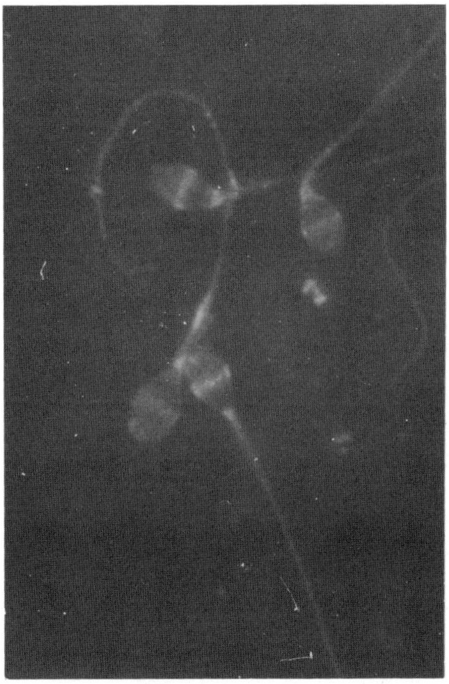

Fig. 1. Immunofluorescence staining of human sperm. Sections were incubated with YWK-II ascitic fluid (diluted 1:100) and FITC-conjugated IgG fraction of goat anti-mouse IgG (diluted 1:100). Note moderate staining at the equatorial region of head, midpiece and tail, x1800.

## DISCUSSION

Sera from mice immunized with human sperm membrane proteins interacted with authentic CEA, and the hybridoma cell line prepared from the spleen cells of one of these immunized mice produced antibodies that interacted with three different preparations of purified CEA. The physicochemical properties of the sperm immunoreactive CEA-like substance are being determined. CEA contains 50-60% carbohydrates and its estimated mol. wt. is 200,000 (8,9).

A substance reacting in the RIA for CEA was detected in human seminal plasma (10,11) and prostate gland (12,13). The seminal plasma substance is a large molecule exceeding 200 kDa since it is eluted in the Vo fraction on gel filtration through Sephadex G-200 and probably originates from the prostate gland (12,13).

The present finding that the YWK-II antibodies localized to the equatorial region of the human sperm head is of interest. One of the monoclonal antibodies raised against human sperm by Isahakia and Alexander (14), designated as MA5 and belonging to the IgM class, showed similar localization. The estimated mol. wt. of the sperm protein interacting with MA5 antibodies was 71 kDa. The MA5 antibodies depressed sperm motility (sperm immobilization) without inducing agglutination, resembling the monoclonal antibodies raised by Shigeta _et al_. (15). The antigen interacting with the sperm immobilizing antibodies is a sperm coating protein and is present in seminal plasma. The Mr of this antigen is about 15 kDa (16). Based on these results, the sperm proteins interacting with the YWK-II, MA5 (14) and sperm immobilizing (15,16) antibodies are probably different antigens.

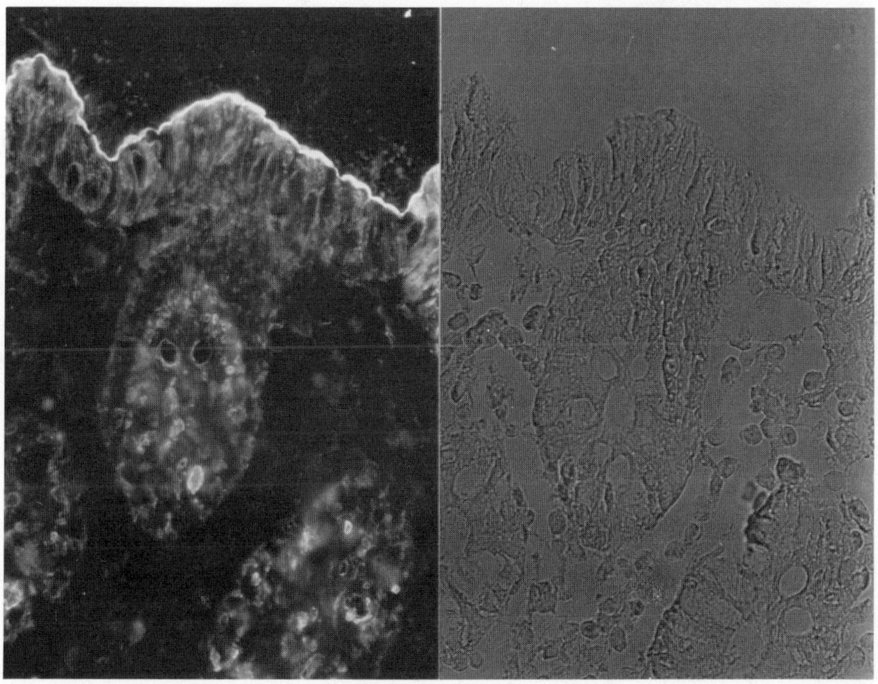

Fig. 2. Immunofluorescence staining of colon adenocarcinoma. (A) Well-differentiated adenocarcinoma of colon. Glycocalyx and cytoplasm of tumor cells show strong staining reaction (left); phase contrast (right), ×400.

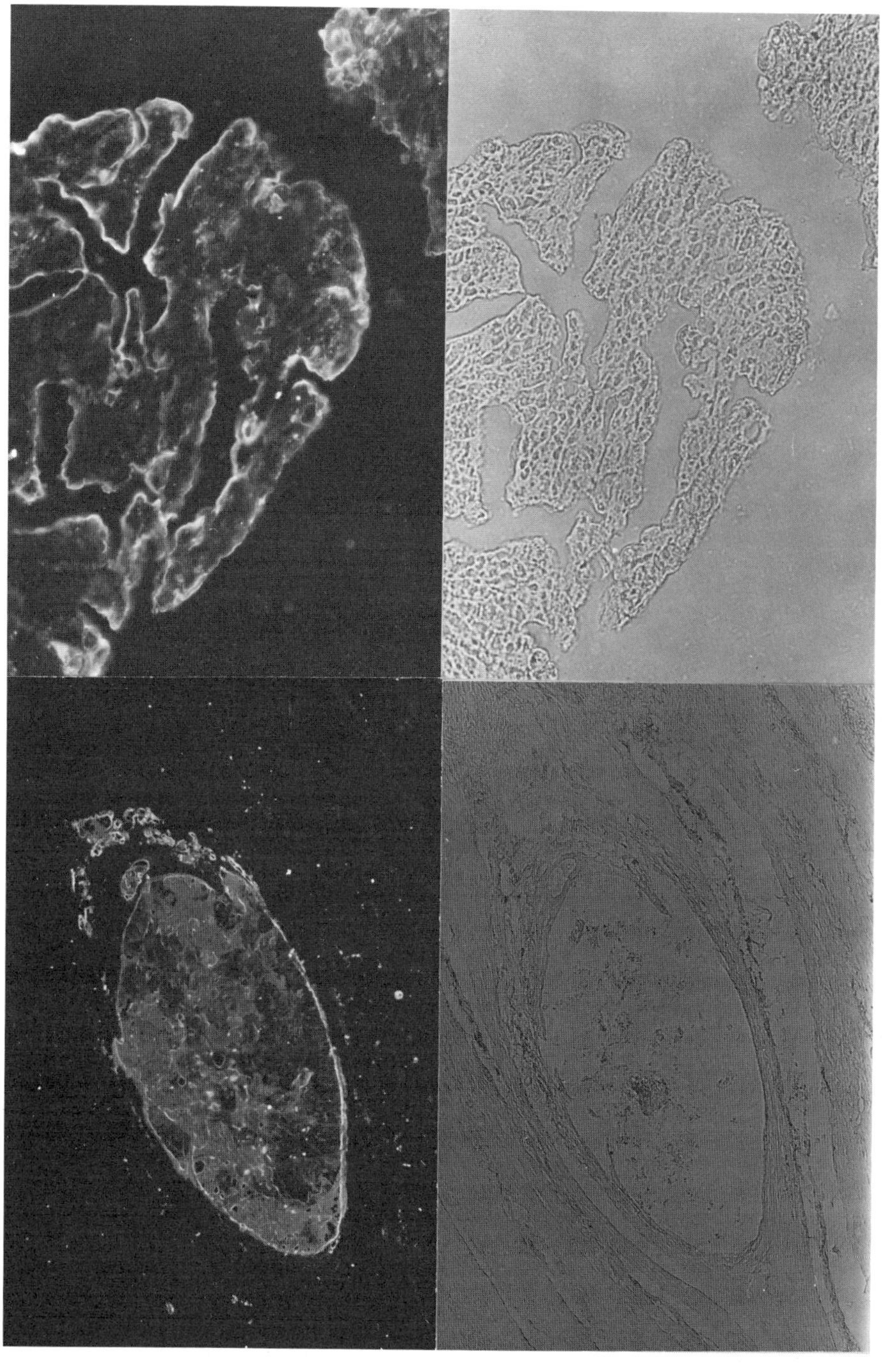

Fig. 2. (B) Papillary area of adenocarcinoma of colon. Luminal lining shows strong positive staining (left); phase contrast (right), x 400. (C) Cystic tumor gland of colon adenocarcinoma. Positive staining of lining of cystically dilated tumor gland and cellular debris in lumen (left); phase contrast (right, x400.

The cellular distribution of the immunoreactive antigen in colon adenocarcinoma was determined by an indirect immunofluorescence method using the YWK-II antibodies. The observed distribution of the antibodies was strikingly similar to the immunolocalization of CEA (17-20). In the reported studies, positive staining for CEA occurred at the glycocalyx of the surface of epithelial cells of the mucosa of normal colon and apical cytoplasm and luminal content of well-differentiated and moderately differentiated colorectal carcinoma cells. There was pronounced linear staining of the apical pole of cells lining the glandular epithelium and mucosal surface. The lining and intraglandular luminal content of cystically dilated tumor glands also stained intensely.

Several antigens have been purified that cross-react with antibodies to CEA. These antigens include the nonspecific cross-reacting antigens (NCA) (21,22) normal fecal antigens (NFA) (23) and biliary glycoprotein (24). They are glycoproteins. With the use of monoclonal antibodies immunological heterogeneity of CEA was demonstrated (25-29). The immunological heterogeneity is due to separate epitopes on CEA (28). At least four separate antigenic determinants can be differentiated on colonic cancer CEA. One of the antigenic determinants is shared by CEA, NCA and NFA or meconium antigen. Of these antigens the sperm protein interacting with YWK-II antibodies most closely resembles NCA. The tissue and cellular localization of the immunocytochemical staining with YWK-II antibodies and with the monoclonal antibodies designated as NP-1 are strikingly similar (26-28). The NP-1 antibodies cross-react with NCA and stain neutrophils. Leucocytes are known to synthesize NCA but not CEA (30,31). Since macrophages stained positively with YWK-II antibodies, the interacting antigen is a NCA-related substance rather than CEA. NCA sediments at 3S to 4S corresponding to an estimated mol. wt. of 40-50 kDa (21). The present findings suggest that NCA and YWK-II antigen are related proteins.

ACKNOWLEDGEMENTS

Y.C.Y and L.F.W. were postdoctoral fellows on the Rockefeller Foundation. Human semen specimens were obtained from Dr. D. Phillips, The Population Council, and Dr. S. Leto, Washington Fertility Study Center. We are grateful to Dr. J. Krupey for the generous gift of authentic CEA. This study was supported by a grant from The Mellon Foundation.

REFERENCES

1. Jones, W.R. Immunologic infertility: Fact or fiction?. Fertil. Steril. 33:577-586 (1980).

2. Franklin, R.R. and Dukes, C.D. Antispermatozoa antibody and unexplained infertility. Acta Obstet. Gynecol. Scand. 89:6-9 (1964).

3. Haas, G.G., Cines, D.B., and Schreiber, A.D. Immunological infertility: Identification of patients with antisperm antibody. New Engl. J. Med. 303:722-727 (1980).

4. Menge, A.C. Clinical immunologic infertility: Diagnostic measure, incidence of antisperm antibodies, fertility and mechanisms. In: D.S. Dhindsa and G.F.B. Schumacher (eds) Immunological Aspects of Infertility and Fertility Regulation. Elsevier/North Holland, New York, pp 205-224 (1980).

5. Hargreave, T.B. Incidence of sperm agglutinating and immobilizing sperm antibodies in infertile couples. Int. J. Fertil. 27:90-94 (1982).

6. Yan, Y.C., Wang, L.F., Sato, E., and Koide, S.S. Monoclonal antibody inducing human sperm agglutination. Am. J. Reprod. Immunol. 4:111-115 (1983).

7. Goding, J.W. Antibody production by hybridomas. J. Immunol. Meth. 39:285-308 (1980).

8. Gold, P. and Freedman, S.O. Specific carcinoembryonic antigens of the human digestive system. J. Exp. Med. 122:467-481 (1965).

9. Krupey, J., Gold, P., and Freedman, S.O. Physicochemical studies of the carcinoembryonic antigens of the human digestive system. J. Exp. Med. 128:387-398 (1968).

10. Krause, W. The occurrence of carcinoembryonic antigen-like immunoreactivity in human semen. Andrologia 12:130-134 (1980).

11. Eneroth, P., Lizana, J., Moberg, P., and Bygdeman, M. Carcinoembryonic antigen (CEA) immunoreactivity in human seminal plasma. Scand J. Clin. Lab. Invest. (Abstract 142/Suppl. 152) 39:51 (1979).

12. Williams, R.D., Bronson, D.L., Myl, A.D., Vandevoorde, J.P., and Elliot, A.Y. Carcinoembryonic antigen-like substance derived from human prostate. Cancer Res. 39:2447-2450 (1979).

13. Lizana, J., Moberg, P.J., and Eneroth, P. Beta-microglobulin, carcinoembryonic antigen and prostatic acid phosphatase in split ejaculates and urine voided before and after massage of the prostate. Arch. Androl. 11:225-232 (1983).

14. Isahakia, M. and Alexander, N.J. Interspecies cross-reactivity of monoclonal antibodies detected against human sperm antigens. Biol. Reprod. 30:1015-1026 (1984).

15. Shigeta, M., Watanabe, T., Maruyama, S., Koyama, K., and Isojima, S. Sperm-immobilizing monoclonal antibody to human seminal plasma antigens. Clin. Exp. Immunol. 42:458-462 (1980).

16. Isojima, S., Koyama, K., and Fujiwara, N. Purification of human seminal plasma No. 7 antigens by immunoaffinity on bound monoclonal antibody. Clin. Exp. Immunol. 49:449-456 (1982).

17. Dawson, P.A. and Filipe, M.I. An ultrastructural and histochemical study of the mucous membrane adjacent to and remote from carcinoma of the colon. Cancer 37:2388-2398 (1976).

18. Sharkey, R.M., Hagihara, P.F., and Goldenberg, D.M. Localization by immunoperoxidase and estimation by radioimmunoassay of carcinoembryonic antigen in colonic polyps. Br. J. Cancer 35:179-189 (1977).

19. O'Brien, M.J., Zamcheck, N., Burke, B., Kirkham, S.E., Saravis, C.A., and Gottlieb, L.S. Immunocytochemical localization of carcinoembryonic antigen in benign and malignant colorectal tissues. Amer. J. Clin. Path. 75:283-290 (1981).

20. Goldenberg, D.M., Sharkey, R.M., and Primus, F.J. Immunocytochemical detection of carcinoembryonic antigen in conventional histopathology specimens. Cancer 42:1546-1553 (1978).

21. VonKleist, S., Chavanel, G., and Burtin, P. Identification of an antigen from normal human tissue that cross- reacts with carcinoembryonic antigen. Proc. Natl. Acad. Sci. USA 69:2492-2494 (1972).

22. Burtin, P., Chavanel, G., and Hirsch-Marie, H. Characterization of a second normal antigen that cross-reacts with CEA. J. Immunol. 111:1926-1928 (1973).

23. Kuroki, M., Koga, Y., and Matsuoka, Y. Purification and characterization of carcinoembryonic antigen-related antigens in normal adult feces. Cancer Res. 41:713-720 (1981).

24. Svenberg, T., Hammarstrom, S., and Hedin, A. Purification and properties of biliary glycoprotein 1 (BGPI) Immunochemical relationship to carcinoembryonic antigen. Mol. Immunol. 16:245-252 (1979).

25. Primus, F.J., Clark, C.A., and Goldenberg, D.M. Immunoperoxidase localization of carcinoembryonic antigen in normal intestinal mucosa. J. Natl. Cancer Inst. 67:1031-1039 (1981).

26. Primus, F.J., Freeman, J.W., and Goldenberg, D.M. Immunological heterogeneity of carcinoembryonic antigen: Purification from meconium of an antigen related to carcinoembryonic antigen. Cancer Res. 43:679-685 (1983).

27. Primus, F.J., Kuhns, W.J., and Goldenberg, D.M. Immunological heterogeneity of carcinoembryonic antigen: Immuno-histochemical detection of carcinoembryonic antigen determinants in colonic tumors with monoclonal antibodies. Cancer Res. 43:693-701 (1983).

28. Primus, F.J., Newell, K.D., Blue, A., and Goldenberg, D.M. Immunological heterogeneity of carcinoembryonic antigen: Antigenic determinants on carcinoembryonic antigen distinguished by monoclonal antibodies. Cancer Res. 43:686-692 (1983).

29. Stahli, C., Miggiano, V., LeDain, M., Ianelli, D., Fessler, R., Haring, P., Schmidt, J., and Staehelin, T. Distinction and characterization by monoclonal antibodies of epitopes on four proteins of clinical interest. Res. Monogr. Immunol. 3:201-208 (1981).

30. Bordes, M., Knobel, S., and Martin, F. Carcinoembryonic antigen (CEA) and related antigens in blood cells and hematopoietic tissues. Europ. J. Cancer 11:783-786 (1975).

31. Burtin, P., Quan, P.C., and Sabine, M.C. Nonspecific crossreactivity antigen as a marker for human polymorphs, macrophages and monocytes. Nature 235:714-716 (1975).

# MOLECULAR GENETICS OF THE MOUSE ZONA PELLUCIDA: IMPLICATIONS FOR FERTILIZATION AND EARLY DEVELOPMENT

Jurrien Dean, Maurice Ringuette, Donna A. Sobieski
Iain J. East and Steven Chamow

Laboratory of Cellular and Developmental Biology
Building 6, Room B1-07
NIADDK
National Institutes of Health
Bethesda, Maryland 20205

## INTRODUCTION

Pre-implantation development in mammals begins with the one-cell zygote and continues through to the formation of the blastocyst which ultimately implants on the wall of the uterus. The maternal genome plays an important role in gene expression not only during oogenesis but also during early development. There are few genes which are specific to this period of embryogenesis (4-6,19) and even fewer with known biological functions. However, the genes that code for proteins of the mouse zona pellucida are an exception. They are expressed during oogenesis in a coordinate manner and the production of their protein products is turned off as the oocyte matures even though biological roles of the zona proteins persist into pre-implantation development. By studying the genes coding for the zona proteins we hope to learn more about mechanisms that control gene expression during oogenesis and early embryogenesis.

The murine zona pellucida is comprised of three sulfated glycoproteins designated ZP-1, ZP-2, and ZP-3 (1,18). These proteins are synthesized by the maturing oocyte and secreted to form an extracellular matrix which surrounds the growing oocyte, ovulated egg and pre-implantation embryo. Mouse ZP-3 has an average molecular weight of 85,000 daltons and has been reported to mediate the sperm-egg interaction at fertilization via O-linked oligosaccharide side chains (2,12). ZP-2 with an average molecular weight of 140,000 daltons is modified during fertilization and may play a role in the post-fertilization block to polyspermy (3). The third zona protein, ZP-1, (200,000 daltons) is thought to cross-link ZP-2 and ZP-3 in the extracellular matrix (13).

Immunocontraception based on the antigenicity of the zona pellucida has been reported using passive immunization of anti-zona antisera as well as active immunization with zona components (for review see reference 15). Both of these approaches suffer from the heterogeneity of the injected material. The advent of monoclonal antibody technology now allows the isolation of homogeneous antibody populations directed not only against individual zona proteins but to specific antigenic determinants within each protein. Passive immunization with these antibodies can then be tested to determine their effect on fertilization and early

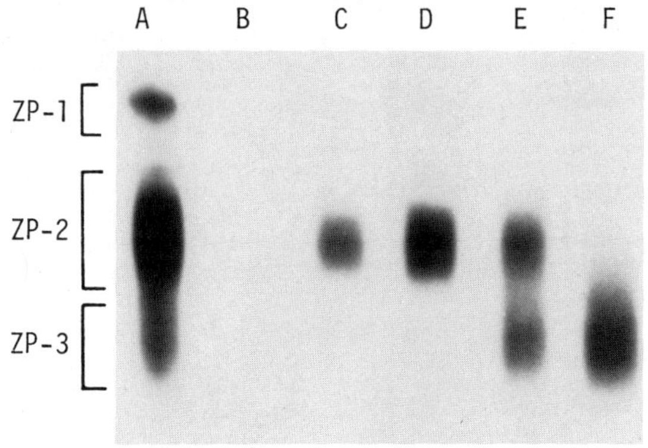


Figure 1. Autoradiograph of SDS-PAGE of Immunoprecipitation. Isolated $^{125}$[I]-Bolton-Hunter labeled zonae pellucidae ($3 \times 10^4$ cpm) (A) alone, or after immunoprecipitation with: (B) control ascites fluid; (C) monoclonal antibody IE-1; (D) IE-3; (E) IE-4; and (F) IE-10 (see reference 7).

development and, thus, identify regions of zona proteins important for biological function (7). Using this data and recombinant DNA techniques, the DNA coding for the antigenic determinants important in fertilization can be cloned and expressed as fusion proteins. After purification these zona proteins can be used as vaccines to test their effect on fertilization and early development.

## MONOCLONAL ANTIBODIES

We have produced a series of rat monoclonal antibodies specific for ZP-2, ZP-3 and one which reacts with both ZP-2 and ZP-3 (Figure 1). Three criteria have been used to substantiate that these antibodies are, indeed, monoclonal. Each cell line has been subcloned by limiting dilution three times. Each expressed an IgG of a single sub-type and, finally, chromatographically purified immunoglobulins from each cell line had a single and unique light chain as determined by two-dimensional gel electrophoresis (8,9). These antibodies have been used to demonstrate that the zona proteins are found uniquely in the ovary (Figure 2) where they surround oocytes in the growth and maturation phase of development (10,11). Ovulated eggs stained with monoclonal antibodies show a reticulated pattern reminescent of earlier studies of the zona with scanning electron microscopy. Binding studies show that the monoclonal antibodies bind to eggs with dissociation constants between $3 \times 10^{-9}$ and $6 \times 10^{-10}$ mol $l^{-1}$. Antibodies to ZP-2 bind to roughly $3 \times 10^8$ sites, or 2-3% of all available ZP-2 molecules in the mouse zona pellucida (8). Thus, it was of interest to determine if the presence of the antibody perturbed any of the known functions of the zona pellucida in early development.

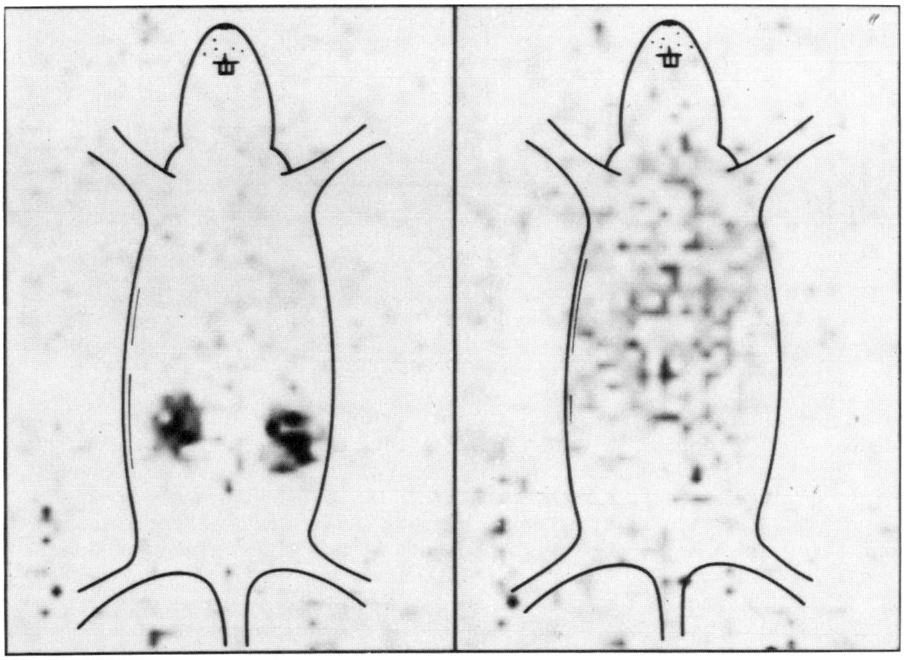

Figure 2. Immunoscintophotographs of Mice. NIH Swiss mice were injected with 2.7 μCi of [$^{125}$I]-labeled monoclonal antibody specific to ZP-2 and sacrificed 22 days later. Scintophotographs were obtained with a ventral gamma camera. Female mouse with both ovaries clearly visible is on the left and a male mouse with non-specific body background radioactivity is on the right (see reference 11).

## EFFECTS ON EARLY DEVELOPMENT

When immunized with 250 μg of anti-zona monoclonal antibodies, 100% of female mice mated with males were infertile. Furthermore, it appeared that antibodies specific to either ZP-2 or ZP-3 were equally effective in blocking the formation of 2-cell embryos (Figure 3) and this block was associated with antibodies coating the surface of the zona pellucida (9,10). *In vitro* fertilization studies demonstrated that fertilization was 50% inhibited by 20 ng/ml of anti-ZP-2 or 185 ng/ml of anti-ZP-3 monoclonal antibodies (Figure 4). The presence of the antibody did not perturb sperm function and neither ZP-2 nor ZP-3 antibodies effectively prevented sperm attaching and binding to mouse eggs. However, the presence of the antibody did inhibit sperm penetration of the zona and was, thus, a potent block to fertilization (9). This contraceptive effect in continuously mated animals was of long duration lasting an average of 64 days, although there was considerable variation, (44-117 days) among animals (Figure 5). Furthermore, the block was reversible with sufficient time following antibody treatment and eventually all of the animals had litters which were of the same size and weight as control animals. When subsequently remated, the treated animals gave birth to litters at a rate similar to control animals (Figure 5). This reversibility was associated with the loss of the monoclonal antibody from the zonae of intraovarian oocytes (10).

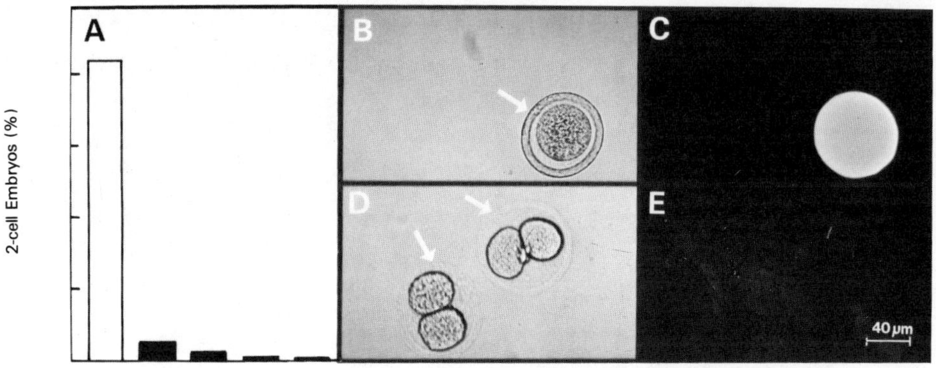


Figure 3. Inhibition of 2-cell Embryo Formation by Antibodies. (A) Percentage of 2-cell embryos formed after passive immunization of female mice with pre-immune serum (control), monoclonal antibodies specific to: ZP-2 (IE-1, IE-3); to ZP-3 (IE-10); or to both ZP-2 and ZP-3 (IE-4). (B) Light microscopy of egg from mouse after passive immunization with anti-ZP-2 and stained with FITC-conjugated sheep anti-rat Ig antibodies. Arrow indicates outer diameter of zona pellucida. (C) Fluorescence microscopy of egg from (B). (D) Light microscopy of 2-cell embryo from mouse treated with preimmune rat serum and stained with FITC-conjugated sheep anti-rat Ig antibodies. Arrow indicates outer diameter of translucent zona pellucida. (E) Fluorescence microscopy of embryos from (D) (see reference 7).

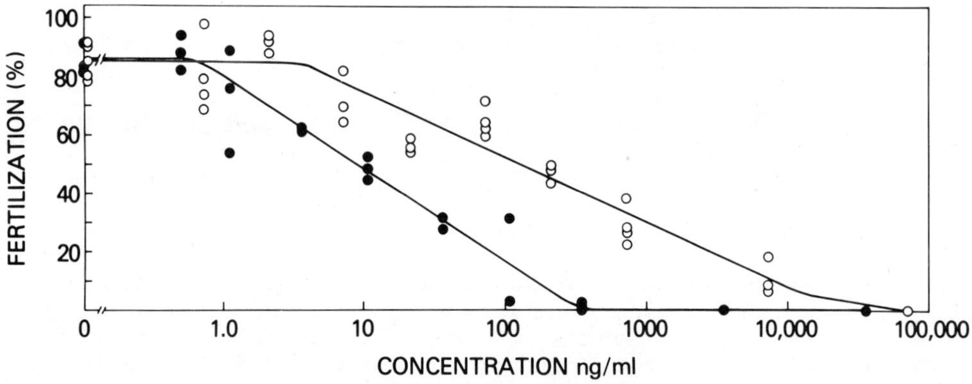


Figure 4. *In vitro* Fertilization. Percentage of superovulated eggs from B6C3 $F_1$ hybrid females fertilized *in vitro* with sperm from ZBW $F_1$ males in the presence of increasing concentration of ●—● anti-ZP-2 monoclonal antibody (IE-3) or o—o anti-ZP-3 monoclonal antibody (IE-10) (see reference 9).

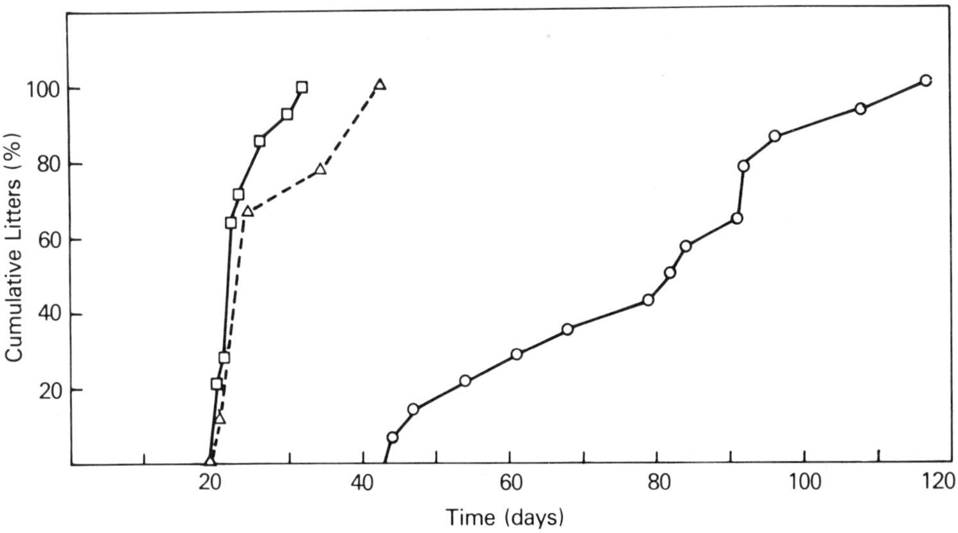


Figure 5. Reversibility of Block to Fertility. Cummulative liter (%) over time of groups of 14 mice continuously mated after administration of saline (□) or 250 µg of anti-ZP-2 monoclonal antibody (o). Nine mice from the antibody-treated group remated after the resumption of fertility (Δ). Days are numbered from time that males were caged with females (see reference 10).

Thus, the passive immunization of mice with anti-zona monoclonal antibodies results in localization of the antibody to maturing intra-ovarian oocytes. When ovulated, these eggs can not be fertilized due to a block to sperm penetration of the zona pellucida. As all of the antibody coated oocytes are ovulated, new oocytes are recruited into the growth and maturation pool and in the absence of circulating antibodies, their zonae are not coated. Thus, after ovulation, they can be fertilized which accounts for the reversibility of the contraceptive effect. We have observed no other perturbation of early *in vivo* or *in vitro* development induced by monoclonal antibodies either to ZP-2 or to ZP-3 (7-11). These antibodies did not react to the zona pellucida of other mammalian species (9).

## ORGANIZATION OF THE ZP-3 GENE

An alternative approach to immunocontraception is active immunization with zona protein. However, due to the difficulty in obtaining sufficient quantities of biological material, it is not feasible to test the efficacy of native mouse zona components. Recently, recombinant DNA techniques have allowed us to clone ZP-3, the sperm receptor, and express it as a fusion protein. This fusion protein expresses an epitope recognized by a monoclonal antibody which blocks fertilization and is specific for ZP-3. Thus, the fusion protein may be a prime candidate to test as a contraceptive vaccine.

We first constructed a cDNA library from poly $A^+$ mRNA isolated from ovarian tissue (16). These cDNAs were ligated into the unique EcoRI site near the 3' end of the β-galactosidase gene in the expression vector λgt11. We identified a clone coding for ZP-3 which, a) expressed a fu-

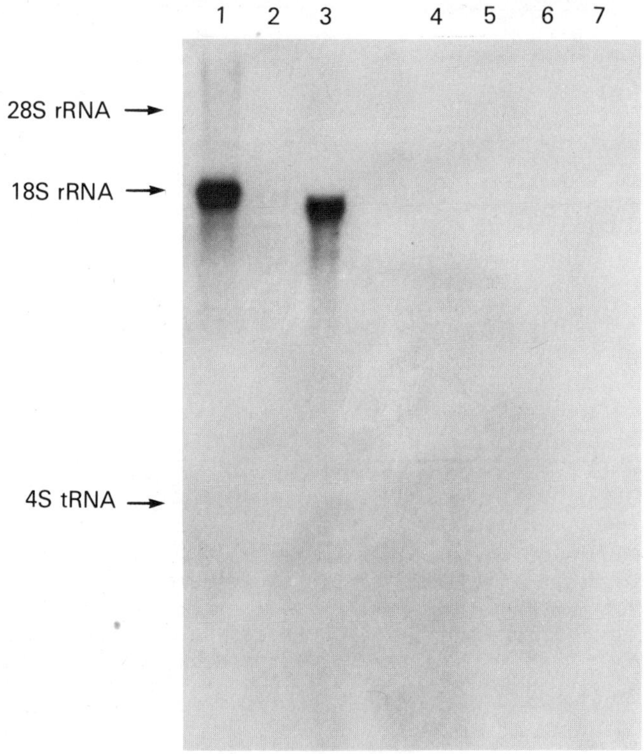


Figure 6. Northern Blot Analysis of Tissue Specific RNA. An insert from plasmid pZP-3.1 containing the cDNA coding for ZP-3 was labeled with [$^{32}$P] and used to probe: (1) ovarian poly A$^{+}$ mRNA; (2) ovarian poly A$^{-}$ mRNA; (3) total ovarian RNA; (4) total liver RNA; (5) total heart RNA; (6) total brain RNA; and (7) total testes RNA (see reference 16).

sion protein recognized by monoclonal antibodies specific to ZP-3; b) detected transcription of a homogeneous 1.7 kb polyadenylated mRNA only in ovarian tissue (Figure 6); and c) hybrid selected a mRNA that codes for a 44 kd protein which is the molecular weight of the core protein of ZP-3 (17).

This cDNA clone was subsequently used as a probe in examining the genomic organization of ZP-3. DNAs from brain, liver and ovarian tissues were restricted separately with four different enzymes, blotted according to Southern and probed with [$^{32}$P]-labeled ZP-3 cDNA. The pattern among the three tissue DNAs was unique for each enzyme but identical among tissues (Figure 7) and the simplicity of the patterns suggests that the ZP-3 gene exists in the mouse genome as a low-copy-number gene. Furthermore, it appears that the coding regions of ZP-3 are spread out over 13-18 kb of mouse genomic DNA. Using an isoschizomer pair which differ in ability to recognize sites containing methylated cytosines, we have shown that the DNA in and around the ZP-3 locus is hypomethylated in ovarian tissue (where it is expressed) in comparison to non-expressing tissue such as brain and liver (16).

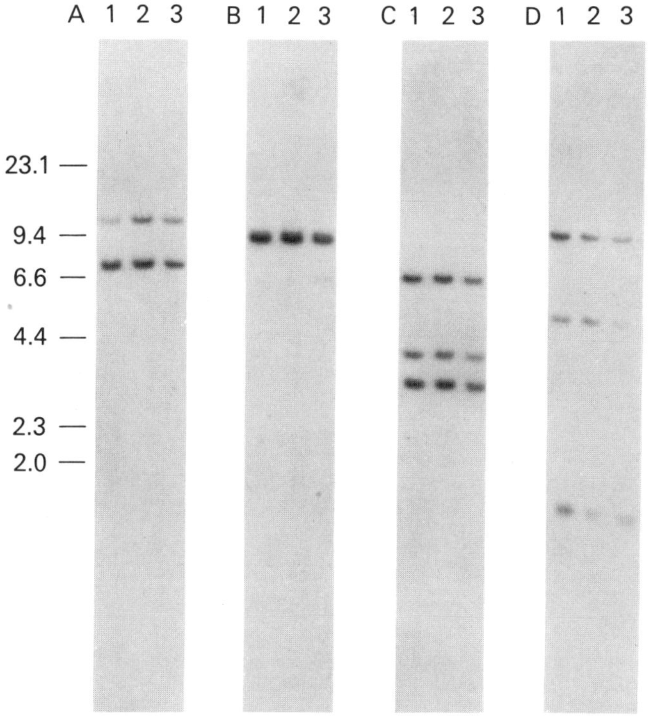


Figure 7. Southern Blot Analysis of ZP-3 Gene. Genomic DNAs from (1) liver, (2) brain and (3) ovarian mouse tissue were restricted with (A) Bam HI, (B) Hind III, (C) Sst I and (D) Pst I. After hybridization with [$^{32}$P]-labeled cDNA coding for ZP-3, the blots were washed with .1 x SSC at 50°C (see reference 16).

ZP-3 mediates a relatively species-specific reaction and, therefore, each species may have a unique ZP-3 protein. Indeed, using monoclonal antibodies to at least five different epitopes on the zona pellucida, we have detected no immunological cross-reactivity among a variety of mammals. Thus, it was of interest to determine the degree of homology on a DNA level among mammalian species. The mouse ZP-3 cDNA clone cross-hybridized with genomic DNA from rat, dog, cow and human under conditions where one would expect to detect sequence of greater than 80% homology (Figure 8A). Rabbit and pig DNA hybridized poorly at this stringency. However, when the wash conditions allowed hybrids of 55% homology to remain bound, rabbit and pig DNA showed homology to the mouse clone (Figure 8B). The Southern blot patterns of each mammals' DNA differed from mouse and from each other indicating sequence divergence in this genomic region among mammals (16).

## IMPLICATIONS FOR CONTRACEPTIVE VACCINES

The zona proteins represent a set of genes that are functionally related, developmentally controlled and expressed during oogenesis in the absence of cell division. Monoclonal antibodies specific to five different epitopes on the zona pellucida can act as effective, long-term but ultimately reversible contraceptive agents. We have cloned the epitope

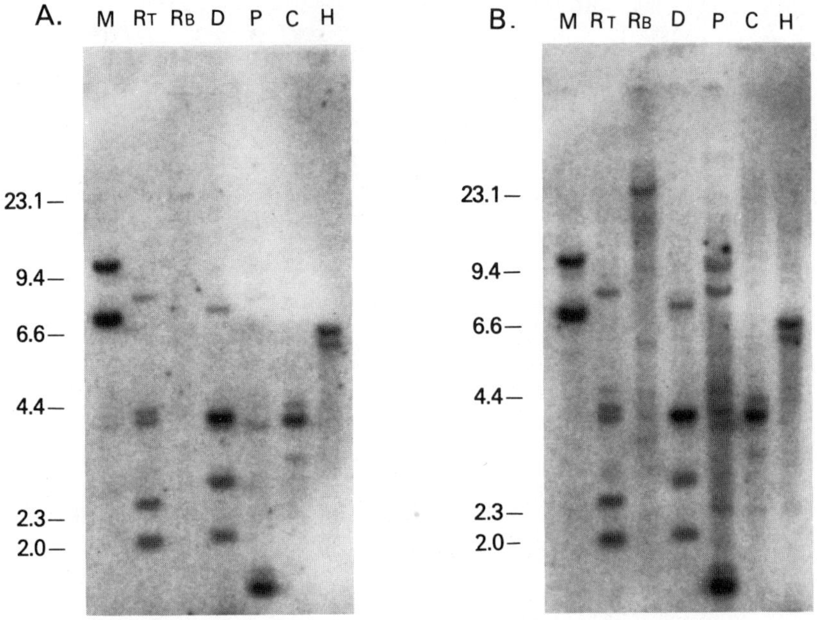


Figure 8. Cross Hybridization of ZP-3 Among Mammals. Genomic DNAs from (M) mouse, (RT) rat, (RB) rabbit, (D) dog, (P) pig, (C) cow and (H) human were digested with Bam HI, and hybridized with [$^{32}$P]-labeled cloned ZP-3 cDNA. The blot in A was washed with .1 X SSC at 50°C. In B, the blot was washed under reduced stringency with 2 x SSC at 50°C.

on ZP-3 recognized by one of these antibodies. This clone expressed the ZP-3 epitope as a portion of a β-galactosidase-containing fusion protein. We now plan to actively immunize mice with this fusion protein to determine its effect on fertilization and early development. Furthermore, the mouse ZP-3 clone is homologous to the DNA of a variety of mammalian species including man. Thus, using recombinant DNA technology we can clone the ZP-3 gene from a number of mammals, express that clone as a fusion protein and, ultimately, test its efficacy as a contraceptive vaccine. Although as yet these are model systems, contraception based on the zona proteins may play an important role in our armamentarium for effective fertility control.

ACKNOWLEDGEMENTS

We appreciate the critical reading of the manuscript by Dr. R.T. Simpson and thank Mrs. B. Richards for expert typing.

REFERENCES

1. Bleil, J.D. and P.M. Wassarman, Structure and function of the zona pellucida: Identification and characterization of the protein of the mouse oocyte's zona pellucida, Dev. Biol., 76: 185 (1980).

2. Bleil, J.D. and P.M. Wassarman, Mammalian sperm-egg interaction: Identification of a glycoprotein in mouse egg zonae pellucidae possessing receptor activity for sperm, Cell, 20: 873 (1980).
3. Bleil, J.D., C.F. Beall and P.M. Wassarman, Mammalian sperm-egg interaction: Fertilization of mouse eggs triggers modification of the major zona pellucida glycoprotein, ZP-2, Dev. Biol., 86:189 (1981).
4. Braude, P., H. Pelham, G. Flach and R. Lobatto, Post-transcriptional control in the early mouse embryo, Nature (Lond.), 282:102 (1979).
5. Cascio, S.M. and P.M. Wassarman, Program of early development in the mammal: Post-transcriptional control of a class of proteins synthesized by mouse oocytes and early embryos. Dev. Biol., 89:397 (1982).
6. Cullen, B., K. Emigholz and J. Monahan, The transient appearance of specific proteins in one-cell mouse embryos, Dev. Biol., 76:215 (1980).
7. Dean, J. and I.J. East, Effects of anti-zona pellucida monoclonal antibodies on fertilization and early development, in: "The Molecular and Cellular Biology of Fertilization," J.L. Hedrick, ed., Plenum Press, New York, in press.
8. East, I.J. and J. Dean, Monoclonal antibodies as probes of the distribution of ZP-2, the major sulfated glycoprotein of the murine zona pellucida. J. Cell Biol., 98:795 (1984).
9. East, I.J., B.J. Gulyas and J. Dean, Monoclonal antibodies to the murine zona pellucida protein with sperm receptor activity: Effects on fertilization and early development, Devel. Biol., 109:268 (1985).
10. East, I.J., D.R. Mattison and J. Dean, Monoclonal antibodies to the major protein of the murine zona pellucida: Effects on fertilization and early development. Devel. Biol., 104:49 (1984).
11. East, I.J., A.M. Keenan, S.M. Larson and J. Dean, Scintigraphy of normal mouse ovaries with monoclonal antibodies to ZP-2, the major zona pellucida protein, Science, 225:938 (1984).
12. Florman, H.M. and P.M. Wassarman, O-linked oligosaccharides of mouse egg ZP-3 account for its sperm receptor activity, Cell, 41:313 (1985)
13. Greve, J.M. and P.M. Wassarman, Mouse extracellular coat is a matrix of interconnected filaments possessing a structural repeat, J. Mol. Biol., 181:253 (1985).
14. Johnson, M.H., The molecular and cellular basis of pre-implantation mouse development, Biol. Rev., 56:463 (1981).
15. Jones, W.R., Immunization against the oocyte, in: "Immunological Fertility Regulation," Blackwell, Oxford (1982), pp. 147-174.
16. Ringuette, M., D.A. Sobieski, S. Chamow and J. Dean, Molecular cloning of ZP-3: Sperm receptor of the mouse zona pellucida submitted for publication.
17. Salzmann, G.S., J.M. Greve, R.J. Roller and P.M. Wassarman, Biosynthesis of the sperm receptor during oogenesis in the mouse. EMBO J., 2:1451 (1983).
18. Shimizu, S., M. Tsuji and J. Dean, In vitro biosynthesis of three sulfated glycoproteins of murine zonae pellucidae by oocytes grown in follicle culture. J. Biol. Chem., 258:5858 (1983).
19. Van Blerkom, J., Structural relationship and posttranslational modification of stage specific proteins synthesized during preimplantation development in the mouse, Proc. Natl. Acad. Sci. U.S.A., 78:7629 (1981).

# SPECIES VARIATION IN THE ZONA PELLUCIDA

S.M. Skinner and B.S. Dunbar

Department of Cell Biology
Baylor College of Medicine, One Baylor Plaza
Houston, Texas 77030

## INTRODUCTION

The mammalian fertilization process is an intricate one which involves many aspects of species specificity. Before the fusion of gamete membranes occurs and fertilization is achieved, a number of closely synchronized events must take place. In order to monitor and ultimately to control this process, it is necessary to understand the fundamental nature as well as the timing of these events. Central to the success of fertilization is the ovulation of a mature ovum which is surrounded by a unique extracellular matrix, the zona pellucida (ZP). This glycoprotein matrix surrounds the mammalian oocyte at a time early in follicular development and remains intact until the eventual implantation of the fertilized ovum. After ovulation, the sperm must attach to and penetrate the ZP. Over the past decade, much attention has been brought to studies which have demonstrated that immunization with ZP glycoproteins results in a dramatic reduction in fertility. In order for us to appreciate the mechanisms by which this immunologically induced infertility occurs, it is essential to understand the biochemical and functional properties of the ZP throughout ovarian follicular development.

## BIOLOGICAL ROLES OF THE ZONA PELLUCIDA

### ZP Formation During Follicular Development

The role of formation of the ZP during early stages of the growth and development of the oocyte is only now beginning to be fully appreciated. Recent studies have been carried out using immunocytochemical localization to demonstrate that the formation of the rabbit ZP is initiated just prior to differentiation of the granulosa cells (Wolgemuth et al., 1984).

In these studies, the appearance of ZP glycoproteins was first observed in the oocyte at the time when its growth was first apparent. Following the extracellular appearance of a thin, continuous layer of ZP protein around the oocyte, the first layer of granulosa epithelial cells differentiates from flat to cuboidal cells. At the stage at which the follicle is composed of 3-4 cell layers, intense staining of ZP protein is observed in the inner layer of follicle cells. This staining disappears as the follicle matures to the antral stage. While immunocytochemical localization of specific proteins is not direct proof of synthesis, these studies strongly suggest that the formation of the ZP of some species is complex and may involve dual cell types. The role of the ZP as an extracellular matrix which may act in regulating the differentiation of granulosa cells is also implied by these studies. Additional studies which would support this role demonstrate that heteroimmunization of rabbits with porcine ZP glycoprotein results in abnormal follicular development, ultimately causing reduction in or cessation of ovulation (Skinner et al., 1984). The obligatory role of the ZP in the successful development of the ovum is further discussed below.

## Interaction of Spermatozoa with the ZP

A major function of the ZP in fertilization involves the attachment or "binding" of the spermatozoan to the zona surface (see reviews by Dunbar and Wolgemuth, 1984; Dunbar, 1983a,b; Hartman and Gwatkin, 1971; Hartman et al., 1972; Hartman and Hutchinson, 1974; Saling et al., 1978). Recently, many studies have been carried out to elucidate the mechanisms by which the sperm passes through the cells of the cumulus oophorus to contact the ZP (Yanagimachi and Phillips, 1984; Talbot and DiCarlantonio, 1984a; Talbot and DeCarlantonio, 1984b; Green and Purves, 1984) and the mechanism by which the sperm adheres to and subsequently penetrates the ZP (Talbot and DeCarlantonio, 1984a; Gaddum-Rosse et al., 1984; Stambaugh and Nicosia, 1984; Huang and Yanagimachi, 1984; Crozet and Dumont, 1984; Kuzan et al., 1984; Urch et al., 1985; Bleil and Wassarman, 1980b; Florman and Wassarman, 1985; Dunbar et al., 1985; East et al., 1985). Although the majority of the detailed studies in this area have been done in rodent systems, it has recently been shown that marked species variations are observed in these phases of the fertilization process, particularly at the stage of sperm-ZP interaction (see reviews by Dunbar, 1983; Dunbar and Wolgemuth, 1984).

The sperm presumably binds to the ZP via species specific sperm "receptor sites" which are thought to play important roles in the species specificity of sperm-egg interaction. Investigation into the nature of this interaction has shown that treatment with a variety of enzymes alters binding properties of sperm. Those "receptors" of the hamster ZP, for example, are sensitive to trypsin, chymotrypsin, and trypsin-like acrosin preparations from hamster, ram and boar sperm (Gwatkin et al., 1973; Gwatkin et al., 1977). Sperm receptors of the rabbit (Overstreet and Bedford, 1975) or the mouse zona (Aitken and Richardson, 1980) are not destroyed by such treatment. However, Oikawa et al. (1975) have demonstrated that treatment of hamster eggs with these enzymes does modify zona glycopeptides. More recently, investigations have been carried out to analyze ZP molecules which are associated with sperm "receptor" activity. These studies indicate that the carbohydrates of a specific ZP glycoprotein are involved in sperm zona interaction (Bleil and Wassarman, 1980b; Shur and Hall, 1982; Florman and Wassarman, 1985). Recent studies in the mouse system suggest that one of the ZP glycoproteins (ZP3) is associated with penetraton but not surface "binding" of the sperm to the ZP (East et al., 1985). The molecular mechanisms of sperm-zona interaction in other species remain to be elucidated and appear to be more complex since some, such as the rabbit and pig, lack species specificity of sperm recognition (Swenson and Dunbar, 1982; Bedford, 1977). Interspecies sperm/ZP associations were investigated recently by O'Rand et al. (1985) in *in vitro* studies in which sperm proteins from a variety of mammals were blotted onto nitrocellulose paper. Characteristic binding to these by zona proteins both within and between species was demonstrated. Other studies have been carried out which suggest that sperm "binding" activity may be associated with a particular glycoprotein component of the pig ZP (Sacco et al., 1984). The intricacy of sperm/ZP interaction in this species was further demonstrated in studies by Dunbar et al. (1985) showing that porcine sperm acrosin specifically proteolyzes particular integral glycoproteins of the porcine ZP, leaving the native ZP matrix intact.

In some mammalian species, the sperm-binding properties of the ZP are altered following fertilization. This is known as the block to polyspermy. Furthermore, the ZP's resistance to proteolytic digestion is altered (Gwatkin et al., 1973; Austin and Braden, 1956; Barros and Yanagimachi, 1971, 1972; Gianfortoni and Gulyas, 1985; Florman and Wassarman, 1985). These changes, referred to as the 'zona reaction' (Braden et al., 1954), are thought to be induced by the release of components of cortical granules after sperm-oocyte plasma membrane fusion (Austin and Braden, 1956; Barros and Yanagimachi, 1972; Gwatkin et al., 1973; Yanagimachi, 1977).

Finally, the ZP remains intact after fertilization, ensuring proper embryo development and embryo movement in the oviduct (Modlinski, J.A., 1970), and possibly preventing embryo fusion within the oviduct (Mintz, B., 1962).

## ANALYSIS OF ZONA PELLUCIDA GLYCOPROTEINS

### Isolation

Because of the availability of large numbers of invertebrate and amphibian gametes, it has long been possible to carry out studies on the molecular basis of sperm-egg interaction in these species (Glabe and Vacquier, 1977; Aketa, 1973; Kinsey and Lennarz, 1981). Recently, improved procedures for the collection of large numbers of mammalian eggs and their ZP have made it possible to purify the constituent ZP glycoproteins for use in detailed molecular studies of structure and function. Recent collection methods, previously reviewed (Dunbar et al., 1980; Dunbar and Raynor, 1980; Wood et al., 1981), allow isolation of up to 400,000 porcine ZP or 30,000 rabbit ZP, resulting in a preparation estimated to be 93% pure. Unfortunately, it has not been possible to adapt these procedures to the smaller and more fragile rodent zonae.

### Physical Properties

*Molecular composition of the ZP.* The analysis of the molecular structure of the mammalian ZP was an early target of biochemical investigation. The ZP of different species vary in size with respect to their oocytes (Dunbar, 1983a). In general, the ZP of rodent species are smaller than those of most other mammalian species. However, scanning electron microscopy has shown them to be markedly similar with respect to their fenestrated external surface and their somewhat smoother inner surface (Dudkiewicz et al., 1976; Gwatkin et al., 1976; Jackowski and Dumont, 1979; Philips and Shalgi, 1980). The differential permeability of the ZP to a variety of substances (Sellens and Jenkinson, 1975) appears not to be related to their molecular weight, but rather to the

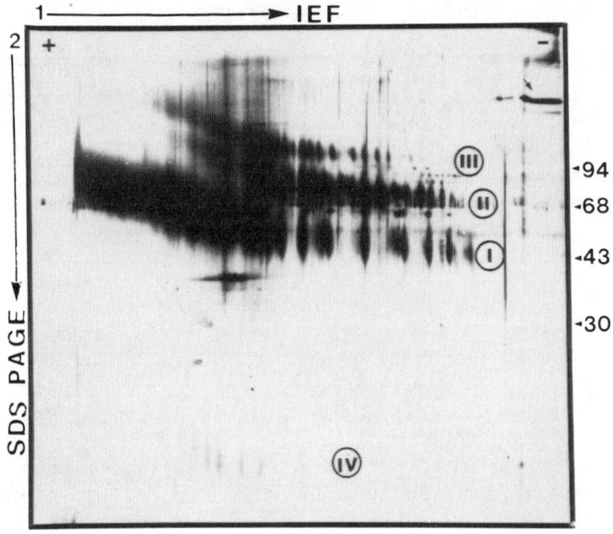


Fig. 1 High-resolution two-dimensional polyacrylamide gel electrophoresis separation of porcine zona pellucida glycoproteins showing isoelectric focusing (IEF) in the first dimension and SDS-polyacrylamide gel electrophoresis (SDS-PAGE) in the second dimension. The color-based silver staining procedure allows visualization of the four major glycoprotein families (I, II, III, IV) in which extensive size and charge heterogeneity is apparent. A variety of minor proteins are observed in this sample because this was of an intact ZP preparation which is known to contain minor contaminants. This preparation is used for immunoblotting studies to ensure that antibodies are not directed against these minor components.

molecular configuration or charge properties of the substance in question.

Histological staining techniques (Baranska et al., 1975; Wolgemuth and Gavin, 1981) as well as the use of plant lectins which bind carbohydrate residues (Dunbar, 1980) have shown the ZP to be composed of morphologically distinct layers. Asymmetrical regional distribution of several of these bound lectins convincingly illustrates the biological heterogeneity of the ZP (Dunbar et al., 1980; Nicholson et al., 1975; Watanabe et al., 1981; Dunbar, 1980).

Early cytochemical studies suggested that the ZP was mucopolysaccharide in nature. However, recent investigations show the ZP to be composed of glycoprotein (Dunbar, 1980; Dunbar et al., 1981; Sacco et al., 1981, 1984; Bleil and Wassarman, 1980b). Specifically, the porcine ZP consists of 71% protein, 19% neutral hexose, 2.7% sialic acid and

2.4% sulfate. As would be expected from the obvious difference in their size, the porcine ZP (30 ng/ZP) contains almost seven times the protein of mouse ZP.

Solubilization of the ZP. To further investigate the structural nature of the ZP, it became necessary to solubilize this matrix. Light microscopic, as well as biochemical analyses have demonstrated that dissolution of ZP of different species varies according to their susceptibility to such agents as acid, base, heat or proteolytic enzymes (Dunbar et al., 1980; Dunbar 1983b). Rodent ZP have been found to be much more sensitive to chemical and enzymatic solubilization than are the ZP of larger species, such as the pig, rabbit, cow, or human (Dunbar, 1983b) (see below). Successful dissolution of the ZP depends upon time, temperature, and pH (Dunbar et al., 1980).

## Purification of ZP Glycoproteins

Further biochemical investigation of ZP structure and function was impossible without the isolation and purification of the ZP glycoproteins themselves. Because of their extreme size and charge heterogeneity, one-dimensional sodium dodecyl sulfate polyacrylamide gel electrophoresis (SDS-PAGE) produced only smears, making detailed analysis of specific proteins difficult (Dunbar et al., 1980; Gwatkin et al., 1980; Dunbar, 1980; Bleil and Wassarman, 1980b). High-resolution 2D-PAGE has proven to be the most valuable technique for analyzing ZP proteins (Dunbar et al., 1981; Sacco et al., 1982). The porcine ZP pattern obtained using 2D-PAGE analysis is that of three major glycoprotein families (Figure 1), each of which has extensive charge and molecular weight heterogeneity. The apparent molecular weights of the three proteins are (I) 42-120K, (II) 69-110K, and (III) 90-120K. Such charge heterogeneity is typical of proteins which have undergone extensive post-translational modification such as glycosylation (Anderson and Anderson, 1977; Dunbar et al., 1981). Rabbit zonae give a similar pattern of three major protein families. They are less well resolved on 2D-PAGE, and their apparent molecular weights are (I) 68-125K, (II) 81-100.5K, and (III) 100-132K (Dunbar et al., 1981).

Using 2D-PAGE analysis, recent studies have been undertaken to deglycosylate the porcine and rabbit ZP with endoglycosidase F (Endo F) (Elder and Alexander, 1982) or with trifluoromethanesulfonic acid (TFMS) (Karp et al., 1982). Such treatment reduces the molecular weight and charge heterogeneity of all three major porcine and rabbit ZP glycoproteins (Figure 2). If the conformation is altered such that the cleavage site is exposed, Endo F may be used to cleave glycans from N-linked glycoproteins (Anderson and Anderson, 1977). Additional removal of carbohydrates may then be achieved by acid hydrolysis of glycosidic bonds using TFMS (Karp et al., 1982). The apparent molecular weights of the three major porcine ZP glycoproteins after either treatment are (I) 35K, (II) 55K, and (III) 70K (Drell et al., 1984). One-dimensional SDS-PAGE was used by Florman and Wassarman (1985) to analyze the results of enzyme treatments of mouse ZP glycoprotein 3. They concluded that O-linked oligosaccharides present in ZP3 are necessary for "sperm receptor" activity.

The color-based silver stain developed by Sammons et al. (Sammons et al., 1981) has recently been used to analyze ZP proteins. This detection procedure will stain proteins a variety of colors, the basis for which is not yet clearly understood. Such staining heterogeneity

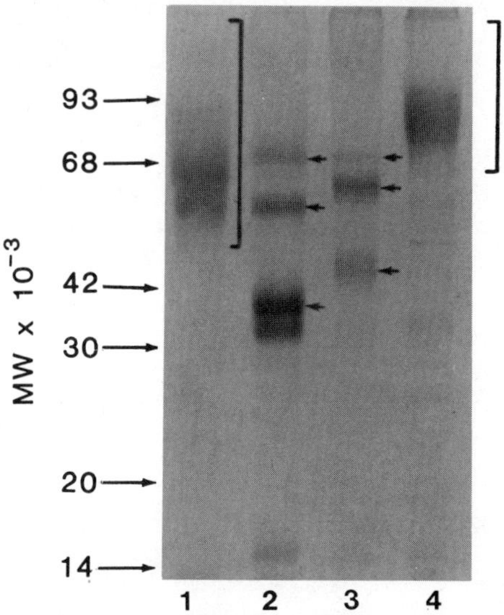


Fig. 2 One-dimensional polyacrylamide gel electrophoresis (1D-PAGE) showing the size heterogeneity of the ZP glycoproteins from pig and rabbit ZP (columns 1 and 4, respectively). Following deglycosylation with trifluoromethane sulfonic acid (TFMS), zona proteins of the pig and rabbit can be resolved as discrete proteins (columns 2 and 3, respectively).

has been useful in identifying two distinct components of the enzymatically treated major glycoprotein train I of porcine ZP. When native porcine ZP matrices are treated with trypsin or with the boar sperm enzyme, they remain morphologically intact under light microscopy. The protein pattern obtained on 2D-PAGE analysis shows, however, that the molecular composition of these ZP is dramatically altered (Dunbar, 1985). The major ZP protein family I is separated into two peptides, designated Ia and Ib, which differ in color, yet the apparent molecular weight range appears the same as before digestion. Porcine ZP glycoprotein II is more sensitive to proteolysis than protein I, while train III is completely eliminated under the conditions which proteolyze train I (Dunbar et al., 1985). Such studies have provided valuable information on the structure and function of specific domains of the ZP matrix which may be involved in the fertilization process.

## IMMUNOCHEMICAL APPROACHES TO THE STUDY OF ZP FUNCTION

The techniques developed for analysis of ZP glycoproteins have also served to identify specific antibodies which have now been used to further investigate the role of the ZP in fertilization. Early studies carried out on the immunogenicity of isolated porcine zonae in rabbits and of rabbit zonae in rabbits and guinea pigs (Dunbar and Raynor, 1980; Dunbar, 1983a,b) have shown that the immunogenicity of the porcine zona is complex. The immunological response depends upon the amount of ZP immunogen used, as well as on the solubilization conditions used in its preparation.

## Antibody Detection and Characterization

To date, the most critical factor limiting the evaluation of the effects of anti-ZP antibodies on fertility has been development of dependable assays for antibody detection and characterization. Most early studies, as well as some current ones, have relied upon the use of immunofluorescence as their method of choice (see review by Dunbar, 1983a). This use of immunofluorescence assays has led to controversy concerning the presence of anti-ZP antibodies in human sera (Nishimoto et al., 1980; Nayuda et al., 1982a; Sacco and Moghiss, 1979; Kamada et al., 1984; Mhasker et al., 1984). Other inconsistencies have appeared among studies on the inhibition of fertility in animal models (Nayuda et al., 1982; Isojima et al., 1984). Studies have shown that immunofluorescence methods do not necessarily correlate with other more specific and sensitive assays such as radioimmunoadsorption assays (Gerrity et al., 1981), enzyme-linked immunoassays, or immunoelectrophoresis methods (Dunbar, unpublished observations). It is important to note that the ZP is a complex extracellular matrix which can easily trap Ig molecules (such as immune complexes formed from Fc aggregation). Because it is difficult to wash the ZP free of these antibodies, non-specific fluorescence of non-immune sera frequently results. Such assays must therefore be interpreted with great caution and must be supported by alternative methods of antibody detection.

Immunoelectrophoresis methods including rocket and crossed immunoelectrophoresis have been used to demonstrate that multiple antigens are associated with the ZP (Dunbar and Raynor, 1980; Sacco et al., 1983a; Surneva-Nakova et al., 1982). Because the ZP antigens give heterogeneous immunoprecipitation patterns, it becomes difficult to determine the precise numbers of antigens associated with the ZP. These studies do indicate, however, that as many as four porcine ZP-specific antigens can be demonstrated using rabbit antisera to intact or heat-solubilized zonae (Dunbar et al., 1980). These studies further suggest that antibodies which recognize a conformational determinant are induced when intact zonae are used as the immunogen. Such conformational determinants have been described for the H3-H4 complex of calf thymus histones, as well as for other protein conformations (Habeeb, A.F.S.A., 1977; Cinader, B., 1977). Additional evidence that antibodies to ZP recognize a conformational determinant has emerged with the use of radioimmunoassay (Gerrity et al., 1981). The more recent development of specific and sensitive assays such as the RIA's (Gerrity et al., 1981; Sacco et al., 1981), the enzyme-linked immunoassays (ELISA) (Drell and Dunbar, 1984; Surneva-Nakova et al., 1984), and 2D-PAGE immunoblotting methods (Dunbar and Wolgemuth, 1984; Drell et al., 1984; Skinner et al., 1984) have allowed greater sensitivity and identification of specific ZP antigens. Using these specific assay methods, both species specific and species cross-reactive antigenic determinants can easily be detected and analyzed. It also becomes obvious that both the immunogenicity and the antigenicity of ZP glycoproteins varies among species (Dunbar, 1983a; Dunbar et al., 1981; Dunbar and Wolgemuth, 1984; Drell et al., 1984; Skinner et al., 1984), and that polyclonal antibodies developed against

Table 1. Use of Monoclonal Antibody to Probe Nature of Zona Pellucida Antigenic Determinants[a]

| | Subcloned Cell Lines Tested | Species Specific | Species Cross-Reactive | Conformational Determinant | Sequential Determinant |
|---|---|---|---|---|---|
| McAb to Pig Zonae: | 6 | + | - | + | - |
| McAb to Rabbit Zonae: | 6 | + | - | + | - |
| | 1 | - | + | - | + |

[a]Summarized from Drell and Dunbar, 1984.

purified as well as total porcine ZP proteins do not recognize determinants on rodent ZP (Drell et al., 1984; Sacco et al., 1982).

## Hybridoma Technology/The Use of Monoclonal Antibodies

Advances in hybridoma technology for producing monoclonal antibodies (Kohler and Milstein, 1975; Kennett et al., 1980) have allowed the production of antibody to specific ZP antigenic determinants (Drell and Dunbar, 1984; East and Dean, 1984; Isojima et al., 1984; East et al., 1985). The results of one of these recent studies show that there are species specific as well as shared antigenic determinants associated with the ZP of the pig and the rabbit. This is summarized in Table 1. Monoclonal antibody recognizes an antigenic determinant associated with all charge species, the major low molecular weight porcine ZP glycoprotein I (Drell and Dunbar, 1984) as well as the rabbit glycoprotein I. Given that specific domains of such a protein are involved in particular functions, it should be possible to use specific antibodies such as these to probe the functional domains of the zona glycoproteins. Recent use of such antibody probes in murine systems implicated zona glycoprotein components in sperm attachment, penetration, and the block to polyspermy seen in this species (East et al., 1984, 1985).

## Synthesis and Localization of ZP Glycoproteins

The ZP is formed during specific stages of oogenesis. Evidence, most of which was collected in rodent systems, supports an oocyte origin of ZP glycoproteins, a follicular cell origin, or a dual cell origin from these two very different cell types (Bleil and Wassarman, 1980a; Greve et al., 1982; Shimizu et al., 1983; Wolgemuth et al., 1984). The signal responsible for the initiation of zona production is unknown and could occur at the level of post-translational modification, translation, transcription or genomic organization.

Studies on zona synthesis have used ultrastructural, histochemical, and immunocytochemical procedures as well as radiochemical techniques for the analysis of protein synthesis. These have been extensively reviewed (Dunbar, 1983a,b; Dunbar and Wolgemuth, 1984). Recently, antibodies to rabbit ZP proteins electrophoretically purified from 2D-PAGE gels were used to localize zona antigens immunocytochemically using peroxidase-labeled antibodies (Wolgemuth et al., 1984). Extensive characterization showed these antibodies to be highly specific, and high antisera dilutions coupled with this visualization technique provided great sensitivity and resolution. The precise localization of ZP glycoproteins within ovarian cells showed a non-uniform distribution in rabbit oocytes with a more intense binding observed early in the process of zona formation at the inner and outer peripheries than was seen in the center region of the ZP. The antisera used in these studies appear to recognize protein rather than carbohydrate antigens since they react with deglycosylated proteins and with peptides of ZP proteins (Dunbar, unpublished observations).

Immunocytochemical localization studies using enzymatically labeled second antibodies have also been used to demonstrate the presence of specific zona antigens in the oocyte cytoplasm of the rabbit (Wolgemuth et al., 1984) and pig (Hedrick and Fry, 1980). Such antigens also appear in follicle cell cytoplasm at certain stages of follicular development. This localization in both cell types may well reflect the biological variation in the cellular origin of zona components among species.

Studies on the cellular origin of mouse ZP components involved the incorporation of labeled precursors into macromolecules known by their electrophoretic or immunologic properties to be associated with the zona (Greve et al., 1982). These in vitro studies have shown that growing mouse oocytes and intact follicles can synthesize glycoproteins having similar relative mobilities to ZP proteins which have been resolved using non-reducing, one-dimensional SDS-PAGE (Bleil and Wassarman, 1980; Shimizu et al., 1983). Moreover, one of these proteins can be immunoprecipitated with an antiserum prepared against a major mouse ZP protein (Greve et al., 1982). At some point, these proteins may prove valuable as biosynthetic markers for the study of oocyte growth and development. However, two major problems remain with respect to the mouse system. Among laboratories using this model, characterization of the mouse ZP proteins has varied depending upon the type of electrophoretic methods used (Sacco et al., 1982; Dunbar, 1983a; Bleil and Wassarman, 1980; Shimizu et al., 1983). Furthermore, the morphological, immunochemical and physicochemical properties of the mouse ZP proteins, as well as their 2D-PAGE patterns (Sacco et al., 1982; Dunbar, 1983b) differ markedly from those of larger mammals, including the human (Drell et al., 1984; Sacco et al., 1981 Wolgemuth et al., 1982). For these reasons, biosynthetic studies, so far done only in the mouse system, are not likely to give results which would be directly applicable to the very different zona structures of larger mammals.

## PASSIVE IMMUNIZATION WITH ANTIBODIES TO ZONA PELLUCIDA ANTIGENS

Prior to 1980, many studies showed that immunization with heteroantisera raised to ovarian tissue, to isolated oocytes, or to ZP could reduce fertility (Dunbar, 1983a). As with most early studies, lack of adequate antibody characterization meant that antibody specificity could not be properly evaluated. More recent studies, however, using a monoclonal antibody to mouse ZP have shown that passive immunization of mice resulted in reduced fertility (East et al., 1984a). Similarly, passive immunization of rabbits with monoclonal antibodies specific for rabbit ZP was shown to reduce fertility (Gibson et al., 1985). Anti-ZP IgG was seen to accumulate only in ovarian tissue at two and three weeks post-injection. The fertility rate of immunized animals in these studies was less than half that of controls. This reduction was found to be dependent upon the amount of immunogen used and upon the time of Ig administration before mating. Much work remains to be done to ascertain the usefulness of such a method for contraceptive purposes.

## ACTIVE IMMUNIZATION WITH ZONA PELLUCIDA PROTEINS

A variety of attempts to study the effects of active immunization with ovary tissues or ZP upon fertility have been extensively reviewed (Dunbar, 1983a). Ovarian homogenates used in many studies did result in reduced fertility, although the identities of the true immunogens responsible for the reaction were not obvious. Later work (Wood et al., 1981; Skinner et al., 1984) showed a dramatic and consistent reduction in fertility when zonae from a heterologous species were used, and when these were solubilized in such a way that the conformational or "structural" determinant was conserved.

Recently, large scale studies using heat-solubilized porcine ZP as the immunogen in rabbits have demonstrated that this conformational determinant not only eliminates fertility, but does so in a manner that interferes dramatically with follicular growth and differentiation (Skinner et al., 1984) (Figure 3C). Follicles entering their growth phase at the time when measurable antibody titers were achieved were prevented from further development. Estrogen secretion by these cells became insufficient to inhibit LH and FSH secretion into the peripheral plasma. Growing ova, together with their surrounding zonae, disappeared from the ovary. In their place were found granulosa-like cells grouped in uneven clusters of varying size and shape (Figure 4). Ovulation, of course, did not occur in response to any attempted stimulation, physical or hormonal. With the demise of earlier corpora lutea, ovarian progesterone secretion ceased. Long-term sterility ensued along with greatly altered hormonal function. It is interesting to note that this dramatic effect is achieved without resort to booster injections of any kind. Antibody titers remain high indefinitely as a result of one primary immunization with approximately 10,000 heat-solubilized pig zonae. Antisera were extensively characterized using a radioimmunoadsorbent assay (Gerrity et al., 1981), an enzyme-linked immunoassay (Batnaghar et al., 1985), and immunoblotting methods (Skinner et al., 1984). The immunoblot characterization is illustrated in Figure 3A, showing the pattern achieved when such antiserum is applied to nitrocellulose paper bearing the porcine ZP glycoprotein pattern adsorbed from a 2D-PAGE gel such as that shown in Figure 1. Antibodies to heat-solubilized ZP were seen to recognize all three of the major glycoprotein families of the porcine zona immunogen and were specific for ZP antigenic determinants.

Studies carried out recently in dogs (Mahi-Brown and Yanagimachi, 1985) and in cynomolgus monkeys (Gulyas et al., 1983) used porcine ZP as the immunogen, but used a different isolation procedure than the one described above, and included no characterization of the antigen in either case. (Although detailed characterization of the identity and specificity of the immunogen(s) and antibodies developed in these animals were not provided, evidence of cyclic interference and of inconsistent interruption of fertility was given).

Although it is plain that the molecular relationship of the three zona glycoprotein families to one another is important for the immunogenicity of the heat-solubilized preparation (Wood et al., 1981; Skinner et al., 1984), it is not known which of the three proteins or interac-

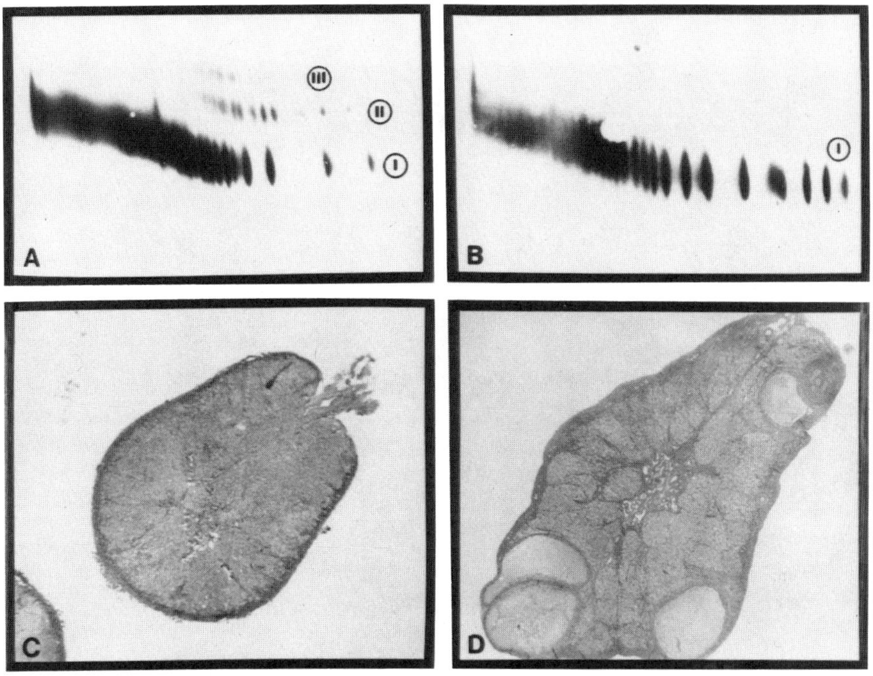


Fig. 3 Results of immunization of rabbits with heat-solubilized porcine ZP (A,C) or with ZP protein alone isolated from a 2D-SDS-PAGE separation procedure (B,D).

Panel A shows the results of an immunoblot using rabbit anti-HSPZ antiserum upon porcine ZP proteins separated by 2D-PAGE. Antibodies were identified by $^{125}$I-Protein A. Antigenic determinants on all three glycoprotein families are recognized by antisera from all animals in this group.

Panel B shows a similar immunoblot carried out with antisera from rabbits immunized with the single glycoprotein train I species isolated from Coomassie blue stained 2D-PAGE gels.

Panel C shows a histological section of an organ from a rabbit immunized with heat-solubilized pig ZP. The animal had been treated with hCG 10-12 hours before the ovary was removed. Follicular growth and ovulation has been completely eliminated and disorganized clusters of follicle-like cells (see Fig. 4) replace normal growing follicles.

Panel D shows a PAS-stained ovarian section taken from a rabbit immunized with the purified ZP glycoprotein train I. After several booster injections over a nine month period, the animal was treated with hCG and the ovary taken 10-12 hours later. Extensive follicular activity remains, with some diminution of growing follicles and the presence of a few disorganized cell clusters.

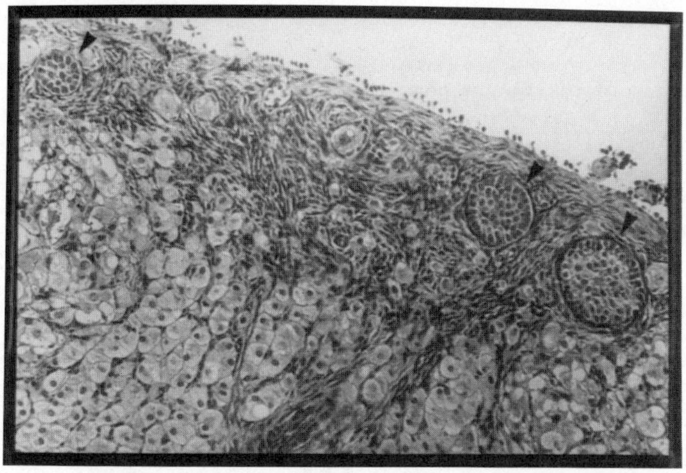

Fig. 4 Shows a higher magnification of a Periodic Acid Schiff-stained ovarian section equivalent to that shown in Fig. 3, Panel C. Follicles beyond the primordial stage have disappeared. Clusters of follicle-like cells in asymmetric groupings occur throughout the thin, inactive ovarian cortex. None of these clusters contains an intact ovum or ZP as revealed by extensive serial sectioning.

tions among these contributes to the infertility observed in these studies. To address this question, a series of active immunization studies have been carried out using as the immunogen each of the purified, denatured glycoprotein families recovered after 2D-PAGE separation. Control preparations have shown no response to the Coomassie blue stain and the acrylamide inherent in such material. It was further noticed that a number of booster injections were necessary to reach a significant antibody titer in response to such an immunogen. Even with these additional booster injections, the antibody level previously achieved with the entire heat-solubilized zona complex was never approached. Immunoblot characterization using this antiserum (Figure 3B) shows that these anti-ZP antibodies recognize only porcine zona glycoprotein train I, the original antigen. Furthermore, trials using this purified glycoprotein train I have resulted in normal gonadotrophin secretion patterns and apparently normal ovarian histology (Figure 3D) (unpublished observations). Similar studies of the other two glycoprotein components are in progress.

Studies using the chromatographically purified porcine ZP glycoprotein I in squirrel monkeys have been carried out by Sacco et al. (1983b). A reduced number of oocytes were recovered by laparoscopy, but no report is yet available on the hormonal status of these animals.

SPECIES VARIATION

The ZP is now known to be an extremely complex biomatrix composed of extensively sulfated glycoproteins. The relative molecular weights, as well as the nature and extent of sulfation or other modification of these proteins is seen to vary dramatically from species to species. In the grossest functional sense, the molecular composition of the ZP dictates the degree of structural integrity it may maintain in the presence of sperm enzymes. The ZP structure may even change to accomodate the path of the penetrating sperm cell.

In a more basic, developmental sense, the ZP is directly involved in the maintenance of the ovum and in the growth and differentiation of its ovarian follicle. These processes lie at the heart of the exquisitely timed series of events culminating in ovulation. Development of any acceptable means of human fertility control requires a much more complete understanding of these events than we currently have. However, much headway has been made in this regard through the use of highly specific immunological probes drawn from the ZP and its constituent macromolecules.

Since heteroimmunization of several species with ZP proteins results in ovarian dysfunction with attendant hormonal irregularities, it is necessary to carry out systematic experiments to determine which of the three major glycoproteins, variants of which are seen in every species so far investigated, induces antibodies responsible for the resulting infertility. Since every species may vary in its response to such immunization, it will be important initially to use primates immunized with the heat-solubilized complex of all three zona proteins, including the conformational or "structural" determinants which appear to be critical for their unique immunogenicity. These studies have been initiated using the rhesus monkey. Once antibodies are identified which correlate with infertility, these can be characterized and the molecules of interest purified for use in fertility studies. Species-specific and species cross-reactive determinants can be more fully explored and the question of species specific differences in fertilization events can be more directly addressed.

Although passive immunization approaches can lead to greater understanding of the mode of action of the antibodies in question, these techniques require large amounts of IgG for larger animal models. Active immunization, requiring only small amounts of antigen, appears a more feasible technique for large scale studies, is suitable for animals of any size, and opens up this approach for a wide range of animal models.

Since it is not feasible to isolate and purify sufficient quantities of ZP protein for use as a practical source of immunogen for large scale clinical use, it will eventually be necessary to turn to recently developed methods of genetic engineering to produce recombinant DNA molecules for use in immunogen production.

Once the antigenic determinants of the ZP glycoproteins are more fully understood, these molecules should be invaluable in probing those mechanisms involved in successful fertilization. Most importantly, such probes will allow, for the first time, in depth exploration of the early events of mammalian follicular differentiation and development. It is this process, necessary to successful ovulation in all species, which offers the best opportunity for safe, effective and acceptable intervention in the fertilization process.

## REFERENCES


Aitken, R.J., and Richardson, D.W., 1980, Immunization against zona pellucida antigens, in "Immunological Aspects of Reproduction and Fertility Control," J.P. Hearn, ed., Lancaster, U.K.: MTP Press Ltd.

Aketa, K., 1973, Physiological studies on the egg surface components responsible for sperm-egg binding in sea urchin fertilization. I. Effect of sperm-binding protein on the fertilizing capacity of sperm, Exp. Cell Res., 70: 439.

Anderson, N.L., and Anderson, A.G., 1977, High-resolution two-dimensional electrophoresis of human plasma proteins, Proc. Natl. Acad. Sci. USA, 74:5421.

Austin, C.R., and Braden, A.W.H., 1956, Early reactions of the rodent egg spermatozoan penetration, J. Exp. Biol., 33:358.

Baranska, W., Konwinski, M., and Kuwaja, 1975, Fine structure of the zona pellucida of unfertilized egg cells and embryos, J. Exp. Zool., 192:193.

Barros, C., and Yanagimachi, R., 1971, Induction of zona reaction in golden hamster eggs by cortical granule material, Nature, 233:258.

Barros, C., and Yanagimachi, R., 1972, Polyspermy-preventing mechanisms in the golden hamster egg, J. Exp. Zool., 180:251.

Batnagar, P., Skinner, S.M., and Dunbar, B.S., 1985, Antigenicity and immunogenicity of anti-zona pellucida antibodies, (in preparation).

Bedford, J.M., 1977, Sperm/egg interaction: The specificity of human spermatozoa, Anat. Rec., 188:477.

Bleil, J.D., and Wassarman, P.M., 1980a, Synthesis of zona pellucida proteins by denuded and follicle-enclosed mouse oocytes during culture in vitro, Proc. Natl. Acad. Sci. USA, 77:1029.

Bleil, J.D., and Wassarman, P.M., 1980b, Structure and function of the zona pellucida: Identification and characterization of the proteins of the mouse oocyte zona pellucida, Dev. Biol., 76:185.

Braden, A.W.H., Austin, C.R., and David, H.A., 1954, The reaction of the zona pellucida to sperm penetration, Austral. J. Biol. Sci., 7:391.

Cinader, B., 1977, Enzyme-antibody interactions, in "Methods in Immunology and Immunochemistry," Vol. 44, C.A. Williams and M.W. Chase, eds., New York: Academic Press, 313.

Crozet, N., and Dumont, M., 1984, The site of the acrosome reaction during in vivo penetration of the sheep oocyte, Gam. Res., 10:97.

Drell, D.W., and Dunbar, B.S., 1984, Monoclonal antibodies to rabbit and pig zonae pellucidae distinguish species specific as well as shared antigenic determinants, Biol. Reprod., 30:435.

Drell, D.W., Wood, D.M., Bundman, D.S., and Dunbar, B.S., 1984, Immunological comparison of antibodies to porcine zonae pellucidae in rats and rabbits, Biol. Reprod., 30:455.

Dudkiewicz, A.B., Shivers, C.A., and Williams, W.L., 1976, Ultrastucture of hamster zona pellucida treated with zona-precipitating antibody, Biol. Reprod., 14:175.

Dunbar, B.S., 1980, Model system to study the relationship between antibodies to zonae and infertility. Comparison of rabbit and porcine zonae pellucidae, Proc. Int. Cong. Anim. Reprod. Artif. Insem., II:191.

Dunbar, B.S., and Raynor, B.D., 1980, Characterization of porcine zona pellucida antigens, Biol. Reprod., 22:941.

Dunbar, B.S., Wardrip, N.J., and Hedrick, J.L., 1980, Isolation, physicochemical properties and the macromolecular composition of the zona pellucida from porcine oocytes, Biochemistry, 19:356.

Dunbar, B.S., Liu, C., and Sammons, D.W., 1981), Identification of the three major proteins of porcine and rabbit zonae pellucidae by high-resolution two-dimensional gel electrophoresis: Comparison with follicular fluid, sera, and ovarian cell proteins, Biol. Reprod., 24:1111.

Dunbar, B.S., 1983a, Antibodies to zonae pellucidae antigens and their role in fertility, in "International Congress on Reproductive Immunology," T. Wegmann and T. Gills (eds.), London: Oxford University Press, 505.

Dunbar, B.S., 1983b, Morphological, biochemical and immunochemical characterization of the mammalian zona pellucida, in "Mechanism and Control of Animal Fertilization," J. Hartmann (ed.), Academic Press, New York, 139.

Dunbar, B.S., and Wolgemuth, D.J., 1984), Structure and function of the mammalian zona pellucida, a unique extracellular matrix, in "Modern Cell Biology," B. Satir (ed.), Alan R. Liss, Inc., New York, 3:77.

Dunbar, B.S., Dudkiewicz, A.B., and Bundman, D.S., 1985, Proteolysis of specific porcine zona pellucida glycoproteins by boar acrosin, Biol. Reprod., 32:619.

East, I.J., and Dean, J., 1984, Monoclonal antibodies as probes of the distribution of ZP-2, the major sulfated glycoprotein of the murine zona pellucida, J. Cell Biol., 98:795.

East, I.J., Mattison, D.R., and Dean, J., 1984a, Monoclonal antibodies to the major proteins of the murine zona pellucida: effects on fertilization and early development, Devel. Biol., 104:49.

East, I.J., Keenan, A.M., Larson, S.M., and Dean, J., 1984b, Scintography of normal mouse ovaries with monoclonal antibodies to ZP-2, the major zona pellucida protein, Science, 225:(4665), 938.

East, I.J., Gulyas, B.J., and Dean, J., 1985, Monoclonal antibodies to the murine zona pellucida protein with sperm receptor activity: effects on fertilization and early development, Devel. Biol., 109:268.

Elder, J.H., and Alexander, S., 1982, Endo-N-acetylglucoaminidase F: Endoglycosidase from flavobacterium meningosepticium that cleaves both high mannose and complex glycoproteins, Proc. Natl. Acad. Sci. USA, 79:4540.

Florman, H.M., and Wassarman, P.M., 1985, O-linked oligosaccharides of mouse egg ZP3 account for its sperm receptor activity, Cell, 41:313.

Gaddum-Rosse, P., Blandau, R.J., Langley, L.B., and Barraglia, D.E., 1984, In vitro fertilization in the rat: observations on living eggs, Fertil. Steril, 42(2):285.

Gerrity, M., Niu, E., and Dunbar, B.S., 1981, A specific radioimmunoassay for evaluation of serum antibodies to zona pellucida antigens, J. Reprod. Immunol., 3:59.

Gianfortoni, J.G., and Gulyas, B.J., 1985, The effects of short-term incubation (aging) of mouse oocytes on in vitro fertilization, zona solubility, and embryonic development, Gam. Res., 11:59.

Gibson, R.E., Spilman, C.H., Skinner, S., and Dunbar, B.S., 1985, Passive immunization with polyclonal and monoclonal (McAb) antibodies to zonae pellucidae, Biol. Repr., (submitted).

Glabe, C.G., and Vacquier, V.D., 1977, Isolation and characterization of the vitelline layer of sea urchin eggs, J. Cell Biol., 75:410.

Green, D.P.L., and Purves, R.D., 1984, Mechanical hypothesis of sperm penetration, Biophys. J., 45:659.

Greve, J.M., Salzman, G.S., Roller, R.J., and Wassarman, P.M., 1982, Biosynthesis of the major zona pellucida glycoprotein secreted by oocytes during mammalian oogenesis, Cell, 31:749.

Gulyas, B.J., Gwatkin, R.B.L., and Yuan, L.C., 1983, Active immunization of cynomalgus monkeys (Macaca fascicularis) with porcine zona pellucida, Gam. Res., 7(4):299.

Gwatkin, R.B.L., Williams, D.T., and Anderson, O.F., 1973, Zona reaction of mammalian eggs: properties of the cortical granule protease (Cortin) and its receptor substrate in hamster eggs, J. Cell Biol., 59:128a.

Gwatkin, R.B.L., Carter, H.W., and Patterson, H., 1976, Association of mammalian sperm with the cumulus cells and the zona pellucida studied by scanning electron microscopy. Part IV, "Proceedings of the Workshop on SEM in Reproductive Biology," O. Johari and R.P. Becker, eds., Chicago: IITRES. Inst. Vd., 379.

Gwatkin, R.B.L., Williams, D.T., and Carlo, D.J., 1977, Immunization of mice with heat-solubilized hamster zonae: production of anti-zona antibody and inhibition of fertility, Fertil. Steril., 28:871.

Gwatkin, R.B.L., Anderson, O.F., and Williams, D.T., 1980, Large scale isolation of bovine, and pig zonae pellucidae: chemical, immunological, and receptor properties, Gamete Res., 3:217.

Habeeb, A.F.S.A., 1977, Influence of conformation on immunochemical properties of proteins, in: "Immunochemistry of Proteins," Vol. 2, M.Z. Atassi, ed., New York: Plenum Press, 163.

Hartmann, J.F., and Gwatkin, R.B.L., 1971, Alteration of sites on the mammalian sperm surface following capacitation, Nature, 234:479.

Hartmann, J.F., Gwatkin, R.B.L., and Hutchison, C.F., 1972, Early contact interactions between mammalian gametes *in vitro*: evidence that the vitellus influences adherence between sperm and zona pellucida, Proc. Natl. Acad. Sci. USA, 69:2767.

Hartmann, J.F., and Hutchison, C.F., 1974, Nature of pre-penetration contact interaction between hamster gametes *in vitro*, J. Reprod. Fertil., 36:49.

Hedrick, J.L., and Fry, G.N., 1980, Immunocytochemical studies on the porcine zona pellucida, J. Cell Biol., 87:136a.

Huang, T.T.F., and Yanagimachi, R., 1984, Fucoidin inhibits attachment of guinea pig spermatozoa to the zona pellucida through binding to the lunar acrosomal membrane and equatorial domains, Exp. Cell Res., 153:363.

Isojima, S., Koyama, K., Hasegawa, A., Tsunoda, Y., and Hanadu, A., 1984, Monoclonal antibodies to porcine zona pellucida antigens and their inhibitory effects on fertilization, J. Reprod. Immun., 6(2):77.

Jackowski, S., and Dumont, J.N., 1979, Surface alterations of the mouse zona pellucida and ovum following *in vitro* fertilization: correlation with cell cycle, Biol. Reprod., 20:150.

Kamada, M., Hasebe, H., Milrahara, T., Kinoshita, T., Naka, O., and Mori, T., 1984, Detection of anti-zona pellucida activities in human sera by the passive hemagglutination reaction, Fertil. Steril., 41(6):901.

Karp, D.R., Atkinson, J.P., and Shreffler, D.C., 1982, Genetic variation in glycosylation of the fourth component of murine complement, J. Biol. Chem., 257(13):7330.

Kennett, R.H., McKearn, T.J., and Bechtol, K.B., 1980, "Monoclonal antibodies. Hybridomas: A new dimension in biological analyses," Plenum Press, New York.

Kinsey, W.H., and Lennarz, W.J., 1981, Isolation of a glycopeptide fraction from the surface of the sea urchin egg that inhibits sperm-egg binding and fertilization, J. Cell Biol., 91:325.

Kohler, G., and Milstein, C., 1975, Continuous cultures of fused cells secreting antibody of predefined specificity, Nature, 256:495.

Kuzan, F.B., Fleming, A.D., and Seidel, G.E., 1984, Successful fertilization *in vitro* of fresh, intact oocytes by perivitelline (acrosome-reacted) spermatozoa of the rabbit, Fertil. Steril., 41(5):766.

Mahi-Brown, C.A., and Yanagimachi, R., 1985, Effect of immunization with porcine zona pellucida on ovarian cycles in the bitch, In press (Biol. Reprod.).

Mhasker, A., Buckshee, K., and Talwar, G.P., 1984, Autoantibodies to zona pellucida in tubectomized women, Contraception, 29(i):75.

Mintz, B., 1962, Experimental study of the developing mammalian egg: removal of the zona pellucida, Science, 138:594.

Modlinski, J.A., 1970, The role of the zona pellucida in the development of mouse eggs in vivo, J. Embryol. Exp. Morph., 23:539.

Nayuda, P.L., Freeman, L.E., and Trounson, A.O., 1982a, Zona pellucida antibodies in human sera, J. Reprod. Fertil., 65:77.

Nayuda, P.L., Freeman, L.E., and Trounson, A.O., 1982b, A quantitative indirect immunofluorescent assay for zona pellucida antibodies, J. Reprod. Fertil., 65:67.

Nicholson, G.L., Yanagimachi, R., and Yanagimachi, H., 1975, Ultrastructural localization of lectin-binding sites on the zonae pellucidae and plasma membranes of mammalian eggs, J. Cell Biol., 66:263.

Nishimoto, T., Mori, T., Yamada, I., and Nishimura, T., 1980, Autoantibodies to zona pellucida in infertile and aged women, Fertil. Steril., 34:522.

Oikawa, T., Nicholson, G.L., and Yanagimachi, R., 1975, Trypsin-mediated modification of the zona pellucida glycopeptide structure of hamster eggs, J. Reprod. Fertil., 43:133.

O'Rand, M.G., Matthews, J.E., Welch, J.E., Fisher, S.J., 1985, Identification of zona binding proteins of rabbit, pig, human and mouse spermatozoa on nitrocellulose blots, J. Expl Zool., (in press).

Overstreet, J.W., and Bedford, J.M., 1975, The penetrability of rabbit ova treated with enzymes or anti-progesterone antibodies: a probe into the nature of mammalian fertilization, J. Reprod. Fertil., 44:273.

Phillips, D.M., and Shalgi, R.M., 1980, Surface properties of the zona pellucida, J. Exp. Zool., 213:1.

Sacco, A.G., and Moghiss, K.S., 1979, Anti-zona pellucida activity in human sera, Fertil. Steril., 31:503.

Sacco, A.G., Subramanian, G., and Yurewicz, E.C., 1981, Application of a radioimmunoassay (RIA) for monitoring immune response to porcine zona pellucida, Proc. Soc. Expt. Biol. Mod., 167:318.

Sacco, A.G., Subramanian, M.G., and Yurewicz, E.C., 1981, Active immunization of mice with porcine zonae pellucidae: immune response and effect on fertility, J. Exp. Zool., 218:405.

Sacco, A.G., Yurewicz, E.C., Subramanian, M.G., and DeMayo, F.J., 1982, Zona pellucida composition: Species crossreactivity and contraceptive potential of antiserum of a partially purified pig zona antigen, Biol. Reprod., 25:997.

Sacco, A.G., Yurewicz, E.C., and Zhang, S., 1983a, Immunoelectrophoretic analysis of the porcine zona pellucida, J. Repr. Fertil., 68:21.

Sacco, A.G., Subramanian, M.G., Yurewicz, E.C., DeMayo, F.J., and Dukelow, W.R., 1983b, Heteroimmunization of squirrel monkeys (Saineri sciureus) with a purified porcine zona antigen: Immune response and biological activity of antiserum, Fertil. Steril., 39:350.

Sacco, A.G., Subramanian, M.G., and Yurewicz, E.C., 1984, Association of sperm receptor activity with a purified pig zona antigen (PPZA), J. Rep. Immunol., 6:89.

Saling, P.M., Storey, B.T., and Wolf, D.P., 1978, Calcium-dependent binding of mouse epididymal spermatozoa to the zona pellucida, Devel. Biol., 65:515.

Sammons, D.W., Anderson, L.D., and Nishiawa, E.E., 1981, Ultrasensitive color-based silver staining of polypeptides in polyacrylamide gels, Electrophor., 2:135.

Sellens, M.H., and Jenkinson, E.J., 1975, Permeability of the mouse zona pellucida to immunoglobulin, J. Reprod. Fertil., 42:153.
Shimizu, S., Masahiro, T., and Dean, J., 1983, In vitro biosynthesis of three sulfated glycoproteins of murine ZP by oocytes grown in follicle culture, J. Biol. Chem., 258(9):5858.
Shur, B.D., and Hall, N.G., 1982, A role for mouse sperm galactosyltransferase in sperm binding to the egg zona pellucida, J. Cell Biol., 95(2):574.
Skinner, S.M., Mills, T., Kirchick, H.J., and Dunbar, B.S., 1984, Immunization with zona pellucida proteins results in abnormal ovarian follicular differentiation and inhibition of gonadotropin-induced steroid secretion, Endocrin., 115(b):2418.
Stambaugh, R.L., and Nicosia, S.V., 1984, Localization of tubulin and microtubules of in vitro fertilized rabbit oocytes, J. Androl., 5:259.
Surneva-Nakova, T., and Nakov, L.S., 1982, Immunoelectrophoretic characterization of antigens of porcine zona pellucida, Comptes rendus de l'Academie blugare des sciences, Tome 35(9):1307.
Surneva-Nakova, N., Nakov, L.S., Kyurkchiev, S.D., Gancheva, S.D., and Yalumov, O.I., 1984, Study on the specificity of pig zona pellucida by enzyme-linked immunoadsorbent assay (ELISA), Comptes rendus de l'Academi bulgare des Sciences, 37(7):975.
Swenson, C.E., and Dunbar, B.S., 1982, Specificity of sperm-zona interaction, J. Exp. Zool., 219:97.
Talbot, P., and DiCarlantonio, G., 1984a, The oocyte-cumulus complex: ultrastructure of the extracellular components in hamsters and mice, Gam. Res., 10:127.
Talbot, P., and DiCarlantonio, G., 1984b, Ultrastructure of opossum oocyte investing coats and their senstivity to trypsin and hyaluronidase, Devel. Biol., 103:159.
Urch, U.A., Wardrip, N.J., and Hedrick, J.L., 1985, Limited and specific proteolysis of the zona pellucida by acrosin, J. Exper. Zool., 233:479.
Watanabe, M., Muramatsu, T., Shirne, H., and Ugai, K., 1981, Discrete distribution of binding sites for dolichos biflorus agglutinin (DBA) and for peanut agglutinin (PNA) in mouse organ tissues, J. Histochem. Cytochem., 29:779.
Wolgemuth, D.J., and Gavin, B.J., 1981, Ultrastructural and biochemical characterization of gene expression on follicular oocytes in neonatal and prepubertal rats, in "Proceedings of the Fifth Workshop on Development and Function of the Reproductive Organs," Byskov, A.G. (ed.), Amsterdam: Excerpta Medica, 289.
Wolgemuth, D.J., Gavin, B.J., Wood, D.M., Celenza, J.L., and Dunbar, B.S., 1982, Differences in crossreactivity of zona pellucida antigens among mammals, J. Cell Biol., 95(2):8032.
Wolgemuth, D.J., Celenza, J., Bundman, D.S., and Dunbar, B.S., 1984, Formation of the rabbit zona pellucida and its relationship to ovarian follicular development, Devel. Biol., 106:1.
Wood, D.M., Liu, C., and Dunbar, B.S., 1981, The effect of alloimmunization and heteroimmunization with zonae pellucidae on fertility in rabbits, Biol. Reprod., 25:439.
Yanagimachi, R., 1977, Specificity of sperm-egg interaction, in: "Immunobiology of Gametes," M. Edidin and M.H. Johnson (eds.), Cambridge: Cambridge University Press, 187.
Yanagimachi, R., and Phillips, D.M., 1984, The status of acrosomal caps of hamster spermatozoa immediately before fertilization in vivo, Gam. Res., 9:1.

# IMMUNOHISTOLOGICAL STUDIES DURING IMMUNIZATION OF PRIMATES WITH PORCINE ZONA PELLUCIDA: PRELIMINARY OBSERVATIONS[1]

S.K. Gupta[2], P. Bhatnagar[3], B.S. Dunbar[3] and S. Sehgal[2]

Department of Immunopathology[2]
Postgraduate Institute of Medical Education and Research
Chandigarh, India, and
Department of Cell Biology[3]
Baylor College of Medicine
Houston, Texas 77030 USA
Indo-U.S. Collaborative Project[1]

## INTRODUCTION

Oocytes of nearly all mammals are surrounded by a highly complex structure composed of glycoproteins, referred to as zona pellucida (ZP). It not only preserves the integrity of the oocytes but also plays a pivotal role in sperm-egg interaction and prevention of polyspermy (Wood et al., 1981; Ownby and Shivers, 1972; Gwatkin et al., 1977; Yanagimachi, 1977). Since sperm must adhere to and penetrate the ZP, interruption of this binding or penetration is possible using anti-ZP antibodies. Attempts have therefore been made to exploit immunization with ZP antigens as a possible mode of immuno-contraception. Earlier studies by Sacco et al. (1981), Dunbar et al. (1984), and Wood et al. (1981) have highlighted the effects of allo-immunization and hetero-immunization on fertility in rabbits and rodents. In these studies, high-resolution two-dimensional gel electrophoresis was used to demonstrate that the porcine ZP consists of 3 major families of glycoproteins. These proteins exhibit both charge as well as molecular weight heterogeneity due to extensive post-translational modification. More recently, studies by Skinner et al. (1984) have indicated that immunization with ZP proteins of porcine origin leads to serious impairment of follicular maturation in the rabbit ovary. In the present study, porcine ZP antigens have been used to immunize rhesus monkeys to assess the cross-reactivity of porcine ZP proteins with the primate ZP proteins and to determine the type of ZP antibodies generated during the course of such immunization.

## METHODS

Porcine ovaries were obtained from Health Products Inc. (South Haven, Mich.). They were minced in an apparatus with circular cutting blades and the oocytes isolated using serial seiving procedure (Wood et al., 1981). The oocytes were heat-solubilized in 0.4 mM bicarbonate buffer, pH 9.0, for a period of 1 hr at 60°C. Preparations were monitored by two-dimensional polyacrylamide gel electrophoresis. The protein content of the supernatant was adjusted to a final concentration of 1 mg/ml. Rhesus monkeys obtained from the Indian Animal House, Lucknow, were kept on a standard laboratory diet and observed for a period of 3-4 weeks before immunization. All the monkeys were tested for tuberculin reaction and found to be negative. Basal haematological investigations including haemoglobulin, total and differential leukocyte counts, packed cell volume, etc., were also conducted. After acclimatization, they were immunized with 250 μg of ZP protein mixed with 0.5 ml of complete Freund's adjuvant (CFA, Group-I). The animals were observed for cyclicity and serial vaginal smears were taken for hormone assessment. The animals were bled sequentially at an interval of 2-3 weeks and the sera subjected to the following tests:

1. Anti-zona antibodies using counter electrophoresis. The test was conducted in a continuous buffer system using 1% agarose in 0.01 M barbital buffer, pH 8.4. A current of 6 mA was applied to each microscopic slide for a period of 1-1/2 hrs.

2. Rocket electrophoresis was performed using 10-20 μg of heat-solubilized porcine zonae antigen and 10% monkey serum was incorporated in the agar gel. Electrophoresis was carried out using the LKB flat bed apparatus for 18 hrs at 2.5 volts/$cm^2$ at 20°C and the gels were stained with 0.05% Coomassie Brilliant Blue. Another set of six monkeys were immunized with the same amount of ZP protein without CFA (Group-II).

### Indirect Immunofluorescence

Anti-zona antibodies were also detected by the indirect immunofluorescence procedure using rabbit, porcine and primate ovaries. Briefly, 5 μ thick sections were cut in a cryostat and left overnight at -70°C. This step prevented the sections from floating during the process of staining. Sera from immunized monkeys were allowed to interact with the sections for a period of 45 minutes at room temperature in a humid chamber. Sections were washed with several changes of phosphate buffered saline (PBS), pH 7.4, and layered with 1/16 dilution of anti-human immunoglobulins IgG, IgA, and IgM labeled with fluorescein (Nordic Pharmaceuticals Limited) for a period of another hour. The slides were washed in PBS, mounted in buffered glycerine and viewed in a Zeiss 16 research microscope. The intensity of fluorescence was arbitrarily graded from + to ++++.

### Antibody Titers Using Avidin Biotin Assay

A modification of the enzyme-linked immunoassay described by Drell et al. (1984) was used. ZP protein (50 ng/well) was plated into micro-ELISA plates and the Vectastain kit (Vector Laboratories) was used to analyze antibodies. Rabbit anti-baboon IgG was used as the second antibody and was a gift from Dr. Vern Stevens (Ohio State University).

### In Vivo Binding of Antisera ZP Using Immunoperoxidase

Rabbit and primate ovaries were processed in cold according to the method advocated by Saint Marie (1962). Small blocks of tissues were placed in chilled alcohol at 4°C for a period of 2 hr and transferred to fresh chilled alcohol for a period of another 20 hrs. Tissues were dehydrated in 4 changes of 100% alcohol for a period of 1 hr each; cleared in 3 changes of cold xylene for 1 hr each and embedded in paraffin. Five micron thick sections were cut and stained with peroxidase antiperoxidase method as advocated by Sternberger (1975).

Zona Pellucida Dissolution by Pronase

The methods previously described by Drell and Dunbar (1984) were used to determine if antibodies against ZP will protect it from dissolution by pronase. For this study, ZP were incubated with 0.3% pronase and were analyzed microscopically to determine the time required to cause dissolution of the ZP matrix.

RESULTS

Monkeys immunized with ZP emulsified with CFA revealed an exponential rise of antibody titers until 12 weeks after which there was a marginal decline. During this period, however, there was no interruption of cyclicity despite the rise in antibody titers. This was substantiated by serial vaginal smear examinations. After April, the majority of monkeys entered a phase of summer amenorrohea as is usual in tropical climates, therefore, cyclicity could not be monitored. Figure 1 illustrates the antibodies in monkey no. 5 as detected by rocket electrophoresis against porcine ZP antigens.

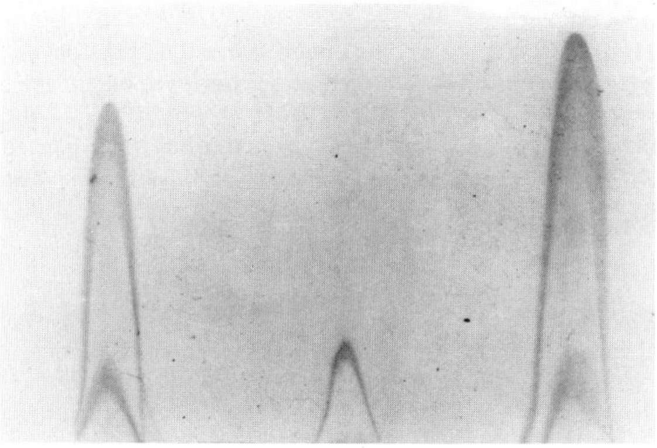

10 5 15 ug

Fig. 1: Rocket immunoelectrophoresis. Different concentrations of porcine ZP protein were added to wells and electrophoresis was carried out using antisera from a monkey immunized with porcine ZP. Agarose contains 10% sera.

The antibody titers detected by avidin-biotin ELISA assay, were not detectable by 4 weeks in Group II as compared to Group I, all of which gave antibody titers of greater than 1:64,000. The results of zona dissolution assay corroborated the ELISA assay. Table 1 shows that while 0.03% pronase caused a complete lysis of zonae within 5-10 minutes, addition of immune sera obtained throughout the period of observation delayed dissolution of zonae by more than 3 hrs.

Table I

Zona Pellucida Dissolution Assay (Group I)

| Monkey No. | Pre-Immune Sera | Time Taken for ZP Dissolution (in minutes) 4 weeks sera | 12 weeks serum | 16-20 week serum (1:50 dilution) |
|---|---|---|---|---|
| M1 | 23 | 55 | > 180 | > 200 |
| M2 | 25 | 60 | > 180 | > 200 |
| M3 | 30 | 60 | > 180 | > 200 |
| M4 | 20 | 70 | > 180 | > 200 |
| M5 | 18 | 75 | > 180 | > 200 |
| M6 | 28 | 40 | > 180 | > 200 |

Control: Zona dissolution in five to twelve minutes in the absence of sera.

It is evident from the indirect immunofluorescence studies on rabbit and monkey ovaries that there is cross-reactivity between rabbit, pig, and monkey zonae. Furthermore, the majority of antibody belonged to the IgG class as judged by immunofluorescence since only a faint staining reaction was observed with anti-IgM and the anti-IgA reaction was negative (Table 2).

Table IIa

Indirect Immunofluorescence with Immune Monkey Sera

(Substrate: Porcine Ovaries)

| Monkey No. | IgG | IgM | IgA | BiC[a] |
|---|---|---|---|---|
| M1[b] | ++ | - | - | - |
| M2 | ++ | ± | - | - |
| M3 | ++ | + | - | - |
| M4 | ++ | - | - | - |
| M5 | ++ | ± | - | - |
| M6 | ++ | - | - | - |

[a]BiC = β-immune complement C.

[b]Group I sera tested after 3 months.

Table IIb

Indirect Immunofluorescence with Immune Sera
( Using Monkey Ovaries as Substrate)

| Monkey No./Months | IgG | IgA | IgM |
|---|---|---|---|
| M1/4 | ++ | - | - |
| M2/5 | ++ | - | ± |
| M3/5 | ++ | - | + |
| M4/5 | ++ | - | - |
| M5/5 | ++ | - | ± |
| M6/5 | ++ | - | - |
| M7/1* | - | - | - |
| M8/1 | - | - | - |
| M9/1 | - | - | - |
| M11/1 | - | - | - |
| M12/1 | - | - | - |

*Monkeys Nos. 7-12 immunized without CFA.

All the control sera and sera from monkeys immunized without CFA showed no staining.

Results of the immunoperoxidase studies showed that antibodies were also generated against antigenic determinants shared with monkey zonae. Figure 2 illustrates intensely brown staining of homologous monkey zona pellucida with the serum of an immunized monkey.

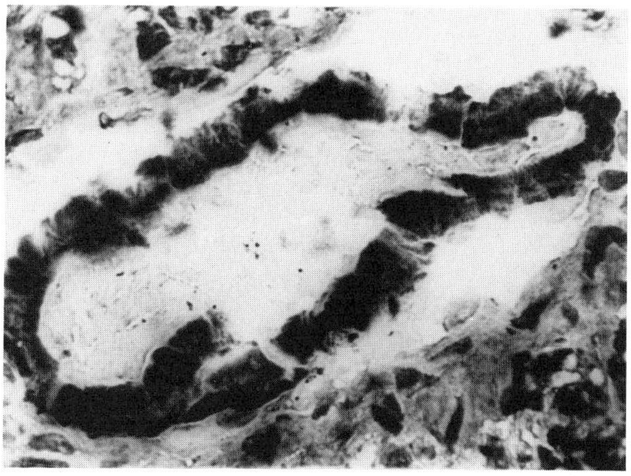

Fig. 2: Peroxidase anti-peroxidase reaction ( counter stain H&E x880 mag.) using serum from monkey immunized with porcine ZP and a thin section of monkey ovary. The intensely positive stained zona pellucida demonstrates the cross-reactivity between the porcine and monkey ZP.

There was no difference in the intensity of reaction with rabbit, porcine or monkey ovaries. In the maturing follicles, follicular cells in the immediate vicinity of ZP also gave a positive peroxidase reaction. This is similar to observations made in the rabbit ovary (Wolgemuth et al., 1984). Antibodies raised against follicular cells failed to detect staining of the ZP (Figure 3).

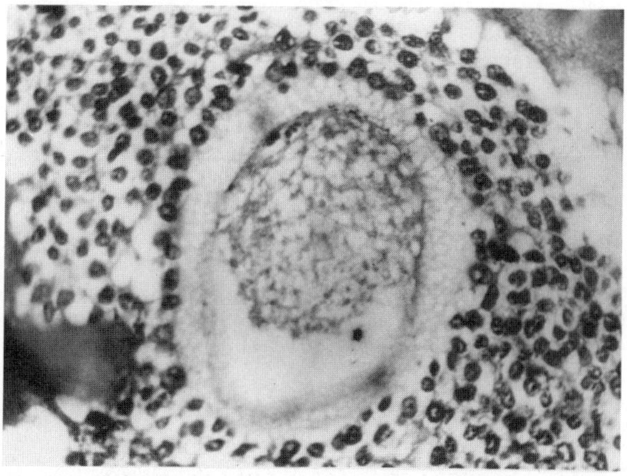

Fig. 3: Antibodies raised against porcine follicular cells in rabbits fail to stain monkey zona pellucida (peroxidase anti-peroxidase x 680).

DISCUSSION

Immunization of monkeys with heat-solubilized porcine zonae results in the generation of high titers of antibodies as detected by different assay systems. These antibodies, as is evident from indirect immunofluorescence assay, belong primarily to the IgG class of antibodies. It has been stated earlier that immunofluorescence is not the method of choice since it is likely to give non-specific reactions. In the present study, however, it has been observed that while the ZP of intact oocytes have the capacity to bind antibodies non-specifically, such a phenomenon is not observed in situ, i.e., if thin, frozen sections of ovaries are used. Similarly, recognition of blood group antigens is also minimized if frozen sections of the ovary are used.

There appears to be a long latent period between generation of significant anti-zonae antibodies and interruption of cyclicity in monkeys as the animals continued to cycle until 14 weeks after immunization despite high titers of antibodies. Further, there appears to be an imperfect correlation with the antibody titers and impairment of cyclicity. It is difficult to be categorical about the state of follicular maturation after 16 weeks as summer normally imposes amenorrohea in monkeys. Monkeys immunized with porcine zonae generate antibodies that react with porcine, rabbit and monkey ovaries with equal intensity. The immunohistochemical study revealed that porcine zonae are capable of evoking significant antibody titers which react in a homologous system, i.e., with rhesus zonae.

The antibodies do not show cross-reactivity with other components of the ovarian tissue. The staining of adjacent layers of granulosa cells could be explained on the basis of synthesis of zona pellucida glycoproteins by these cells in maturing follicles as has earlier been suggested by Wolgemuth et al. ( 1984). Follow up studies in these animals will allow us to determine whether a single dose of the total ZP immunogen can cause an immunological response which will result in the arrest of follicular maturation as has been documented by Skinner et al. ( 1984) in rabbits. These studies will further allow us to determine if ZP protein are immunogenic if used in the absence of complete Freund's adjuvant.

REFERENCES


1. Drell, D.W., and Dunbar, B.S. (1984) Monoclonal antibodies to rabbit and pig zonae pellucidae distinguish species specific and shared shared antigenic determinants. Biol. Reprod. 30, 445-457.
2. Dunbar, B.S., and Wolgemuth, D.J. ( 1984) Structure and function of the mammalian zona pellucida, a unique extracellular matrix. Modern Cell Biology 3, 77-111.
3. Dunbar, B.S., and Raynor, B.D. ( 1980) Characterization of porcine zona pellucida antigen. Biol. Reprod. 22, 941-954.
4. Gwatkin, R.B.L., and Williams, D.T. ( 1977) Receptor activity of the hamster and mouse solubilized zona pellucida before and after the zona reaction. J. Reprod. Fertil. 49, 55-59.
5. Ownby, C.L., and Shivers, C.A. ( 1972) Antigens of the hamster ovary and effects of anti-ovary serum on eggs. Biol. Reprod. 6, 310-318.
6. Sacco, A.G., Subramanian, M.G., and Yurewicz, E.C. ( 1981) Active immunization of mice with porcine zonae pellucidae: immune response and effect on fertility. J. Exp. Zool. 218, 405.
7. Saint Marie ( 1962) A paraffin embedding technique for studies employing immunofluorescence. J. Histochem. Cytochem. 10, 250-256.
8. Skinner, S.M., Mills, T., Kirchick, H.J., and Dunbar, B.S. ( 1984) Immunization with zona pellucidae proteins results in abnormal ovarian follicular differentiation and inhibition of gonadotropin-induced steroid secretion. Endocrinology 115( 6), 2418-2432.
9. Sternberger, L.A. ( 1979) Immunocytochemistry. J. Wiley & Sons, Inc.
10. Wolgemuth, D.J., Celenza, J., Bundman, D.S., and Dunbar, B.S. ( 1984) Formation of rabbit zonae pellucidae and its relationship to ovarian follicular development. Develop. Biol. 105.
11. Wood, D.M., Liu, C., and Dunbar, B.S. ( 1981) The effect of allo-immunization and heteroimmunization with zona pellucida on fertility in rabbits. Biol. Reprod. 25, 439-450.
12. Yanagimachi, R. ( 1971) Specificity of sperm-egg interaction. In "Immunology of Gametes," (M. Editdin and M.H. Johnson, eds.), pp. 187-207, Cambridge University Press, London/New York.

# ANTIGENIC PROFILE AND IMPACT OF IMMUNIZATION WITH ZONA PELLUCIDA ANTIGENS IN PRIMATES

Anthony G. Sacco, Marappa G. Subramanian, Edward C. Yurewicz, Donna L. Pierce[1] and W. Richard Dukelow[1]

Wayne State University School of Medicine, Department of Obstetrics and Gynecology, C. S. Mott Center for Human Growth and Development, Detroit, MI and Michigan State University[1], Endocrine Research Center, East Lansing, MI

## INTRODUCTION AND BACKGROUND

Within the past 10-12 years numerous studies have been published which describe the investigation of zona pellucida antigens for immunocontraceptive purposes (for reviews see Sacco, 1981; Dunbar, 1983). The earliest of these studies primarily used antigens associated with rodent zonae as immunogens and involved the use of antisera developed against total zona proteins. These early *in vitro* experiments and passive immunization studies clearly demonstrated the contraceptive potential of antibodies produced against the zona pellucida. When the immunologic similarity of antigens present in porcine and human zona was demonstrated (Sacco, 1977), the porcine zona became a prime candidate for consideration as a target antigen for the development of a human contraceptive vaccine. The availability of large numbers of porcine ovaries as a source of zonae made this species particularly attractive for immunocontraceptive studies.

Within the past five years, numerous advances in the area of the zona pellucida and immunocontraception have been made. Such advances have been primarily in three areas which include: (1) the application of new methodologies to the zona system. Examples are improved zonae collection and concentration techniques (Oikawa, 1978; Wood, et al., 1981), sensitive zona radioimmunoassays (Palm, et al., 1979; Subramanian, et al., 1981; Sacco, et al., 1981a; Gerrity, et al., 1981) and ELISA procedures (Fox, et al., 1981; Gulyas, et al., 1983a) for antibody quantitation, the application of 2-dimensional polyacrylamide gel electrophoresis (2-D PAGE; Bleil and Wassarman, 1980; Subramanian, et al., 1981; Dunbar, et al., 1981) and 2-dimensional immunoelectrophoresis (Wood and Dunbar, 1981; Sacco, et al., 1983a) to zona macromolecules and the production of monoclonal antibodies to zona antigens (Isojima, et al., 1981; Drell and Dunbar, 1984); (2) advances in knowledge regarding zona pellucida biochemistry (Bleil and Wassarman, 1980; Subramanian, et al., 1981; Dunbar, et al., 1981; Yurewicz, et al., 1983); and (3) fertility studies involving the active immunization of females from various species with porcine zona pellucida proteins.

The recent fertility investigations have included the active immunization of dogs (Shivers, et al., 1981; Mahi-Brown, et al., 1982, 1985), rabbits (Wood, et al., 1981; Dietl, et al., 1982; Skinner, et al., 1984), squirrel monkeys (Sacco, et al, 1983b) and cynomolgus monkeys (Gulyas, et al., 1983b). Collectively, data from these studies indicate that immunization with porcine zona results in a dramatic inhibitory effect upon fertility, thus again emphasizing the contraceptive effectiveness of this approach to fertility regulation. Furthermore, such active immunization studies also vividly emphasize that the antibodies developed against porcine zonae do possess sufficient in situ cross-reactivity with the zonae material of the immunized species (i.e., the heterologous species) to successfully inhibit fertility. However, several of these studies also noted alterations in normal ovarian physiology and/or cycle irregularities following such active immunization. Histological examination of ovaries from actively immunized rabbits indicated that the antibodies to zona were likely interfering with normal ovarian follicular development (Skinner, et al., 1984). Thus, a major revelation of these most recent studies was, that at least in some cases, the infertility observed following active immunization of females with porcine zona material may be primarily induced by zona antibodies inhibiting normal ovarian function rather than sperm-egg interaction. Thus, it appears that zona antibodies can inhibit fertility by disrupting two major reproductive processes: (1) follicular development/differentiation and (2) sperm-egg interaction.

As indicated in this symposium, several laboratories are currently engaged in immunocontraceptive studies involving the active immunization of primates with total porcine zona material or with purified porcine zona macromolecules. Such primates include the bonnet monkey, rhesus monkey, squirrel monkey and baboon. These studies are designed to evaluate primate immune response to different porcine zona immunogens, immune responses following use of various adjuvants, effect of immunization on fertility, mechanism of action of zona antibodies in producing any observed infertility and to observe immunized animals for possible adverse side effects. Within the next few years, considerable data should become available to adequately evaluate the efficacy of active immunization of primates with porcine zona pellucida material.

The purpose of this chapter is to describe an ongoing immunocontraceptive study which involves the active immunization of female squirrel monkeys (Saimiri sciureus). This investigation is presently unique because it represents the first primate study which utilizes a large number (50) of immunized animals as well as a homogeneous, well characterized porcine zona pellucida macromolecule (the 55K glycoprotein family) as immunogen. Monkeys were immunized in July, 1984 and consequently the available data at this time are very preliminary. Nonetheless, certain trends are evident, even at this early date, which may influence methodologies and experimental designs chosen for future immunocontraceptive studies which utilize porcine zona macromolecules.

## ACTIVE IMMUNIZATION OF SQUIRREL MONKEYS (SAIMIRI SCIUREUS) WITH PORCINE ZONAE

### Species Selection

It has been known for several years that antiserum produced against zonae pellucidae of one species will cross react in varying degrees with zonae from other species. Therefore, common or similar antigens/epitopes must be shared by the zonae of a number of different animals. For immunocontraceptive purposes involving active heteroimmunization, the degree or level of this cross reaction and zona antigenic similarity becomes paramount. Unfortunately, in our consideration of the porcine zona as the basis for contraceptive vaccine development, antisera produced against porcine zonae antigens react very poorly with zona from rodent

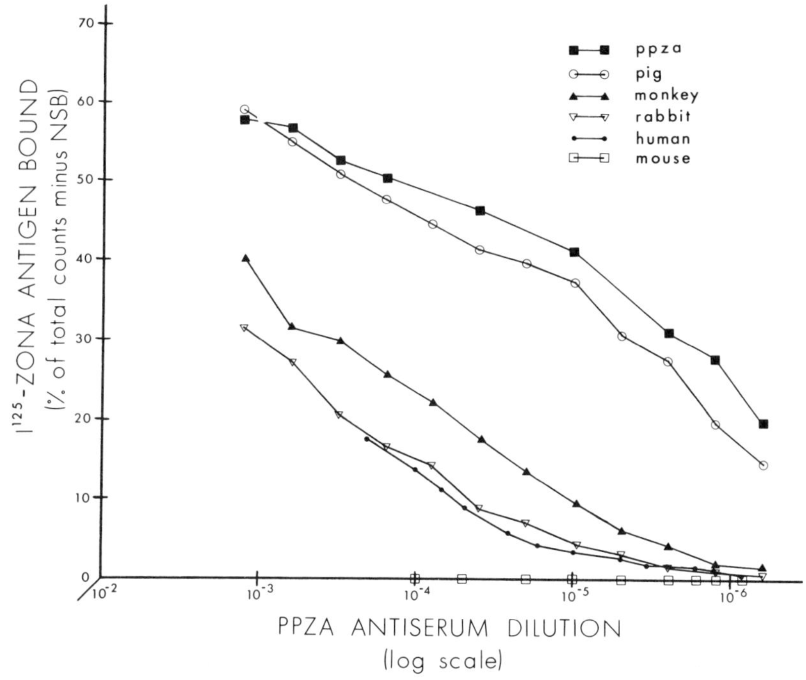


Fig. 1 Rabbit anti-PPZA binding profiles to $I^{125}$-labeled PPZA and $I^{125}$ SIZP (heat-solubilized isolated zonae pellucidae) preparations from the pig, squirrel monkey, human, rabbit and mouse. The low level of cross-reactivity in the mouse system is typical of rodents in general. (From Sacco, et al., 1981c).

species (Fig. 1). Consequently, common laboratory animals such as the mouse, rat, hamster, etc., cannot be considered for use in fertility investigations designed to evaluate the contraceptive efficacy of active immunization using porcine zona antigens (Sacco, et al., 1981b, c). Although the level of cross reactivity of antibodies to pig zonae and rabbit zonae appears adequate (Fig. 1), antibodies to pig zonae fail to inhibit homologous sperm-zona interaction in the rabbit system (Sacco, et al., 1981c). On the basis of these types of data, the non-human primate appeared to be the best test system to consider for the evaluation of a porcine zona pellucida contraceptive vaccine. Because of our preliminary data using the squirrel monkey, we selected this species for our immunocontraceptive investigations.

Antigen Selection

The porcine zona pellucida is biochemically and antigenically complex. As resolved by 2-dimensional polyacrylamide gel electrophoresis (2-D PAGE), it consists of four major families of charge heterogeneous acidic glycoproteins (Subramanian, et al., 1981; Sacco, et al., 1981a, c; Dunbar, et al., 1981; Hedrick and Wardrip, 1981) with apparent molecular weights of 82K (ZP1), 61K (ZP2), 55K (ZP3) and 21K (ZP4) (Fig. 2A). In our consideration of the porcine zona for use in contraceptive vaccine development, our approach is to ultimately utilize the smallest component of the porcine zona which is capable of eliciting antibodies possessing contraceptive properties. Along these lines, as our first candidate, we selected the 55K (ZP3) glycoprotein macromolecule for the following reasons:

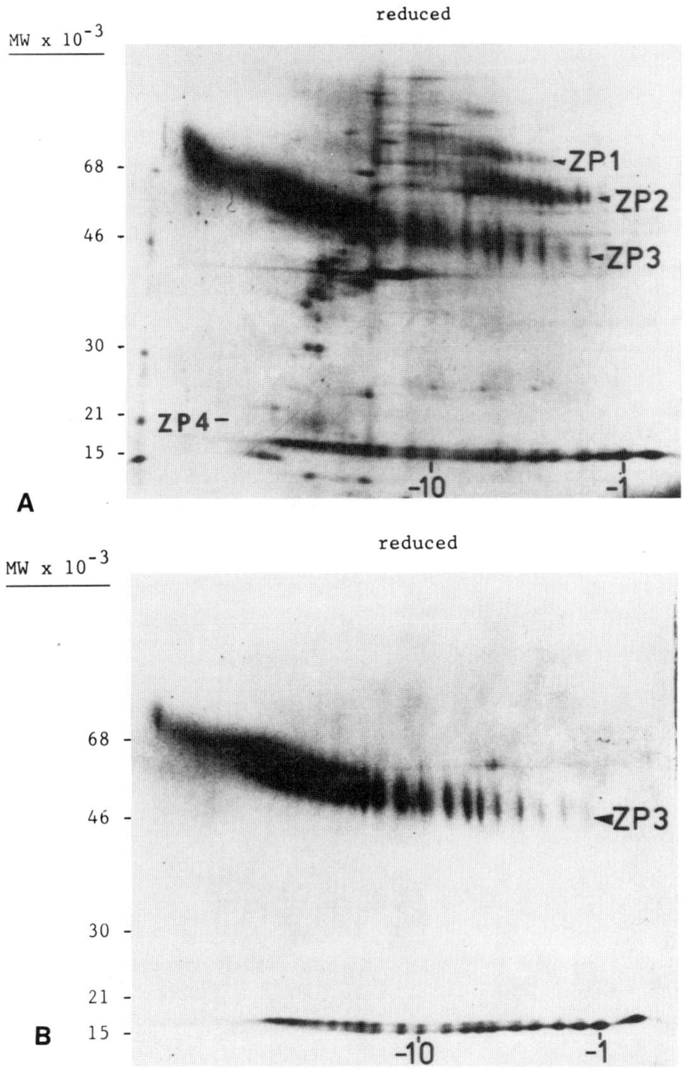


Fig. 2 Two-dimensional polyacrylamide gel electrophoresis (2-D PAGE) of porcine zona pellucida. Isoelectric focusing is represented in the horizontal dimension (acidic end to the left) and SDS-PAGE is represented in the vertical dimension (migration from top to bottom). Gels were stained with Coomassie blue. (A) SIZP (heat solubilized isolated zonae pellucidae, reduced). (B) purified ZP3 glycoprotein family, reduced.

(1) preliminary data indicated it represented the best prospect for successful purification by chromatographic procedures, (2) it represents the most predominant glycoprotein comprising approximately 60% of the pig zona, (3) data indicate it appears to be the most immunogenic glycoprotein (Sacco, et al., 1983a) and, (4) studies suggested that it may be biologically significant and possess sperm receptor activity (Sacco, et al., 1984).

Our first attempts to purify the 55K (ZP3) component resulted in a preparation which was not totally homogeneous but was free of the other major porcine zona pellucida macromolecules (i.e. ZP1, ZP2 and ZP4; Yurewicz, et al., 1983). This preparation was referred to as PPZA (purified pig zona antigen) and consisted primarily of the 55K (ZP3) component and represented the first purified porcine zona macromolecule used to immunize squirrel monkeys (Sacco, et al., 1983b). Recently, our laboratory has been successful in chromatographically purifying the 55K (ZP3) component to electrophoretic homogeneity (Yurewicz, et al., 1984a, b). This preparation is referred to as ZP3 (Fig. 2B) and has been used in one pilot immunization study involving 6 squirrel monkeys and in a large scale fertility study. For the purposes of this chapter the 55K component = PPZA = ZP3 and these terms will be used interchangeably.

## ANTIGENIC PROFILE

### Antiserum Titration

Three squirrel monkey active immunization studies have been undertaken to date and are summarized in Table 1.

TABLE 1. Summary of Studies Involving Active Immunization of Squirrel Monkeys (Saimiri sciureus) with Porcine Zona Pellucida Antigens

| Study Number | No. of Animals | Date Immunized | Antigen | Dose Range |
|---|---|---|---|---|
| 1 | 6 | 12/80 | PPZA | 0.5 - 2.0 mg |
| 2 | 6 | 4/83 | ZP3 | 100 - 400 μg |
| 3 | 50 | 7/84 | ZP3 | 200 μg |

They include two pilot immunization programs involving 6 animals each and a large scale study consisting of 50 ZP3-immunized animals, 25 Freund's adjuvant injected animals and 25 uninjected controls. The purpose of the pilot studies was two-fold: (1) to evaluate the immunogenicity of a purified porcine zona macromolecule (i.e., the 55K glycoprotein referred to initially as PPZA and later as ZP3) in a primate system and (2) to monitor the immune response (i.e., titration profiles) of the immunized monkeys. Because of the limited number of animals involved, no fertility experiments were attempted in these two pilot investigations. The third study involved 50 immunized animals and included fertility investigations.

In the first pilot study, each of two female monkeys was injected with a total of either 0.5, 1.0 or 2.0 mg PPZA, respectively. One-half of the indicated total dosage was given to each monkey over a series of 4 injections spaced one week apart. The remaining material was given in a single booster injection once peak titers, as established by RIA, had been attained. Freund's complete adjuvant was used with the first injection and Freund's incomplete adjuvant was used for all other injections. For the second pilot study, immunogen dosage was significantly reduced. The homogeneous preparation of the 55K macromolecule (ZP3) was available at this time and was used in this study. Each of two female monkeys was injected with a total of either 100, 200 or 400 ug ZP3 respectively. Immunizations were conducted as described for the first pilot study except that the initial series of injections was reduced from four to three. A dosage of 200 ug ZP3 was selected for the large scale study.

RIA titration profiles for each of the three studies are presented in Fig. 3. A rapid rise in titer was detected immediately following the initial injection series, followed by a leveling in response. After the

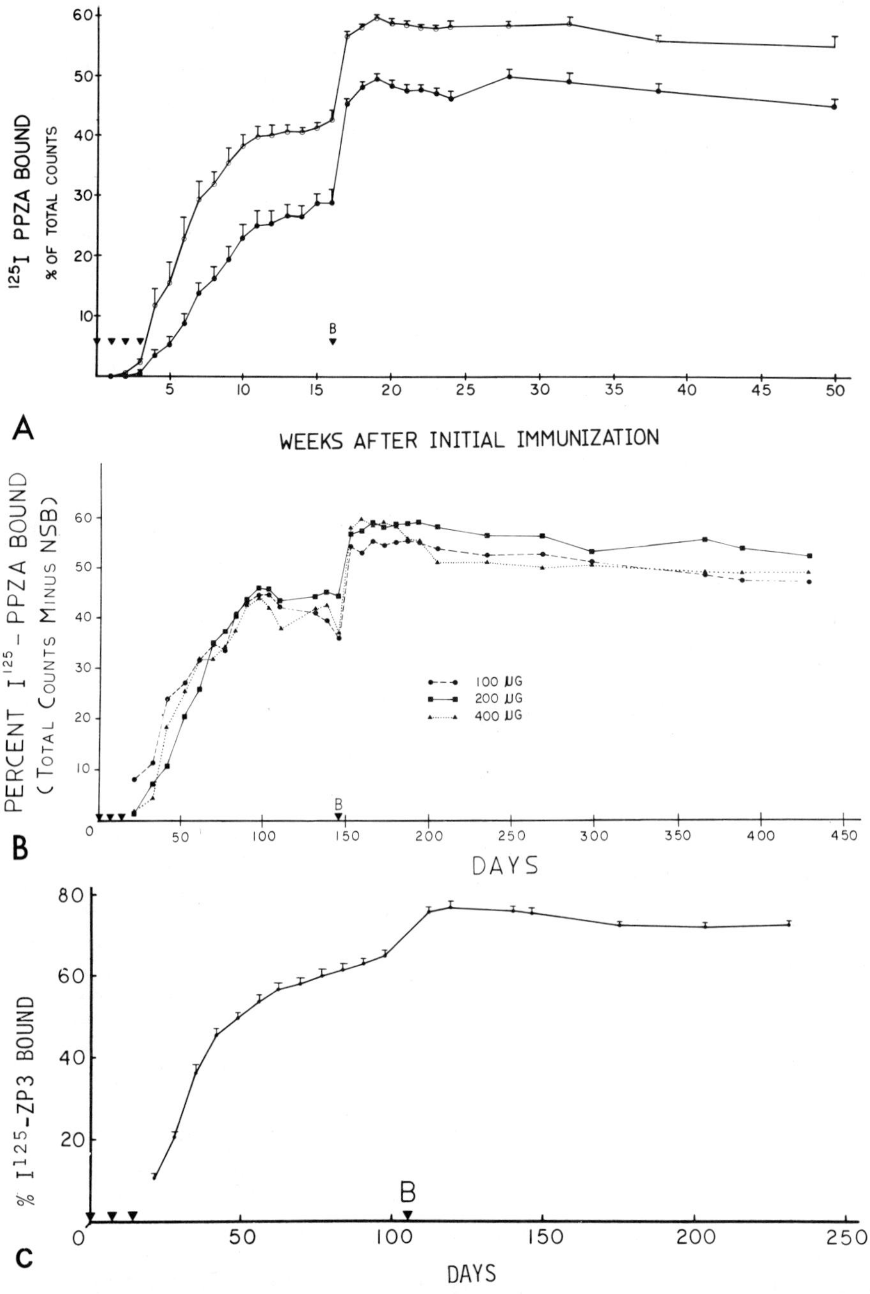


Fig. 3 Radioimmunoassay (RIA) titration profiles of squirrel monkey antisera prepared against PPZA or ZP3. Arrows indicate the initial series of injections and the single booster (B) injection. (A) Collective titration profile (mean ± SE) of the six monkeys injected in the first pilot immunization study. Titers were estimated at two serum dilutions: -0-, 1:000; -●-, 1:5000. (From Sacco, et al., 1983b).
(B) RIA titration profiles of the six monkeys injected in the second pilot immunization study. Note no significant dose-response difference among the three dosage levels. Each curve represents pooled data from two monkeys injected with same dosage.
(C) Collective titration profile (mean ± SE) of the 50 monkeys immunized with ZP3 in the large scale fertility study.

single booster immunization, a second rapid and significant increase in antibody activity occurred, which peaked in approximately 2-3 weeks, followed by a plateau and then a gradual decline. From these results, three major conclusions were drawn: (1) Based upon the binding levels obtained, the 55K macromolecule (PPZA, ZP3) represents a potent immunogen; (2) on the basis of the chosen immunization schedule, the resulting immune response, even in the absence of additional boosters, is of long term duration; (3) no significant dose response differences were detected in the two pilot studies. In respect to the latter, in the first pilot study (Fig. 3A) titration profiles for each of the immunogen dosage levels were similar to those presented in Fig. 3B.

### In Vitro Contraceptive Potential of Antiserum to ZP3

Antisera obtained from representative monkeys from each of the three immunization studies has been tested for its ability to produce a precipitation layer on zona from the pig, squirrel monkey and human and also tested for its ability to inhibit homologous sperm attachment in each of these species. Representative examples are presented in Fig. 4. All antisera tested regardless of immunogen, dosage, monkey or bleeding used, produced a precipitate on the zona surface indicating antibody cross-reactivity with a native zona component present in the intact zona from each of the three species. The intensity of the precipitate, however, did vary depending upon the species tested. Antisera treatment of intact pig zonae, representing the homologous antigen, produced a dense precipitate on the zona surface (Fig. 4A). Treatment of squirrel monkey zonae produced a moderately dense precipitate (Fig. 4C), while treatment of human zonae resulted in a faint to moderately dense precipitate (Fig. 4E). Exposure of such antibody pretreated zonae from each of the various species to homologous sperm preparations resulted in the total inhibition of sperm attachment to such antibody-treated zonae (Fig. 4B,D,F). Such findings unequivocally demonstrate the *in vitro* contraceptive potential of squirrel monkey antisera to porcine zona in the pig, monkey and human systems.

## IMPACT OF IMMUNIZATION

### Egg Yields

To evaluate possible adverse effects of immunization on normal ovarian function, attempts were made to recover follicular eggs from immunized and control monkeys using previously described procedures for hormonally induced ovum maturation and laparoscopic egg recovery in the squirrel monkey (Ariga and Dukelow, 1977). In our initial attempt, monkeys from the first pilot immunization study were utilized. As previously reported (Sacco, et al., 1983b) significantly fewer oocytes were obtained from immunized monkeys when compared with comparably hormone-stimulated non-immunized controls (0.1 versus 1.8 oocytes per monkey, respectively). Furthermore, at the time of laparoscopy, as compared to the controls, the ovaries of the immunized monkeys appeared somewhat smaller in size, contained fewer visible follicles and looked generally unresponsive to the exogenous hormone treatment.

A similar study has recently been repeated on a more extensive basis. Approximately four months following initial immunization and just at the onset of the breeding season 50 ZP3-injected monkeys, 25 Freund's adjuvant-injected monkeys and 25 untreated monkeys were hormonally stimulated and subjected to laparoscopy at which time ovaries were viewed and follicles aspirated for oocyte retrieval. Results are summarized in Table 2.

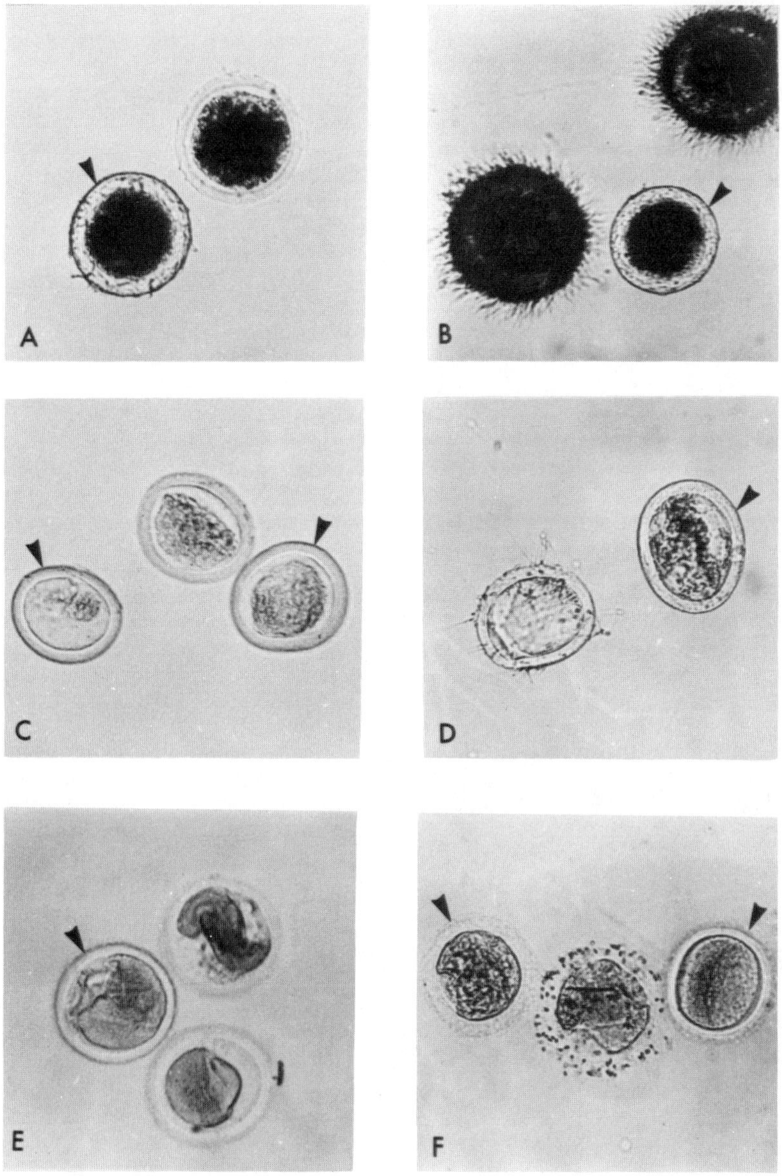


Fig. 4 Inhibition of sperm-zona binding by squirrel monkey antisera to PPZA. Oocytes from pig (A,B), squirrel monkey (C,D) and human (E,F) were treated with either squirrel monkey anti-PPZA serum (arrows) or squirrel monkey preimmune serum (unlabeled). Plates A,C,E demonstrate the formation of the precipitation layers on the zona surface of the antiserum treated eggs. Preimmune serum treated eggs have no precipitation layer. Plates B,D,F demonstrate the inhibition of homologous sperm attachment to oocytes pretreated with antiserum. Numerous sperm bind to preimmune treated oocytes (From Sacco, et al., 1983b).

TABLE 2. Follicles Observed and Oocytes Retrieved in ZP3-Injected, Adjuvant-Injected Control and Untreated Control Monkeys

| GROUP | N | WT (gms) | Follicles S < 1mm | M 1-2mm | L > 2mm | Oocytes Monkey |
|---|---|---|---|---|---|---|
| UT | 25 | 636 | 7.5 | 6.2 | 1.1 | 2.1 |
| Adj Cont | 25 | 625 | 11.8 | 6.2 | 3.1 | 3.1 |
| ZP3 Inj | 50 | 591 | 3.6 | 0.45 | 0.4 | 0.4 |

These recent data confirmed our earlier findings and again indicated that the number of follicles present and the number of oocytes retrieved were significantly reduced in the ZP3-immunized animals as compared to the controls. While these findings strongly suggest that ZP3 immunization is influencing normal ovarian function, at least at 4 months, this effect is not absolute since some monkeys are still responding to exogenous hormone stimulation and producing oocytes.

## Ovarian Histology

Ovaries have been obtained and prepared for histological examination from each of two monkeys from the ZP3-immunized group and the adjuvant-immunized group (total 4 monkeys) of our most recent study. Death in each case occurred approximately 6-7 months following initial immunization and was attributed to infection of open sores at the booster injection site (monkey's back) and not directly to antigen injected. Ovaries were removed and fixed in Bouin's solution as soon as possible after the deaths were discovered and sections were stained with hematoxylin and eosin.

Normal ovarian histology was presented in tissue sections obtained from both the adjuvant and ZP3 injected animals (Fig. 5). However, sections from one of the ZP3 immunized animals (Fig. 5C) contained very few large preovulatory follicles although numerous oocyte containing primary follicles as well as small growing follicles and several corpora lutea were present. The ovaries from this animal may reflect very early signs of ovarian dysfunction but, obviously, further studies involving examination of additional sections from this animal and material from other animals must be carried out.

## Hormonal Profiles

An initial series of daily blood samples were obtained from randomly selected ZP3-injected, adjuvant-injected and untreated monkeys and estradiol ($E_2$) and progesterone (P) levels measured by RIA. These particular samples were obtained just at the onset of the squirrel monkey breeding season in Michigan (November-April). Although cyclical trends of $E_2$ and P levels were observed in these daily samples, none of the monkeys in the three groups was exhibiting ovulatory cycles as judged by the peak $E_2$ and P levels obtained (Diamond, et al., 1984). Maximum $E_2$ and P levels detected in these daily samples are presented in Table 3. On the basis of these preliminary hormone analyses the following comments can be made: (1) Maximum $E_2$ and P levels obtained from representative monkeys in each of the three treatment groups at the onset of the breeding season indicated that none of the monkeys tested was exhibiting an ovulatory cycle at that time; (2) $E_2$ secretion, as judged by the maximum $E_2$ levels obtained, appeared to be lower in the ZP3-injected and adjuvant-injected groups as compared to the untreated group; and (3) P levels in the untreated and adjuvant-injected control groups were relatively comparable, whereas P levels in the ZP3-injected group were extremely variable.

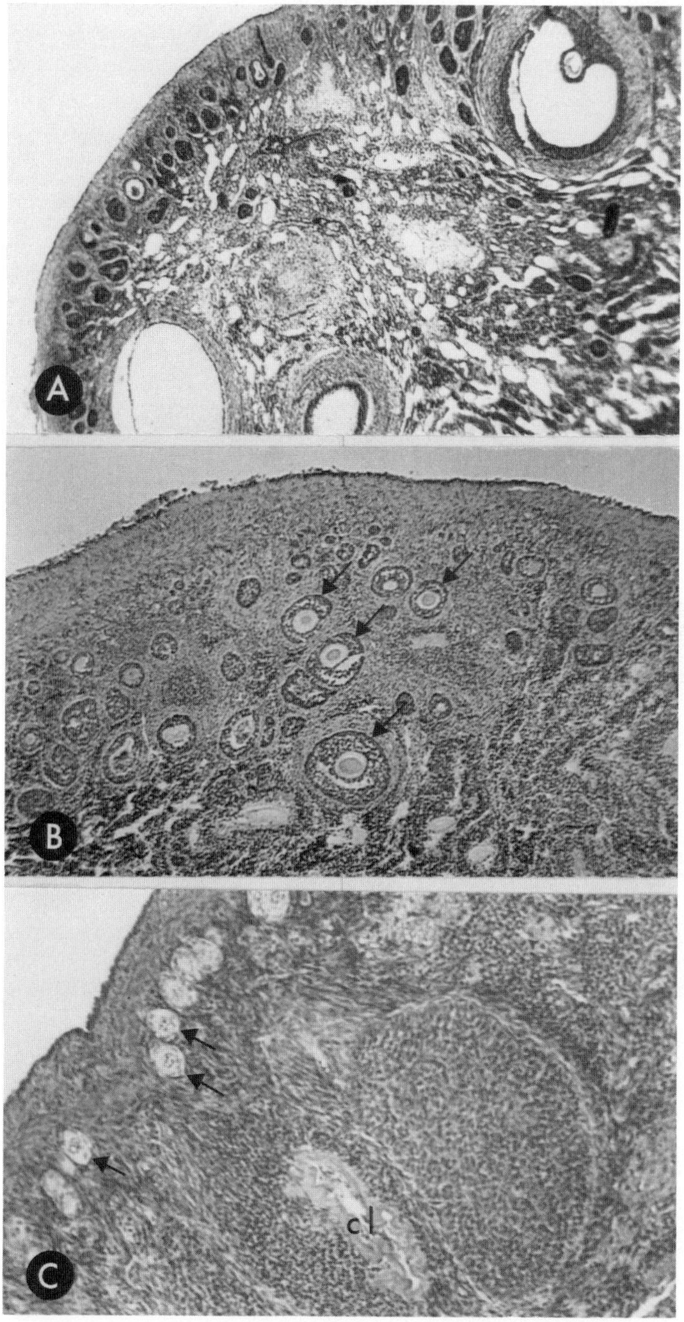


Fig. 5 Ovarian histology of squirrel monkeys immunized with either ZP3 plus Freund's adjuvant or with Freund's adjuvant alone. A., Tissue section from monkey immunized with Freund's adjuvant alone. B., Section from monkey immunized with ZP3. Arrows designate follicles containing oocytes. C., Section from second monkey immunized with ZP3. Arrows designate oocyte containing follicles. cl = corpus luteum.

TABLE 3. Maximum Estradiol ($E_2$) and Progesterone (P) Levels Detected in Daily Blood Samples Collected from Squirrel Monkeys at the Onset of the Breeding Season

| Untreated | | | Adjuvant-Injected | | | ZP3 Injected | | |
|---|---|---|---|---|---|---|---|---|
| Monkey# | $E_2$(pg/ml) | P(ng/ml) | Monkey# | $E_2$ | P | Monkey# | $E_2$ | P |
| 1 | 41 | 2.35 | 1 | 26 | 4.70 | 1 | 0 | 19.50 |
| 2 | 99 | 2.49 | 2 | 50 | 1.86 | 2 | 32 | 4.52 |
| 3 | 94 | 6.54 | 3 | 46 | 1.74 | 3 | 0 | 4.52 |
| 4 | 101 | 1.62 | 4 | 24 | 3.54 | 4 | 32 | 28.46 |
| 5 | 50 | 0.90 | 5 | 28 | 0.80 | 5 | 7 | 7.66 |
| | | | | | | 6 | 0 | 6.54 |
| | | | | | | 7 | 72 | 69.92 |
| X | 77 | 2.78 | | 35 | 2.53 | | 20.4 | 20.2 |
| ±SE | 13.0 | 0.98 | | 5.5 | 0.70 | | 10.0 | 9.0 |

E2 and P levels were also measured in representative samples collected at three monthly intervals around the midpoint of the breeding season. These samples were primarily obtained for titer and pregnancy determination. Daily samples were not collected at this time because monkeys were involved in the fertility portion of the investigation. From these hormone analyses, the following observations were made: (1) Both $E_2$ and P levels, on an average, appeared to be lower in samples obtained from the ZP3-injected and adjuvant-injected groups as compared to the untreated group; (2) the maximum $E_2$ and P levels in all three treatment groups were definitely greater than those obtained in the initial series of daily samples collected at the onset of the breeding season.

## Fertility Data

Preliminary results during the first half of the breeding season indicate 4 pregnancies (16%) in the untreated group and 0 pregnancies in the adjuvant-injected and ZP3-injected groups.

## COMMENTS AND CONCLUSIONS

As indicated previously, studies involving the active immunization of female dogs (Mahi-Brown, et al., 1982, 1985), rabbits (Skinner, et al., 1984) and cynomolgus monkeys (Gulyas, et al., 1983b) with porcine zona material have demonstrated a dramatic inhibitory effect upon fertility. Such findings provide much optimism for continued investigation of this approach for fertility regulation. These studies, however, have also revealed cycle disturbances in these immunized animals which suggests that, *in vivo*, antibodies to zona may be exerting their primary effect at the level of the ovary rather than at the level of sperm-zona interaction as previously presumed. Whether this interference with normal follicular development/differentiation by zona antibodies can be obviated by using purified zona macromolecules as immunogens is as yet unresolved. Promising results from preliminary investigations do provide considerable encouragement (Mahi-Brown, et al., 1985; Skinner and Dunbar, 1984).

Our preliminary squirrel monkey findings, the egg yield, hormonal and possibly the histological data suggest that ZP3 immunization is having an effect on normal ovarian function. However, to this point in the investigation, individual monkey responses have been extremely variable and consistent effects of comparable magnitude have not been detected in all animals within a given treatment group. One obvious conclusion even at this early point in these squirrel monkey studies is that the situation in the primate system regarding active immunization with porcine zona material is not identical to that recently reported in the rabbit (Skinner, et al., 1984). Based upon our current information, the suspected effects on ovarian function in the squirrel monkey following active immunization with ZP3 do not appear to be (at least initially) as severe and, possibly require a longer time period to materialize as compared to the rabbit. These differences may be a reflection of our use of the purified ZP3 macromolecule and provide further support for continued investigation using purified porcine zona macromolecules as immunogens. Upcoming data from these squirrel monkey studies as well as the other primate investigations discussed in this symposium will ultimately reveal whether the intact ZP3 macromolecule will remain a viable candidate as an immunocontraceptive target antigen.

An unexpected finding in the squirrel monkey studies was the possible adverse influence of Freund's adjuvant alone on normal hormonal profiles. Studies are in progress to clarify this issue. If new data support these findings then use of Freund's adjuvant in upcoming or planned immunocontraceptive primate investigations should not be considered.

In summary, early immunocontraceptive investigations as well as the more recent active immunization studies have emphasized the contraceptive effectiveness of antibodies directed against zona pellucida macromolcules. Although some of these most recent immunization experiments have resulted in alterations in normal ovarian function using current porcine zona target antigens, a host of other potential porcine target antigens remains to be investigated. Among these would be the ZP1, ZP2 and ZP4 glycoprotein families as well as modified forms (e.g. deglycosylated, enzyme digests, peptide fragments, etc.) of the ZP3 macromolecule. Any of these porcine zona candidates possesses the potential to elicit antibodies which exert their contraceptive effect only at the level of sperm-zona interaction.

## REFERENCES


Ariga, S. and Dukelow, W.R. (1977). Nonsurgical (laparoscopic) uterine flushing and egg recovery techniques in the squirrel monkey (Saimiri sciureus). Primates 18:453.

Bleil, J.D. and Wassarman, P.M. (1980). Mammalian sperm-egg interaction: identification of a glycoprotein in mouse egg zonae pellucida possessing receptor activity for sperm. Cell 20:873-882.

Diamond, E.J., Aksel, S., Hazelton, J.M., Jennings, R.A. and Abee, C.R. (1984). Seasonal changes of serum concentration of estradiol and progesterone in Bolivian squirrel monkeys (Saimiri scireus). Amer. J. Primatol. 6:103-113.

Dietl, J., Freye, J. and Mettler, L. (1982). Fertility inhibition using low-dose immunization with porcine zona pellucida. A.J.R.I. 2:153-156.

Drell, D.W. and Dunbar, B.S. (1984). Monoclonal antibodies to rabbit and pig zonae pellucidae distinguish species-specific and shared antigenic determinants. Biol. Reprod. 30:445-457.

Dunbar, B.S. (1983). Antibodies to zona pellucida antigens and their role in fertility. In: Immunology of Reproduction, T. Wegmann, T. Gill, C. Cumming and E. Nisbet-Brown, eds., Oxford University Press, pgs. 506-534.

Dunbar, B.S., Liu, C., and Sammons, D.W. (1981). Identification of three major proteins of porcine and rabbit zonae pellucidae by high resolution two-dimensional gel electrophoresis: comparison with serum, follicular fluid, and ovarian cell proteins. Biol. Reprod. 24:1111-1124.

Fox, L.L, Gengozian, N., Shivers, C.A., and Sieg, P. (1981). Marmoset response to immunization with porcine zonae pellucida. J. Med. Primatol. 10:205-211.

Gerrity, M., Niu, E., and Dunbar, B.S. (1981). A specific radioimmunoassay for evaluation of serum antibodies to zona pellucida antigens. J. Reprod. Immunol. 3:59-70.

Gulyas, B.J., Yuan, L.C., Gwatkin, R.B.L., and Schmell, E.D. (1983a). Response of monkeys to porcine zona pellucida as detected by a solid-phase radioimmunoassay. J. Med. Primatol. 12:332-342.

Gulyas, B.J., Gwatkin, R.B.L. and Yuan, L.C. (1983b). Active immunization of cynomolgus monkeys (Macaca fascicularis) with porcine zona pellucidae. Gamete Research 4:299-307.

Hedrick, J.L. and Wardrip, N. (1981). Microheterogeneity in the glycoproteins of the zona pellucida is due to the carbohydrate moiety. J. Cell Biol. 91:77a.

Isojima, S., Koyama, K., and Hasegawa, A. (1981). Production of monoclonal antibodies to zona pellucida from porcine oocytes. Acta. Obst. Gynaec. Jpn. 33:1995-1996.

Mahi-Brown, C.A., Huang, T.T.F. and Yanagimachi, R. (1982). Infertility in bitches induced by active immunization with porcine zonae pellucidae. J. Exp. Zool. 222:89-95.

Mahi-Brown, C.A., Yanagimachi, R., Hoffmann, J.D., and Huang, T.T.F. (1985). Fertility control in the bitch by active immunization with porcine zonae pellucidae: use of different adjuvants and patterns of estradiol and progesterone levels in estrous cycles. Biol. Reprod. 32:761-772.

Oikawa, T. (1978). A simple method for the isolation of a large number of ova from pig ovaries. Gamete Res. 1:265-267.

Palm, V.S., Sacco, A.G., Syner, F., and Subramanian, M.G. (1979). Tissue specificity of porcine zona pellucida antigen(s) as tested by radioimmunoassay. Biol. Reprod. 21:709-713.

Sacco, A.G. (1977). Antigenic cross-reactivity between human and pig zona pellucida. Biol. Reprod. 16:164-173.

Sacco, A.G. (1981). Immunocontraception: consideration of the zona pellucida as a target antigen. In: Obstetrics and Gynecology Annual, R.M. Wynn, ed., Vol. 10:1-26.

Sacco, A.G., Subramanian, M.G., and Yurewicz, E.C. (1981a). Application of a radioimmunoassay (RIA) for monitoring immune response to porcine zonae pellucidae. Proc. Soc. Exp. Biol. Med. 167:318-326.

Sacco, A.G., Subrmanian, M.G., and Yurewicz, E.C. (1981b). Active immunization of mice with porcine zonae pellucidae: immune response and effect on fertility. J. Exp. Zool. 218:405-418.

Sacco, A.G., Yurewicz, E.C., Subramanian, M.G., and DeMayo, F.J. (1981c). Zona pellucida composition: species cross reactivity and contraceptive potential of antiserum to a purified pig zona antigen (PPZA). Biol. Reprod. 25:997-1008.

Sacco, A.G., Yurewicz, E.C., and Zhang, S. (1983a). Immunoelectrophoretic analysis of the porcine zona pellucida. J. Reprod. Fert. 68:21-31.

Sacco, A.G., Subramanian, M.G., Yurewicz, E.C., DeMayo, F.J., and Dukelow, (1983b). Heteroimmunization of squirrel monkeys (Saimiri sciureus) with a purified porcine zona antigen (PPZA): immune response and biologic activity of antiserum. Fertil. Steril. 39:350-358.

Sacco, A.G., Subramanian, M.G., and Yurewicz, E.C. (1984). Association of sperm receptor activity with a purified pig zona antigen (PPZA). J. Reprod. Immunol. 6:89-103.

Shivers, C.A., Sieg, P.M., and Kitchen, H. (1981). Pregnancy prevention in the dog: Potential for an immunological approach. J. Amer. An. Hosp. Assoc. 17:823 828.

Skinner, S.M. and Dunbar, B.S. (1984) Comparison of immunization using a purified zona pellucida (ZP) protein or total ZP protein on ovarian follicular development. Biol. Reprod. 30 (Supplement 1): 73.

Skinner, S.M., Mills, T., Kirchick, H.J., and Dunbar, B.S. (1984). Immunization with zona pellucida proteins results in abnormal ovarian follicular differentiation and inhibition of gonadotropin-induced steroid secretion. Endocrinology 115:2418-2432.

Subramanian, M.G., Yurewicz, E.C., and Sacco, A.G. (1981). Specific radioimmunoassay for the detection of a purified porcine zona pellucida antigen (PPZA). Biol. Reprod. 24:933-943.

Wood, D.M. and Dunbar, B.S. (1981). Direct detection of two cross-reactive antigens between porcine and rabbit zonae pellucidae by radioimmunoassay and immunoelectrophoresis. J. Exp. Zool. 217:423-433.

Wood, D.M., Lui, C., and Dunbar, B.S. (1981). Effect of alloimmunization and heteroimmunization with zonae pellucidae on fertility in rabbits. Biol. Reprod. 25:439-450.

Yurewicz, E.C., Sacco, A.G., and Subramanian, M.G. (1983). Isolation and preliminary characterization of a purified pig zona antigen (PPZA) from porcine oocytes. Biol. Reprod. 29:511-523.

Yurewicz, E.C., Sacco, A.G. and Subramanian, M.G. (1984a). Purification and characterization of glycoprotein antigens of the porcine zona pellucida. Fed. Proc. 43:2039.

Yurewicz, E.C., Sacco, A.G. and Subramanian, M.G. (1984b). Structure of the porcine zona pellucida: isolation and properties of the major glycoprotein family. J. Cell Biol. 99:73a.

# EFFECT OF IMMUNIZATION OF PRIMATES AGAINST PORCINE ZONAE ON FERTILITY AND HORMONE PROFILES

Suman, A.K. Bamezai*, C. Das and G.P. Talwar*

Department of Biochemistry, All India Institute of Medical Sciences, *National Institute of Immunology
New Delhi, India

## INTRODUCTION AND BACKGROUND

Zona pellucida, the acellular glycoprotein envelope which surrounds the mammalian oocyte, has attracted attention as a possible antigen for immuno-contraceptive purposes. This interest is based on the demonstration that the zona pellucida contains at least one tissue specific antigen, as observed by immuno-diffusion and immunofluorescence (Sacco and Shivers 1978; Sacco 1981), SDS gel electrophoresis (Dunbar and Raynor 1980; Dunbar et al. 1981) and radio-immunoassay (Palm et al. 1979; Subramanian et al. 1981; Sacco et al. 1981; Gerrity et al. 1981).

Although zona antigens are tissue specific, they are not species specific (Sacco 1981) and antibodies produced against zona from one species can cross react to varying degree with zona of other species. Since pig and human zonae contain a cross-reactive antigen (Sacco 1977; Shivers and Dunbar 1977; Trounson et al. 1980), pig zonae has been employed for experimental studies. Reports on occurrence of anti zona pellucida antibodies in cases of natural infertility aroused much interest initially but are controversial (Sacco and Moghissi 1979; Mori et al. 1978; Kurachi et al. 1984). However immunization of animals with zonae has been demonstrated to lead to infertility. Immunization with cumulus-free ova (Tsunoda 1977) and isolated murine free zonae pellucidae (Tsunoda and Chang 1978; Aitken and Richardson 1981) were observed to be effective in control of fertility. Techniques have been standardized for large scale isolation of zonae pellucidae. Mice immunized with hamster zonae (Gwatkin et al. 1977), rabbits with bovine (Gwatkin and Williams 1978), porcine (Gwatkin et al. 1980; Wood et al. 1981) or rabbit zonae (Wood et al. 1981) and monkeys immunized with porcine zonae (Gulyas et al. 1983 ; Sacco et al. 1983; Suman thesis 1985) had significantly reduced fertility.

Passive immunization with antisera to mouse zonae or $\gamma$-globulin preparations of antisera was effective in mice (Tsunoda and Chang 1978; Suman thesis 1980), rat (Tsunoda and Chang 1978) as was antisera to cow zonae in cows (Tsunoda et al. 1981a) and porcine zonae antisera in pigs, sheep, cows, rabbits and mice (Tsunoda et al. 1981b). In these experiments zona antibodies were located by immunofluorescence on the zonae of eggs recovered from immunized animals.

These diverse observations indicate the possibility of fertility control in various species of animals. A point of concern however is the undesirable consequences reported by Wood et al. (1981) in rabbits immunized with intact or heat solubilised porcine zona pellucida. No eggs were found after ovulation in the former group while ovulation had not occurred in the latter set. Further studies showed that rabbits had abnormal follicular development, and failed to form a functional corpus luteum in response to hCG administration, as evidenced by absence of elevated serum progesterone and persistantly high FSH and LH levels in serum. The effects were apparent within twenty weeks of the primary injection. Histological examination of the ovaries showed only a few growing follicles after twenty-three weeks of immunization and the follicles did not contain oocytes (Skinner et al. 1984). It is not clear whether these changes are peculiar to rabbit or to the mixture of antigens in the crude preparation used for immunization.

The present studies had the objective of determining the effects of immunization with porcine zona pellucida in primates. In particular the questions asked were the following :

1. Does immunization of monkeys with porcine zonae block the fertility?
2. Is immunization accompanied by changes in sex steroids?
3. Is the effect reversible?

## ACTIVE IMMUNIZATION OF RHESUS AND BONNET MONKEYS (MACACCA MULLATA AND RADIATA) WITH INTACT PORCINE ZONAE

Monkeys cycling normally and of proven fertility were chosen and used for immunization.

Zona pellucida has a complex composition and is composed of at least three families of glycoproteins. At the time that the studies were initiated, no clear cut information was available on the component(s) inducing infertility. It is further not clear whether solubilization of the zona at 60°C under conditions of alkaline pH does not change the native conformation of the antigens. Thus, in the present study total intact zonae were employed as the antigen.

These were prepared by slightly modified procedure of Dunbar et al. (1981). Briefly, ovaries were sliced with ganged razor blades in 0.15M saline. Oocytes released from follicles were collected on metallic screens of progressively smaller mesh size. Oocytes and zonae retained on 75µ screen were transferred to a glass petri-dish and manually picked under stereo-microscope. Oocytes and zonae were washed twice with fresh saline and subjected to mechanical stress by passing through a drawn micro-pipette of a smaller diameter than the oocyte (approximately 40 to 50µ in size), thus breaking the zonae at one or more points and separating the vitellus and the free zonae. These were again passed through fresh saline and zonae picked under stereo-microscope. Lots of $6X10^3$ zonae in 1.5 to 2.5 ml of saline were stored at 4°C till further use.

### Immune Response

Studies were carried out in twenty two monkeys, four rhesus and eighteen bonnet monkeys. Table 1 gives the immunization protocol. Primary immunization consisted of one injection of $3X10^3$ zonae with indicated adjuvant given intradermally at multiple sites. In the groups receiving SPLPS, two injections were given at four weeks interval.

Table 1. Immunization Protocol

| Study No. | No. of monkeys | Date Immunized | Species of monkeys used | Primary Immunization Adjuvant | Secondary Immunization Adjuvant |
|---|---|---|---|---|---|
| 1. | 4 | 02/1982 | M.Mullatta | CFA | IFA*,LBA |
| 2. | 3 | 02/1983 | M.Radiata | BCG | LBA |
| 3. | 4 | 07/1983 | " | BCG+SPLPS | " |
| 4. | 2 | 12/1983 | " | SPLPS | " |
| 5. | 9 | 03/1984 | " | CFA | IFA |

*First booster with IFA, rest with LBA.

The antibodies were detectable at 4-6 weeks after initial injection. The peak titers were usually attained at 16 weeks with decline at 27 weeks. Booster injections were given with the indicated adjuvant in the declining phase of the antibodies.

Antibody titers were determined by two different assays. (1) Solid phase enzyme linked immunoassay (Bamezai et al. 1985) and (2) Inhibition of zona lysis by proteolytic enzymes (Sacco and Shivers 1978), the only modification being the use of 0.33% crude trypsin (Difco grade 1:250) in some experiments instead of 0.1% pronase.

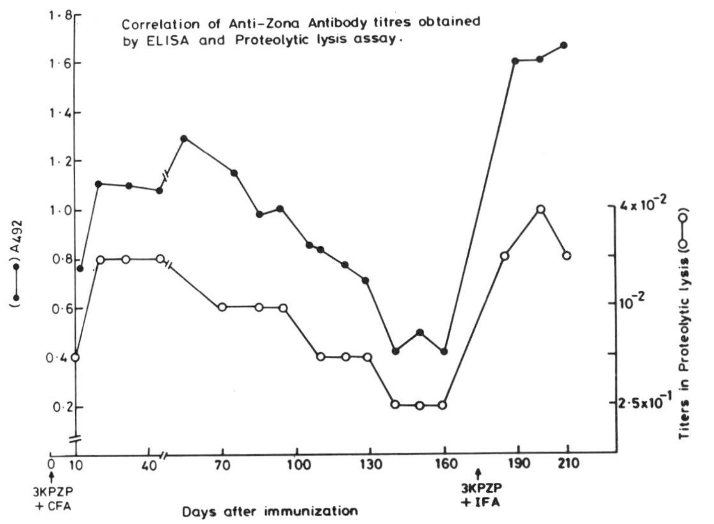


Fig. 1. Comparison between titers obtained by ELISA and inhibition of zona lysis by proteolytic enzymes.

Data in Figure 1 shows the correlation between the titers obtained by the two assay systems. ELISA is no doubt more sensitive but inhibition of proteolytic lysis of zona is believed to reflect the bioefficiency of the antibodies (Tsunoda and Sugie 1978; Sacco et al.1983).

Table 2. Antibody Titers of Monkeys Immunized with Porcine Zonae and Different Adjuvants

| Group No. | No. of Animals | Adjuvant used | No. of Injections | Peak titers obtained* |
|---|---|---|---|---|
| 1a. | 9 | CFA | 2 | 1:100 - 1:400 |
| 1b. | 4 | CFA | 3-4 | 1:550 - 1:1300 |
| 2. | 3 | BCG | 4 | 1:100 - 1:120 |
| 3. | 4 | BCG+SPLPS | 3 | 1:80 - 1:120 |
| 4. | 2 | SPLPS | 2 | 1:50 - 1:60 |

*Titers estimated by inhibition of zona lysis by proteolytic enzymes. The figures give the range of titers of individual monkeys in the group.

Table 2 gives the highest titers obtained in monkeys immunized with zonae using different adjuvants. Animals immunized with Freund's complete adjuvant had higher titers than those immunized with other adjuvants and were of the same order as reported by Sacco et al.(1983). The titers with other adjuvants were about six fold lower. Mahi-Brown et al. (1985), noted a difference of about ten fold in titers of dogs immunized with CFA and other adjuvants.

## IN VITRO CONTRACEPTIVE POTENTIAL OF ANTISERA

Sera of monkeys having a titer of 1:100 or above gave a precipitin reaction with zonae of pig eggs. When these eggs were incubated with homologous sperms prepared by the method of Sacco et al. (1983) few or none got attached to the surface (Figure 2). The antisera had similar effect on zonae of human eggs.

## EFFECT OF IMMUNIZATION ON FERTILITY OF THE ANIMALS

Monkeys were mated between days 9 to 14 of the menstrual cycle. Some of the bonnet monkeys were also mated on a continuous basis by caging with a male partner of proven fertility. In eighteen bonnet monkeys, out of 92 matings only 6 pregnancies took place. In the colony the pregnancy rate of non-immunized animals is 50%. The antibody titers of monkeys in the month that they became pregnant were between 1:25 and 1:50. Most of the animals, except one, carried the pregnancy to term. Pups were delivered normal with no perceptible anatomical abnormality. Two pups died soon after birth, the death of one followed the demise of the mother and the other was diagnosed by autopsy to have died due to pneumonia.

Four rhesus monkeys used in the studies have been followed for over three years. They were given three booster injections over the period of study. They were mated 50 times without resultant pregnancies. In the colony the pregnancy rate of non-immunized monkeys is 65%. Matings were continued in these monkeys after the decline of circulating antibodies. Two of the four monkeys became pregnant. The pups born were normal after normal gestation period. One monkey in this group has become amenorrhic and failed to regain ongoing cyclicity after inductive treatment with steroids. This animal had a peak antibody titer of 1:1300 and continues to have circulating antibody titers of 1:200.

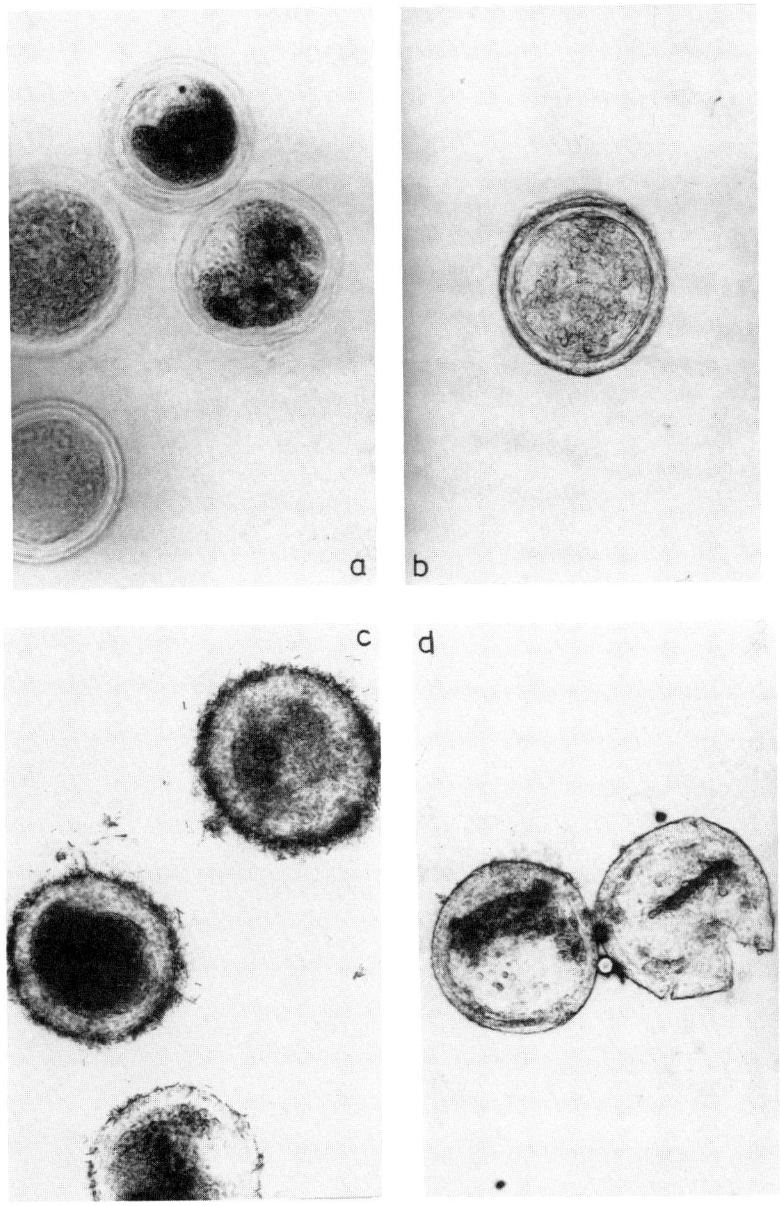


Fig. 2. Inhibition of sperm egg binding by monkey antisera to ZP. (a) Pig oocytes treated with preimmune monkey serum. (b) Pig oocytes treated with monkey anti ZP serum. Note the precipitation layer on the zona. (c) Numerous sperms bind to preimmune treated oocytes in contrast to lack of sperms binding to the antiserum treated oocytes(d).

## EFFECT ON STEROID HORMONE PROFILES

The period of high antibody titers ($>$1:100) was accompanied by serious disturbances in menstrual cycles. Animals became anovulatory as judged by low estrogens and progesterone profiles. Normal cyclicity was not immediately resumed on decline of antibody titers. However, almost all animals, except one, became ovulatory in course of time. Prior to establishment of normal ovulatory cycles the animals had a period of elevated estradiol during follicular phase without adequate rise of progesterone in the luteal phase of the cycle. Evidence for ovulatory cycles and return of fertility is furnished by eight animals becoming pregnant. The pregnancy resulted at an average of one to two months after decline of titers to below 1:50. Out of 22 immunized animals titers declined in 10 to below 1:50 and 8 of these got pregnant. Two animals died and could not be followed up. The remaining 12 with titers >1:100 will be checked for fertility status in the next breeding season.

## OVARIAN HISTOLOGY

Wedge biopsies were performed by laprotomy in several animals to determine the effect of immunization on follicular development. In most monkeys with titers between 1:100 to 1:200, there was a complete absence of large antral or growing follicles indicating the inhibition of follicular development. Wedge biopsy of monkey No. 503, which developed peak titers of 1:1300 and continues to have titers above 1:200 showed gross abnormalities of the resting follicles. The oocytes appeared to be dead with aggregated golgi bodies, abnormal looking mitochondria and a discontinuous and patchy zona layer. It remains to be seen whether this animal would ever regain fertility. There appears to be an irreversible damage to the follicles.

## CONCLUDING COMMENTS

These studies carried out in two strains of monkeys demonstrate the control of fertility by active immunization with porcine zonae. Whole zonae and not the heat solubilized zonae were used as antigen. Nearly half of the animals were immunized with complete Freund's adjuvant, an adjuvant also used by other investigators, but antibody titers high enough to impede fertility were also obtained with alternate adjuvants, such as sodium pthalate derivative of lipopolysaccharide (SPLPS) and/or BCG. The use of latter category of adjuvants induced by and large moderate titers, which start declining after 8 to 10 weeks. Disturbances in menstrual cycle were observed in monkeys soon after attainment of high antibody titers (>1:100). Estradiol and progesterone levels were markedly low and cycles were anovulatory. It is not unlikely that the antifertility effect of immunization with zonae pellucidae may in part be due to these factors, even though the antibodies were effective *in vitro* in preventing the binding of sperms to the oocytes.

Wedge biopsy of ovaries indicated inhibition of follicular development in animals with moderate titers but one monkey with sustained high titers had gross abnormalities and atresia of the follicles. It seems that continuous presence of high titer antibodies may be undesirable in contrast to a short exposure to antibodies which are enough to coat the zonae pellucidae and/or other cells of the follicle. This coating could inhibit the communication of the oocyte with its surrounding corona radiata cells and thus impede or stop oocyte growth. It has been shown that the nutrients used by ovarian oocytes are passed to them through the follicle cells in intimate contact with the oocyte via gap junctions (Herlands and Shultz 1984).

With the decline of antibodies in circulation, a number of animals specially those with moderate titers, became ovulatory. The process appears to be gradual with high estrogens unaccompanied by adequate luteal progesterone in initial cycles. Eight animals out of twenty-two initially immunized, did become pregnant and gave birth to normal pups. Two pups died after birth but the reason was the death of the mother in one case and pneumonia in the other. These animals had peak titers betwee 1:100 to 1:800, which lasted for 6 to 8 weeks and then declined. Gulyas et al. (1983b) found that cynamolgous monkeys immunized with porcine zonae pellucidae (heat solubilized) failed to ovulate, had depressed levels of steroid hormones and after an infertile period, recovered fertility. Sacco et al. (1983) also reported recovery of fewer eggs from squirrel monkeys immunized with purified zona antigen (PPZA) as compared to the recovery from non-immunized monkeys. They found that the eggs recovered from immunized monkeys were degenerated and abnormal. The extent of damage to the follicles may bear relation with the antibody titer and with the time duration over which the antibody is in circulation. High titers could well lead to follicular atresia and ovarian dysfunction.

The present studies confirm the antifertility potential of immunization with porcine zona pellucida in primates. Hyper-immunization may be expected to cause sterilization of animals, as high titers could lead to follicular atresia and ovarian dysfunction. Moderate degree of immunization may however not cause a permanent loss of fertility. Hormonal and menstrual disturbances noted during the period that antibodies are in circulation may not be acceptable in a contraceptive vaccine. Further studies are necessary to dissect the mosaic of antigens composing the zona pellucida and to see whether antigens inducing antibodies with potential of preventing the sperm binding to oocytes can be obtained without disturbances of hormone profiles.

## REFERENCES


Aitken, R.J., and Richardson, D.W., 1981, Measurement of the sperm binding capacity of the mouse zona pellucida and its use in the estimation of the anti-zona antibody titers. J. Reprod. and Fert. , 63:295.

Aitken, R.J., Rudak, E.A., Richardson, D.W. et al., 1981, The influence of anti-zona and antisperm antibodies on sperm-egg interactions. J. Reprod. and Fert., 62:597.

Bamezai, A.K., Suman, and Talwar, G.P., 1985, An enzyme immunoassay for zona pellucida antigens and antizona antibodies. Ind. J. Exp. Biol., Communicated.

Dunbar, B.S., and Raynor, B.D., 1980, Characterization of porcine zona pellucida antigens. Biol. Reprod., 22:941.

Dunbar, B.S., Liu, C., and Sammons, D.W., 1981, Identification of the three major proteins of porcine and rabbit zonae pellucidae by high resolution two-dimensional gel electrophoresis : comparison with serum, follicular fluid, and ovarian cell proteins. Biol. Reprod., 24:1111.

Gerrity, M., Niu, E., and Dunbar, B.S., 1981, A specific radioimmunoassay for evaluation of serum antibodies to zona pellucida antigens. J. Reprod. Immunol. 3:59.

Gulyas, B.J., Gwatkin, R.B.L., and Yuan, L.C., 1983b, Active immunization of cynomolgus monkeys (Macaca fascicularis) with porcine zona pellucidae. Gamete Research, 4:299.

Gwatkin, R.B.L., Williams, D.T., and Carlo, D.J., 1977, Immunization of mice with heat-solubilized hamster zonae : production of anti-zona antibody and inhibition of fertility. Fertil. Steril., 28:871.

Gwatkin, R.B.L., and Williams, D.T., 1978, Immunization of female rabbits with heat-solubilized bovine zonae. Production of anti-zona antibody and inhibition of fertility. Gamete Research, 1:19.

Gwatkin, R.B.L., Anderson, O.F., and Williams, D.T., 1980, Large scale isolation of bovine and pig zonae pellucidae. Chemical, immunological and receptor properties. Gamete Research, 3:217.

Herlands, R.L., and Schultz, R.M., 1984, Regulation of mouse oocyte growth : probable nutritional role for intercellular communication between follicle cells and oocytes in oocyte growth. J. Exp. Zool., 229(2):317.

Kurachi, H:, Wakimoto, H., Sakumoto, T. et al., 1984, Specific antibodies to porcine zona pellucida detected by quantitative radioimmunoassay in both fertile and infertile women. Fertil. Steril., 41:265.

Mahi-Brown, C.A., Yanagimachi, R., Hoffmann, J.D., and Huang, T.T.F., 1985, Fertility control in the bitch by active immunization with porcine zonae pellucidae : use of different adjuvants and patterns of estradiol and progesterone levels in estrous cycles. Biol. Reprod., 32:761.

Mori, T., Nishimoto, T., Kitagawa, M. et al., 1978, Possible presence of autoantibodies to zona pellucida in infertile women. Experientia, 34:797.

Sacco, A.G., 1977, Antigenic cross-reactivity between human and pig zona pellucida. Biol. Reprod. , 21:709.

Sacco, A.G., Shivers, C.A., 1978, Immunologic inhibition of development, in :"Methods in Mammalian Reproduction", J.C. Daniel, Jr., ed., Academic Press, New York.

Sacco, A.G., and Moghissi, K.S., 1979, Anti-zona pellucida activity in human sera. Fertil. Steril., 31:503.

Sacco, A.G., 1981, Immunocontraception : consideration of the zona pellucida as a target antigen, in :"Obstetrics and Gynecology Annual", R.M. Wynn, ed., Appleton-Century-Crofts, New York.

Sacco, A.G., Subramanian, M.G., Yurewicz, E.C. et al., 1983, Heteroimmunization of squirrel monkeys (Saimiri sciureus) with a purified porcine zona antigen (PPZA) : immune response and biologic activity of antiserum. Fertil. Steril., 39:350.

Shivers, C.A., and Dunbar, B.S., 1977, Autoantibodies to zona pellucida. A possible cause for infertility in women. Science , 197:1187.

Skinner, S.M., Mills, T., Kirchick, H.J. et al., 1984, Immunization with zona pellucida proteins results in abnormal ovarian follicular differentiation and inhibition of gonadotropin-induced steroid secretion. Endocrinology, In press.

Subramanian, M.G., Yurewicz, E.C., and Sacco, A.G., 1981, A specific radioimmunoassay for the detection of a purified porcine zona pellucida antigen (PPZA). Biol. Reprod., 24:933.

Suman, 1980, Quantitative studies on amount of anti-mouse zona pellucida antibodies required for blocking fertility in mouse. Thesis submitted for the degree of Masters in Biochemistry awarded by AIIMS, New Delhi.

Suman, 1985, Immunological properties and efficacy of Immunoglobulins induced by hetero-species zona pellucida antigen for blocking fertility in primates. Thesis submitted for award of Ph.D. degree in Biochemistry, to AIIMS, New Delhi.

Trounson, A.O., Shivers, C.A., McMaster, R., and Lopata, A., 1980, Inhibition of sperm binding and fertilization of human ova by antibody to porcine zona pellucida and human sera. Arch. Androl.,4:29.

Tsunoda, Y., 1977, Inhibitory effect of anti mouse egg serum on fertilization in vitro and in vivo in the mouse. J. Reprod. Fertil., 50(2):353.

Tsunoda, Y., and Chang, M.C., 1978, Effect of antisera against eggs and zona pellucida on fertilization and development of mouse eggs in vivo and in culture. J. Reprod. Fertil., 54:233.

Tsunoda, Y., and Sugie, T., 1978, Inhibitory effect on fertilization in vitro and in vivo by zona pellucida antibody and the titration of this antibody, in : "Recent Advances in Reproduction and Regulation of Fertility", G.P. Dalway, ed., Elsevier/North Holland Biomedical Press, Amsterdam.

Tsunoda, Y., Soma, T., and Sugie, T., 1981a, Inhibition of fertilization in cattle by passive immunization with anti-zona pellucida serum. Gamete Research, 4:133.

Tsunoda, Y., Soma, T., Jinbu, M. et al., 1981b, Effect of anti-pig zona pellucida serum on fertilization in several mammals. Gamete Research, 4:231.

Wood, D.M., Lui, C., and Dunbar, B.S., 1981, Effect of alloimmunization and hertoimmunization with zonae pellucidae on fertility in rabbits. Biol. Reprod., 25:439.

# PROSPECTS FOR CONTROL OF FERTILITY IN THE FEMALE DOG BY ACTIVE IMMUNIZATION WITH PORCINE ZONA PELLUCIDA PROTEINS

Cherrie A. Mahi-Brown

Department of Anatomy and Reproductive Biology
John A. Burns School of Medicine
University of Hawaii
Honolulu, Hawaii 96822, USA

## INTRODUCTION

Overpopulation of domestic dogs is a serious problem both in the United States and in many other countries. In the City and County of Honolulu alone, 21,614 dogs and cats were euthanized by the Humane Society from July 1983 through June 1984 simply because they were unwanted. That constituted 87.5% of the animals they took in (figures from Hawaiian Humane Society). Obviously, birth control technology is not the entire solution to this problem, because the best technology will not work unless owners of dogs can be motivated to use it. However, if humane organizations will do their job of educating people to control their pets' fertility, it will be our job to provide a variety of contraceptive strategies to meet the variety of anticipated needs.

When we began this study several years ago, most of the zona pellucida immunization work had been done with rodents. Rats, mice and hamsters had all been immunized either passively with anti-ovary antibodies prepared in rabbits (Jilek and Pavlok, 1975; Oikawa and Yanagimachi, 1975; Tsunoda and Chang, 1976) or actively with ovaries or zonae of other rodents (Gwatkin et al., 1977; Aitken and Richardson, 1981). Inhibition of fertilization in vitro and in vivo was reported uniformly. No side effects of immunization had been reported. Because it seemed like such a simple and specific approach to fertility control, we decided to develop the approach for use in the bitch.

The bitch is not a great model for most reproductive studies because the estrous cycle is so long (5-8 mos) (Evans and Cole, 1931; Jochle and Anderson, 1977; Sokolowski et al., 1977) and ovulation is difficult to time accurately (Wildt et al., 1979). However, the dog is a target species for contraceptive development (Anon, 1983) and does offer the advantage that in vitro fertilization is rather easily accomplished (Mahi and Yanagimachi, 1976, 1978).

## STUDIES OF ANTI-ZONA PELLUCIDA IMMUNIZATION WITH THE BITCH

After finding that rabbit antisera against extracts of canine ovaries would strongly inhibit penetration of canine zonae pellucidae by spermatozoa in vitro (Mahi and Yanagimachi, 1979), we tested rabbit antisera against zonae of hamsters, cows and pigs to see which would best cross-react with canine zonae. The antisera against porcine zonae were extremely effective in vitro. This was fortunate because techniques for isolating large quantities of porcine zonae had already been published (Oikawa, 1978; Dunbar et al., 1980; Gwatkin et al., 1980). Thus we chose porcine zonae for active immunization of bitches.

In our preliminary study (Mahi-Brown et al., 1982), we immunized three bitches with isolated and solubilized porcine zonae pellucidae (crude preparation, cPZP) and two with canine zonae prepared the same way (procedure of Gwatkin et al., 1980). Based on the studies of others (Gwatkin et al., 1977; Wood et al., 1981) we did not think alloimmunization would be effective, but we tried it anyway. Control bitches were given PBS without zonae. Each bitch was immunized with 2000 (primary immunizations) or 1000 zonae (boosts) at monthly intervals until they entered proestrus, so they received 4-6 injections or a total of 5000 - 7000 zonae. Freund's adjuvants (complete for primary immunization, incomplete for boosts) were used to enhance the immune response. Sera collected from the bitches 10-14 days after each injection were assayed by indirect immunofluorescence (IIF). We used this technique and continue to use it because (1) it seems to provide consistent results, (2) it provides information as to where on the zona antibodies are binding, and (3) it does not require any equipment we do not have. We also tested the sera to see whether zonae treated with them were penetrable by spermaotzoa in vitro.

As we expected, immunization with canine zonae was ineffective. The bitches did produce low titers of anti-zona antibodies, but these were insufficient to inhibit feritility in vitro or in vivo. In contrast, bitches immunized with cPZP produced high titers and were infertile. Their antisera inhibited zona penetration in vitro also (Mahi-Brown et al., 1982).

Based on these results, it would seem that active immunization with porcine zonae has very strong contraceptive potential for the bitch. However, all three bitches immunized with cPZP had abnormal estrous cycles. Two had prolonged vaginal bleeding (usually associated only with proestrus and estrus) well into metestrus, and the third had prolonged estrus with full receptivity. We kept two of these bitches and bred them at every cycle. The bitch with prolonged estrus finally conceived at her third cycle after immunization. By this time her cycle had returned to normal. The other bitch was bred repeatedly for 2 years without conceiving. By this time her serum antibody titer was quite low, but she nevertheless remained infertile.

About the same time we were doing our preliminary study, Shivers et al. (1981) and Gwatkin et al. (1980) immunized dogs in independent studies. Gwatkin et al. (1980) immunized just one dog of unspecified sex with bovine zonae. The dog produced high anti-zona titers, but they apparently did not test its fertility. Shivers et al. (1981) used a protocol quite similar to ours. One of the three bitches they immunized remained fertile, however. Also they reported no side effects at all.

Since this first test, we have devoted most of our effort to characterizing the response of bitches to anti-zona immunization and trying to prevent unwanted side effects. Six additional bitches were immunized with the original cPZP and 6 with porcine zonae purified somewhat (pPZP) by gel filtration and ion exchange chromatography using the methods published by Yurewicz et al. (1983). Most bitches were given 3 injections with 0.4 - 0.5 mg protein per injection at monthly intervals, and alum or a synthetic lipid amine adjuvant was used instead of the previously used Freund's adjuvants.

Table 1. Response of Bitches to Immunization with Crude (cPZP) or Partially Purified (pPZP) Porcine Zonae Pellucidae.

| Antigen | No. Bitches | Ave Titer By IIF[a] | Ave % Zona Penetration[b] | No. Fertile (No. Bred) | Cycles[c] |
|---|---|---|---|---|---|
| cPZP | 3 | 1: 2,000 | 13.4 | 0 (3) | 3N |
| cPZP | 3 | 1:10,000 | 7.4 | 0 (2) | 3A |
| pPZP | 6 | 1: 2,000 | 11.0 | 1 (6) | 5N, 1A |

[a]Indirect immunofluorescence; the titer is the highest dilution at which fluorescence distinctly greater than the control can be detected on canine zonae treated with dilutions of antisera followed by FITC-labeled protein A.
[b]Canine oocytes were treated with undiluted antisera from immunized bitches and rinsed thoroughly before insemination in vitro.
[c]N, normal estrous cycles; A; abnormal estrous cycles, either prolonged vaginal bleeding, prolonged proestrus, or prolonged estrus (see text for details).

The results are summarized in Table 1. Based on their responses, the bitches immunized with cPZP could be divided into two groups. Those with moderate titers (arbitrarily set at 1:1000 - 1:2000) and normal estrous cycles and those with high titers (greater than 1:4000) and abnormal estrous cycles. The abnormal estrous cycles varied from bitch to bitch. One was normal except for vaginal bleeding throughout metestrus, one entered prolonged proestrus, and one entered prolonged estrus. The ovarian steroids, estradiol 17$\beta$ and progesterone, were assayed during proestrus, estrus and metestrus in a number of these bitches in all categories using a standard RIA (Nett et al., 1975; Nelson et al., 1978)). The bitches with normal cycles, i.e., those with moderate titers had steroid patterns close to those of control cycles (Figs. 1a, 1b). Those with abnormal cycles, on the other hand, had grossly abnormal patterns (Fig. 1c). Interestingly, the patterns were very similar even though the bitches all had different types of abnormal cycles. Estradiol rose during proestrus as it should, but then instead of falling during estrus, it remained high for an extended period of time. Progesterone patterns are even more dramatic though. There was no rise in progesterone at all. Except for the bitch that was in persistent proestrus, all these bitches were bred, but this should not even matter because the corpus luteum is activated and maintained spontaneously in the bitch regardless of whether or not she is bred. These results reported recently by Mahi-Brown et al. (1985) strongly suggest that ovulation failed.

Examination of the ovaries of these bitches confirmed this conclusion. Most of the bitches with normal cycles had completely normal ovaries (Mahi-Brown et al., 1984). One of the bitches though had small follicular cysts along with other normal structures appropriate to metestrus. The bitches with abnormal cycles and failure of progesterone secretion had grossly abnormal ovaries. Two had large follicular cysts (Fig. 2a) and two had loss of oocytes from most of their follicles (Fig. 2b). In the latter, there was even loss of primordial follicles that would not yet be expected to be secreting zona proteins (Wolgemuth et al., 1984). The follicular cysts were as large as 1.5 cm and were usually lined with folded theca interna (Fig. 2c). There was partial luteinization in some cases.

The bitches immunized with pPZP (Table 1) all produced moderate titers

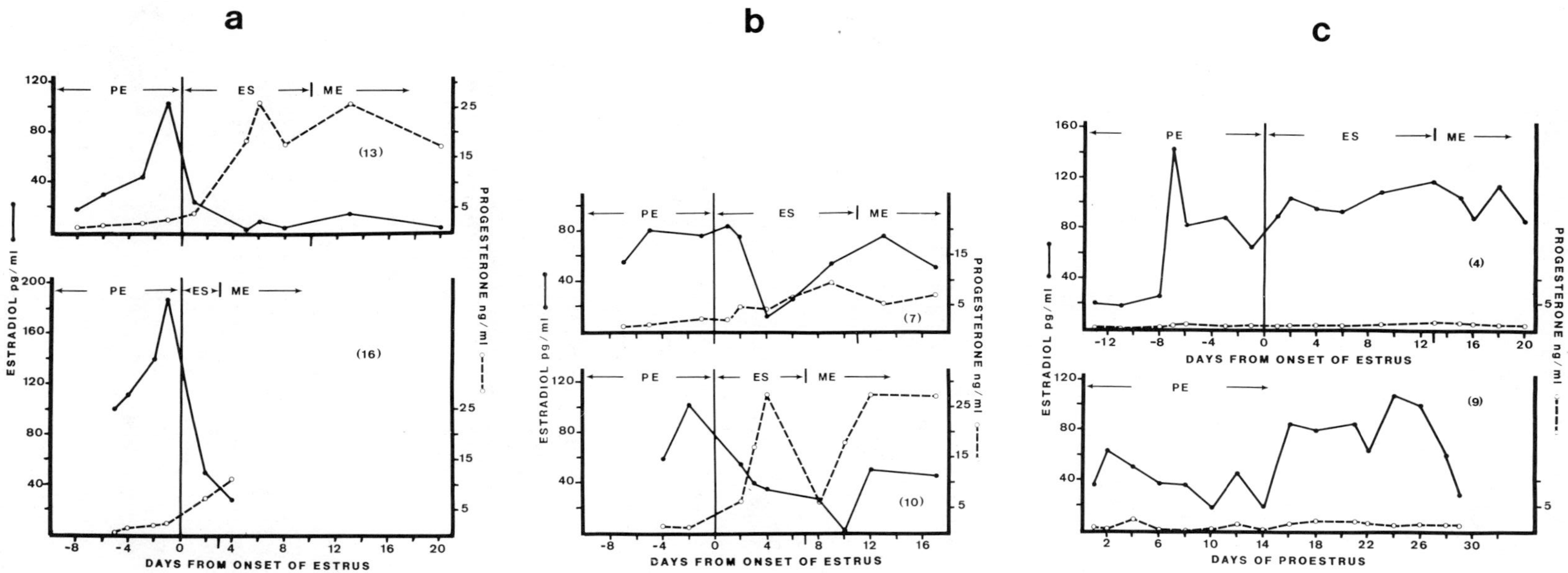


Fig. 1. Patterns of estradiol (solid lines) and progesterone (broken lines) during proestrus, estrus and early metestrus in control bitches (a) and in bitches immunized with cPZP (b, c). Bitches in b had moderate titers (1:1000) and normal cycles, while those in c had high titers (greater than 1:4000) and abnormal cycles. Day 0 in each figure is the day of onset of behavioral estrus except for bitch 9 in Fig. 1c. Since she did not enter estrus, day 0 is the day of onset of proestrus. From Mahi-Brown et al., (1985) with permission.

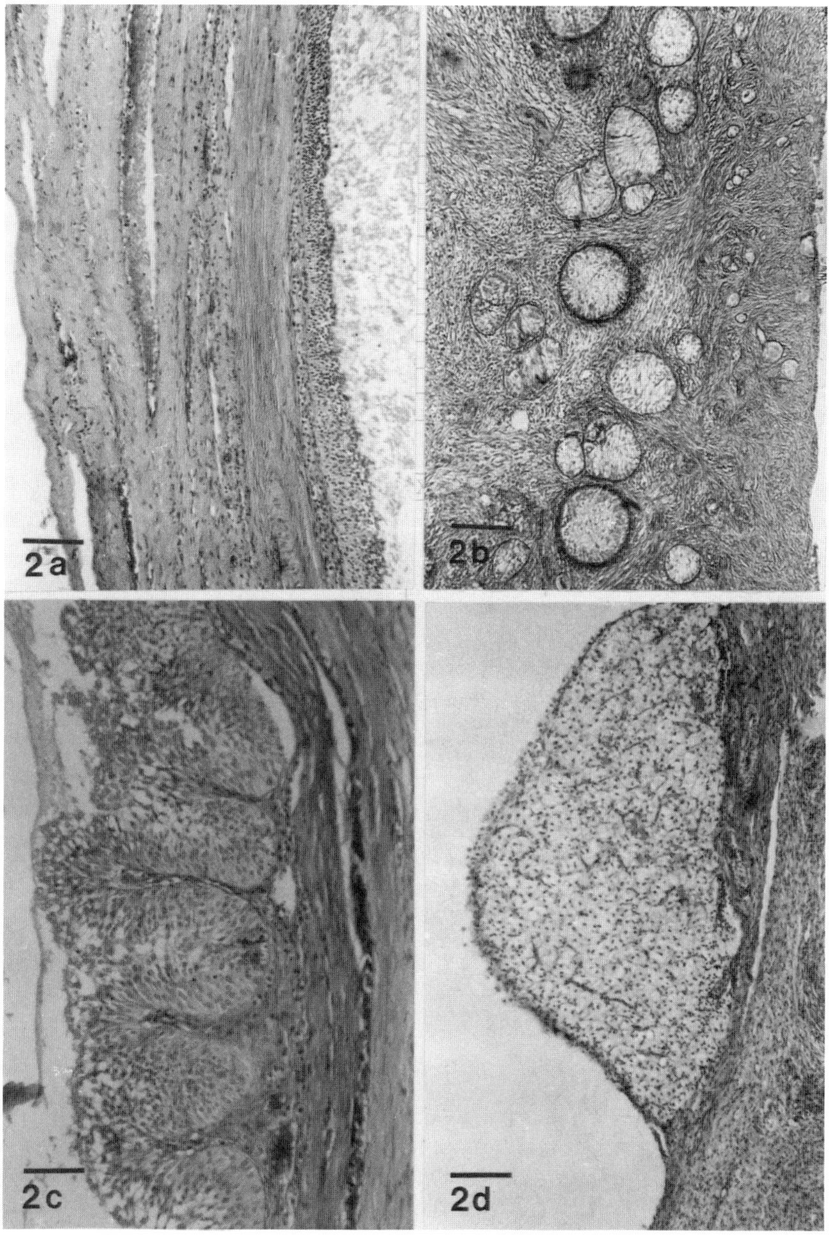


Fig. 2. Sections of ovaries from bitches immunized with crude (a, b and c) and partially purified (d) porcine zonae pellucidae. In Fig. 2a, a large cyst (on the right) is surrounded by a connective tissue capsule (bar = 117 m). In 2b, the ovarian cortex is occupied by follicles without oocytes (bar = 117 m). The folded thecal lining of a follicular cyst is shown in 2c (bar = 80 m). Fig. 2d illustrates a clump of luteinized cells in a cyst lacking a cellular lining in other areas (bar = 75 m). Hematoxylin and eosin.

of antizona antibodies and all but one were infertile at the first cycle after immunization. Five of these bitches were normal at the first cycle after immunization (Fig. 3), but one had an abnormal cycle with prolonged estrus and a failure of progesterone secretion at her second cycle (Fig. 3, bitch 13b). She had been given a total of 6 injections with 2 given between the first and second cycles in contrast to the 3 injections given the other bitches. The sixth bitch had an abnormal first cycle after immunization with prolonged bleeding into metestrus (Mahi-Brown, unpublished observations). Unfortunately, we were not able to assay her ovarian steroids, but the condition of her ovaries clearly indicated that she had not ovulated. At 6 weeks of metestrus, there were no corpora lutea. Furthermore, both ovaries contained small follicular cysts (Fig. 2d). These cysts differed from those in the bitches immunized with cPZP in that they lacked a lining of granulosa cells or the granulosa layer was sloughing away, and there were clumps of luteinized cells. Small cysts like these were also found in the ovaries of the other bitches immunized with pPZP.

Duration of infertility varied considerably in these studies. Shivers et al. (1981) noted infertility for only one cycle in the bitches they immunized. In our studies (Mahi-Brown et al., 1982, 1985), the bitches immunized with cPZP were infertile for at least 2 cycles and one bitch did not regain fertility at all even after 2 years. The absence of follicles in her ovaries suggests that she would never have regained fertility. In bitches immunized with pPZP, on the other hand, infertility appeared to last for only 1 cycle if the bitches were given a standard immunization protocol of three monthly injections. The bitch immunized 6 times, however, remained infertile at her third cycle after immunization (she was not followed longer).

## PROSPECTS FOR USE OF ANTIZONA IMMUNIZATION AS A CONTRACEPTIVE IN BITCHES

The results outlined above strongly suggest that caution will have to be used in applying a zona immunization approach to contraception in the bitch. Although there is undeniable inhibition of fertility, the side effects are not acceptable. Prolonging symptoms of proestrus or estrus will not be acceptable to the owners of pets and the development of follicular cysts is unacceptable from a medical standpoint. The loss of oocytes from follicles can be viewed two ways. If the owner wants to delay conception in his pet for a cycle or two then breed later, loss of oocytes is obviously not acceptable. On the other hand, the animal shelters would like to have a canine (and feline) contraceptive that could be administered easily by a technician to large numbers of animals that would guarantee that offspring of these animals would not be forthcoming after the animals were adopted by new owners (Anon, 1983). If we could specifically identify what is causing oocyte loss in some of the bitches and develop techniques that would cause oocyte loss in absence of other ovarian pathology, this would be a useful technology. It may be that in order to remove oocytes without causing cyst development, bitches may have to be immunized as puppies. Clearly, further studies are required along this line.

This loss of oocytes closely resembles the condition seen in rabbits immunized with porcine zonae (Wood et al., 1981; Skinner et al., 1984). Furthermore, immunized rabbits fail to ovulate in response to exogenous hCG and do not secrete progesterone. Thus the rabbit may be a cheaper model for study of this approach. The loss of oocytes from follicles and general follicular atresia seen in rabbits and bitches immunized with PZP resemble the experimental autoimmune oophoritis seen mice as a result of deletion of supressor T-cells (Sakaguchi et al., 1985) or immunization against whole mouse ovary (Ivanova et al., 1984), except that autoimmune oophoritis is characterized by inflammation with an infiltration of mononuclear cells

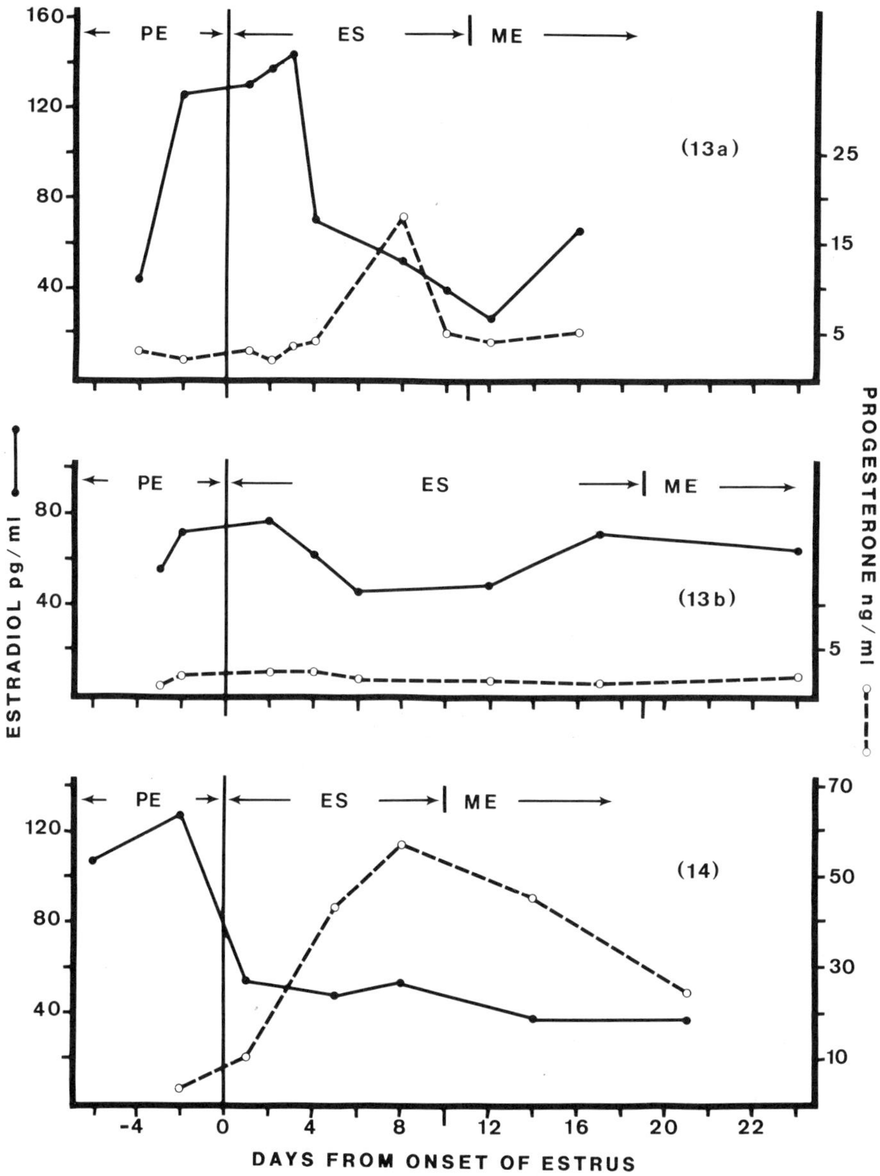


Fig. 3. Patterns of estradiol (solid lines) and progesterone (broken lines) during proestrus, estrus and early metestrus in two bitches immunized with pPZP. Note the abnormal second cycle in bitch 13 (13b). Day 0 is the day of onset of behavioral estrus. From Mahi-Brown et al. (1985) with permission.

into the ovary. No evidence of inflammation has ever been reported in zona immunized animals, so it is not clear whether loss of oocytes in the latter case is comparable to autoimmune oophoritis.

Unlike the rabbit, most bitches immunized with porcine zonae pellucidae develop follicular cysts, even when a partially purified zona preparation is used. This has not been reported in any other species studied and may be unique to the bitch. Follicular cysts of the type seen in bitches immunized with pPZP have been reported to occur naturally in about 4% of laboratory beagles (Andersen and Simpson, 1973) and pound bitches (Marchevsky et al., 1983). Although this seems a high incidence in natural populations, it should be noted that in most cases cysts are seen in older bitches (Andersen and Simpson, 1973). Most of the bitches we studied were less than 4 years of age (Mahi-Brown et al., 1982, 1985). The etiology of ovarian cysts in bitches is not well understood and we do not have any light to shed on this pathology. Perhaps the zona-immunized bitch could serve as a model for the study of ovarian cysts since they seem to occur quite predictably.

The future of anti-zona contraception will, I believe, depend on our developing an understanding of the causes of unwanted side effects and on techniques for isolating very pure preparations of zona proteins that have not lost their immunogenicity. The bitch fits in to the future direction of this research because she responds well to antizona immunization in terms of developing infertility, she develops a number of characteristic side effects of immunization, and the dog is a species with a need for a variety of contraceptive technologies.

## REFERENCES


Aitken, R. J., and Richardson, D. W., 1981, Active immunization of rats with cumulus-free mouse ova: induction of infertility and antibody titers, J. Exp. Zool., 216:149.

Andersen, A. C., and Simpson, M. E., 1973, "The ovary and Reproductive Cycle of the Dog (Beagle)," Geron-X, Los Altos, CA.

Anonymous, 1983, "Report of Canine Birth Control Panel," Morris Animal Foundation, Englewood, CO.

Dunbar, B. S., Wardrip, N. J., and Hedrick, J. L., 1980, Isolation, physicochemical properties, and macromolecular composition of zona pellucida from porcine oocytes, Biochemistry, 19:356.

Evans, H. M., and Cole, H. H. (1931). An introduction to the study of the oestrous cycle in the dog, Mem. Univ. Calif., 9:65.

Gwatkin, R. B. L., Williams, D. T., and Carlo, D. J., 1977, Immunization of mice with heat-solubilized hamster zonae: production of anti-zona antibody and inhibition of fertility, Fertil. Steril., 28:871.

Gwatkin, R. B. L., Andersen, O. F., and Williams, D. T., 1980, Large scale isolation of bovine and pig zonae pellucidae: chemical, immunological and receptor properties, Gamete Res., 3:217.

Ivanova, M., Bourneva, V., Gitsov, L., and Angelova, Z., 1984, Experimental immune oophoritis as a model for studying the thymus-ovary interaction: 1. Morphological studies, Amer. J. Reprod. Immunol., 6:99.

Jilek, F., and Pavlok, A., 1975, Antibodies against mouse ovaries and their effects on fertilization in vitro and in vivo in the mouse, J. Reprod. Fertil., 42:377.

Jochle, W., and Andersen, A. C., 1977, The estrous cycle of the dog: a review, Theriogenology, 7:113.

Mahi, C. A., and Yanagimachi, R., 1976, Maturation and sperm penetration of canine oocytes in vitro, J. Exp. Zool., 196:189.

Mahi, C. A., and Yanagimachi, R., 1978, Capacitation, acrosome reaction and egg penetration by canine spermatozoa in a simple defined medium, Gamete Res., 1:101.

Mahi, C. A., and Yanagimachi, R., 1979, Prevention of in vitro fertilization of canine oocytes by anti-ovary antisera: a potential approach to fertility control in the bitch, J. Exp. Zool., 210:129.

Mahi-Brown, C. A., Huang, T. T. F., and Yanagimachi, R., 1982, Infertility in bitches induced by active immunization with porcine zonae pellucidae, J. Exp. Zool., 222:89.

Mahi-Brown, C. A., Nelson, M. L., and Yanagimachi, R., 1984, Aberrant ovarian histology of bitches immunized with porcine zona pellucida, Biol. Reprod., 30 (Suppl. 1):105.

Mahi-Brown, C. A., Yanagimachi, R., Hoffmann, J. C., and Huang, T. T. F. Jr., 1985, Fertility control in the bitch by active immunization with porcine zonae pellucidae: use of different adjuvants and patterns of estradiol and progesterone levels in estrous cycles, Biol. Reprod., 32:761.

Marchevsky, R. S., Nascimento, E. F., and Chquiloff, M. A. G., 1983, Alteracoes morfologicas no ovario e corno uterino de cadela. I. Cistos ovaricos, Arq. Bras. Med. Vet. Zoot., 35:381.

Nelson, M. L., Cullin, A-M., and Hoffmann, J. C., 1978, Circadian rhythms of serum estradiol and corticosterone and related organ weight changes in the prepubertal female rat, Biol. Reprod., 18:125.

Nett, T. M., Akbar, A. M., Phemister, R. D., Holst, R. A., Reichert, L. E. Jr., and Niswender, G. D., 1975, Levels of luteinizing hormone, estradiol and progesterone in serum during the estrous cycle and pregnancy in the beagle bitch, Proc. Soc. Exp. Biol. Med., 148:134.

Oikawa, T., 1978, A simple method for the isolation of a large number of ova from pig ovaries, Gamete Res., 1:265.

Oikawa, T., and Yanagimachi, R., 1975, Block of hamster fertilization by anti-ovary antibody, J. Reprod. Fertil., 45:487.

Sakaguchi, S., Fukuma, K., Kuribayashi, K., and Masuda, T., 1985, Organ-specific autoimmune diseases induced in mice by elimination of T cell subset, J. Exp. Med., 161:72.

Shivers, C. A., Sieg, P. M., and Kitchen, H., 1981, Pregnancy prevention in the dog: potential for an immunological approach, J. Am. Anim. Hosp. Assoc., 178:823.

Skinner, S. M., Mills, T., Kirchick, H. J., and Dunbar, B. S., 1984, Immunization with zona pellucida proteins results in abnormal ovarian follicular differentiation and inhibition of gonadotropin-induced steroid secretion, Endocrinology, 115:2418.

Sokolowski, J. H., Stover, D. G., and Van Ravenswaay, F., 1977, Seasonal incidence of estrus and interestrous interval for bitches of seven breeds, J. Amer. Vet. Med. Assoc., 171:271.

Tsunoda, Y., and Chang, M. C., 1976, Effect of anti-rat ovary antiserum on the fertilization of rat, mouse and hamster eggs in vivo and in vitro, Biol. Reprod., 14:354.

Wildt, D. E., Panko, W. B., Chakraborty, P. K., and Seager, S. W. J., 1979, Relationship of serum estrone, estradiol-17$\beta$ and progesterone to LH, sexual behavior and time of ovulation in the bitch, Biol. Reprod., 20:648.

Wolgemuth, D. J., Celenza, J., Bundman, D. S., and Dunbar, B. S., 1984, Formation of the rabbit zona pellucida and its relationship to ovarian follicular development, Devel. Biol., 106:1.

Wood, D. M., Liu, C., and Dunbar, B. S., 1981, Effect of alloimmunization and heteroimmunization with zonae pellucidae on fertility in rabbits, Biol. Reprod., 25:439.

Yurewicz, E. C., Sacco, A. G., and Subramanian, M. G., 1983, Isolation and preliminary characterization of a purified pig zona antigen (PPZA) from porcine ovaries. Biol. Reprod., 29:511.

# ANTI-GnRH MONOCLONALS : PITUITARY AND EXTRAPITUITARY ACTIONS IN CONTROL OF FERTILITY

C. Das, S.K. Gupta*, A. Malik and G.P. Talwar*

Department of Biochemistry, All India Institute of Medical Sciences, New Delhi-110029 and *National Institute of Immunology, New Delhi-110 029, India

## INTRODUCTION

The decapeptide gonadotropin releasing hormone (GnRH) has a pivotal role in control of both male and female fertility. It is one of those molecules which has been conserved through evolution. The primary amino acid sequence of the hormone from ovine and porcine sources is identical to that of human. The peptide controls the secretion of luteinizing hormone (LH) and follicle stimulating hormone (FSH) from the pituitary and the same molecule is biologically active in a large number of species (Schally et al, 1973).

Immunoneutralization of GnRH by active immunization causes inhibition of ovulation in rodents (Fraser & Baker, 1978; Takahashi et al, 1978; Kawakami & Higuchi, 1979; Okon et al, 1980), sheeps (Clarke et al, 1978; Jeffcoate et al, 1978), marmoset monkeys (Hodges & Hearn 1977; 1979), rhesus monkeys and baboons (Shastri et al, 1981; Talwar et al, 1983). While the effects of active immunization against the decapeptide leads to a long term inhibition, short term inhibition can be achieved by passive transfer of anti-GnRH antibody (Fraser & Gunn, 1973). Passive immunization, however, demands large amounts of antibodies of requisite specificity with consistent characteristics. The technology of somatic cell hybridization to generate antibodies of predefined specificity as illustrated by Kohler & Milstein (1975) has made it possible to obtain antibodies in unlimited amount. However, one of the possible problems of repeated administration of mouse monoclonals in humans may be the sensitization and production of antibodies against mouse immunoglobulins. To overcome this, human monoclonals are desirable. Koprowski (1983) has, however, treated patients suffering from cancer by employing a regime of mouse monoclonal antibody where only one out of the seven patients got sensitized. Further studies are required to clarify the tolarizing dose of the mouse monoclonals employed in the humans. If true, this would obviate the necessity of human hybridomas for repeated therapeutic use of the hitherto available mouse monoclonals. A risk common to both mouse and human monoclonals will, however, persists namely the production of anti-idiotype (unless these are also suppressed by the Koprowski regime) and the pros and cons of formation of such antibodies has to be carefully evaluated.

In this communication, we report the bioneutralization capability of mouse monoclonal anti-GnRH antibody. The use of these monoclonals has enabled the delineation of two distinct stages at which the anti-GnRH antibodies can interfere with fertility namely i) at the hypothalamic-pituitary axis and ii) directly at the placental level.

## GENERATION AND CHARACTERISTICS OF MONOCLONAL ANTI-GnRH ANTIBODIES

Fusion of SP2/O mouse myeloma cells with splenocytes obtained from mouse immunized with GnRH coupled to tetanus toxoid (TT) has led to the development of hybrid cell clones secreting antibodies binding to GnRH (Gupta & Talwar, 1983). Three stabilized clones are available with us the products of which are highly specific for GnRH (Gupta et al, 1985). The antibodies are totally devoid of reactivity with thyroid stimulating hormone (TSH) as tested in competitive radioimmunoassay. The association constant (Ka) for binding with GnRH ranged from 1.09 to 2.94 x $10^9$ liters/mole as calculated by Scatchard plot. The antibodies are of $IgG_{2a}$ class with kappa light chain.

The monoclonals secreted from one of the clones $P_8 16_{62}$ reacted optimally with the native hormone. Substitution of amide by a carboxyl group at the C-terminal end, decreased the immunoreactivity by a factor of 100 (Talwar et al, 1985). The antibodies recognized the amino acid sequences 4-6, 7-10 and 4-10 to a variable degree suggesting that the antigenic epitope has a conformation involving the entire molecule. The monoclonals reacted 387 fold less with D-ser $(Bu^t)^6$des $Gly^{10}$ GnRH ethylamide and 608 fold less with Bnz-$his^6$-GnRH agonists (Gupta et al, 1985).

## BLOCK OF ESTRUS CYCLE AND OVULATION IN RODENTS

Antibodies raised against hormones are not necessarily of the bioneutralizing type. Failure of antibodies, otherwise immunoreactive in radioimmunoassay to inhibit the biological action of the hormone *in vivo* has been reported for antibodies against carboxy terminal peptides of β-hCG (Louvet et al, 1974; Matsuura et al, 1979); β-TSH (Beall et al, 1973) and steroids (Vacsei et al, 1979). It was, therefore, important to find out whether monoclonal anti-GnRH antibodies have the ability to intercept the biological action of the hormone

Ovulation being dependent on the luteinizing hormone surge induced by GnRH, the effect of monoclonals on ovulation in rats was investigated. Adult female rats having 2-3 consecutive regular estrus cycles were administered with the monoclonals on the morning of proestrus. A single intraperitoneal injection of 0.5ml ascites fluid obtained by growing hybrid cell clone $P_8 16_{62}$ blocked ovulation in all the animals tested. Control group of animals receiving an equivalent amount of ascites, devoid of anti-GnRH antibody had a range of ova released in the oviduct in the morning of estrus (Table I).

Table I : Effect of passive administration of monoclonal anti-GnRH antibody on ovulation in rats.

| Treatment | No. of ovulating/ total | No.of ova (mean $\pm$ SEM) |
|---|---|---|
| Control | 6/6 | 5.8 $\pm$ 0.5 |
| $P_8 16_{62}$ | 0/6 | 0 |

Ascites fluid (0.5ml) of clone $P_8 16_{62}$ was injected i.p. at 9.00 A.M. on proestrus. Control group received an equivalent amount of ascites fluid devoid of anti-GnRH antibody.

GnRH by acting at the pituitary level also plays an important and crucial role in the regulation of estrus cycle in rodents. Single intraperitoneal injection of 0.2ml ascites at diestrus to regularly cycling BALB/c mice disrupted the estrus cycle (Fig. 1). Duration of diestrus was extended for about 28 to 30 days and was related to the amount of monoclonals injected (Gupta et al, 1985). Animals returned to regular cycles after the decline in the circulating anti-GnRH antibody levels.

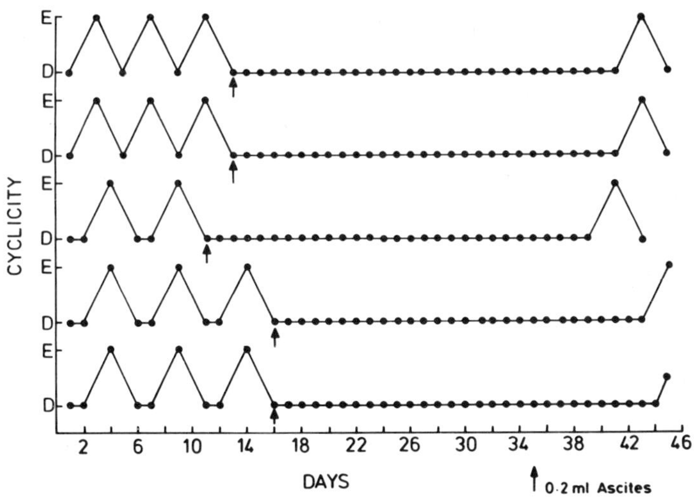


Fig. 1 : Effect of administration of monoclonal anti-GnRH antibody on cyclicity in mice. 0.2 ml of ascites fluid obtained from $P_8 16_{62}$ clone was injected subcutaneously on 1st day of diestrus.E, estrus; D, diestrus (Data from Gupta et al, 1985).

## BLOCK OF ESTRUS IN BITCHES

Some animal species such as the dog, have periodic estrus. The reproductive endocrinology of these animals is only partially understood. Experiments were conducted to see if the highly specific and bio-neutralizing type of anti-GnRH monoclonal antibodies influence the onset of estrus in bitches and thereby illustrate the presence and crucial role of GnRH in regulation of estrus in this species.

A single intravenous injection of 3ml of ascites at proestrus in a female dog suppressed the progression of estrus as indicated by the change in behavioral pattern of the animal in terms of its receptivity to the male, appearance of leucocytes in vaginal smear within 24-48 hrs after administration of the monoclonals and suppression of the rise in circulating plasma levels of progesterone and estradiol typical of normal estrus (Talwar et al, 1975). Animals receiving an equivalent amount of ascites fluid devoid of anti-GnRH antibody showed normal progression of estrus. These experiments provide indirect evidence for the involvement of the GnRH in induction of estrus in this species.

## TERMINATION OF PREGNANCY

The efficacy of mouse monoclonals against GnRH to terminate pregnancy was investigated in two species namely the mouse and the baboon.

### a) Mouse

Female BALB/c mice were mated with males of proven fertility and pregnancy was confirmed by exploratory laparotomy on day 6 by taking day 1 on which vaginal plugs were present. Single injection of 0.1ml of ascites fluid obtained from mouse myeloma (SP2/0)or hybrid cell line ($P_8 16_{62}$) was given intra-peritoneally on various days of pregnancy. Embryos were resorbed in the test animals when the antibodies were injected on days 7, 8 or 9 of pregnancy (Table II). Antibodies injected

Table II : Effect of monoclonal anti-GnRH on pregnancy and its reversal by exogenous progesterone in mice.

| Treatment[a] | Day of[c] anti-GnRH injection | No.of Animals | Days of[c] progesterone administration | Viable[c] Embryos (Mean±SEM) Day14 |
|---|---|---|---|---|
| Control | - | 10 | - | 6.5±0.2 |
| Anti-GnRH | 7 | 15 | - | 0 (Partially resorbed in 2 mice, mean=6) |
| Anti-GnRH | 8 | 7 | - | 0 |
| Anti-GnRH | 9 | 8 | - | 0 |
| Anti-GnRH | 10 | 5 | - | 7.0 ±0.4 |
| Anti-GnRH | 12 | 6 | - | 7.5 ±0.2 |
| Anti-GnRH + Progesterone[b] | 8 | 5 | 7,8,9, 10,11,12 | 8 ±0.7 |

[a] 0.1ml of ascites was given i.p. on indicated days of pregnancy. Control group received an equivalent amount of SP2/0 ascites on day 7 of pregnancy.[b] 2mg progesterone divided in two equal doses was injected s.c. daily in the morning and evening.[c] day of pregnancy.

during mid gestation days 10 or 12, however, did not interfere in the progression of pregnancy. The administration of ascites from SP2/0 cell line did not affect pregnancy in the control group of animals. The pregnancy terminating action of anti-GnRH monoclonals could be overcome by progesterone administered daily from days 7 to 12 of pregnancy at a dose of 2mg per day given subcutaneously in two equally divided doses.

b) Baboons

Using a superactive GnRH agonist, we had earlier observed that thrice daily injection of the agonist given to a pregnant baboon during the peri-implantation period can abrogate pregnancy in these animals (Das & Talwar, 1983). Further experiments were conducted wherein instead of repeated injection of the agonist, bio-neutralizing monoclonal anti-GnRH antibodies were administered to the pregnant baboons. Two injections of the antibodies of 2ml each were given at 24hr interval on the grounds that the rise in chorionic gonadotropin (CG) is steep in early pregnancy and the hormonal support has to be nullified for at least 48hrs to influence pregnancy. Soon after the administration of the anti-GnRH antibodies, a drop in the (CG) level was perceptible which was accompanied by a decrease in progesterone followed by bleeding and termination of pregnancy in three out of five baboons tested (Fig. 2).

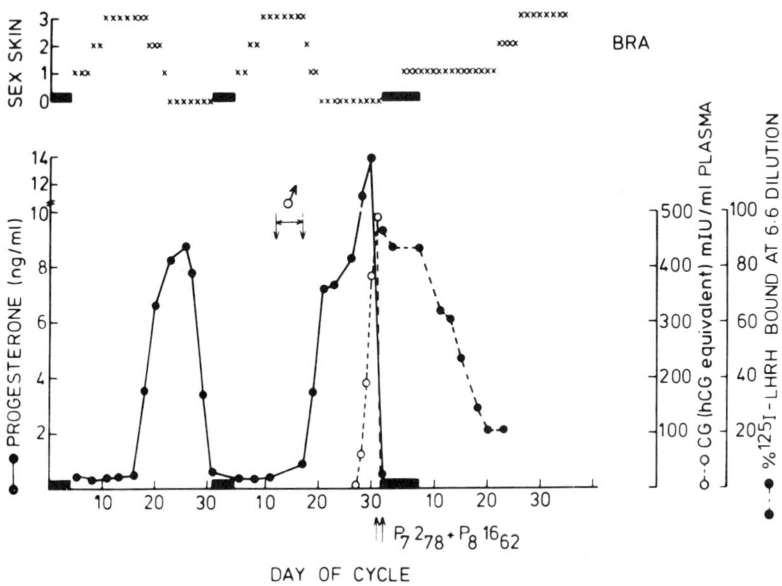


Fig. 2 : Termination of pregnancy in a baboon by anti-GnRH monoclonals. Two injections of 2ml ascites fluid were given intravenously on days 28 and 29 of the cycle. Antibody caused a steep decline in CG and progesterone levels followed by bleeding (black rectangles). Circulating antibody levels measured by RIA are represented by triangles. Progesterone profile of the premating cycle is also given (Data from Das et al, in press).

Out of the two baboons which failed to abort, one animal aborted on the 50th day after LMP. In this animal plasma progesterone levels remained low inspite of increasing levels of CG (Das et al, in press). The second animal which failed to abort after two consecutive injections of the antibodies, was given another injection of 5ml ascites fluid four days later. At this time (CG) levels had started increasing and higher amounts of antibodies was ineffective in suppressing either CG levels or progesterone secretion. Pregnancy in this animal continued uneventfully to term. On careful analysis, the CG levels in this baboon was found to be much higher than the four other animals in which pregnancy was terminated. After regaining her menstrual cycles the baboon was rendered pregnant again and this time 5ml ascites fluid was given on two consecutive days following the same protocol as that of previous experiments. A sharp fall in circulating progesterone and CG levels was observed after the administration of the antibodies and the animal aborted two days later.

Time of injection of the antibodies seem to be very critical, as injected few days later, they do not cause any adverse effect on pregnancy.

MECHANISM OF ACTION OF ANTI-GnRH MONOCLONALS

The mechanism by which the GnRH antibodies act in termination of pregnancy can be either by abrogation of the pituitary support or by interference with placental function (Fig. 3). It is believed that in rodents, pregnancy is

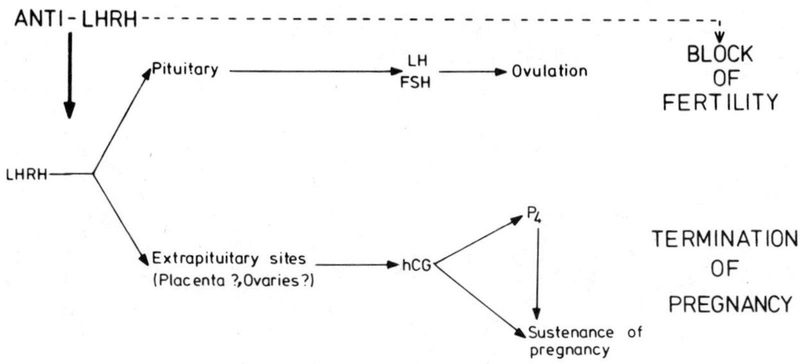


Fig. 3 : Schematic diagramme to illustrate the possible sites of action of monoclonal anti-GnRH antibody in regulation of fertility.

dependent on pituitary support till about mid gestation days. Using anti-ovine luteinizing hormone (oLH) antibodies cross-reactive with rat LH Madwa Raj and Moudgal (1970) were successful in abolishing pregnancy in rats if administered upto day 12 of pregnancy. This is consistent with the present findings in which anti-GnRH antibodies were competent to intercept pregnancy if given earlier than day 10 of pregnancy. In view of the fact that the pregnancy terminating action of monoclonal anti-GnRH antibody could be reversed by progesterone, it may be surmised that intervention by this antibody is at steps leading to steroidogenesis, more precisely the production of progesterone from the ovary under the influence of LH.

However, the presence of GnRH has also been demonstrated in extrahypothalamic sites e.g. ovary (Hsuch & Erickson, 1979, Ying et al, 1981) and placenta (Khodr & Siler & Khodr, 1980). Human placental villi cultured in vitro secreted GnRH which was biologically active and immunologically indistinguishable from hypothalamic GnRH (Siler-Khodr and Khodr, 1979). These observations were further substantiated by studies demonstrating the ability of human placentae to incorporate radioactive amino acids into a material having chromatographic, immunologic and biologic activity identical to hypothalamic GnRH (Khodr & Siler-Khodr, 1980).

The role of GnRH in the placenta in relation to hCG is not fully clear. More than one laboratory has demonstrated the stimulation of hCG production in the human placenta. Siler-Khodr and Khodr (1981) showed that synthetic GnRH can stimulate the release of immunoreactive hCG and its subunits by human placenta _in vitro_ in a dose dependent manner. Macaron and associates (1978) demonstrated an increase in hCG in some but not all trophoblast disease patients following injection of GnRH. This has been independently confirmed by Kim et al (1984) who observed an increase in hCG levels following administration of GnRH in patients with trophoblastic tumour under remission or under chemotherapeutic treatment.

Maintaining human placental villi in culture, we have observed a dose dependent increase in hCG as well as progesterone production by GnRH (Fig. 4).

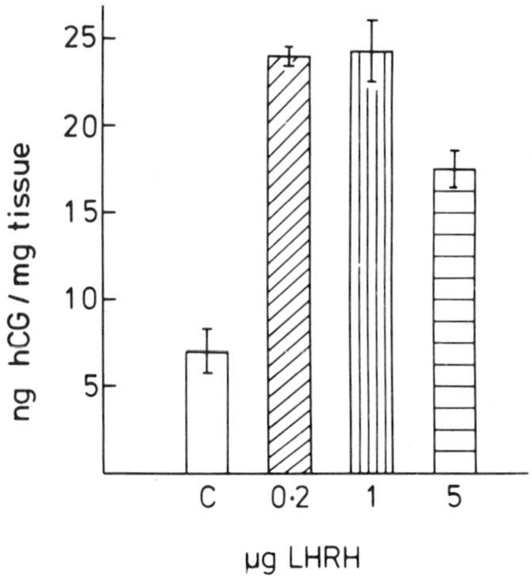


Fig. 4 : Effect of GnRH on hCG production by the human placental villi _in vitro_. Villi were separated out from placenta of 8-10 week gestation and cultured in DMEM under 5% $CO_2$+95% air at 37°C for 24 hrs.

Higher concentration of GnRH had an inhibitory effect on both the parameters (Das, in press). The suppression of placental function at higher concentration of the decapeptide may be ascribable to the well known down regulatory phenomenon of the receptors on the plasma membrane. Monoclonal GnRH antibodies at a dilution of $10^4$ completely blocked the stimulatory effect of GnRH on the gonadotropin as well as the steroid production by the placental villi (Fig. 5a,b).

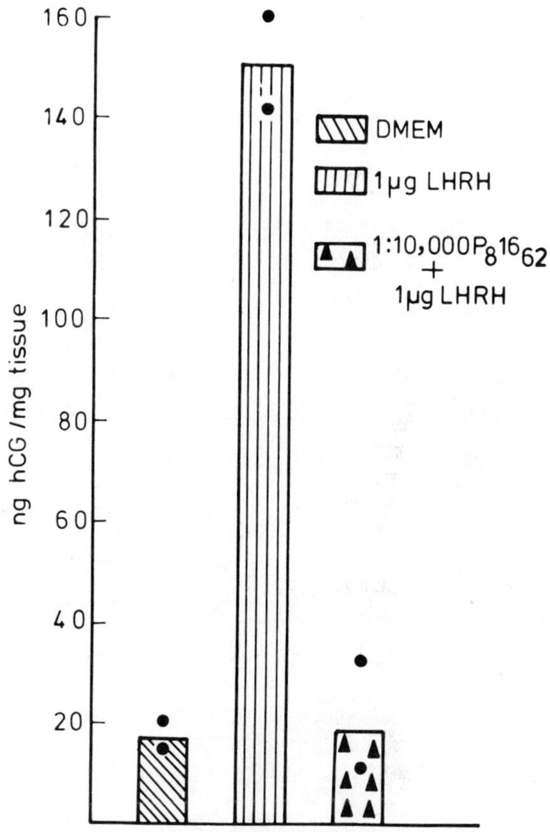


Fig. 5a: Effect of a monoclonal antibody ($P_816_{62}$) on the GnRH induced production of hCG by the human placental villi in vitro. The monoclonal antibody at a dilution of $10^4$ completely blocked the stimulatory effect of GnRH on hCG secretion in 24 hrs culture.

Using pregnant bonnet monkeys as a model for testing the activity of LHRH agonists and antagonists Rao et al (1984) have observed an increase in circulating CG levels by GnRH. Administration of GnRH antibodies, product of the clone $P_816_{62}$ had a suppressive effect on the gonadotropin secretion. These data indicate that the primate placenta not only contains GnRH but is also responsive to the stimulation of GnRH and possibly anti-GnRH antibodies by intercepting this action bring about termination of pregnancy.

CONCLUDING COMMENTS

A monoclonal antibody devoid of reactivity with TRH was generated against GnRH. The antibody reacted optimally with

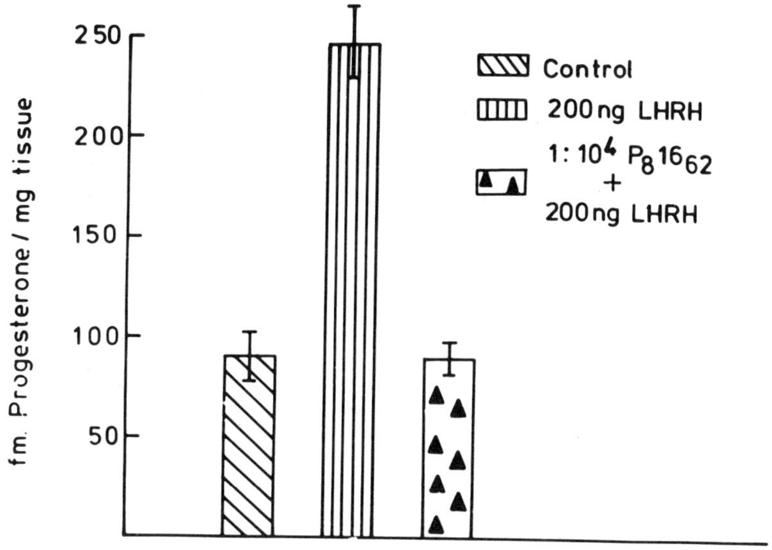


Fig. 5b : Effect of monoclonal antibody ($P_8 16_{62}$) on the GnRH induced production of progesterone by the human placental villi in vitro. The monoclonal antibody at a dilution of $10^4$ completely blocked the stimulatory effect of GnRH on progesterone secretion in 24 hrs culture.

the native hormone. It recognised GnRH with carboxyl group instead of amide at the COOH terminus and shorter peptides with the amino acid sequences 4-6, 7-10 and 4-10 to a variable degree thereby suggesting that the epitope has a conformation involving the entire molecule.

Monoclonal antibody against GnRH was competent to neutralize the in vivo bioactivity of the hormone as evident by the block of estrus and ovulation in rodents. They also bring about termination of pregnancy in mice. Pregnancy terminating action of monoclonals could be prevented by administration of progesterone. Monoclonals against GnRH are effective in suppression of estrus in dogs. Anti-GnRH antibodies administered to baboons in early pregnancy bring about a sharp decrease in blood CG and progesterone levels, which is followed by termination of pregnancy.

Immunointerception by monoclonal antibody directed against GnRH has an effect at two distinct stages in control of fertility. One is at the hypothalamic-pituitary axis by blocking the action of GnRH at the pituitary level and thereby inhibiting the secretion of gonadotropins. Direct and collateral evidence is now available to demonstrate the presence of this decapeptide in other tissues namely placenta. GnRH stimulates the secretion of hCG and progesterone from human placental villi cultured in vitro. Monoclonal antibody blocked the GnRH mediated stimulation of hCG and progesterone from placenta thereby suggesting the other possibility of a direct action at placental level.

## ACKNOWLEDGEMENT

Hybridomas were developed during the tenure of Jawaharlal

Nehru Fellowship by GPT. Other researches receive support from Indian Council of Medical Research, the Family Planning Foundation of India , Rockefeller Foundation and the International Development Research Centre of Canada.

REFERENCES

Beall, G.N., Chopra, I.J., Solomon, D.J., Pierce, J.C. and Cornel, J.S., (1973), Neutralizing and non-neutralizing antibodies to bovine thyroid stimulating hormone and its subunits, J. Clin. Invest., 52 : 2979.

Clarke, I.J., Fraser, H.M. and Mc Neilly, A.S., (1978), Active immunization of ewes against luteinizing hormone releasing hormone and its effects on ovulation and gonadotropin, prolactin and ovarian steroid secretion, J. Endocrinology, 78 : 39.

Das, C. and Talwar, G.P., (1983), Pregnancy terminating action of an LHRH agonist D-ser $(But)^6$ des $Gly^{10}$ ProEA in baboons, Fertil. Steril., 39 : 218.

Das, C., Effect of LHRH and monoclonal antibodies against LHRH during peri-implantation in baboons. India J. Med. Res. (In Press).

Das, C., Gupta, S.K. and Talwar, G.P., Pregnancy interfering action of LHRH agonists and anti-LHRH antibodies J. Steroid Biochem. (In Press).

Fraser, H.M. and Gunn, A., (1973), Effects of antibodies to luteinizing hormone releasing hormone in the male rabbit and on the rat oestrous cycle., Nature, 244 : 160.

Fraser, H.M. and Baker, T.G., (1978), Changes in the ovaries of rats after immunization against luteinizing hormone releasing hormone., J. Endocrinol. 77 : 85.

Gupta, S.K. and Talwar, G.P., 1983, Hybridomas as source of antibodies for immunoassays-monoclonals against LHRH and their detection by EIA, in : Non-Isotopic Immunoassays and their Applications, G.P. Talwar ed. Vikas Publishing House, New Delhi, India.

Gupta,S.K., Singh, O. and Talwar, G.P., 1985, Characteristics and bio-efficacy of monoclonal anti-gonadotropin releasing hormone antibody, Am. J. Reprod. Immunol. Microbiol., 7 : 104.

Hodges, J.K. and Hearn, J.P., (1977), Effects of immunization against lutenizing hormone releasing hormone on reproduction of the marmoset monkey, callithrix jacchus, Nature, 265 : 746.

Hodges, J.K. and Hearn, J.P., (1979), Long term suppression of fertility by immunization against LHRH and its reversibility in female and male marmoset monkeys. In : "Recent Advances in Reproduction and Regulation of Fertility", G.P. Talwar, ed., Elsevier/North Holland Biomedical Press, Amsterdam.

Hsueh, A.J.W. and Erickson, G.F., (1979), Extrapituitary action of gonadotropin releasing hormone : direct inhibition of ovarian steroidogenesis, Science, 204 : 854.

Jeffcoate, J.A., Foster, J.P. and Crighton, D.B., (1978), Effect of active immunization of ewes against synthetic luteinizing hormone releasing hormone, Theriogenology, 10 : 323.

Kawakami, M. and Higuchi, T., (1979), Effects of active and passive immunization with LH-RH on gonadotropin secretion and reproductive function in female rats, Acta Endocrinol., 91 : 616.

Khodr, G.S. and Siler-Khodr, T.M., (1980), Placental LRF and its synthesis, Science, 207 : 315.

Kim, S.J., Kang, B.C., Jung, J.K. and Lee, J.W. (1984), LRH injection test as a remission criterion in trophoblastic disease patients, in : Advances in Experimental Medicine and Biology, volume 176, R.A. Pattillo and R.O. Hussa eds, Plenum Press, New York.

Kohler, G. and Milstein, C.,(1975), Continuous cultures of fused cells secreting antibody of predefined specificity, Nature, 256 : 495.

Koprowski, H., (1973), Mouse Monoclonal antibodies in vivo In : "Monoclonal Antibodies and Cancer", B.B. Boss, R. Longman, I. Trowbridge and R. Dulbecco eds., Academic Press, New York.

Louvet, J.P., Ross, G.T., Birken, S., and Canfield, R.E., (1974), Absence of neutralization effect of antiserum to the unique structural region of human chorionic gonadotropin. J. Clin. Endocrinol. Metab., 39 : 1155.

Macaron, C., Freinkel, N., Brewer, J. Wilber, J.F., Kahan, B. and Halpern, B., (1976), GnRH stimulation of hCG release in trophoblastic disease, Clin. Res., 24 : 274.

Madhwa Raj, H.G. and Moudgal, N.R., (1970), Hormonal control of gestation in the intact rat., Endocrinology, 86 : 874.

Matsuura, S., Ohashi, M., Chen, H.C. and Hodgen, G.D., (1979), An hCG specific antiserum against synthetic peptide analogs to the C-terminal peptide of its B-subunit, Endocrinology, 104 : 396.

Okon, E., Livni, N. and Koch, Y.C., (1980), Immunization against gonadotropin-releasing hormone : histopathological and hormonal changes in the female rat, Br. J. Exp. Pathol, 61 : 579.

Rao, A.J., Mathialagan, N., Kotagi, S.G. and Moudgal, N.R., (1984), Studies on regulation of chorionic gonadotropin secretion in primates, J. Biosc., 6 : 97.

Schally, A.V., Arimura, A.and Kastin, A.J., (1973), Hypothalamic regulating hormones, Science., 179 : 341.

Shastri, N., Manhar, S.K. and Talwar, G.P. (1981), Important role of the carrier in the induction of antibody response without Freund's Complete Adjuvant against a "self" peptide luteinizing hormone-releasing hormone (LHRH). Am. J. Reprod. Immunol., 1 : 262.

Siler-Khodr, T.M. and Khodr, G.S., (1979), Extra hypothalamic luteinizing hormone-releasing factor (LRF) release of immunoreactive LRF *in vitro*, Fertil. Steril., 32 : 294.

Siler-Khodr, T.M. and Khodr, G.S. (1981), Dose response analysis of GnRH stimulation of hCG release from human term placenta, Biol. Reprod., 25 : 353.

Takahashi, M., Ford, J.J., Yoshinaga, K. and Greep, R.O., (1978), Active immunization of female rats with luteinizing hormone releasing hormone (LHRH), Biol. Reprod., 17 : 754.

Talwar, G.P., Gupta, S.K., Singh, O., Singh, V. and Das, C., (1983), New approaches to contraceptive vaccines, in : "Advances in Immunopharmacology", J. Hadden P. Muller, L. Chedid and F. Spreafico eds., Pergamon Press, New York.

Talwar, G.P., Gupta, S.K., Singh, V., Sahal, D., Iyer, K.S.N. and Singh, O. (1985), Bioeffective monoclonal antibody against the decapeptide gonadotropin releasing hormone : Reacting determinant and action on ovulation and estrus suppression. Proc. Natl. Acad. Sci. (USA) 82 : 1228.

Vecsei, P., Haack, D. and Gless, K.H.,(1979), Antagonism of of steroid hormones by specific antibodies, in : "Antihormones", M.K. Agarwal ed., Elsevier/North Holland, Amsterdam.

Ying, S.Y., Ling, N., Bohlen, P., Guillemin, R. (1981), Gonadotropins peptides in ovarian follicular fluid stimulating the secretion of pituitary gonadotropins, Endocrinology, 108 : 1206.

PURIFICATION OF HUMAN GAMETE ANTIGENS RELEVANT TO ANTIBODY PRODUCTION: APPLICATION OF MONOCLONAL ANTIBODIES

Shinzo Isojima[1], Koji Koyama[1], Minoru Shigeta[1], Akiko Hasegawa[1], Stanimir D. Kyurkchiev[1], Kinu Kameda[1], Yukio Tsunoda[2] and Takashi Nagai[2]

[1]Department of Obstetrics & Gynecology, Hyogo Medical College, Nishinomiya & [2]National Institute of Animal Industry, Tsukuba, Japan

## ANTIBODIES TO PORCINE ZONA PELLUCIDA (P-ZP) IN HUMANS

Since Shivers and Dunbar[1] reported the presence of antibodies cross reactive to P-ZP in some sterile women, Mori et al.[2] and others[3,4,5,6] also reported similar results even after absorption with porcine red blood cells (rbc). However, several contradictory results were obtained by Sacco et al.[7], Dakhno et al.[8], Dietle et al.[9] and others[10,11]. Therefore, we studied to confirm these questions.

### Is antibodies to porcine ZP present in human sera ?

In our studies, sera from sterile women, pregnant women and healthy men were examined for staining activities of P-ZP by immunofluorescence after successive absorptions with porcine tissues. The first absorption was carried out with porcine rbc, the second was with porcine kidney and liver and the third was with porcine ovarian tissues. Before absorption with porcine rbc, most sera were positive, but after absorption the positive sera were in 12 of 47 sterile women (25.5%), 28 of 84 pregnant women (33.3%) and 13 of 45 healthy men (28.8%) when FITC-conjugated $F(ab')_2$ of rabbit anti-human Ig (FITC-Ig) was used for staining as the second antibody. On the other hand, when FITC-conjugated $F(ab')_2$ of rabbit anti-human IgG (FITC-IgG) was used for staining as the second antibody, 9 of 47 sterile women (19.1%), 15 of 84 pregnant women (17.9%) and 9 of 45 healthy men (20.0%) showed positive (Table 1). These results did not indicate higher incidence of positive sera in the group of sterile women than in the other two control groups. After further absorption of positive sera with porcine liver and kidney tissues, the incidence of sera to stain P-ZP dropped to 3 of 47 sterile women (6.4%), 11 of 84 pregnant women (13.1%) and 2 of 45 healthy men (4.4%) when FITC-Ig was used as the second antibody, and also dropped to 2 of 47 sterile women (4.3%), 5 of 84 pregnant women (5.9%) and one of 45 healthy men (2.2%) when FITC-IgG was applied as the second antibody. After the second absorption, all positive sera stained P-ZP were completely lost the ability of staining P-ZP after further absorption with porcine ovarian tissues. After the second absorption, only two sera could stain both P-ZP and human ZP by using FITC-Ig as the second antibody. One of two sera was from a pregnant woman and the other was from a man. No

Table 1. Incidence of positive human sera to porcine zona pellucida by immunoflouorescence after successive absorption with various tissues

| After successive absorption with porcine tissues | Infertile women | | Pregnant women | | Healthy men | |
|---|---|---|---|---|---|---|
| | Ig (%) | IgG (%) | Ig (%) | IgG (%) | Ig (%) | IgG (%) |
| RBC | 12/47 (25.5) | 9/47 (19.1) | 28/84 (33.3) | 15/84 (17.9) | 13/45 (28.8) | 9/45 (20.0) |
| Liver & Kidney | 3/47 (6.4) | 2/47 (4.3) | 11/84 (13.1) | 5/84 (5.9) | 2/45 (4.4) | 1/45 (2.2) |
| Ovary | 0/47 (0) | 0/47 (0) | 0/84 (0) | 0/84 (0) | 0/45 (0) | 0/45 (0) |

Ig : FITC-F(ab')$_2$ of rabbit anti-human Ig was used as 2nd Ab.
IgG: FITC-F(ab')$_2$ of rabbit anti-human IgG was used as 2nd Ab.

serum from sterile women remained the ability to stain human ZP after the second absorption (Table 2). It was also proved that the IgG fraction from a man whose serum stained human ZP after the second absorption did retain the ability to stain human ZP. The two sera which stained human ZP were examined for blocking effect on human in vitro fertilization (IVF). Human oocytes obtained from surgical specimens were pre-incubated in BWW culture medium containing 3% human serum albumin for 48 hrs in 5% $CO_2$ incubator, and γ-globulin from each patient's serum was added to medium at the concerntration of 10 mg/ml and incubated for 60 min. at 37°C. Then the capacitated human sperm suspension which was pre-incubated in BWW medium for 5 hrs in 5% $CO_2$ incubator was adjusted at the concentration of 2 x $10^6$ per ml and the pre-incubated human oocytes were added to the sperm suspension, and then incubated for 18 hrs in 5% $CO_2$ incubator at 37°C. The number of bound and penetrated spermatozoa on/in human ZP were counted to evaluate the fertilization. The results indicated that there was no blocking effect by each serum IgG on human IVF, when compared with the control human serum IgG. From these results, it could be concluded that women and men have the same antibodies corresponding to P-ZP but these antibodies were not specific to sterile women. These kinds of antibodies were raised to one of antigens in porcine ovaries, but it may be assumed that some antigenic substances in outer milieu common with P-ZP as bacteria, viruses or foods, might stimulate human to produce antibodies, because men also possessed the same kind of antibody.

Table 2. Number of positive human sera to porcine and human zonae pellucidae by immunofluorescence after 2nd absorption

| Positive staining to | No. of positive sera by immunofluorescence | | |
|---|---|---|---|
| | Infertile women | Pregnant women | Healthy men |
| Porcine ZP | 3/47 | 11/84 | 2/45 |
| Human ZP | 0/47 | 1/84 | 1/45 |

2nd absorption : Absorbed with porcine RBC, liver & kidney tissues

Attempts purifying porcine zona pellucida (P-ZP) by using monoclonal antibodies (Mabs) raised to P-ZP

Purification and characterization of murine ZP have been studied by Wassarman's group [12, 13, 14, 15] but the isolation of P-ZP was attempted mainly by Sacco et al.[16, 17, 18] and Dunbar et al.[19, 20, 21]. These investigators used gel-filtration, ion-exchange chromatography and 2 dimension-PAGE of heat solubilized P-ZP (HS-P-ZP), but we attempted to use immunoaffinity chromatography which bound Mab against HS-P-ZP as purifucation procedure. For this purpose, we established three hybridomas (3A4, 1D5, 1F2) corresponding to HS-P-ZP which secreted Mab only reacting to porcine and human ZPe proved by immunofluorescence[22]. All Mabs did not react with other porcine tissues such as liver, kidney, ovary, testis and rbc. The blocking effect of these Mabs on sperm binding to ZP was not shown in human IVF. The procedures of human IVF is described in our previous paper[22]. Briefly, the oocytes obtained from surgical specimens were pre-incubated in mKRB medium, pH 7.4 containing 7% inactivated human serum for 40-48 hrs at 37°C in a 5% $CO_2$ incubator, and then incubated with Mab-$\gamma$-globulin for 30 min. at 37°C. After washing with mKRB medium, these oocytes were transfered to 0.2ml of sperm suspension ($1 \times 10^6$/ml) under liquid paraffin. The sperm suspension was prepared by washing ejaculated human spermatozoa twice with mKRB medium containing 0.1% BSA and pre-incubated with the same culture medium for 3 hrs at a concentration of 1-5 x $10^7$/ml and the sperm concentration was adjusted to $1 \times 10^6$/ml with mKRB with 7% human serum before use. The inseminated oocytes were incubated for 15 hrs at 37°C in a 5% $CO_2$ incubator and then sperm binding and penetration were observed. The immunofluorescence procedures are described in our previous paper[23].

When goat anti-mouse $\gamma$-globulin serum was added as the 2nd antibody, the fertilization blockings occurred in cases of Mabs 3A4 and 1D5 in human IVF. In order to characterize antigen of HS-P-ZP corresponding to Mab 3A4, HS-P-ZP was iodinated with $^{125}$I and the labelled proteins were fractionated by immunoaffinity chromatography on Sepharose 4B which bound Mab 3A4 and the binding activity of each fraction was examined. It was found that the fraction eluted with glycine HCl buffer pH 2.5 indicated twenty-three times higher binding activity to Mab 3A4 than the Mab unbound fraction. Then the immune precipitate of Mab bound fraction which was formed with Mab 3A4 and rabbit anti-mouse $\gamma$-globulin was applied on SDS-PAGE. The gel was cut with Gilson's gel cutter and the radioactivities of all cut sections were counted. The radioactivity showed three peaks in the zones of 92Kd, 65Kd and 23Kd shown in Fig. 1.

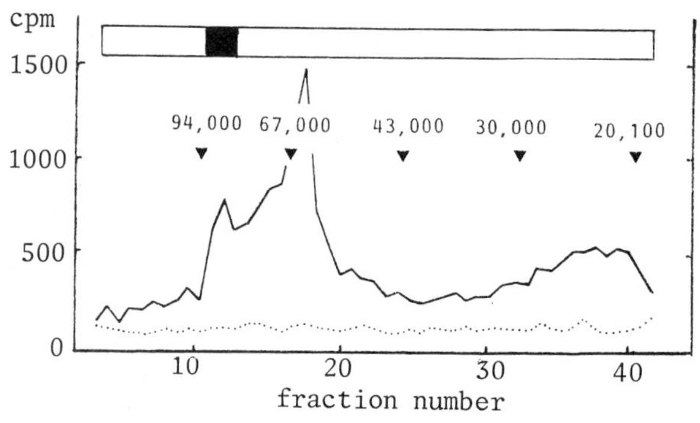


Fig. 1. SDS-PAGE of $^{125}$I HS-P-ZP* immunoprecipitated with Mab 3A4 and reactive epitope after Western blotting

*HS-P-ZP: Heat solubilized porcine zona pellucida

In order to examine the presence of antigenic epitope to Mab 3A4 in these three bands, 200μg of HS-P-ZP was applied on SDS-PAGE and transblotted to nitrocellulose membrane, and then the antigenic epitope transblotted was examined with Mab 3A4 and enzyme(peroxidase)-conjugated goat anti-mouse γ-globulin. It was found that only 92Kd portion of molecules transblotted to nitrocellulose membrane showed antigenicity to Mab 3A4. On the other hand, antigenic molecules which react to Mabs 1D5 and 1F2 were not observed by Western blotting after SDS-PAGE of HS-P-ZP.

Purification of 92Kd fraction for immunization and characterization of antigenic epitope corresponding Mab 3A4: The lyophylized HS-P-ZP (1mg in PBS containing 0.05% SDS) was applied to Sepharose 4B bound Mab 3A4 (20mg Mab/10ml bed volume), washed with PBS containing 0.05% SDS and then eluted with 3M NaSCN in PBS. In order to obtain enough amount of antigen for immunization, NaSCN was used for elution, because most proteins of HS-P-ZP was precipitated by glycine HCl buffer at pH 2.5, due to their isoelectric point. The antibody bound fraction was collected and applied to SDS-PAGE. The band of 92Kd in SDS-PAGE was cut and extracted in 5mM $NaHCO_3$ containing 0.1% SDS, and kept overnight with room temp. and used for immunization. The characteristics of antigenic epitope corresponding to Mab 3A4 in HS-P-ZP was examined and found that it was lost by pronase, trypsin, mixed glycosidase digestions and periodic acid treatment, but was resistant to endoglycosidase D or H by examining inhibitory activity for ELISA system. Therefore, the antigenic epitope seemed to be composed of some kind of glycoprotein. The antigenic epitope corresponding to Mab 3A4 was not a receptor antigen of human ZP, but might be one of the receptor associated antigens because Mab itself did not block fertilization in human IVF, even though it interfered with porcine sperm binding/penetration to porcine oocytes. However, Mab 3A4 was able to block human IVF with goat anti-mouse γ-globulin.

Effect of polyclonal antibodies to partially purified 92Kd molecule of HS-P-ZP: We assumed that the 92Kd molecule of HS-P-ZP must contain sperm receptor-associated antigen which binds Mab 3A4, because Mab 3A4 could block human IVF with goat anti-mouse γ-globulin. For this reason, we immunized BALB/c mice with partially purified 92Kd molecule of HS-P-ZP, and bled to obtain the serum. Antibody titer increased to 1:2000 examined by immunofluorescence. The antibody obtained did not react with various tissues such as liver, kidney, spleen and ovary except ZP in pigs and humans. However, this polyclonal antibody to 92Kd molecule blocked sperm binding to oocytes in human, with precipitin layer over ZP (Table 3). It is interesting that this antibody reacted not only to

Table 3. Effect of anti-3A4-92kd[1] antiserum on human sperm penetration to zona pellucida

| Antibody | No. of examined eggs | No. of bound ± S.D. sperm/egg | No. of penetrated ± S.D. sperm/egg |
|---|---|---|---|
| NMS[2] | 4 | 68.8±36.9 (28-100) | 6.2±4.6 (5-13) |
| anti-HS-P-ZP[3] | 3 | 1.3±1.5 (0-3) | 0.0±0.0 (0) |
| anti-3A4-92kd | 13 | 7.4±6.0 (1-20) | 0.3±0.6 (0-2) |

1. anti-3A4-92kd: Polyclonal antibodies against 92kd molecule of HS-P-ZP reacting to Mab 3A4.
2. NMS: Normal mouse serum.
3. anti-HS-P-ZP: Mouse anti-heat solubilized porcine zona pellucida.

porcine and human ZP but also to hamster ZP examined by immunofluorescence, though Mab 3A4 did not react to hamster ZP. This antibody reacted not only with 92Kd molecule, but also with wide range of molecules after SDS-PAGE of HS-P-ZP. These results clearly showed that the 92Kd molecule purified by immunoaffinity chromatography bound Mab 3A4 and SDS-PAGE still contained a small amount of contamination from other antigenic epitopes. In 1980, we established 5 hybridomas producing different kinds of Mab to P-ZP[23]. Among them, Mab B11C8 which reacted only to P-ZP could block the boar sperm binding to P-ZP. Even Fab fragment of Mab B11C8 IgG strongly blocked boar sperm binding/penetration to P-ZP (Table 4). Mab G10G5 which stained both porcine and hamster Zpe did not block fertilization in pigs and hamsters but when anti-mouse γ-globulin was added as the 2nd antibody, fertilization in hamster was moderately blocked with precipitin layer over ZP. Mab 3A4 which stained both porcine and human ZPe by immunofluorescence could block boar sperm binding to P-ZP, but did not interfere with the human fertilization. However, the goat anti-mouse γ-globulin was added, it could block the human fertilization with precipitin layer on ZP as in case of Mab G10G5 in hamster. From these results, it could be assumed that the antigenic epitope of receptor might be species specific. We can make Mab against receptor which block fertilization only in isologous system but not in heterologous system. The fertilization blocking by antibodies other than ZP receptor antibody was probably due to the steric hindrance with immune precipitates over the receptors. It would be very difficult to make antibodies to human receptor antigen from P-ZP. Therefore, for the contraceptive vaccine program, there will be only a possibility to make antibodies to human receptor associated antigens from P-ZP. However, we have to be very careful for a trace amount of contamination which is cross reactive to other human tissues.

## ANTIGENS AND ANTIBODIES TO HUMAN SPERMATOZOA AS THE CANDIDATE OF CONTRACEPTIVE VACCINE

### Purification of human seminal plasma (HSP) specific antigens using Mab:

Sperm antigens are the most hopeful target to prepare the contraceptive vaccine, because we have many sterile women due to anti-sperm antibodies. In our studies for many years, we recognized the heterogeneity of anti-sperm antibodies in women. Some women produced antibodies to sperm membrane antigens but the other raised antibodies to seminal plasma components. Attempting to purify antigens, we focused the target to human seminal plasma as the source of antigenic material, because antigens

Table 4. Effect of Mab B11C8 IgG and F(ab') fragment of Ig on in vitro fertilization of porcine eggs matured in culture

| Antibody | No. of eggs | No. (%) of eggs penetrated | | | Mean No. of sperm/egg |
|---|---|---|---|---|---|
| | | total | with enlarged sperm head | with both pronuclei | |
| anti-P-ZP IgG* | 15 | 2 (13.3) | 2 | 0 | 1.0 |
| Control IgG** | 15 | 15(100.0) | 14 | 1 | 3.0 |
| Mab B11C8 IgG | 30 | 0 (0.0) | 0 | 0 | 0 |
| Fab | 26 | 4 (15.4) | 4 | 0 | 0 |

*Anti-porcine zona pellucida antibody IgG (mouse)
**Control mouse serum IgG

were already solubilized and not necessary to extract from sperm membrane. After several trials of biochemical and physicochemical procedures[24], getting pure antigens was found to be difficult. Therefore, we attempted to purify them by immunoaffinity chromatography which bound Mab raised to HSP antigen. In 1980, we first succeeded in establishing the hybridoma 1C4 which produced a strong sperm immobilizing Mab to HSP antigen[25]. However, this Mab was found to be raised against HSP No.7 antigen (Ferrisplan) which cross reacted to human milk protein[26]. This means that Mab 1C4 was not useful for purification of HSP antigen as contraceptive vaccine, we then tried to establish other Mabs specific to HSP-antigens, and as a result, the hybridoma 2C6 was established by fusing spleen cells of BALB/c mice immunized with HSP and mouse myeloma cell P3U1. The Mab 2C6 was HSP-specific and IgM(κ). It possessed very strong sperm immobilizing and agglutinating activities and also had a blocking effect on human IVF. This stained acrosome regions of human spermatozoa by immunofluorescence. The purification was carried out first by Sephacryl S-300 after salting out pooled azoospermic semen with saturation of $(NH_4)_2SO_4$. The antigenic activity to Mab 2C6 was fractionated in near void volume and the M.W. of fraction seemed to be more than $400 \times 10^3$. The purification of antigen was examined by inhibitory activity for sperm-Mab 2C6 ELISA system. After procedure of Sephacryl S-300, the purity of first main fraction (A1) increased 3.2 times. In the second, the fraction A1 was applied to DEAE Sephacell chromatography and the eluted major fraction around 0.2M NaCl (A2) showed 1.8 times increase as antigenic purity. In the third procedure, the fraction A2 was applied to immunoaffinity chromatography (Sepharose 4B gel) bound Mab 2C6. The antibody bound fraction (A3) was eluted with glycine HCl buffer pH2.5 and its purity went up 4.8 times. Therefore, the purity of A3 fraction was 29 times compared with original HSP. By these purification procedures, the increase of purity was rather low compared with antigen corresponding to Mab 1C4 which increased the purity 196 times (Table 5). The partially purified A3 antigen was analysed and we discovered that the antigenic activity was lost by the treatment of periodic acid, mixed glycosidase, pronase and partially by trypsin, but was not by lipase, when inhibitory activity of fractions was examined by sperm-Mab 2C6 ELISA system and micro sperm immobilization test. Iodination of fraction A3 was also difficult by several methods, thus we assumed that the content of tryosine residue in peptide chain might be sparse. The cleavage of S-S bond by DTT (dithiothreitol) and

Table 5. Characteristics of Mabs to HSP

| Mabs | Ig Subclass | Ag Specificity | Ab to sperm | Purification of corresponding Ag SIA/protein | Nature of Corresponding Ag |
|---|---|---|---|---|---|
| 1C4 | IgM | HSP<br>HM | Immobil.(+++)<br>Aggl.(±) | 196 | glycoprotein |
| 2C6 | IgM | HSP | Immobil.(+++)<br>Aggl.(++)<br>Fertil. block (+) | 29 | glycoprotein |
| 2E5 | $IgG_3$ | HSP | Immobil.(++)<br>Aggl.(+) | N.D. | glycoprotein |

HSP: Human seminal plasma Mab: Monoclonal antibody N.D.: not determined
HM: Human milk Immobil.: immobilization Ag: Antigen
Aggl.: Agglutination SIA: Sperm immobilizing activity Ab: Antibody

alkylation (by iodoacetamide) in the molecule of A3 did not affect antigenic epitope. The purification of this fraction is being studied biochemically but it has many difficult problems because the antigenic epitope may be composed of glycoprotein. Mab 2E5 was also produced from the established hybridoma 2E5 and its Ig subclass was IgG3(κ). This Mab 2E5 also possessed strong sperm immobilizing and moderate agglutinating activities, but did not block human IVF. The inhibitory activity of spermatozoa for sperm-Mab 2E5 ELISA system was lost by the treatment of spermatozoa with periodic acid, mixed glycosidase, neuraminidase, pronase but not with lipase, trypsin, β-endoglycosidase. The summarized results of biochemical natures of the antigens corresponding to Mabs 2C6 and 2E5 are shown in Table 6. Unfortunately, the sperm immobilizing antibodies in patients' sera did not interfere with the reaction between these partially purified antigens and corresponding Mab system which was examined by ELISA. Therefore, there are following two possibilities. First, these Mabs were possibly produced by recognizing xenogenic epitopes of human spermatozoa and might be different from the antibodies in patients which were produced by recognizing tissue specific epitopes of spermatozoa. Second, the binding affinity of human antibody to spermatozoa may be much weaker than heterologous mouse antibody. From these results, we attempted to establish the human-mouse hetero-hybridomas which produce human immunoglobulin by using peripheral lymphocytes of patients who possessed strong sperm immobilizing antibodies.

## Production of human-mouse hybridoma to HSP

The peripheral blood lymphocytes (PBL, 7 x $10^6$) from sterile women with high titer of sperm immobilizing antibodies were isolated by Ficoll-Conray density gradient centrifugation, and suspended with washed husbands' spermatozoa (3-4 x $10^6$) in 5ml of RPMI 1640 medium containing PWM (1:100) and 10% fetal calf serum, and cultured for 5-6 days after distributing 0.5 ml of each in 10 wells. The pre-cultured PBL were collected and fused with SP 2/0 mouse myeloma cells in the presence of PEG 1000 (fusion ratio 1:1) following by a modified Butler's method[27]. The fused cells were distributed in the Corning plate (No.25860) at a concentration of 44 x $10^3$ cells per well. Culture medium was changed to HAT medium 24 hrs later, and the supernatant of medium growing hybridoma were tested for the production of human γ-globulin by sandwich ELISA, 21 days later. The cell growings were observed in 214 of 632 wells and 21 among 214 hybridoma in the wells showed productions of human immunoglobulins (Ig) which were proved by Sandwich ELISA. The sperm-immobilization and

Table 6. Biochemical natures of the antigens corresponding to Mabs 2C6 and 2E5

| Biochemical natures | 2C6 antigen | 2E5 antigen |
|---|---|---|
| 1. Molecular size | macromolecule (>400 Kd) | macromolecule |
| 2. Lectin (LcH) affinity | + | + |
| 3. Antigenecity after treatment with | | |
| Pronase | decreased | unchanged |
| Trypsin | decreased | unchanged |
| α-Chymotrypsin | decreased | unchanged |
| Lipase | unchanged | unchanged |
| Glycosidase (mixed) | decreased | decreased |
| Neuraminidase | not tested | decreased |
| periodic acid | decreased | decreased |
| 4. Extraction by chloroform-methanol | interface | aqueous layer |

Table 7. Reactivity and stability of human-mouse hybridomas producing anti-human sperm antibodies

| Hetero-hybridoma | Ig class | Production of human immuno-globulins | Reactivity against human sperm | | Stability |
|---|---|---|---|---|---|
| | | | Micro-SIT[2] | Aggl.[3] | |
| H2-3H1 | N.T.[1] | 100 ng/ml | - | + | unstable <40 days |
| H3-1B12 | N.T.[1] | 10 μg/ml | ± | + | unstable <40 days |
| H3-1B5 | IgM(κ) | 100 μg/ml | - | + | >90 days |

1. N.T.: not tested
2. Micro-SIT: micro-sperm immobilization test
3. Aggl.: sperm agglutination
4. Sperm agglutination titer; 1:16

agglutination tests were carried out for all human Ig positive hybridomas, and three hybridomas were selected due to positive sperm-immobilizing or agglutinating antibody production. The characteristics of three human-mouse hybridomas, H2-3H1, H3-1B12 and H3-1B5 are shown in Table 7. Although cloning by limiting dilution was carried out immediately after the detection of Ig production, the hybridomas H2-3H1 and H3-1B12 lost the antibody secretion within 40 days after cell fusion. However, the hybridoma H3-1B5 preserved antibody production after two consecutive clonings and kept stable condition for more than 90 days in the culture. The Ig subclass of Mab produced by hybridoma H3-1B5 was IgM (κ). The hybridoma H3-1B5 began to decrease antibody production after three months. The Mab H3-1B5 did not react to human other tissues and its sperm agglutionation titer was 1:16 as determined by microagglutination test. This Mab also stained post nuclear cap of human spermatozoa. The fluorescent intensity of stained spermatozoa was analyzed by EPICS cell sorter and it was shown that spermatozoa treated with Mab H3-1B5 indicated the specific binding of antibody compared with the negative control (Fig. 2). The Mab H3-1B5 was absorbed only with HSP and human spermatozoa but not with human serum and milk protein. This was the first successful production of a human-mouse hybridoma which secreted human sperm agglutinating antibody, because Herr et al.[28] did not describe any biological activities of human Mab on spermatozoa though, very recently, they succeeded in obtaining mouse-human heterohybridoma secreting human γ-globulin which bound to spermatozoa. However, human chromosomes will be preferentially lost in human-mouse hybridomas, thus the maintenance of these hybridomas will be difficult. In order to obtain antigenic molecules corresponding to anti-sperm antibody in sterile women, the establishment of human hybridoma is neccessary to follow the process of purifying antigens. If we could produce human Mab to human sperm specific antigens, they may also be utilized for passive immunization of women to induce infertility. This study showed us a direction for future research for making a contraceptive vaccine designed for human.

## Acknowledgement

These works were supported by the research grants from the Ministry of Education, Japanese Government and the Japanese Foundation for Promotion of Private School.

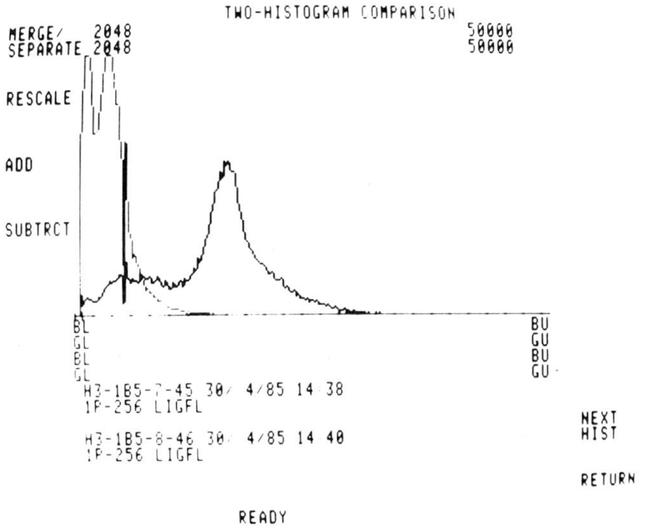


Fig. 2. Fluorescent intensity of spermatozoa (EPICS cell sorter) reacted to Mab H3-1B5 IgG and normal human serum IgG*

*Washed human spermatozoa were incubated with Mab H3-1B5 IgG or normal human serum IgG and then FITC-conjugated rabbit anti-human IgG was mixed for fluorescent staining.

## REFERENCES

1. Shivers, C. A., Dunbar, B. S. Autoantibodies to zona pellucida: A possible cause for infertility in women. Science, 197:1082-1084, 1977.
2. Mori, T., Nishimoto, T., Kohda, H., Takai, I., Nishimura, T. Oikawa, T. A method for specific detection of autoantibodies to the zona pellucida in infertile women. Fertil. Steril., 32:67-72, 1979.
3. Trounson, A. D., Shivers, C. A., McMaster, R., Lopata, A. Inhibition of sperm binding and fertilization of human ova by antibody to porcine zona pellucida and human sera. Arch. Androl., 4:29-36, 1980.
4. Bousquet, D., St-Jacques, S., Roberts, K. D., Chapdelaine, A., Bleau, G. Zona pellucida antibodies in a group of women with idiopathic infertility. Am. J. Reprod. Immunol., 2:73-78, 1982.
5. Kamada, M., Hasebe, H., Inahara, M., Kinoshita, T., Naka, O., Mori, T. Detection of anti-zona pellucida antibodies in human sera by the possitive hemagglutination reaction. Fertil. Steril., 41:901-906, 1984.
6. Singh, J., Mhaskar, A. M. Enzyme-linked immunosorbent determination of autoantibodies to zona pellucida as a possible cause of infertility in women. J. Immunol. Meth., 79:133-141, 1985.
7. Sacco, A. G., Moghissi, K. S., Anti-zona pellucida activity in human sera. Fertil. Steril., 31:503-506, 1979.
8. Dakhno, F. V., Hjort, T., Grischenko, V. I. Evaluation of immunofluorescence on pig zona pellucida for detection of anti-zona antibodies in human sera. J. Reprod. Immunol., 2:281-291, 1980.
9. Dietle, J., Knop, G., Mettler, L., The frequency of serological

anti-zona pellucida activity in males, females and children. J. Reprod. Immunol., 4:123-131, 1982.

10. Najudu, P. L., Freeman, L. F., Trounson, A. O. Zona pellucida antibodies in human sera. J. Reprod. Fertil., 65:77-84, 1982.
11. Kurachi, H., Wakimoto, H., Sakumoto, T., Aono, T., Kurachi, K. Specific antibodies to porcine zona pellucida detected by quantitative radioimmunoassay in both fertile and infertile women. Fertil. Steril., 41:265-269, 1984.
12. Bleil, J. D., Wassarman, P. M. Structure and function of the zona pellucida; identification and characterization of the proteins of the mouse oocyte's zona pellucida. Develop. Biol., 76:185-203, 1980.
13. Bleil, J. D., Wassarman, P. M. Mammalian sperm-egg interaction: Identification of a glycoprotein in mouse egg zonae pellucidae possessing receptor activity for sperm. Cell, 20:873-882, 1980.
14. Bleil, J. D., Wassarman, P. M. Synthesis of zona pellucida proteins by denuded and follicle enclosed mouse oocytes during culture in vitro. Proc. Natl. Acad. Sci. U.S.A., 77:1029-1033, 1980.
15. Greve, J. M., Salzmann, G. S., Roller, R. J., Wassarman, P. M. Biosynthesis of the major zona pellucida glycoprotein secreted by oocytes during mammalian oogenesis. Cell, 31:749-759, 1982.
16. Sacco, A. G., Yurewicz, E. C., Subramanian, M. G., De Mayo, F. J. Zona pellucida composition: Species cross reactivity and contraceptive potential of antiserum to a purified pig zona anti(PPZA). Biol. Reprod., 25:997-1008, 1981.
17. Yurewicz, E. C., Sacco, A. G., Subramanian, M. G. Isolation and preliminary characterization of a purified pig zona antigen (PPZA) from porcine oocytes. Biol. Reprod., 29:511-523, 1983.
18. Sacco, A. G., Subramanian, M. G., Yurewicz, E. C., Dukelow, W. R. Heteroimmunization of squirrel monkey (Saimiri Sciureus) with a purified porcine zona antigen (PPZA); immune response and biological activity of antiserum. Fertil. Steril., 39:350-358, 1983.
19. Dunbar, B. S., Liu, C., Sammons, D. W. Identification of the three major proteins of porcine and rabbit zonae pellucidae by high resolution two dimentional gel electrophoresis: Comparison with serum, follicular fluid, and ovarian cell proteins. Biol. Reprod., 24:1111-1124, 1981.
20. Shinner, S. M., Mills, T., Kirchick, H. J., Dunbar, B. S. Immunization with zona pellucida proteins results in abnormal ovarian follicular differentiation and inhibition of gonadotropin-induced steroid secretion. Endocrinology, 115:2418-2432, 1984.
21. Drell, D. W., Dunbar, B. S. Monoclonal antibodies to rabbit and pig zonae pellucidae distinguish species-specific and shared antigenic determinants. Biol. Reprod., 30:445-457, 1984.
22. Koyama, K., Hasegawa, A., Tsuji, Y., Isojima, S. Production and characterization of monoclonal antibodies to cross-reactive antigens of human and porcine zonae pellucidae. J. Reprod. Immunol. (In press), 1985.
23. Isojima, S., Koyama, K., Hasegawa, A., Tsunoda, Y., Hanada, A. Monoclonal antibodies to porcine zona pellucida antigens and their inhibitory effects on fertilization. J. Reprod. Immunol., 6:77-87, 1984.
24. Isojima, S., Koyama, K., Tsuchiya, K. The effect on fertility in women of circulating antibodies against human spermatozoa. J. Reprod. Fertil., Suppl., 21:125-150, 1974.
25. Shigeta, M., Watanabe, T., Maruyama, S., Koyama, K., Isojima, S. Sperm-immunobilizing monoclonal antibody to human seminal plasma antigens. Clin. exp. Immunol., 42:458-462, 1980.
26. Isojima, S., Koyama, K., Fujiwara, N. Purification of human seminal

plasma No.7 antigen by immunoaffinity chromatography on bound monoclonal antibody. Clin. exp. Immunol., 49:449-456, 1982.
27. Butler, J. L., Lane, H. C., Fauci, A. S. Delineation of optimal conditions for producing mouse-human heterohybridomas from human peripheral blood B cells of immunized subjects. J. Immunol., 130:165-168, 1983.
28. Herr, J. C., Flowler, J. E., Jr., Howards, S. S., Sigman, M., Sutherland, W. M., Koons, D. J. Human antisperm monoclonal antibodies constructed postvasectomy. Biol. Reprod., 32:695-711. 1985.

# CHARACTERISTICS OF ANTI-ZONA MONOCLONAL ANTIBODIES

A.K. Bamezai, Suman and G.P. Talwar

National Institute of Immunology & Department of Biochemistry

A.I.I.M.S., P.O. Box No. 4922, New Delhi-110029, India

Zona pellucida (ZP) is one of the potential target antigen for immunocontraception (1,2). Conventional antibodies raised against ZP inhibit sperm-zona interaction in vitro (3-6) and block fertility in various species on active and passive immunization (7-10). Most studies have focussed on porcine ZP, in view of its immunological reactivity with human zonae. Moreover heterospecies antigen is also expected to be more immunogenic. Indeed immunization of rabbits with porcine zonae resulted in production of high antibody titres and block of fertility in contrast to rabbit zonae which were not as effective.

Porcine zona pellucida is a complex antigenic mass. It is composed of three families of glycoproteins heterogenous with respect to charge and molecular weight. These aspects will be discussed by Dr. Dunbar and Dr. Sacco in the symposium. This presentation provides information on the characteristics of a number of monoclonals generated against the porcine zona pellucida. Some determinants inducing highly reactive antibodies as determined by immunofluorescence and enzyme immunoassays may not be of immunocontraceptive interest as these antibodies do not prevent the binding of the sperm with egg nor inhibit the lysis of the zonae by proteolytic enzymes. The diversity of the antigenic determinants is highlighted. The monoclonals may help in sifting of the bioeffective determinants from others, such as those which are involved in arrest of the follicular development. An acceptable vaccine based on zonae would seek to use only those antigens which produce antibodies interfering with fertility, but not producing undesirable side effects. Zona has tissue specific as well as antigens cross-reactive with other organs. Invariably the conventional antibodies raised against the whole zonae or originating from infertile patients deemed to have antizona antibodies are absorbed with homologous or heterologous erythrocytes to eliminate most of the cross-reactive antibodies. Monoclonals specific to zonae provide a means to distinguish the tissue specific from cross-reactive antigens. Several other pertinent questions can also be answered by an adequate library of monoclonals. These include the identity of zona antigens reactive with ovarian follicular cells.

Table 1. Dissociation between the EIA titres and ability to inhibit the lysis of zona by proteolytic enzymes

| No. | MoAb | Immunofluorescence | EIA titre | Titres* upto which inhibitory in zona lysis assay |
|---|---|---|---|---|
| 1. | $A_2$ | 4 + (thick precipitin-rim) | $1 \times 10^{-5}$ | + upto $10^{-3}$ |
| 2. | $A_6$ | 3 + (thin rim) | -do- | -do- |
| 3. | $C_{10}$ | 4 + (Patchy) | -do | -do- |
| 4. | $G_8$ | 3 + (thin rim) | -do- | -do- |
| 5. | $H_9$ | 3 + (thin rim) | -do- | -do- |
| 6. | $D_{10}$ | 3 + (thin rim) | -do- | -do- |
| 7. | $C_3F_7$ | 3+ | -do- | -do- |
| 8. | $D_7F_{10}$ | 3+ | -do- | not inhibitory |
| 9. | $G_6B_{10}$ | 3+ | -do- | not inhibitory |
| 10. | $E_{12}$ | | -do- | not inhibitory |

* Dilution at which lysis delayed for three times the control

Ten stable hybrid cell clones were developed by fusion of splenocytes immunized with intact porcine zonae (11). The clones were selected by solid phase enzyme immuno-assay using solubilized zonae as an antigen. The cells grow as ascites in the mouse peritoneum and ascites fluid was used as source of antibody.

All monoclonals gave a clear immunofluorescence reaction with porcine zonae. The pattern varied and is described in Table 1.

The EIA titres of all the monoclonals used were the same e.g. $1 \times 10^{-5}$. The antibodies were tested for their ability to inhibit the lysis of zona by proteolytic enzyme. The assay was initially proposed by Dr. C.A. Shivers (12). It is recognized that the blastocyst sheds off the zona before implantation. This important event is considered to be brought about by a proteolytic enzyme (13) originating either from the blastocyst (14) or from the uterus (15,16). Interestingly the anti-zona antibodies render the zona relatively resistent to the action of even a powerful proteolytic enzyme such as pronase. All monoclonals did not confer the resistance to zona lysis even though all of them were immuno-reactive with zona antigens in EIA and immunofluorescence (Table 1). Assuming that this property may be relevant to the bioefficacy of antibodies for control of fertility, the determinants corresponding to monoclonals $D_7F_{10}$, $G_6B_{10}$, $E_{12}$ would not be of interest for contraceptive purposes.

<u>Properties of monoclonal</u> - $A_2$

$A_2$, is an $IgG_1$, k antibody. It gives a thick precipitation rim around

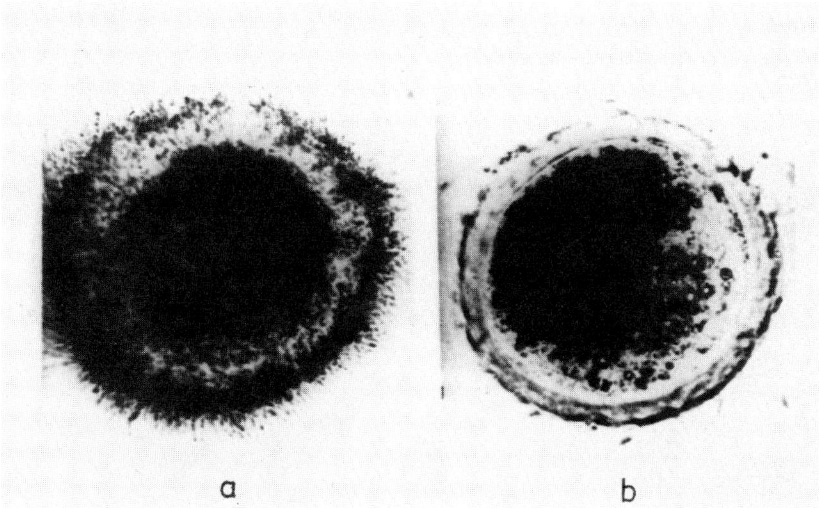

Fig. 1. Prevention of the sperm binding to porcine zona pelucida by MoAb-$A_2$. Eggs aspirated from mature follicles were incubated with 1:100 dilution of ascites fluid and the binding of the sperm was checked by the method described elsewhere (11). Eggs were incubated (a) with $Sp^2/0$ ascites and (b) with MoAb-$A_2$ ascites.

the zona as seen by immunofluorescence. It inhibits the lysis of zona by pronase. Its action on binding of porcine epididymal sperm to egg was studied essentially by following the method described elsewhere (11). The antibody did not prevent the attachment of the sperm to the egg. However when the eggs were pipetted in and out of the Pasteur pipette, the loosely attached sperm were dissociated, while those more firmly bound to the egg remained attached. Eggs treated with MoAb-$A_2$ for 2 hr at room temperature ($\sim 25^\circ C$) did not have the sperm firmly bound (Fig 1b) in comparison to controls (Fig 1a).

## Species restriction of zona antigens

MoAb-$A_2$ gives a strong immunofluorescent reaction with porcine zonae but was found devoid of similar reactivity with human zona, with egg of bonnet monkey, cat, dog, hamster, rat and mouse zonae. The reactivity with canine zonae was examined by Dr. Mahi-Brown and with human eggs by Dr. S. Isojima. These observations point out to the existence of species restricted determinants on zona, besides those which may be cross reactive amongst zona of various species. MoAb $A_6$, $C_{10}$ was cross-reactive with cannine zonae. MoAb-$C_{10}$ had also a weak cross reaction with human zonae.

## Reactivity of monoclonals with ovarian follicular cells

The monoclonals $A_2$, $C_{10}$, $A_6$ are directed to an antigenic determinant which is not present on the porcine erythrocytes (Fig 2a). A major problem in development of antizona vaccines is the inhibitory effect of the antibodies on follicular development. This is expressed in either the disturbances of sex steroid hormonal profiles and lack of normal follicular development in primates (as will be discussed by Suman et al and Dr. Sacco in the symposium) or in irreversible atresia of follicles in rabbits (8). MoAb-$A_2$ has several interesting properties such as the inhibition of zona

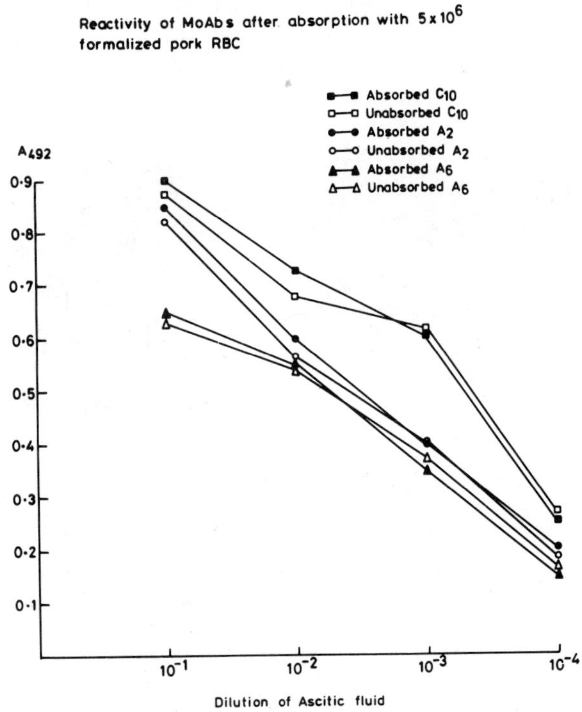


Fig.2a. Lack of cross reactivity of MoAb with porcine erythrocytes; the ascites fluids containing antibodies at indicated dilution were absorbed with $5 \times 10^6$ cells at 4°C for 16 hrs. The immunoreactivity of the absorbed and unabsorbed MoAbs was determined by ELISA.

lysis by proteolytic enzymes and prevention of sperm binding to egg. The reactivity of this antibody (as also was of two other monoclonals) with porcine follicular cells were determined by the more sensitive enzyme immunoassay. The antibody was absorbed with follicular cells and its activity in EIA determined. Data in Fig. 2b indicates the absence of reactivity with follicular cells.

Antigen to which MoAb-$A_2$ is directed

Heat solubilized porcine zonae were run on a SDS-polyacrylamide gel along with molecular weight markers, revealed by Coomasie staining. Immunoreactivity of the MoAb-$A_2$ as well as the monkey polyvalent antibody raised against the intact porcine ZP or against purified $ZP_3$ from Dr. Sacco was determined by Western blots. Results are given in Fig.3. The monkey serum against the intact zonae pellucidae had a broad reactivity with several components of the zonae. The monkey serum against purified $ZP_3$ was with a glycoprotein of average molecular weight of 55K. The MoAb-$A_2$ reacted also with a single antigenic moiety migrating in these gels near about the same region as $ZP_3$. It is however difficult to conclude that antigenic determinant of this antibody is in $ZP_3$ as the above analytical methods do not have high enough resolution. Further studies are required to elucidate the delineate the antigen carrying MoAb-$A_2$ binding epitope.

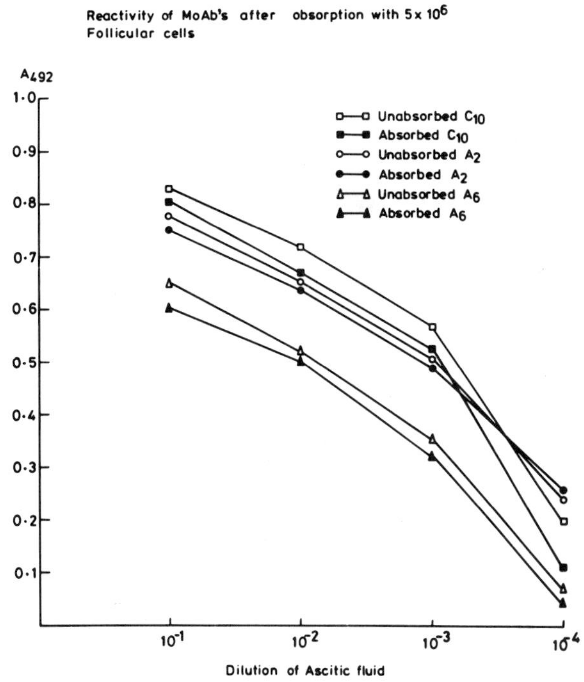


Fig.2b. Reactivity of MoAb's before and after absorption with 5 x $10^6$ ovarian follicular cells (For Method see legend Fig. 2a).

The extensive studies have been carried out by Dr. Sacco and his group on impact of immunization of Squirrel monkey with purified $ZP_3$ reported in another paper in this volume. We are extending the studies on the same antigen in bonnet monkeys. It is also intended to purify by affinity chromatography the antigens binding with MoAb-$A_2$ and other monoclonals with properties of inhibiting the zona lysis and sperm binding to eggs.

## Concluding comments

Zona as a target for immuno-interception was an attractive proposition on the belief that antibodies directed against zona antigens would act by prevention of sperm-ovum interaction and thus provide a pre-fertilization block of fertility. Initial experimental studies in rodents and other species were encouraging and demonstrated the impairment of fertility in animals immunized with this antigen. However follow up investigations reveal the complexity of zona antigens which are composed of a variety of glycoproteins. Immunization was not bereft of undesirable consequences. A major task is to avoid reactions leading to practically the sterilization in rabbits and serious abberations of sex steroid hormonal profiles and diminished incidence of ovulation in primates. Moderate immunization of primates has no irreversable consequences and regain of fertility has been observed in course of time (Suman et. al. presentation in the symposium). Even in this study, during the period of high antibody titres, oestrogen and progesterone are markedly depressed. It is obvious that unless

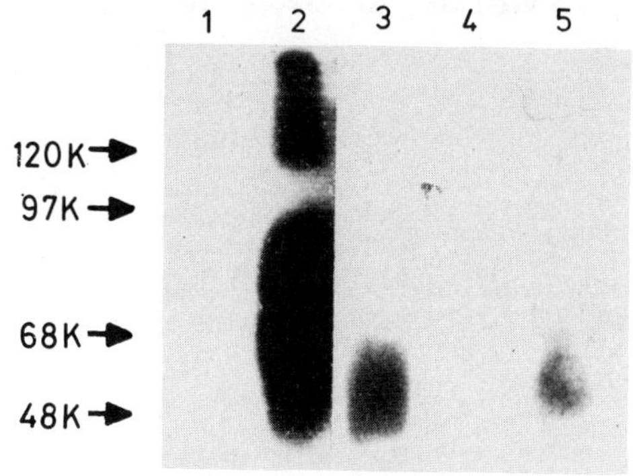


Fig.3. Western blots of heat solubilized porcine zona pellucida after 1D SDS-PAGE. (1) Normal monkey serum, (2) Monkey anti-porcine ZP (polyclonal), (3) Monkey anti-$ZP_3$ polyclonal, (4) $Sp^2/0$ ascites, (5) MoAb-$A_2$ ascites. The antibodies were put in evidence after incubation with $I^{125}$-Protein A and exposed to ORWO X-ray film at -70°C for 6-24 hrs.

dissociation can be affected between antigens capable of imparting infertility from those responsible for undesirable side effects, zona may not be a preferred antigen for birth control vaccine. This task demands molecular dissection of the mosaic of antigens comprising ZP. Molecular genetics and monoclonal antibodies provide useful approaches to determine whether the desired goal is achievable.


## Acknowledgement

This work was supported by grants from the Rockefeller Foundation and the National Coordinated project of ICMR and cooperation under Indo-US programme.


## References


1. A.G. Sacco, Immunocontraception : Consideration of the zona pellucida as a target antigen, in : "Obstetrics and Gynecology Annual", R.M. Wynn, ed., 10:1 (1981).

2. B.S. Dunbar, and D.J. Wolegemuth, Structure and function of the mammalian zona pellucida, a unique extracellular matrix, in : "Modern cell Biology". B. Satir, ed., Alan R. Liss, Inc., New York, 3 : 77 (1984).

3. C.A. Shivers, A.B. Dudkiewicz, L.E. Franklin, and E.N. Fussel, Inhibition of sperm-egg interaction by specific antibody, Science, 178 : 1211 (1972).

4. A. Garavagno, J. Posada, C. Barros, and C.A. Shivers, Some characteristics of the zona pellucida antigen in the hamster, J. Exp. Zool. 189 : 37 (1974).

5. F. Jilek, and A. Pavlok, Antibodies against mouse ovaries and their effect on fertilization in vitro and in vivo in mouse, J. Reprod. Fertil. 42 : 377 (1975).

6. R. Yanagimachi, J. Winkelhake, and G.L. Nicolson, Immunological block to mammalian fertilization : Survival and organ distribution of immunoglobulin which inhibits fertilization in vivo. Proc. Natl. Acad. Sci, USA. 73 : 2405 (1976).

7. R.J. Aitken, and D.W. Richardson, in : "Immunological aspects of reproduction and fertility control" J.P. Hearn, ed. MTP press, limited UK p. 173 (1980).

8. D.M. Wood, C. Lui, and B.S. Dunbar, Effect of alloimmunization and heteroimmunization with zonae pellucidae on fertility in rabbits, Biol. Reprod. 25 : 439 (1981).

9. C.A. Mahi-Borwn, T.T.F. Huang, and R. Yanagimachi, Infertility in bitches induced by active immunization with porcine zona pellucida, J. Exp. Zool. 222 : 89 (1982).

10. A.G. Sacco, M.G. Subramanian, E.C. Yurewicz, F.J. DeMayo, and W.R. Dekelow, Heteroimmunization of sequirrel monkeys (Saimiri schivreus) with purified porcine zona antigens (PPZA) : Immune response and biologic activity of antigserum, Fertil. Steril, 39 :350 (1983).

11. A.K. Bamezai, A. Bhattacharya, A.H. Band, Suman, G.P. Talwar, Diversity of antigenic determinants of porcine zona pellucida revealed by monoclonal antibodies, J. Biosci. 7 :105 (1985).

12. C.A. Shivers, Immunological interference with fertilization in : "Karolinska Symposium on research methods in reproductive endocrinology", 7th Symposium Immunological approaches to fertility control", p. 223 (1974).

13. H.W. Denker, Role of proteinases in implantation, Prog. Reprod. Biol. 7 : 28 (1980).

14. Z. Dickmann, Shedding of zona pellucida, Adv. Reprod. Physiol. 4 : 187 (1969).

15. A. McLaren, A note on zona pellucida in mice, Adv. Reprod. Physiol. 4 : 207 (1969).

16. A. McLaren, The fate of zona pellucida in mice, J. Embryol. Exp. Morph. 23 :1 (1970).

# AGGRESSIVE AND PROTECTIVE IMMUNOLOGICAL REACTIONS OF THE PREGNANT MOTHER TO THE CONCEPTUS

Guy André Voisin

Centre d'Immuno-Pathologie et d'Immunologie Expérimentale (INSERM U 23, UA 289 CNRS, C 12 Ass.C.Bernard; Hôp.St-Antoine 75571 Paris Cédex 12, France

In order to clearly analyze the immune processes involved in gestation, five established points must be stated and accepted from the beginning.

- Point number one : the pregnant mother has been found immunologically aware of the presence of the conceptus in each tested species.

As a consequence, she reacts specifically towards the naturally grafted semi-allogenic conceptus. However, the reaction does not result in the conceptus rejection.

- Point number two : the immune reaction mounted by the pregnant mother towards the conceptus-borne foreign antigens is clearly weaker than and different from the one induced by an allograft : it does not induce an accelerated rejection of a graft of paternal or embryonal origin ; even, on the contrary, a tumoral allograft of paternal strain (but not of an unrelated strain) may not be rejected or be rejected in a delayed way.

This indicates an efferent mechanism of decreased rejection reaction and/or a central mechanism of immune deviation from an active rejection reaction to an active favorable reaction.

- Point number three : An artificial immunization of a pregnant mother against paternal antigens injected either before or during the pregnancy induces in the mother a state of transplantation immunity (including cytotoxic T cells) resulting in an accelerated rejection of a surgical graft of paternal or embryonal origin. The *in situ* conceptus, however, remains unaffected.

This indicates the presence of an immunologically protective barrier at the interface level, especially placenta and decidua, *i.e.* an efferent protection against an established rejection reaction.

- Point number four : at each step of the maternal immune reaction, i.e. afferent induction, central reaction and efferent expression, the role of the placenta (especially the trophoblast) appears to be crucial both locally and through released substances.

- Point number five : the conceptus antigens towards which the pregnant mother reacts are conceptus-borne paternal antigens and conceptus-proper antigens.

. The conceptus-borne paternal antigens are encoded in the main histocompatibility complex (MHC) as well as in minor histocompatibility loci.

. The conceptus-proper antigens are especially the trophoblast antigens.

With these five points in mind, one may try to analyse the nature of the immune reactions of the pregnant mother towards its conceptus and the ways by which the latter is favored as compared to a conventional allograft.

A conventional allograft induces and is submitted to a complex immune reaction in which the agents of an immune rejection predominate. However, other specific agents do appear, limiting the excessive development of the rejection reaction (RR). Such regulatory agents, if they were at a high level, might protect the antigen-bearing target and even stimulate it. In the case of a conventional allograft, they are at a relatively low level and remain undetected if not specifically looked for. This protective part of the immune reaction is what we have called the facilitation reaction (FR).

The major components of the RR and the FR are as in Table 1.

Table I

IMMUNE AGENTS OF THE RR AND THE FR

| NATURE OF AGENTS | RR | FR |
|---|---|---|
| Antibodies | . Able to activate C' and/or K cells | . Not able to activate C' |
| | (some lymphocytes, monocytes, granulocytes) | . Immune complexes |
| Lymphocytes | . Tc | . Ts |
| | . $T_{DH}$ able to activate : Macrophages (MAF) NK cells ($IF_{\gamma}$) | |

It is our purpose here : first, to analyze the components of the systemic immune reaction of the mother towards the conceptus ; second to analyze the influence of the placenta (especially the trophoblast), in the balance of the component of that systemic reaction as well as the local role of the trophoblast and finally to take a look at the nature of the antigens involved.

## I - THE COMPONENTS OF THE SYSTEMIC MATERNAL IMMUNE REACTION OF THE PREGNANT MOTHER TO THE CONCEPTUS

To a certain extent, these components may be compared to the ones met in a conventional allograft (with, however, some essential differences) in that they consist in elements of rejection and elements of protection. But, at variance with the conventional allograft, here the protective elements predominate over the ones of the RR and even may prevent the induction of the effector agents - as long as the target antigens are presented in the context of the conceptus and its environment (trophoblast and gestational decidua).

A. Elements of a RR mounted by the mother towards the conceptus.

1. In mammalian normal gestation, these elements are weak and often uneasy to detect : delayed hypersensitivity to the father (Rocklin et al., 1979), secondary type of MLR reactivity (Chaouat and Voisin, 1979), ability to make an anti-paternal GVHR in H-2 compatible strains (see Voisin, 1983a) and, under favorable conditions, capacity of maternal splenocytes to transfer an accelerated graft rejection (Chaouat et al., 1980).

2. However, during normal gestation, this reaction does not spontaneously result in the formation of effector agents of alloimmune rejection : cytotoxic T cells (Chaouat et al., 1982) and C'-activating antibodies (Voisin and Chaouat, 1974 ; Chaouat et al., 1984 ; Bell and Billington, 1980).

3. Still there are cases when immune agents of the RR are elaborated by the pregnant mother : a) in natural cases of non-placental ovoviviparity in salamanders (Chateaureynaud et al., 1979) when maternal spleen cells are able to kill in vitro up to 90 % of embryonal cells. b) In experimental cases of xenogeneic gestation either hybrid as in the mules or completely xenogeneic as in the mus musculus-mus caroli embryo transfer (see Antezak and Allen, 1984 ; Clark, 1985). c) In pathological cases, usually related to spontaneous abortion.

In human gestation, CTLs seem to have been detected (N. Genetêt, personal communications) as well as cytotoxic antibodies absorbable with trophoblast (see Faulk, 1984).

More predominent are the

B. Elements of a FR mounted by the mother towards the conceptus. Such elements are made of regulatory antibodies and cells.

1. Regulatory or enhancing antibodies (especially IgG1 in the mouse) are fixed on the placenta from which they can be eluted. They are specific of the father and enhance the growth of a paternal strain tumor grafted on a maternal strain recipient (Voisin and Chaouat, 1974 ; Chaouat et al., 1980).

2. Regulatory or suppressor T lymphocytes are found in the spleens of pregnant animals. They are active in vitro in MLR (Chaouat and Voisin, 1979) and against induction of CTLs (Chaouat et al., 1982) as well as in vivo in passive transfer of enhancement (Chaouat et al., 1980). They have been found to be Thy1$^+$, Lyt2$^+$, Ia$^+$, MHC-restricted and acting through soluble factors (Chaouat and Voisin, 1981a, 1981b). These cells have some, but weak, activity in blocking effector CTLs (Chaouat et al., 1982). Both enhancing antibodies and suppressor T cells increase with parity.

3. Other signs of a beneficial action of a systemic maternal immune reactivity towards conceptus antigens have been described by several authors :

a) presence of blocking antibodies in normal gestation, often absent in spontaneous abortion (Rocklin et al., 1982, Mc Intyre and Faulk, 1983).

b) Beneficial action of immunization with allogeneic blood cells in human cases of recurrent abortion (Beer, 1984 ; Mowbray et al, 1983).

c) Experimental cases of systemic immunization of CBA/J females by BALB/c male cells, preventing them to have an abnormally high proportions of fetal resorptions after mating with DBA 2/J males (Clark, 1984 ; Chaouat et al., 1983). This success seems to be associated with an increase in non-T suppressor cell activity in the decidua and with an increase in placental factors able to inhibit NK activity (see Clark, 1985). It appears to be transferable by systemic injections of cells as well as antibodies from the immunized mice (see Wegmann, this symposium).

Therefore, various systemic immune agents, humoral and cellular, seem to be associated with the success or the failure of gestation.

## II - IMMUNOLOGICAL ROLE OF THE PLACENTA (ESPECIALLY TROPHOBLAST) IN THE SUCCESS OF GESTATION

This role appears to be crucial both in systemic and in local reactions.

A. In the systemic reaction of the mother towards the conceptus. An artificial model of systemic immune reactions akin gestation has been devised in our laboratory consisting in alloimmunizing a recipient in the presence of isogenic placental substances. This results in a state of immunomodulation of the reactions as compared to those observed in the absence of placental substances : specific abrogation of the second set accelerated rejection (Chaouat et al., 1980) and even enhancement of a specific tumoral allograft increase in T suppressor cells, with a decrease in CTLs, increase in IgG1 enhancing antibodies and decrease (or retardation) in IgG2 cytotoxic ones. Also this state of decreased rejection reactivity can be transfered both passively with serum and adoptively with spleen cells (T lymphocytes IJ$^+$) (Duc et al., 1985).

In another set of experiments, it was shown that spleen cells from CBA mice similarly treated with A/J cells plus CBA placental extracts can no longer increase the stimulation index in a local GVHR made in the foot pad of relevant hybrid mice, reducing it to almost none in a highly significant maner (Voisin et al., 1983).

Other experiments, made in vitro have shown that placental extracts or fractions decrease MLC reactivity (Chaouat et al., 1980) and CTL generation while they increase suppressor T cell generation (Duc et al., to be published).

The results of this artificial immunization are comparable to the ones observed in gestation : decrease of the agents of the RR, increase of the ones of the FR (Voisin, 1983b).

This immunodeviation capacity of trophoblast substances has been shown to apply to other antigens such as sheep red blood cells (SRBC) provided the latter are injected together with the placental substances : there is then a strong decrease in the capacity to form IgM direct plaque forming cells (PFC) due to a 40 KD factor or an increase in that capacity, due to a 60 KD factor (Bobé et al., 1984). The 40 KD factor acts through Lyt2$^+$ suppressor cells ; the 60 KD one through B lymphocytes (Bobé et al., submitted for publication in J. Immunol.). These active substances seem to be localized in the mouse spongiotrophoblast and are absent from the central labyrinth ; they may diffuse to the decidua or some be synthetized by it.

B. In the local protection of the fetus. The role of the placenta (especially the trophoblast) is crucial in many ways :

1. By building barriers (circulatory, cellular and molecular).

2. By decreasing histocompatibility antigen expression : especially class II MHC (Ia) which seem to be permanently absent. As for class I antigens, they are less expressed in general (apparently absent during nidation), but have been detected at some interface sites.

3. By specifically trapping maternal anti-conceptus antibodies, especially class I MHC antigens (Voisin and Chaouat, 1974 ; Singh et al., 1983). This has important consequences : a) the absorbed antibodies do not pass into the fetus, b) they mask the corresponding antigens and might induce antigenic modulation. c) They may act on specific passing-by lymphocytes, activating suppressor cells and inactivating effector ones.

4. By resisting the action of specific CTLs as compared to other targets (Smith, 1983).

5. By elaborating "anti-cytotoxic" substances able to non-specifically inhibit the action of CTLs, K cells acting through ADCC, NK cells and complement-mediated cytotoxicity (see Chaouat, 1984).

6. By establishing functional relations (which need to be clarified) with the maternal decidua in which it is implanted. It seems that the gestational decidua which includes isolated trophoblast cells has immunological properties (such as accepting allogeneic tissue allografts) that are not acquired by the cyclic decidua, in the absence of implantation. These functional relations, not adequately studied yet on an immunological basis, result, among other consequences, in the induction of decidual suppressor cells which are not antigen-specific, non-T, resembling small lymphocytes with cytoplasmic granules and releasing a 100 KD factor antagonizing IL2 activity (Clark et al., 1985). These suppressor cells seem in close correlation with the success of gestation both in the case of Mus caroli/mus musculus embryonal transfer system and in the CBA/J x DBA 2/J combination (Clark, 1984).

## III - NATURE OF THE ANTIGENS INVOLVED IN THE MATERNAL IMMUNE REACTIONS TO THE CONCEPTUS

several if not many antigens seem to be involved. Probably some are yet to be discovered. Their role if not clarified although several points have been more or less firmly established.

In addition to the not enough studied passage in the mother's circulation of fetal cells, the involved antigens are present on (or released by) the placenta (trophoblast). They are of two different kinds : allotypic and organ-specific.

A. Allotypic antigens (with variable degrees of polymorphism) are of three types :

1. MHC antigens, highly polymorphic. Class II antigens are believed not to be expressed at all at the interface, in spite of the existence of anti-Ia-like anti-

bodies described during pregnancy. Class I antigens are puzzlingly expressed at the interface : not at all times, not at all sites, in low density and, possibly, not even with the usual presentation.

These class I antigens are the ones we have met in the mouse and which have allowed us to draw a scheme of systemic immune regulation in particular during gestation. This scheme is valid for other antigens such as minor transplantation antigens (Voisin et al., 1983) and, artificially, for xenoantigens such as sheep red blood cells (Bobé et al., 1984).

2. MHC-linked allotypic antigens are much less polymorphic and of great potential interest. The main trophoblast antigens of that kind are those of the TLX system described in the human species (Faulk and McIntyre, 1983). The Pa antigens of the rat may be an equivalent (Gill, 1983). These antigens behave as class I MHC antigens with restricted specificities shared by many individuals and raise fascinating questions : are they related to the Qa or, conceivably, the T locus (or equivalent) ? Are they modified, less polymorphic expressions of MHC class I antigens ? Have they intrinsic properties allowing them to preferentially induce a protective immune response of the facilitation reaction type (i.e. enhancing antibodies and suppressor cells) ?

3. MHC-independent allotypic antigens also are of great potential interest, especially minor histocompatibility loci antigens.

BALB/c and DBA 2 are two strains of mice of the same $H\text{-}2^d$ haplotype. BALB/c spleen cells do not induce detectable GVHR either systemic in DBA 2 newborns or local in the popliteal lymph nodes of (BALB/c x DBA 2)F1 hybrids, unless BALB/c have been preimmunized with DBA 2 cells or, to a much lesser, but significant, extent if BALB/c are pregnant of DBA 2 (see Voisin, 1983a). On the other hand, if the BALB/c preimmunization to DBA 2 cells has been done in the presence of BALB/c placental extract, the induced capacity of BALB/c cells to mount a GVHR is inhibited either completely in local GVHR or to a great extent in systemic one (Voisin et al., 1983).

Another example is given in the CBA/J pregnant of DBA 2/J when spontaneous fetal resorptions are prevented by BALB/c male immunization (Chaouat et al., 1983 ; Clark, 1984), while immunization with DBA 2 male cells may lead to increased resorptions (Clark, 1985).

These various experiments show the importance of the response to minor histocompatibility loci antigens by the pregnant mother in the issue of gestation.

B. Organ specific antigens, apparently monomorphic. After having been established, homozygous strains of mice do reproduce normally. If the pregnant mothers react immunologically to their isogenic conceptus, this reaction is to be non-allotypic, of an "organ-specific" type (in a broad sense).

Actually, while we have seen (Voisin and Chaouat, 1984 ; Chaouat et al., 1980) anti-H-2 antibodies (enhancing IgG1 fixed on the placentae of semi-allogeneic pregnancies), there was also a degree of fixation of immunoglobulins on the spongiotrophoblast of isogenic pregnancies. These immunoglobulins were devoid of H-2 specificities and are presumed to be anti-trophoblast as such. Evidence increase that antibodies directed to trophoblast or embryo-specific antigens (and presumably differentiation) antigens exist in normal pregnancies both in the mouse (Hull, 1984) and in the human species (Davies, 1985).

On the other hand, we know from previous work of our and other laboratories that organ-specific autoantigens may give rise to a rejection type of reaction and that this may be prevented and counteracted by manipulation of the facilitation reaction (Voisin, 1971, 1980).

All the preceding facts point :

1. to the richness and regulated balance of the pregnant mother immune reactions towards (and not against) the conceptus, some of them being aggressive, more being protective and even enhancing.

2. to the crucial role of placenta (especially the trophoblast) in inducing a favorable (protection and stimulation) type of immune reaction as well as in organizing local defenses.

## REFERENCES


Antczak, D.F. and Allen, W.R., 1984, Invasive trophoblast in the genus equus. Ann. Immunol. (Inst. Pasteur), 135D:325.

Beer, A.E., 1984, How did your mother not reject you ?, Ann. Immunol. (Inst.Pasteur), 135D:315.

Bell, S.C. and Billington, W.D., 1980, Major anti-paternal alloantibody induced by murine pregnancy is non-complement-fixing IgG1, Nature (Lond), 288:387.

Bobé, P., Doric, M., Kinsky, R.G. and Voisin, G.A., 1984, Modulation of mouse anti-SRBC antibody response by placental extracts, Cell. Immunol., 89:355.

Chaouat, G., Chaffaux, S., Duchet-Suchaux, M. and Voisin, G.A., 1980, Immunoactive products of mouse placenta. I - Immuno-suppressive effects of crude and water soluble extracts, J. Reprod. Immunol., 2:127.

Chaouat, G.,Kiger, N., Kolb, J.P., Stanislawski, M. and Wegmann, T.G., 1985, Immunological consequences of vaccination against abortion in mice, J. Immunol., 134:1594.

Chaouat, G., Kiger, N. and Wegmann, T.G., 1983, Vaccination against spontaneous abortion in mice., J. Reprod. Immunol, 5:389.

Chaouat, G., Kolb, J.P. and Rivière, M., 1984, Role of the placental interface and of trophoblast/maternal tissue interactions in the survival of the murine foetal allograft, Ann. Immunol. (Inst. Pasteur),, 135D:302.

Chaouat, G., Monnot, P., Hoffmann, M. and Voisin, G.A., 1982, Regulatory T cells in pregnancy. VI - Evidence for T-cell mediated suppression of CTL generation towards paternal alloantigens, Cell. Immunol., 68:322.

Chaouat, G. and Voisin, G.A., 1979, Regulatory T cell subpopulations in pregnancy. I - Evidence for suppressive activity of the early phase of MLR,J.Immunol. 122:1383.

Chaouat, G. and Voisin, G.A., 1981a, Regulatory T cells in pregnancy. IV - Genetic characteristics and mode of action of early MLR suppressive T cells populations, J. Immunol., 127:1335.

Chaouat, G. and Voisin, G.A., 1981b, Regulatory T cells in pregnancy. V - Allopregnancy induced T cell suppressor factor is H-2 restricted and bears Ia determinants, Cell. Immunol., 62:186.

Chaouat, G., Voisin, G.A., Escalier, D. and Robert, P., 1979, Facilitation reaction (enhancing antibodies and suppressor cells) and rejection reaction (sensitized cells) from the mother to the paternal antigens of the conceptus, Clin.exp.Immunol., 35:13.

Chateaureynaud-Duprat, P., Badet, M.-T. and Voisin, G.A., 1979, Antagonistic immune reactions (rejection and facilitation) to the embryo in the urodele amphibian salamandra salamandra Lin, J. Reprod. Immunol., 1:47.

Clark, D.A., 1984, Local suppressor cells and the success or failure of the "foetal allograft", Ann. Immunol. (Inst. Pasteur), 135D:321.

Clark, D.A., 1985, Materno-fetal relations. Review, Immunol. Lett., 9:239.

Clark, D.A., Chaput, A., Walker, C. and Rosenthal, K.L., 1985, Active suppression of host-vs-graft disease in pregnant mice. VII - Soluble suppressor activity obtained from decidua of allopregnant mice blocks the response to IL2, J. Immunol., 134:1659.

Davies, M., 1985, An ELISA for the detection of maternal anti-trophoblast antibodies in human pregnancy, J. Immunol. Meth., 77:109.

Duc, H.T., Massé, A., Bobé, P., Kinsky, R.G. and Voisin, G.A., 1985, Deviation of humoral and cellular alloimmune reactions by placental extracts, J. Reprod. Immunol., 7:27.

Faulk, W.P., 1984, Humoral keystones in the gestational voussoir, Ann. Immunol. (Inst. Pasteur), 135D:319.

Faulk, W.P. and McIntyre, I.A., 1983, Immunologic studies of human trophoblast : markers, subsets and functions, Immunol. Lett., 75:139.

Gill, T.J. III, 1984, Speculations on the transplantation biology of the maternal-fetal interface, Ann. Immunol (Inst. Pasteur), 135D:307.

Hull, S., 1984, Anti-fetal antibody response in syngeneic pregnancy. B. Sc. thesis, University of Bristol. (Cited in W.D. Billington, Ann. Immunol. (Inst. Pasteur), 1984, 135D:331).

McIntyre, I.A. and Faulk, W.P., 1983, Recurrent spontaneous abortion in human pregnancy : results of immunogenetical, cellular and humoral studies, Amer. J. Reprod. Immunol., 4:165.

Mowbray, J.F., Gibbings, C.R., Sidgwick, A.J., Ruszkiewicz, M. and Beard, R.W., 1983, Effects of transfusion in women with recurrent spontaneous abortion, Transplant. Proc., 15:896.

Rocklin, R.E., Kitzmiller, J.L. and Garvoy, M.R., 1982, Maternal fetal relation. II - Further characterization of an immunologic blocking factor that develops during pregnancy, Clin. Immunol. Immunopath., 22:305.

Rocklin, R.E., Kitzmiller, J.L. and Kaye, M.D., 1979, Immunobiology of the maternal fetal relationship, Annu. Rev. Med., 30:375.

Singh, B., Raghupathy, R., Anderson, D. and Wegmann, T.G., 1983, The placenta as an immunological barrier between mother and fetus, in "Immunology of Reproduction", T.G. Wegmann and T.J. Gill, eds, Oxford University Press., London.

Smith, G., 1983, In vitro susceptibility of murine placental trophoblast to cytotoxic effector cells, J. Reprod. Immunol., 5:39.

Voisin, G.A., 1971, Immunological facilitation, a broadening of the concept of enhancement phenomenon, Progr. Allergy, 15:328.

Voisin, G.A., 1980, Role of antibody classes in the regulatory facilitation reaction. in "Regulation of the immune response by antibodies against the immunogen", Immunol. Rev., 49:3.

Voisin, G.A., 1983a, Immunological interventions of the placenta in maternal immunological tolerance to the foetus, in "Immunology of Reproduction", T.G. Wegmann and T.J. Gill III, eds, Oxford University Press, London.

Voisin, G.A., 1983b, Enhancing antibodies and suppressor cells in pregnancy : role of the placentation, in "Reproductive Immunology", S. Isojima and W.D. Billington, eds, Elsevier Sciences Publ., Amsterdam.

Voisin, G.A. and Chaouat, G., 1974, Demonstration, nature and properties of antibodies fixed on maternal placenta and directed against paternal antigens, J. Reprod. Fertil, Suppl. 21:89.

Voisin, J., Kinsky, R.G. and Voisin, G.A., 1983, Immunodepressive action of placental extracts on allo-immunisation as tested by graft-versus-host reactions (GVHR) in non H-2 histoincompatible strains. In "5th Int. Congress of Immunology", Kyoto, abstract 310-09.

# EFFECTS OF ANTIBODIES TO STEROID HORMONES ON REPRODUCTIVE EVENTS OF SHEEP AND CATTLE

R.M. Hoskinson, R.J. Scaramuzzi, B.K. Campbell,
J.A. Downing, R.J. Welch and B.E. Harrison

C.S.I.R.O, Division of Animal Production
P.O. Box 239, Blacktown, N.S.W., Australia

## INTRODUCTION

This paper is concerned with the effect of androgen immunity on the expression of ovulation rate in the two important domestic ruminants, sheep and cattle. In the case of sheep the paper will review the development of a commercial vaccine (Fecundin®; Polyandroalbumin, Glaxo (Australia) Pty. Ltd.) which increases the numbers of lambs born to treated ewes. In the case of cattle, three experiments that have explored the ovulation rate response to active androgen immunity will be reported. The data will allow for some important comparisons to be made between the two species.

The importance of increasing ovulation rates and lambing percentages as a means of improving the efficiency of sheep production has been widely recognised for many years. Numerous practices have been advocated as a means of achieving this objective including: (i) the skilful management of feeding; (ii) cross breeding programs that utilize maternal heterosis and (iii) hormonal preparations such as pregnant mare serum gonadotrophin (PMSG). While the efficacy of such methods cannot be questioned, none can be regarded as the ideal method of enhancing reproductive efficiency.

While with cattle we believe that the efficiency of beef production would be significantly enhanced by a method that could routinely increase calving rates, there is not universal agreement that this is likely or desirable. The incidence of twin calving in cattle is around 3-5% (Labhsetwar et al., 1963; Scanlon et al., 1973) and there is a belief that if this figure were increased then farmers would be confronted with significant birth-related management problems. This rather pessimistic view is not supported by studies of twin-calving in cattle by non-surgical embryo transfer where twinning rates of 41 percent (Sreenan et al., 1981) and 49 percent (Renard et al., 1979) have been recorded.

## CRITICAL STAGES IN THE DEVELOPMENT OF FECUNDIN® VACCINE FOR INCREASING LAMBING PERCENTAGES IN BREEDING EWES

In 1977 it was reported (Scaramuzzi et al., 1977) that chronic androstenedione immunity in the Welsh Mountain ewe induced a significantly increased ovulation rate. There was a narrow distribution of the additional ovulations between ewes and the length of the oestrous cycle remained unaffected. The possibility now existed for the development of an endocrine-directed vaccine for increasing reproductive efficiency of sheep based on an antibody-mediated increase in lambing percentage.

Of course it had to be demonstrated that the additional eggs shed in response to the effects of anti-androstenedione antibody were functional and that the immune ewe could carry her litter to term. The first such study on a small group of ewes (Van Look et al., 1978) suggested that there was no improvement in lambing percentage despite an increased ovulation rate. Nevertheless, these early results were sufficiently encouraging to justify the conducting of large scale trials to evaluate the practical potential of these findings.

### The "Window of Immunity" Notion

During early investigations it became apparent that the reproductive response to steroid immunity in the ewe was critically dependent upon the mean level of immunity established in the flock (Martin et al., 1979; Cox et al., 1982). Table 1 summarizes data from two separate studies that illustrate this effect. It is emphasized that these were separate experiments in Merino ewes that otherwise differed in respect of antigens used, location and year. Despite this large between-experiment variance, the data illustrate reproductive effects that are observed at low and high levels of antibody titre.

A Note About Antibody Titre. For the most part antibody titres reported here have been measured and defined essentially as described by Abraham (1974). Individual values shown in the Tables are group mean reciprocal steroid-binding antibody titres.

At low antibody titres (around 1:100) it was possible to increase flock ovulation rate without affecting the proportion of ewes that mate and then subsequently produce lambs. However, in such experiments the gain in ovulation rate in immunized flocks was relatively small and at lambing there were no effects on litter size or on total lamb production.

In contrast, at high antibody titres (around 1:30,000) a highly significant increase in ovulation rate was observed in the Merino, in agreement with the initial observations on the Welsh Mountain ewe (Scaramuzzi et al., 1977). Additionally, however, the expression of oestrous behaviour was significantly depressed so that fewer ewes mated. Of those that did mate, a significant proportion failed to deliver a lamb, thereby suggesting a diminished ability of the highly immune Merino to either establish or maintain pregnancy. Of the highly immune Merinos that did deliver lambs, there was a significant increase in litter size compared to untreated ewes but this gain was offset by an increased proportion of barren ewes in the flock of treated ewes.

Taken together, these data pointed to the probability that somewhere between mean flock anti-androstenedione antibody titres of 1:100 and 1:30,000 there was a range of titres that would stimulate ovulation rate but be without a deleterious effect on behavioural

Table 1. Reproductive Responses in Merino Ewe Flocks Having Disparate Levels of Androstenedione Immunity

| | Low-titre study | | High-titre study | |
|---|---|---|---|---|
| | Untreated | Immune | Untreated | Immune |
| N | 39 | 43 | 50 | 50 |
| Titre at mating | - | 100 | - | 30,000 (6,000)§ |
| Oestrus (%) | 77 | 78 | 98 | 78** |
| Ovulation rate | 1.11 | 1.30 * | 1.36 | 1.87* |
| No. of ewes with: | | | | |
| 1 CL | 33 | 29 | 32 | 13 |
| 2 CL | 4 | 10 | 18 | 28 |
| >3 CL | - | 1 | - | 6 |
| Ewes lambed (%) | 87 | 86 | 92 | 58*** |
| No. of ewes with: | | | | |
| 1 lamb | 32 | 31 | 33 | 14 |
| 2 lambs | 2 | 6 | 13 | 15 |
| Lambs born | 36 | 43 | 59 | 44 |
| Lambs born per ewe joined | 0.92 | 1.00 | 1.18 | 0.88* |

*$P<0.05$; **$P<0.01$; ***$P<0.001$ (in each case the immune group is compared with its corresponding control)
§Standard error.

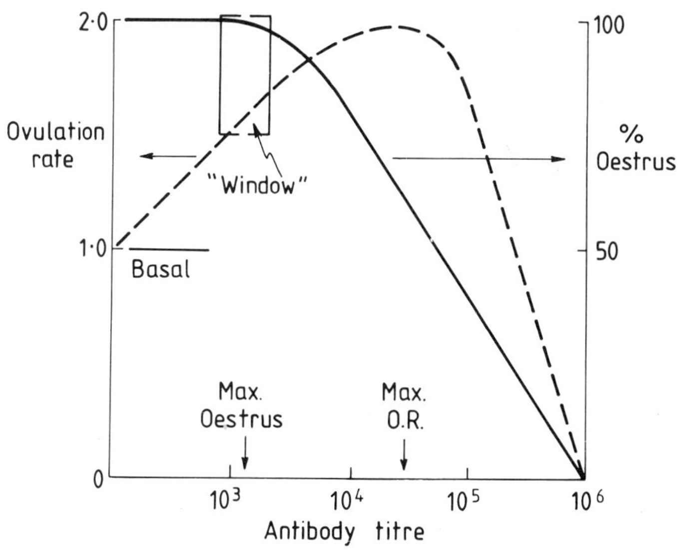


Figure 1. Qualitative effects of anti-androstenedione antibody titre on ovulation rate and oestrus in Merino ewes.

oestrus. We came to regard this critical range of titres as a "window of immunity" which flocks would have to achieve at mating before an increase in lambing percentage due to immunization could be realized.

Recognition of the dimensions of the "window" came about from an appreciation of the independent effects of antibody titre on the ovulatory and oestrus responses.

Figure 1 illustrates that in response to increasing flock antibody titres ovulation rate rises from basal values, reaches a maximum and then declines to sub-basal values as a steadily increasing proportion of the flock become anovulatory. Oestrous behaviour is initially unaffected but eventually commences to decline continuously in response to rising titres. However, the figure is to be interpreted in a qualitative sense only because an exact determintion of the relationships depicted, over a broad titre range, has never been undertaken. The important feature of Fig. 1 is its demonstration that the critical titre "window" is located over a relatively narrow titre range where ovulation rate is still increasing and oestrus expression is maximal.

By empirical experimentation extending over several years, the titre "window" for the Merino ewe was found to be in the range 1:500 to 1:3,000. Table 2 illustrates the reproductive gain achieved in a Merino flock having its mean titre controlled to lie within the "window".

Under these conditions oestrus was unaffected and ovulation rate was increased. The litter size (lambs born per ewe lambing) was increased and the total number of lambs born to the flock of immunized ewes was also increased.

Table 2. Reproductive responses in Merino ewes having a Controlled Level of Androstenedione Antibody Titre.

| Variable | Untreated Flock | Immune Flock |
|---|---|---|
| N | 49 | 50 |
| Titre at mating | - | 1,600 (300)§ |
| Oestrus (%) | 100 | 100 |
| Ovulation rate | 1.45 | 1.86** |
| No. of ewes with: | | |
| 1CL | 27 | 13 |
| 2CL | 22 | 34 |
| >3CL | - | 3 |
| Ewes lambed (%) | 94 | 94 |
| No. of ewes with: | | |
| 1 lamb | 31 | 20 |
| 2 lambs | 15 | 27 |
| Lambs born | 61 | 74 |
| Lambs born per ewe joined | 1.25 | 1.48** |

**P<0.01

§ Standard error.

Of importance to the commercial application of androstenedione immunity to increase lambing percentages is the fact that the increased reproductive response can be confined largely to an increase in the number of ewes producing twins at the expense of single-born lambs. Thus the increase in the number of lambs born can be confined to a litter size that can be managed by the ewe.

## Vaccine Formulation

There exists a great body of knowledge, dealing with many aspects of steroid immunity in animals, using steroid : protein conjugates together with an immunoadjuvant (for a relevant review see Scaramuzzi and Hoskinson, 1984). Rarely, if ever, has there been a requirement to confer a controlled degree of immunity on a population such as is required by the "window" applicable to these lambing studies (Figure 1).

Accumulating data suggested that increases in ovulation rate and lambing percentage could be achieved with either androgen or oestrogen immunity (Smith et al., 1981; Cox et al., 1982). Furthermore other data suggested that the steroid derivative used to form the steroid protein conjugate was not critical to the enhancement of ovulation rate (Hoskinson et al. 1981). Ultimately, the androstenedione derivative reported by Lindner et al. (1972) was used to form androstenedione-7αcarboxyethylthioether:human serum albumin as the immunogenic component of the vaccine. This conjugate can be synthesized readily by a route that starts from androstenedione. It has the characteristic that it provokes androstenedione-specific antibody (Lindner et al., 1972).

The immunoadjuvant selected for the vaccine was DEAE-dextran (Wittman 1970; Cox and Wilson, 1976). This polycation has numerous advantages for use in a vaccine to create short-term immunity, that include:

(i) a relatively weak primary response;

(ii) a secondary response that fades rapidly from peak values (Anderson et al., 1971) and,

(iii) anamnestic characteristics which determine that annual boosts in sensitized animals restore a level of immunity similar to the initial secondary response.

Other polyelectrolytes that have been investigated and found unsatisfactory (R.M. Hoskinson and R.J. Scaramuzzi, unpublished data) include alginic acid, dextran sulfate and polyethyleneimine. A synthetic styrene-maleic anhydride copolymer was of marginal efficacy (M.S.F. Wong et al., submitted for publication).

The vaccine comprising steroid:HSA immunogen and DEAE-dextran is a clear solution effective when administered sub-cutaneously; it induces a transient and very slight local reaction.

## Development of the Vaccination Process to Increase Lambing Percentages in Breeding Ewes

The useful feature of the process to be described here is that it can be applied to non-synchronized flocks kept under extensive farm management conditions. Two important factors that facilitated the development of such a process are:

(i) the titre "window" to be achieved occurs at a relatively low level of immunity;

(ii) the magnitude of the secondary response to the DEAE-dextran based vaccine can be predetermined to some degree by variations in the interval between primary and booster vaccinations.

Figure 2 illustrates schematically how the vaccine is used in practice. Previously untreated ewes are given a primary followed by a booster vaccination 3-4 weeks later. In response to the boost, androstenedione antibody titres rise to peak values and promptly commence to decline. At this time (3-4 weeks post-boost) rams are introduced to the flock and are kept with the ewes for 5-6 weeks in the usual manner. Throughout the breeding period antibody titres in the flock continue to decline through the "window" thereby provoking optimum ovarian stimulation. Throughout the pregnancy androstenedione immunity continues to decline till at lambing only very low titres can be measured in the ewes. In succeeding years a single booster vaccination restores antibody titres and allows the process to be repeated.

Using this process farm trials were conducted in Australia and New Zealand (Scaramuzzi et al., 1983; Geldard, 1984; Geldard et al., 1984). The trials showed that immunization of ewes with Fecundin® increased the number of lambs born by an average of 18 (Merino), 25 (Corriedale), 31 (Border Leicester x Merino) or 40 (Romney-cross) lambs per 100 ewes treated. The economic advantage of achieving these gains in lambing percentages is clearly dependent on commercial considerations; certainly, there now is proof that a substantial part of the ovulation rate gain due to androstenedione immunity in the ewe can be expressed as lambs born.

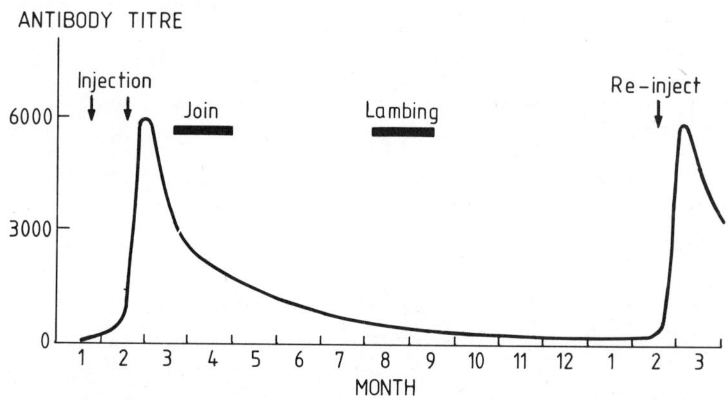


Figure 2. Schematic illustration of the application of the vaccination process to an extensive sheep breeding enterprise using non-synchronized flocks.

No attempt will be made here to elaborate on the many factors known to affect the lambing response to Fecundin® vaccine. Major determinants are: (i) any departure from the nominated vaccination protocol which could leave the breeding flock outside the titre "window"; (ii) bodyweight of the ewe at mating; (iii) breed of ewe; and (iv) the ovulation rate of the flock before treatment. In this respect flocks that are not already yielding at least 70-80 lambs per 100 mated ewes are probably unsuitable because of pre-existing limits to reproduction which Fecundin® will not alleviate. Likewise, flocks already yielding about 170 lambs per 100 mated ewes may also be unsuited because such flocks are likely to produce an increasing proportion of triplets in response to the vaccination.

In this mini review, justice has not been done to the studies of others involving reproductive effects of active (Gibb et al., 1981; Gibb et al., 1982) or passive (Land et al., 1982) steroid immunity in the ewe; nor have mechanistic effects of the immunity on ovarian function been considered (Scaramuzzi, 1979; Scaramuzzi and Hoskinson, 1984; Webb, Land, Pathiraja and Morris, 1984). However, to allow a subsequent comparison with androgen-immune cattle it should be stated that androgen immunity in the ewe has marked effects on the patterns of LH secretion; these patterns are believed to result from disruption of negative feedback mechanisms. During the breeding season mean and basal LH levels were increased by androgen immunity. Pulse frequency was increased during the luteal but not the follicular phase of the oestrous cycle in response to androstenedione antibodies (Scaramuzzi and Hoskinson, 1984). Basal levels, pulse frequency and pulse amplitude of LH were also increased in testosterone-immune ewes (Martensz, Scaramuzzi and Van Look, 1979).

Preliminary investigations of embryo survival in androstenedione-immune ewes suggest that under some circumstances the immunity can result in depressed embryo survival and egg recovery rates (Boland et al., 1984).

## STUDIES OF REPRODUCTIVE RESPONSES IN ANDROGEN-IMMUNE CATTLE

Publications dealing with steroid immunity in cattle have been variously concerned with oestrous cyclicity (Martin et al., 1978), enhancement of ovulation and calving rates (Wise and Schanbacher, 1983), effects on growth rates (Wise and Ferrell, 1984) or enhancement of spermatogenesis in bull calves (Walker et al., 1984). In each case relatively low levels of antibody titre were reported. There appears to be a considerable need to develop protocols for vaccinating cattle against steroid hormones to provide a much broader range of titre responses for application to physiological studies.

Reported here are three experiments concerning the development of androgen immunity in cattle and its effect on oestrus and ovulation. The overall objective has been to explore the potential for a steroid vaccine to stimulate ovulation and calving rates in cattle. It has been assumed that a vaccine with immunogenicity substantially greater than that of Fecundin® would be required because , compared to sheep, cattle show poor immunological responses to the hapten of conventional steroid:protein conjugates.

## Experiment 1: Comparison of the Antibody Responses of Four Androgen : Protein Conjugates and their Effects on the Ovulatory Cycles of Friesian Heifers

The following four immunogens were prepared for this study:

Immunogen 1: Testotsterone-3CMO:human serum albumin (T:HSA) was prepared by the diimide method (Lindner et al., 1972) using tetrahydrofuran as the solvent for steroid activation. Proportions of reactants were testosterone-3CMO (1.0 mM), ethyl dimethylaminopropyl carbodiimide hydrochloride (ECDI 1.0 mM) and human serum albumin (HSA, 0.0056 mM). Conjugation occurred in phosphate buffer (0.05 M, pH 7.8) over 16 hrs at ambient temperature. The tetrahydrofuran was evaporated from the reaction mixture under reduced pressure at 40°C. The residue, comprising both soluble and insoluble products, was lyophilized.

Immunogen 2: Testosterone-3CMO:ovalbumin (T:oval) was prepared by conjugation of the N-hydroxysuccinimide ester of the steroid acid (Horoda et al., 1979) in dimethylformamide with ovalbumin dissolved in 0.05 M phosphate buffer (pH 7.8). Proportions of reactants were: testosterone-3CMO (2.0 mM) and ovalbumin (0.02 mM). Conjugtion occurred over 16 hours at ambient temperature. By-products and buffer salts were removed by dialysis and the lyophilized product contained 21 moles steroid per mole protein.

Immunogen 3: Androstenedione-7α-carboxyethylthioether:human serum albumin (A:HSA) was made similarly to immunogen 1 in dioxan-0.05 M phosphate buffer (1:1 pH 7.8). Proportions of reactants were: steroid acid (0.75 mM) ECDI (0.75 mM) and HSA (0.0055 mM). The conjugate was purified by dialysis and the lyophilized product contained 22 moles steroid per mole HSA.

Immunogen 4: Androstenedione-7-α-carboxyethylthioether:thyroglobulin (porcine) ($A:T_g$) was made similarly to immunogen 1 in tetrahydrofuran-0.05 M phosphate buffer (pH 7.8). Proportions of reactants were androstenedione-7α-carboxyethylthioether (1 mM), ECDI (1 mM) and protein (0.00065 mM). By-products and buffer salts were removed by dialysis and the lyophilized product contained 68 moles steroid per mole protein.

Table 3. Anti-Tetosterone Antibody Titres Occurring in Friesian Heifers

| Day | Immunization Treatment | Antibody titre* with: | |
|---|---|---|---|
| | | T:HSA | T:oval |
| 0 | Primary | - | - |
| 98 | Boost | 3,500 ( 890)§ | 300 ( 50) |
| 105 | | 21,000 (2,900) | 7,600 (4,600) |
| 131 | | 17,000 (4,200) | 6,300 (4,700) |
| 198 | Boost | 3,600 (1,500) | 140 ( - ) |
| 205 | | 5,100 (2,100) | 1,650 ( 340) |
| 224 | Boost | 3,000 (1,500) | 540 ( 150) |
| 236 | | 4,300 (2,000) | 860 ( 220) |
| 242 | | 3,000 (1,300) | 540 ( 170) |

*Mean reciprocal values
§Bracketed values are standard errors.

Table 4. Anti-Androstenedione Antibody Titres Occurring in Friesian Heifers

| Day | Immunization Treatment | Antibody titre* with: | |
|---|---|---|---|
| | | A:HSA | A:Tg |
| 0 | Primary | | |
| 98 | Boost | 50 ( - ) | 600 ( 200)§ |
| 105 | | 2,000 ( 900) | 8,600 (5,700) |
| 131 | | 450 ( 270) | 1,800 (1,350) |
| 198 | Boost | 110 ( 60) | 298 ( 180) |
| 205 | | 2,700 (1,800) | 4,100 (2,500) |
| 224 | Boost | 640 ( 460) | 2,500 (1,400) |
| 236 | | 780 ( 480) | 5,400 (1,850) |
| 242 | | 350 ( 190) | 3,970 (1,200) |

*Mean reciprocal values
§Bracketed values are standard errors.

Experimental Procedure. Heifers (5 per group) were immunized with conjugate (equivalent to 15 mg protein) in an emulsion of Freund's complete adjuvant (6 ml, containing added Arlacel 80 comprising 10% of the oil phase volume), subcutaneously at 3 sites on each side of the neck (day 0). Booster treatments of the same type and by the same routes were given on days 98, 198 and 224 post-primary. Serum for antibody titre measurement was obtained on 8 occasions throughout the treatment period. Laparoscopy under pentothal anaesthesia by the mid-ventral route (Holland et al., 1981) was performed on days 139, 191 and 217 post-primary immunization. Control heifers (7 per group) were untreated.

Results and Discussion. Tables 3 and 4 summarize the antisteroid antibody titres determined throughout the experimental period. In each case there was a small primary and a marked secondary response that declined to about 20% of peak values within 40-100 days. The antibody response to a third or fourth vaccination with any of the steroid: albumin conjugates was poor and failed to restore peak secondary levels of antibody titre. The androstenedione thyroglobulin conjugate was marginally more effective than the corresponding albumin conjugate (A:HSA).

Throughout the experiment 81 ovulatory cycles were examined at laparoscopy. Table 5 shows that overall the main effect of steroid immunity was to increase the number of anovulatory cycles and

Table 5. Summary of Ovulation Responses in Steroid-Immune Friesian Heifers

| Immunity | Total Obser-vations | Distribution of CL§ | | | Mean Ovulation Rate# |
|---|---|---|---|---|---|
| | | 0 | 1 | 2 | |
| Testosterone | 30 | 10 | 17 | 3 | 0.77* |
| Androstenedione | 30 | 11 | 18 | 1 | 0.67** |
| Control | 21 | 2 | 19 | 0 | 0.90 |

§Corpora lutea; #Based on all cows;
*P=0.04; **P=0.02.

significantly depress the mean ovulation rate in the treated heifers.

All immunised heifers responded with local reactions to the vaccination that ranged from mild to severe granuloma development. There were no ulcerative reactions and eventually all reactions regressed.

Analysis of the mean antibody titres (Table 6) in the immune heifers established that these values in the anovulatory animals were greater than those shedding a single egg per ovulatory cycle. However, the difference in mean titres of these two groups of heifers was comparatively small.

This study has provided useful information about: (i) the kinds of steroid-protein conjugates that will yield steroid-specific antibodies in cattle; (ii) the general profile of antibody production in response to a sequence of vaccinations and (iii) preliminary data on the effect of steroid antibodies on the ovulatory cycles of dairy-breed heifers.

From the viewpoint of antigen performance the most promising development derives from the use of the testosterone-3-CMO:HSA conjugate. This conjugate was used in a crude, unpurified form which would be expected to consist of buffer salts, non-immunogenic steroid derivatives as well as steroid protein conjugate. Our purpose was to test the idea that such a crude product could enhance the immune response by local irritation. Whether this effect actually occurred is unknown but certainly the unpurified (non-dialysed) testosterone-3-CMO:HSA conjugate gave significantly greater antibody titres than any of the other three dialysed conjugates studied. To form a stable emulsion of the unpurified testosterone conjugate in Freund's complete adjuvant, it was necessary to increase the Arlacel concentration, an expedient which may have contributed to the tissue reaction to vaccination.

Others have reported (Walker et al., 1984) that cattle do not continue to respond substantially to sequential boosts with a steroid: albumin conjugate. This characteristic of cattle has particular significance to studies of ovulation rate enhancement by steroid immunity. To observe effects on ovarian morphology under conditions of maximum antibody titre it is necessary to observe the ovary at approximately 3-4 weeks following the second in a sequence of two vaccinations. Subsequent boosting with the same antigen will not

Table 6. Mean Antibody Titre and Ovulation Status in Steroid-Immune Friesian Heifers

| Immunity | Titre in Heifers:# | | |
|---|---|---|---|
| | Anovulatory | Single CL§ | Twin CL |
| Testosterone | 6,200** (±2,000) | 1,700 (±600) | 13,000 (±8,200) |
| Androstenedione | 2,100* (±1,100) | 438 (±215) | 630 |

Testosterone: **$P<0.01$ (anovulars vs single);
Androstenedione: *$P<0.05$ (anovular vs single);
§Corpora lutea;
#Reciprocal mean values ± SEM.

restore the antibody titre prevailing at this time. There is a report that a change in the carrier protein does restore peak antibody titres in response to post-secondary boosts (Walker et al., 1984). Clearly, there is much to be learnt about the profiles of antibody response that can be achieved in steroid-immune cattle.

It is notable that in the present experiment the principal response of the ovary to steroid immunity was to become anovulatory rather than to shed an increased number of eggs per ovulatory cycle.

## Experiment 2. Androgen Immunity in Hereford Cattle and Effects on Oestrus and Ovulatory Cycles

Experimental Procedure. Conjugates used for this study were testosterone-3-CMO:HSA and androstenedione-7α-carboxyethylthioether:HSA prepared by the method of immunogen 1 (experiment 1).

Mature multiparous Hereford cows (liveweight (488.2 kg; range 356-634 kg) were vaccinated with an unpurified testosterone-3-CMO:HSA conjugate (N=20) or a comparable unpurified androstenedione-7α-carboxyethylthioether:HSA conjugate (N=9) or were untreated controls (N=18). Conjugates (equivalent to 15 mg protein) were given in Freund's complete adjuvant as in experiment 1. The protocol consisted of primary immunization (day 0), boost (day 91), oestrus synchronization using PRIDS® (Abbott Pty.Ltd.) without the attached oestrogen capsule, days 98 to 110 and administration of 500 μg of a prostaglandin analogue Estrumate®, [ICI (Aust.) Pty. Ltd.] on day 110 followed by oestrus detection commencing on day 110 using Kamar® (Kamar Inc., Steamboat Springs Co., U.S.A.) heat mount detectors and laparoscopy on day 123.

During the induced oestrous cycle, 5 each of control, androstenedione-immune and testosterone-immune cattle were fitted with indwelling jugular catheters, and serially bled at 15 min. intervals for 6 hours during mid-luteal (day 14 after oestrus) and follicular phases (24-30 h after prostaglandin analogue injection) of the cycle. The plasma was used for measurements of LH using an heterologous sheep double antibody radioimmunoassay (Martensz et al., 1976) with NIH-LH-B5 as a standard. Mean values for LH pulse frequency LH pulse amplitude and basal LH concentrations were derived from the LH data.

Results and Discussion. Table 7 shows that the effect of the testosterone immunity in the Hereford cows was to significantly depress both ovulation rate and the expression of oestrous behaviour when compared to untreated control cattle.

Androstenedione immunity was without effect.

Table 7. Ovulation and Oestrus Responses in Androgen-Immune Hereford Cattle

| Immunity | N | No. of CL | | | Ovulation Rate§ | % Oestrus |
|---|---|---|---|---|---|---|
| | | 0 | 1 | 2 | | |
| Testosterone | 20 | 9 | 11 | - | 0.55* | 60** |
| Androstenedione | 9 | - | 8 | 1 | 1.11 | 100 |
| Control | 18 | - | 18 | - | 1.00 | 100 |

*P=0.001; **P=0.002 (compared with controls);
§Based on all cows.

Table 8. Antibody Titres in Immunized Hereford Cattle on Day 98 of Treatment

| Immunity | N | Mean Titre§ |
|---|---|---|
| Testosterone | | |
| all cows | 20 | 3,200 ( 740)# |
| ovulatory cows | 11 | 2,000 ( 570) |
| anovulatory cows | 9 | 4,700 (1,300)* |
| Androstenedione | 9 | 1,600 ( 700) |

§Mean reciprocal values
#Bracketed values are standard errors
*P<0.05 (anovulatory vs ovulatory)

Table 8 summarizes the steroid-specific antibody titres in the immune cows at day 98, corresponding to the peak secondary response. Of interest is the mean anti-testosterone titre which at 1:3,200 is significantly lower than found with the same type of antigen in the Friesian heifers (experiment 1). This difference suggests that there may be breed or age differences in the immune response among cattle.

More relevant to the objectives of the experiment were the antibody titres in the ovulatory compared to anovulatory cattle. Though these titre values (1:2,000 vs 1:4,700) are significantly different the magnitude of the difference is relatively small, reflecting a relationship between immune response and ovulation response similar to that found with the Friesian heifers.

Table 9. Luteinizing Hormone (LH) Profiles in Control and Androgen-Immune Hereford Cows (N=5 per group)

| Immunity | Mid-Luteal Phase | Follicular Phase |
|---|---|---|
| **LH Pulse Frequency (pulses/hr)** | | |
| Control | 0.30 (0.05)# | 0.75 (0.05) |
| Androstenedione | 0.70* (0.11) | 0.77 (0.14) |
| Testosterone | 0.63§ (0.17) | 0.70 (0.10) |
| **LH Pulse Amplitude (ng/ml)** | | |
| Control | 3.09 (0.66) | 3.60 (0.65) |
| Androstenedione | 5.66* (0.91) | 8.15* (1.12) |
| Testosterone | 5.47* (0.40) | 7.00* (0.89) |
| **Basal LH Concentrations (ng/ml)** | | |
| Control | 1.64 (0.34) | 2.41 (0.48) |
| Androstenedione | 3.53§ (0.90) | 3.23 (0.34) |
| Testosterone | 3.04§ (0.92) | 3.81 (0.71) |

#Bracketed values are standard errors
*P<0.05 (compared to control)
§P<0.1 (compared to control)

The failure of androstenedione immunity to induce an increase in ovulation rate is not in agreement with the work of Wise and Schanbacher (1983) who used this treatment to induce an ovulation rate gain of 0.36 in immune pregnant heifers and a potential calving rate gain of 0.27 confirmed by slaughter at approximately day 47 of gestation.

Table 9 shows that androgen immunity results in significant changes to the luteinizing hormone profiles of cattle. During the follicular phase of the cycle, LH pulse amplitude was increased but there were no effects on pulse frequency or basal levels. In contrast, during the mid-luteal phase LH pulse frequency was increased as was LH pulse amplitude and basal levels of LH.

## Experiment 3: Effect of Exogenous hCG Treatment on the Ovulatory Response of Testosterone-Immune Hereford Cows

Experimental Procedure. Seventy cows were used in this study [37 testosterone-immune cows with a previous history of 2 or 3 vaccinations with T:HSA (immunogen 1); 33 controls]. Oestrus synchronization was commenced on day 0 using a PRID® treatment as described for experiment 2. Additionally, a prostaglandin analogue (Estrumate®, 500 µg, i.m.) was given on days 0, 12 and 26. On day 18 the immune cows were given a booster vaccination as described. Oestrus detection using Kamar® heat mount detectors was commenced on day 26 and on day 28 (48 hrs post-prostaglandin) hCG (Chorulon®, Intervet International, Boxmeer, Holland) (2,000 i.u., i.v.) was administered to 20 immune and 15 control cows. Ovulation rates were determined at laparoscopy on day 34.

Results and Discussion. The rationale for this experiment was based on the supposition that the anovulatory steroid-immune Hereford cows in experiment 2 suffered a failure of the oestradiol positive feedback mechanism leading to a failure of the LH surge mechanism and anovulation. It was considered that an appropriately timed exogenous gonadotrophin treatment should compensate and lead to the ovulation of any "mature" follicles. Table 10 shows that this expectation has probably been realized.

Firstly, however, hCG treatment appears to have suppressed oestrous behaviour in control cattle but has had no effect on the ovulation rate of this group. In the immune group there was both a decrease in behavioural oestrus and in the ovulation rate across the group as observed in experiment 2. When hCG was given to testosterone-immune cattle, the number of anovulatory cattle was decreased and the ovulation rate correspondingly increased. However, the combination of steroid immunity and hCG treatment virtually abolished oestrous behaviour in cows given this double treatment. The gain in ovulation rate in immune cattle given hCG does suggest an increase in ovarian follicular development in those animals.

## COMPARISON OF THE REPRODUCTIVE RESPONSES OF SHEEP AND CATTLE TO ANDROGEN IMMUNITY

The foregoing data allow the following conclusions, providing the Hereford breed can be taken to represent cattle generally:

(a) sheep and cattle both become anovulatory and anoestrus at comparable levels of antibody titre.

Table 10. Oestrus and Ovulation Rate Responses in Testosterone-Immune Hereford Cows Given hCG

| Treatment | N | % Oestrus | No. of CL 0 | 1 | 2 | Ovulation Rate |
|---|---|---|---|---|---|---|
| Untreated | 18 | 73 | - | 18 | - | 1.00# (1.00)§ |
| Untreated given hCG | 15 | 53** | 1 | 13 | 1 | 1.00 (1.07) |
| Immune | 17 | 50** | 9 | 7 | 1 | 0.53**(1.13) |
| Immune given hCG | 20 | 10*** | 3 | 12 | 5 | 1.10* (1.29)## |

#All cows; §Ovulatory cows;
* $P<0.05$ (compared to immune);
** $P<0.01$ (compared to untreated);
***$P<0.001$ (compared to immune);
## $P<0.05$ (compared to untreated).

(b) antibody-induced anovulatory individuals in both species can be made to ovulate following administration of an exogenous gonadotrophin stimulus (see also Scaramuzzi and Hoskinson 1984).

(c) the concept of a critical titre "window" in sheep has been recognised as a level of immunity where an ovulation rate gain can be achieved and the expression of oestrous behaviour preserved. If such a "window" exists for cattle it must be characterized by a very narrow range of antibody titre. The present data indicate that androgen-immune cattle prefer to become anovulatory rather than multiple ovulators in response to increasing antibody titre.

(d) both species respond to androgen-immunity with an increase in LH pulse frequency and magnitude during the luteal phase of the oestrous cycle.

We are unable to reconcile our data on Hereford cattle with that of Wise and Schanbacher (1983) who reported an ovulation rate gain in androstenedione-immune crossbred heifers. Their antibody titres were apparently lower than those of our single-ovulating androstenedione- or testosterone-immune Herefords. Perhaps crossbred cattle will be found to be more responsive to the reproductive effects of androgen immunity. It is worth observing that crossbred sheep are more responsive to Fecundin® vaccine than are pure bred lines.

REFERENCES

Abraham, G.E., 1974, Radioimmunoassay of steroids in biological materials, Acta Endocr. (Copenh.), 75, suppl. 183:7.
Anderson, E.C., Masters, R.C., and Mowat, G.N., 1971, Immune response of pigs to inactivated Foot-and-Mouth disease vaccines, Res. Vet. Sci., 12:351.

Boland, M.P., Murray, J.D., Scaramuzzi, R.J., Sutton, R., Hoskinson, R.M., Hazelton, I.G., and Nancarrow, C.D., 1984, Reproductive wastage and chromosomal abnormalities in early embryos from androstenedione-immune and control Merino ewes, in: "Reproduction in Sheep," D.E. Lindsay and D.T. Pearce, ed., Australian Academy of Science, Canberra, p. 137.

Cox, R.I., and Wilson, P.A., 1976, Effects of immunizing sheep to steroid oestrogens and phyto-oestrogens, J. Reprod. Fert., 46:524.

Cox, R.I., Wilson, P.A., Scaramuzzi, R.J., Hoskinson, R.M., George, J.M., and Bindon, B.M., 1982, The active immunization of sheep against oestrone, androstenedione or testosterone to increase twinning. Proc. Aust. Soc. Anim. Prod., 14:511.

Geldard, H., 1984, Field evaluation of Fecundin, an immunogen against androstenedione. Proc. Aust. Soc. Anim. Prod., 15:182.

Geldard, H., Scaramuzzi, R.J., and Wilkins, J.F., 1984, Immunization against polyandroalbumin leads to increases in tailing percentages, N.Z. Vet. J., 32:2.

Geldard, H., Dow, G.J., and Kieran, P.J., 1984, Further developments in fecundity immunization field results, Wool Technol. Sheep Breed., 32:69.

Gibb, M., Thurley, D.C., and McNatty, K.P., 1981, Active immunization of Romney ewes with an androstenedione-protein conjugate, N.Z. J. Agric. Res., 24:5.

Gibb, M., Hudson, N., Kieboom, L., and McNatty, K.P., 1982, Long-term active immunization of Romney ewes with an androstenedione-protein conjugate - effects on oestrus, ovulation and lambing, N.Z. J. Exp. Agric., 125:128.

Holland, E.J., Bindon, B.M., Piper, L.R., Thimonier, J., Cornish, K.A., and Radford, H.M., 1981, Endoscopy in cattle: techniques for ovarian examination by the paralumbar and mid-ventral routes, Anim. Reprod. Sci., 4:127.

Hoskinson, R.M., Cox, R.I., Scaramuzzi, R.J., Hinks, N.J., Hillard, M.A., Turnbull, K.E., and Wong, M.S.F., 1981, Stimulation of ovulation rate in Merino ewes by immunization against steroids, Proc. Aust. Soc. Reprod. Biol., 13:27.

Hosoda, H., Sakai, Y., Yoshida, S., Miyairi, S., Ishii, K., and Nambara, T., 1979, The preparation of steroid N-hydroxysuccinimide esters and their reactivities with bovine serum albumin, Chem. Pharm. Bull. (Tokyo), 27:742.

Labhsetwar, A.P., Tyler, W.J., and Casida, L.E., 1963, Analysis of variation in some factors affecting multiple ovulations in Holstein cattle, J. Dairy Sci., 46:840.

Land, R.B., Morris, B.A., Baxter, G., Fordyce, M., and Forster, J., 1982, Improvements of sheep fecundity by treatment with antisera to gonadal steroids, J. Reprod. Fert., 66:625.

Lindner, H.R., Perel, E., Friedlander, A., and Zeitlin, A., 1972, Specificity of antibodies to ovarian hormones in relation to the site of attachment of the steroid haptens to the peptide carrier, Steroids, 19:357.

Martin, T.E., Rawlings, N.C., Hill, J.R., and Henricks, D.M., 1978, Active immunization of the cow against oestradiol-17β, J. Reprod. Fert., 53:173.

Martin, G.B., Scaramuzzi, R.J., Cox, R.I., and Gheradi, P.B., 1979, Effects of active immunization against androstenedione or oestrone on oestrus, ovulation and lambing in Merino ewes, Aust. J. Exp. Agric. Anim. Husb., 19:673.

Martensz, N.D., Baird, D.T., Scaramuzzi, R.J., and Van Look, P.F.A., 1976, Androstenedione and the control of luteinizing hormone in the ewe during anoestrus, J. Endocr., 69:227.

Martensz, N.D., Scaramuzzi, R.J., and Van Look, P.F.A., 1979, Plasma concentrations of luteinizing hormone and follicle stimulating hormone during anoestrus in ewes actively immunized against oestradiol-17β, oestrone or testosterone, J. Endocr., 81:261.

Renard, J.P., Ozil, J.P., and Heyman, Y., 1979, The use of embryo transfer in the field for increased calf crops in beef and dairy cattle, Anim. Reprod. Sci., 2:353.

Scaramuzzi, R.J., Davidson, W.G., and Van Look, P.F.A., 1977, Increasing ovulation rate in sheep by active immunization against an ovarian steroid, androstenedione, Nature, 269:817.

Scaramuzzi, R.J., 1979, Antibodies to androgens and ovulation in the ewe, J. Steroid Biochem., 11:957.

Scaramuzzi, R.J., Geldard, H., Beels, C.M., Hoskinson, R.M., and Cox, R.I., 1983, Increased lambing percentages through immunization against steroid hormones, Wool Technol. Sheep Breed., 31:87.

Scaramuzzi, R.J., and Hoskinson, R.M., 1984, Active immunization against steroid hormones for increasing fecundity, In: "Immunological aspects of reproduction in mammals," D.B. Crighton, ed., Butterworths, London, p. 445.

Scanlon, P.F., Gordon, I., and Sreenan, J.M., 1973, Multiple ovulations, multiple pregnancies and multiple births in Irish cattle, Irish J. Agr. Fish., 70:45.

Smith, J.F., Cox, R.I., McGowan, L.T., Wilson, P.A., and Hoskinson, R.M., 1981, Increasing the ovulation rate in ewes by immunization, Proc. N.Z. Soc. Anim. Prod., 41:193.

Sreenan, J.M., Diskin, M.G., and McDonagh, T., 1981, Induction of twin-calving by non-surgical embryo transfer: a field trial, Vet. Rec., 109:77.

Van Look, P.F.A., Clarke, I.J., Davidson, W.G., and Scaramuzzi, R.J., 1978, Ovulation and lambing rates in ewes actively immunized against androstenedione, J. Reprod. Fert., 53:129.

Walker, M.P., Thompson, D.L., Godke, R.A., and Honey, P.G., 1984, Active immunization of prepubertal bulls against testosterone: seminal and testicular characteristics after puberty, Theriogenology, 22:269.

Webb, R., Land, R.B., Pathiraja, N., and Morris, B.A., 1984, Passive immunization against steroid hormones in the female, In: "Immunological aspects of reproduction in mammals", D.B. Crighton, ed., Butterworths, London, p. 475.

Wise, T.H., and Schanbacher, B.D., 1983, Reproductive effects of immunising heifers against androstenedione and oestradiol-17β, J. Reprod. Fert., 69:605.

Wise, T., and Ferrell, C., 1984, Effects of immunization of heifers against estradiol on growth, reproductive traits and carcass characteristics, Proc. Soc. Exp. Biol. Med., 176:243.

Wittman, G., 1970, Use of diethylaminoethyl dextran (DEAE-D) as an adjuvant in the immunization of guinea pigs with inactivated foot and mouth disease virus, Zentbl. Bakt. Parasitkde I (Orig.), 213:1.

THE RELATIONSHIP OF EGG PRODUCTION IN THE CHICKEN TO

ITS MAJOR HISTOCOMPATIBILITY COMPLEX

Morten Simonsen

Institute for Experimental Immunology
University of Copenhagen
Nørre Allé 71, DK-2100 Copenhagen Ø, Denmark

I will hasten to make it clearfirst of all that I am not an acricultural scientist; but I am collaborating with people who are. My primary interests are in studies of the roles played by histocompatibility structures and in their evolutionary history. The major histocompatibility complex (MHC) of the chicken, the B-complex (Briles et al., 1982)., is of a 2-fold interest in this connection. First, the B-complex is the best investigated of non mammalian MHCs and, second, it belongs to an animal species of economic importance, which fact permits large-scale experimentation in spite of chickens being more demanding than mice on funds for their maintenance.

The conditions for successful egg production come to the fore in this context. To a large extent, the egg-laying hen of today is a product of human civilization, as witnessed by the wild ancestral form, the Red Jungle-Fowl, from which the <u>Gallus gallus domesticus</u> originated. The Red Jungle-Fowl has a restricted mating season in which to lay its eggs, and the size of the latter are such that no self-respecting grocery store would dream of putting them up for sale.

The success of present day breeds of high egg-laying performance, such as White Leghorn, is a composite of husbandry and genetic selection for desirable traits. Many different genes are probably important in this context; the questions here are whether MHC genes are among those of importance for egg production and, if so, by which mechanism.

## The B-complex

Most of what is known today about the B-complex serves to show its similarity with the 2 best studied of mammalian MHCs, the H-2 of the mouse and the HLA of man (Pink et al, 1977, Crone & Simonsen, 1985). There are, nevertheless, 2 rather distinctive features that should be mentioned here:

a. The firmness of the linkage between class I and class II genes is extreme. Skjødt et al. (1985), who have examined the largest material, failed to find a single recombinant between class I and class II genes and came to a maximum estimate for the map distance of 0.048 cM, based on their own data in addition to those published by others. It would seem that the class I and II genes of the B-complex are extremely closely linked or, alternatively, that no hot-spot for for recombination exists in the chicken MHC.

b. There exists a gene, or a gene family, called B-G which encodes a system as polymorphic as either of the classical MHC genes above (Simonsen et al., 1982) and which is closely linked to either with a recombination frequency of about 1:2000 (Koch et al., 1983). B-G is exclusively expressed in the erythrocytes and their precursors (Longenecker and Mossmann, 1980). It has an interesting adjuvant effect (Hála et al., 1981) in the production of antibodies to class I antigens, which are also expressed in erythrocytes. Thus, there are 2 different MHC-linked and highly polymorphic systems expressed in the chicken erythrocyte, and they are both useful for MHC typing by haemagglutination. The latter method still remains the preferred typing method in chickens. It is, however, important that typing reagents for both of these classes of antigens be used, in particular for the typing of outbred populations. This is because of the fact, that some MHC haplotypes share either class I or B-G alleles in common. For example, the haplotypes known as B2 and B12 have the same B-G allele and can therefore be distinguished in haemagglutination only by class I antisera. In contrast, B4 and B13 have the same class I (and class II) and can be distinguished only by B-G reagents. The internationally recognized B-haplotypes (Briles et al., 1982) are all designated by numbers, and each haplotype comprises an allelic form of both class I (B-F), class II (B-L) and class IV (B-G).

## A Scandinavian selection experiment

As earlier reported (Simonsen et al., 1982), a selection experiment was initiated in Scandinavia in 1969 by the establishment of a common base population of White Leghorn imported from 7 major commercial firms, mostly in North America. The base population was established in Uppsala by systematic intercrossing of the imported birds, and birds of the F2 offspring were subsequently distributed between Denmark, Norway, Finland, and Sweden. In each country, selection lines were developed according to similar criteria, and unselected control lines were kept under identical conditions. After 6 generations of selection for desirable egg production parameters, in particular number and size of eggs, it was decided to type the birds with respect to the B-complex. We found the results of this typing intriguing for 2 reasons.

1). Although upwards of 10 haplotypes were segregating in the control populations, 2 of these, B15 and B19, constituted more than 60 % of the gene pool in these populations, with B21 as number 3 in frequency. These findings suggested to us that these particular haplotypes might have been positively correlated with favourable production traits in the commercial stocks of origin.

2). Nevertheless, when the imported genes were thoroughly mixed in the process of establishing the base population, and selection for productivity was renewed in the Scandinavian setting, B15 and B19 responded differently to the selection pressures applied. B15 was favoured relative to B19, in particular in Norway and Sweden.

The observations prompted new joint experiments in Denmark, Finland, Norway, and Sweden in which selection was made entirely by MHC-typing: For example, B15/19, B15/21, and B19/21 heterozygotes were mated in order to test the segregating offspring for correlations between B-genotype and egg-laying.

In Denmark, an additional experiment was started in which birds of the unselected control line were identified by the criteria of possessing both one common (B13, B15, B19, or B21) and one rare haplotype (the rest). These heterozygotes constituted the parent generation from which were raised both F1 and F2 generations permitting correlation studies of egg-laying with the presence of either 2 common haplotypes, 2 rare ones, or one of each.

The statistical analysis of the very substantial body of data

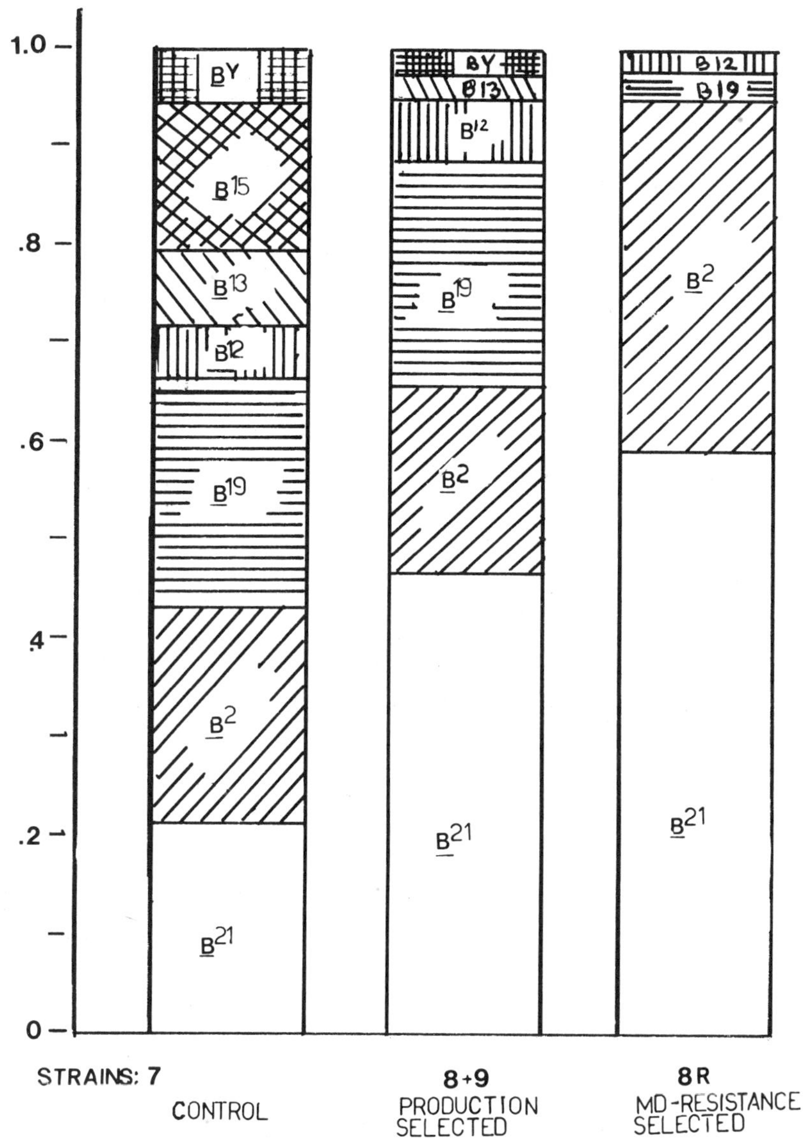


FIG. 1. CUMULATIVE GENE FREQUENCIES OF MHC HAPLOTYPES IN OTTAWA CHICKEN STRAINS, MAY 1983.

generated in these experiments is still in progress, but should be completed during 1985.

## A Canadian selection experiment

Meanwhile, I have been involved in MHC-typing also of birds from a selection experiment conducted by agricultural scientists in Ottawa, Canada (Gavora et al., 1985). As in the Scandinavian experiment, a base population was first established (1958-1960) by crossing reciprocally between commercial hybrids obtained from major companies in North America.

From 1969 onwards, selection lines were established. Lines 8 and 9 were selected on the basis of high egg production as the principal trait, with fertility, hatchability, viability, and egg quality as additional secondary traits. Line 8R was selected for resistance to challenge with Marek's disease (MD) virus in addition to high egg production. Line 7 was the unselected control line. In May, 1983 I received almost 100 blood samples of all 4 lines for MHC-typing by haemagglutination with respect to both the class I and the B-G alleles. The typing was performed blindly and de-coding of the data was made in Canada. A summary of the results is shown graphically in Fig. 1.

It is seen that selection for production traits alone resulted in a doubling of the B21 gene (haplotype) frequency, mostly at the expense of B13 and B15. The most dramatic changes, however, occurred in line 8R, selected also for resistence to MD. Some 95 % of the gene pool now consisted of 2 haplotypes only, namely B2 and B21. These results make very good sense in terms of previous data on the influence of B-haplotypes on the resistance to MD.

## On the associations of Marek's disease with B-haplotypes, and on silent immunological selection

MD, also known as fowl paralysis, is caused by an herpesvirus which is widespread in both domestic and wild chickens. It is extremely contagious and causes a number of pathological lesions including lymphomas in different organs, and demyelination of peripheral nerves. Until the development of an effective vaccine, MD was one of the most dreaded plagues in the poultry industry and, in spite of vaccination, it remains an important problem (Gavora and Spencer, 1979).

Dating back to a report by Hansen et al.(1967), several investigations have confirmed that chickens carrying B21 are relatively resistant to Marek's disease (see review by Setness, 1982). Actually, MD may represent the best example known from any animal species of MHC-control of susceptibility versus resistance to a contagious disease which poses a treat to the species because it carries massive lethality before the age of reproduction.

In a recent study, Briles et al. (1983) made use of birds with a recombinant haplotype possessing the B21 genes for class I and class II in association with the B-G gene of B19. This recombinant haplotype provided as much resistance to MD virus as did the full parental B21 haplotype. Since B19 is a haplotype associated with great susceptibility to the disease, the experiment suggests that B-G is irrelevant, while resistance is carried by the class I and/or the class II genes. This is perhaps not unsuspected, and it leaves unanswered the relative importance of the latter genes.

Another report by Briles et al. (1982) is highly relevant to the findings in the Canadian experiment above. They infected with MD virus some 400 progeny of five heterozygous B-complex genotypes resulting from a cross between two Leghorn lines. The five genotypes shared B21 in common. A standard infective virus dose administered at 3 weeks of age resulted in the following percent incidence (in parenthesis) of MD: B2/21 (5), B5/21 (38), B15/21 (48), B19/21 (50), and BX/21 (48), where X represents a "new" haplotype. The much lower susceptibility (or higher resistance) of B2/21 heterozygotes in comparison with the other heterozygotes is highly significant and indicates that these 2 haplotypes somehow complement each other in conferring resistance to MD virus infection. In fact, the degree of protection they jointly provide is comparable to that given by B21 in the homozygous state.

Going back to Fig. 1, the most important, and at the same time most difficult point for discussion, is the marked increase in the frequency of B21 that occurred in strains 8 + 9, i.e. without deliberate selection for resistance to MD. In view of what has been said already, it seems a distinct possibility that also this increase may in fact have been caused by resistance to MD. This may be so because of the fact that general viability entered the secondary traits on which selection was based, and also because of the possibility that clinically undetected (silent) infection might easily lead to a temporary reduction in the yield of eggs, which parameter formed the primary trait for selection.

In this particular experiment, the latter possibility, which I will refer to as "silent immunological selection", comes easy to mind. However, by extrapolation, silent immunological selection might apply also in other experiments in relation to other haplotypes where disease associations to other infections exist which have not been identified yet.

## Non immunological MHC functions

Having thus paid attention to immunological selection, be it silent or not, of some MHC haplotypes in preference to others, I personally find it premature, and even unwise, to disregard the possibility that non-immunological functions of MHC may also operate in selection for egg-laying.

Since the early 1960ies, Czechoslovakian workers in particular have uncovered an array of H-2 linked parameters in the mouse that would appear to be closer related to endocrinology than to immunology. I have in mind such parameters as testis mass and vesicular gland mass, the level of testosterone-binding protein in the serum, or of cortisol-binding protein in the cytosol, or of cAMP in liver cells. References to these and many other curious H-2 associations were compiled and discussed by Iványi (1978).

More recently, evidence has accumulated in favour of associations between MHC class I molecules and peptide hormone receptors. My favourite example here is the insulin receptor, which we have been studying in collaboration with my Danish colleague, Lennart Olsson and his laboratory (Simonsen et al., 1983, 1985).

What sparked off this work was an original observation by Lennart Olsson of the fact that the human Daudi cell line failed to bind insulin. Now, this line lack MHC class I molecules in its membrane, and the possible causal correlation between this fact and the deficient insulin binding received circumstantial support from the fact that other human cell lines did bind insulin, including lines that were lacking MHC class II. Taking our lead from these observations, we proceeded to try influencing insulin-binding by manipulating the membrane expression of MHC molecules in an insuling-binding human monocytoid cell line, U-937. A considerable number of capping experiments have now been performed by Dr. Claus Due, and these have confirmed the already published findings (Simonsen et al., 1985) that insulin-binding is markedly diminished by capping of MHC class I by antibodies to either its heavy or light chain, but is uninfluenced by the capping of MHC class II molecules.

The most compelling evidence to date of molecular interaction between the insulin receptor and MHC class I comes, however, from the group of Max Fehlman (Brossette et al., 1985). These workers employed an insulin preparation which was labelled both by $^{125}I$ and by a photoaffinity label and still retained a nearly normal ligand function for the receptor. After preparing liver cell membranes from $H\text{-}2^k$ mice, they reacted these membranes with the doubly labelled insulin, activated the photoaffinity label with UV light, solubilized the membranes, and immunoprecipitated the covalent complex of $^{125}I$-labelled insulin + insulin receptor with antibodies to the insulin receptor. The remarkable fact, however, is that a significant amount was also precipitated by monoclonal antibodies to $H\text{-}2K^k$ though not by antibodies to $H\text{-}2D^k$. Appropriate controls ruled out the possibility of an accidental crossreactivity of anti $H\text{-}2K^k$ with the insulin receptor itself. Thus the indication is very strong of an affinity of binding between particular MHC class I molecules and the insulin receptor which is high enough to mediate co-precipitation even of molecules in free solution. This being so, there is all the more reason to assume similar interactions in the intact cell membrane where the extremely narrow space promotes the association of molecules into compounds (Cohen and Eisen, 1977).

Other examples of apparent interactions between peptide hormones or their receptors and MHC class I molecules are provided by glucagon and by the epidermal growth factor (Edidin, 1983) and by gamma-endorphin (Claas and Van Rood, 1985). We have ventured to generalize these and other observations in a theory of compound receptors which attributes to MHC molecules in the membrane a basic regulatory physiological role in reversible interactions with other membrane molecules and visualizes the well-known immunological MHC restriction as a natural consequence of this more basic, general function.

As a final comment on the mechanisms by which MHC polymorphism might possibly influence egg-laying, I would suggest that silent immunological selection will necessarily often appear to be capricious for the simple reason that the microbial selection pressure usually is unknown. A given haplotype may therefore be favoured in one specific setting but not in another. In comparison, I would expect MHC associations due to interactions with physiological peptides, or peptide receptors to be more universally reproducible.

## References


1. Briles, W.E., Bumstead, N., Ewert, D.L., Gilmour, D.G., Gogusev, J., Hála, K., Koch, C., Longenecker, B.M., Nordskog, A.W., Pink, J.R.L., Schierman, L.W., Simonsen, M., Toivanen, A., Toivanen, P., Vainio, O., and Wick, G., 1982, Nomenclature for chicken major histocompatibility (B) complex, Immunogenetics, 15:441.

2. Briles, W.E. and Briles, R., 1982, Breeding and Genetics. Marek's disease resistance of B (MHC) heterozygotes in a cross of purebred Leghorn lines, Poultry Sci., 61:205.

3. Briles, W.E., Briles, R., Taffs, R.E., and Stone, H.E., 1983, Resistance to a malignant lymphoma in chickens is mapped to subregion of major histocompatibility (B) complex, Science, 137:620.

4. Brossette, N., van Obberghen, E., and Fehlmann, M., 1985, Interactions between insulin receptors and major histocompatibility complex antigens in mouse liver membranes, Diabetologia, 27:74.

5. Claas, F.H.J. and van Rood, J.J., 1985, The interaction of drugs and endogenous substances with HLA class-I antigens, Progr. Allergy, 36:135.

6. Cohen, R.J. and Eisen, H.N., 1977, Hypothesis. Interactions of macromolecules on cell membranes and restrictions of T-cell specificity by products of the major histocompatibility complex, Cell. Immunol., 32:1.

7. Crone, M. and Simonsen, M., Avian Major Histocompatibility Complex, 1985, in: Basis and Praxis of Avian Immunology, A. Toivanen and P. Toivanen, eds., CRC Press, Inc., New York, in press.

8. Edidin, M., 1983, MHC antigens and non-immune functions, Immunol. Today, 4:269.

9. Gavora, J.S. and Spencer, J.L., 1979, Studies on genetic resistance of chickens to Marek's disease - a review, Comp. Immun. Microbiol. Infect. Dis., 2:359.

10. Gavora, J.S., Simonsen, M., Spencer, J.L., Fairfull, R.W., and Gowe, R.S., 1985, Changes in the frequency of MHC haplotypes in chickens under selection for both high egg production and resistance to Marek's disease, Zeitschr. für Tierzucht und Züchtungsbiologie, in press.

11. Hála, K., Plachy, J., and Schulmannová, J., 1981, Role of the B-G--region antigen of chicken MHC, Immunogenetics, 14:393.

12. Hansen, M.P., van Zandy, J.N., and Law, G.R.J., 1967, Differences in susceptibility to Marek's disease and chickens carrying two different B locus blood alleles, Poultry Sci., 46:1268.

13. Iványi, P., 1978, Some aspects of the H-2 system, the major histocompatibility system in the mouse, Proc. R. Soc. Lond. B, 202:117.

14. Koch, C., Skjødt, K., Toivanen, A., and Toivanen, P., 1983, New recombinants within the MHC (B complex) of the chicken, Tissue Antigens, 21:129.

15. Longenecker, B.M. and Mossman, T.R., 1980, Restricted expression of an MHC allo-antigen in cells of the erythroid series: a specific marker for erythroid differentiation, J. Supramol. Struct., 13:395.

16. Pink, J.R.L., Droege, W., Hála, K., Miggiano, V.C., and Ziegler, A., 1977. A three-locus model for the chicken major histocompatibility complex, Immunogenetics, 5:203.

17. Settnes, O.P., 1982, Marek's Disease. A common naturally herpes-virus-induced lymphoma of the chicken. A comprehensive review, Nord. Vet. Med., Suppl.II:11-132.

18. Simonsen, M., Crone, M., Koch, C., and Hála, K., 1982, The MHC haplotypes of the chicken, Immunogenetics, 16:513.

19. Simonsen, M., Kolstad, N., Edfors-Lilja, I., Liljedahl, L.-E. and Sørensen, P.,1982, Major histocompatibility genes in egg- laying hens, AJRI, 2:148.

20. Simonsen, M. and Olsson, L., 1983, Possible roles of compound membrane receptors in the immune system. Ann. Immunol. (Inst. Pasteur), 134D:85.

21. Simonsen, M., Skjødt, K., Crone, M., Sanderson, A., Fujita-Yamaguchi, Y., Due, C., Rønne, E., Linnet, K., and Olsson, L., 1985, Compound receptors in the cell membrane: ruminations from the borderland of immunology and physiology, Prog. Allergy, 36:151.

22. Skjødt, K., Koch, C., Crone, M., and Simonsen, M., 1985, Analysis of the chickens for recombination within the MHC (B complex), Tissue Antigens, 25:278.

# BOVINE EMBRYO: DEVELOPMENT, CLONING, SEXING AND TRANSFER OF GENES

N. L. First, E. S. Critser and J. M. Robl

Department of Meat and Animal Science
University of Wisconsin
Madison, WI

## INTRODUCTION

Recent technological advancements in biology including the use of immunological tools have relevance to the livestock industry. These technologies are in support of and expected to contribute most importantly to the cattle artificial breeding and embryo transfer industries. At present nearly 70% of 11 million U.S. dairy cows are mated by artificial insemination. Genetic improvement in dairy cattle through artificial insemination has resulted in a doubling of milk production per cow over the past 30 years. Little progress has been made in genetic improvement by selection of offspring from superior females because a cow produces relatively few calves per year or in a lifetime. To multiply the progeny from an outstanding female or mating, a commercial embryo transfer industry has developed. This industry last year performed approximately 100,000 transfers in the USA and 200,000 in the world of which approximately 25% were with frozen embryos. Its present armament of technologies include the ability to superovulate cows, collect and transfer embryos nonsurgically, store embryos frozen and divide each embryo into two viable embryos. At present 20-30 calves can be produced from one valuable donor cow/year by use of embryo transfer.

Because of segregation and recombination during gametogenesis and low heritabilities for milk and growth traits, sibling embryos are not alike in expected production. This industry is seeking methods for cloning and sexing valuable embryos. Cloning of valuable embryos is needed to increase the number and to establish a tested population of uniform and predictable performance. Cloning of embryos would also provide a phenotypic selection rather than the present inefficient genetic selection. The sexing of embryos is desired because the female is the unit of milk production for dairy cattle. Also transferring two embryos increases the likelihood of pregnancy and sexing would allow placement of embryos of the same sex in a recipient thereby avoiding production of sterile freemartins. Recently developed plasmids are capable of inserting growth hormone and a promoter into the genome of mice. Transgenic mice grew twice as large and more rapidly than normal. This created the exciting possibility that genes affecting growth, milk production or disease resistance might be transferred into the germ line of cattle. If genes are to be introduced into 1-cell embryos methods are needed to develop bovine embryos in vitro.

It is now possible to produce embryos with the inner cell mass and trophoblast derived from separate embryos of the same or differing species. This has been done by replacement of the inner cell mass of the blastocyst (Papaioannov, 1982; Rossant et al., 1983) and by reconstituting an embryo from cells of the 8-cell stage of one species with the 4-cell stage of another (Fehilly et al., 1984). Cells of the more advanced stage tend to become the inner cell mass. These chimeric embryos and micromanipulations with embryos in general could provide immunologists with powerful tools for determining nuclear/cytoplasmic contributions of embryos and fetuses to developing the immune system, identifying genes responsible for developing specific immune responses and for studying the interaction of conceptus and mother in pregnancy recognition and maintenance.

## DEVELOPMENT OF EMBRYOS

The successful application of genetic engineering and micromanipulation techniques to preimplantation mammalian embryos is dependent upon efficient methods for maturing, fertilizing, culturing and developing embryos in vitro.

### Oocyte Maturation

Oocyte maturation may be defined as those events which render the oocyte capable of being fertilized and supporting early embryonic development. This process involves at least three events preceding fertilization: 1) nuclear maturation, 2) cumulus expansion and 3) cytoplasmic maturation. Nuclear maturation, characterized by germinal vesicle breakdown and resumption of meiosis is triggered by the ovulatory hormone LH in vivo but occurs spontaneously when oocytes are removed from the follicle (Leibfried and First, 1979). Maintenance of meiotic arrest may be due to an inhibitory product of the ovarian follicle (oocyte maturation inhibitor, OMI; Tsafriri and Channing, 1975) or terminated by a meiosis inducing factor (MIS; Westergaard et al., 1984). Expansion of the cumulus cells occurs in response to follicle stimulating hormone (FSH; Ball et al., 1980; 1983) triggering the secretion of a hyaluronic acid matrix and leaving the cumulus-oocyte complex sufficiently sticky to be transported into the oviduct (Mahi-Brown and Yanagimachi, 1983). Expansion of the cumulus mass facilitates sperm penetration of the oocyte (Ball et al., 1983) and may play a role in sperm capacitation (Ball et al., 1982; Handrow et al., 1982). A second FSH induced product produced by the cumulus appears to be a peptide which causes hyperactivated sperm motility (Bradley and Garbers, 1983). Cytoplasmic maturation originally described by Thibault et al. (1975) involves the development of cytoplasmic signals essential for completing fertilization and directing early embryonic development. These signals appear to result from translation of maternal mRNA synthesized during oogenesis (Cascio and Wasserman, 1982). Bovine oocytes recovered from small follicles complete nuclear maturation (Leibfried and First, 1979) and cumulus expansion in vitro (Ball et al., 1983) and are capable of being fertilized (Leibfried-Rutledge et al., 1985) but fail to support early embryonic development (Critser et al., unpublished). The acquisition of developmental competence by maturing follicular oocytes appears to depend on hormonally stimulated granulosa cells. Co-culture of ovine granulosa cells and immature ovine oocytes with LH, FSH and estradiol 17ß imparts postfertilization developmental capacity to approximately half the oocytes (Staigmiller and Moor, 1984). Still to be developed for most species are methods for harvesting the large number of immature oocytes of the ovary and for maturing them in vitro such that they are competent to complete embryoic development.

## In Vitro Fertilizaton

Thus far, efficient systems for fertilization of oocytes matured and recovered in vivo have been developed for mice, hamsters, rabbits, cattle, humans, and to a lesser extent nonhuman primates and swine. The most recognized application of in vitro fertilization (IVF) is in the human where world-wide more than 2,000 pregnancies have resulted for otherwise infertile couples. Couples using IVF are mostly those in which the woman has obstructed oviducts (Gold, 1985). For domestic species such as cattle the goal of utilizing oocytes matured in vitro from the large ovarian pool of oocytes or oocytes recovered by laparoscope from preovulatory follicles of superovulated cows makes in vitro fertilization mandatory for their usefulness. Production of embryos by IVF would also be useful for gene transfer and embryo cloning or other manipulations where precise timing of fertilization is needed. It is expected that IVF would also be useful for predicting fertility of males. Successful IVF requires capacitation of the sperm and maturation of the oocyte and is dependent upon proper timing, temperature, gas and media conditions for fertilization. Capacitation involves removal or perturbation of sperm plasma membrane components allowing calcium entry into the sperm and results in the occurrence of the sperm acrosome reaction. The acrosomal enzymes presumed to be involved in fertilization are thus released. A change in sperm motility pattern known as activation also occurs during capacitation.

Bovine sperm can be capacitated by glycosaminoglycans (GAGs) from the oviduct, follicular fluid, and FSH stimulated cumulus cells surrounding the eggs (Lee and Ax, 1984; Lenz et al., 1983; Handrow et al., 1982; Parrish et al., 1985). The most potent of these GAGs is heparin (Fig. 1; Handrow et al., 1982). Highly efficient systems for in vitro fertilization using heparin to capacitate bovine sperm are available (Parrish et al., 1984, 1985). Sperm motility is stimulated by a product of cumulus cells surrounding the eggs, but the product's identity is as yet unknown for mammals (Bradley and Garbers, 1983). The product has characteristics of a protein and is liberated into media by cumulus cells only after FSH stimulated cumulus expansion. In sea urchins increased respiration is caused by a peptide from the egg jelly coat called speract (Hansbrough and Garbers, 1981). Combining capacitated, activated sperm and matured oocytes at body temperature or slightly above in media compatible with survival of the gametes and a gas environment equivalent to the oviduct usually results in fertilization 8-20 hr later.

## Ontogeny of Embryos In Vivo and In Vitro

At present most knowledge concerning early embryonic development comes from studies of invertebrates or from strains of mice whose embryos can be cultured from the 1-cell stage to blastocyst. In murine embryos there appear to be three discrete periods of stage specific proteins. These periods are: from 1-cell to early 2-cell when most proteins are of maternal origin (Braude et al., 1979), from late 2-cell to 8-cell when embryonic RNA synthesis is initiated and a few discrete proteins of embryonic origin are synthesized, and from 16-cell to blastocyst when a new and expanded array of proteins are synthesized (Johnson, 1981; Bolton et al., 1984). It is likely that the developmental events are similar for all mammalian species but timing for transitions from one stage to another differ. For example, transition from maternal to embryonic control of development is early in mice (2-cell stage) but morphological evidence suggests it is later (8-cell stage) in cattle (King et al., 1985) and sheep (Calarco and McLaren, 1976) and more like amphibians where nuclear transfer is feasible. If true, cloning bovine or ovine embryos by exchange of nuclei from 8-cell to 1- or 2-cell stages may be possible.

Reliance on the mouse as a model for mammalian development occurred because embryos of most species are blocked in development during culture in vitro. Embryos from most strains of mice (Johnson, 1981), as well as pigs (Polge, 1982), sheep (Calarco and McLaren, 1976) and cows (Camous et al., 1984; Critser, unpublished) exhibit a block in vitro. The successful exceptions are mice derived from the C57 strain, rabbits and humans. Interestingly, strains of mice whose embryos are incapable of early development in vitro block at the 2-cell stage. This coincides with transition from maternal mRNA regulated protein synthesis to regulation of RNA and protein synthesis by the nucleus of the zygote (Goddard and Pratt, 1983; Bolton et al., 1984). In mice a prolonged cell cycle immediately precedes the onset of embryonic genomic expression (Bolton et al., 1984) and the occurrence of an in vitro block. A prolonged cell cycle also precedes the stage of blocked development in culture for cattle (Eyestone, unpublished) and swine (Polge, 1982).

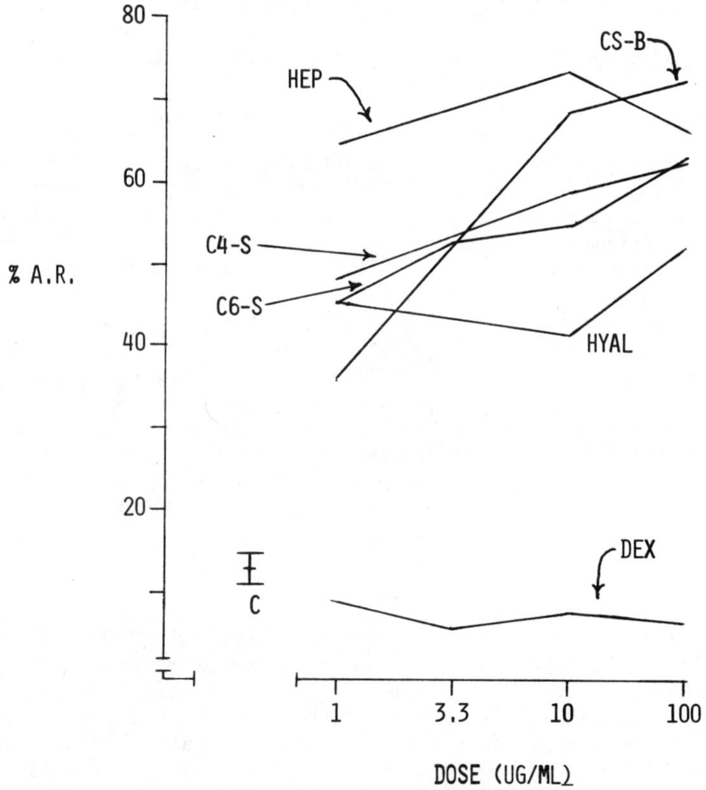


Fig. 1. The relative potency of 5 glycosaminoglycans in causing capacitation and subsequent acrosome reaction of $10^8$ bovine spermatozoa. HEP, heparin; CS-B, dermatan sulfate; C-4-S, Chondroitin-4-sulfate; C-6-S, chondroitin-6-sulfate; HYAL, hyaluronic acid; DEX, dextran sulfate used as a sulfated sugar control; C, control of media only.

Silver staining nucleolar organizing regions (NORs) on the short arms of 5 or 6 chromosomes (humans or mice, respectively) are recognized as morphological markers for the sites of rRNA transcription and development of nucleoli. The first NOR staining activity in murine embryos is in 2-cells (Hansmann et al., 1978) and coincides with the beginning of rRNA synthesis (Knowland and Graham, 1972). The first NOR staining activity for bovine embryos is after the 8-cell stage (King et al., 1985). The presence and number of NORs are morphological indicators of the beginning of embryonic transcriptional activity and at a given stage represent a gross estimate of transcriptional activity. This transition from maternal to zygotic control of development is also known to coincide for murine embryos with a time when murine nucleoli transition from fibrillar to granular nucleoli (Hillman and Tasch, 1969). Interestingly, the transition of nucleolar development from fibrillar nucleoli to granular nucleoli indicating active rRNA synthesis is at the end of the period where murine (Hillman and Tasch, 1969), ovine (Calarco and McLaren, 1976) and porcine (Norberg, 1973) embryos are blocked in development.

In the absence of culture systems capable of developing embryos of domestic animals from 1-cells to blastocysts, embryos can be cultured in vivo. Successful systems for in vivo culture are also useful in understanding causes of blocks to development and in developing in vitro embryo culture. The two in vivo systems shown useful for bulk culture (20 or more) of bovine embryos are isolated embryos placed surgically in rabbit oviducts (Boland, 1984; Sirard et al., 1985a, 1985b) or in agar blocks surgically transferred into oviducts of sheep (Willadsen, 1982; Eyestone et al., 1985). The in vivo cultured blastocysts give reasonably normal pregnancy rates when transferred to recipient cows (63%, Eyestone et al., 1985; 49% Sirard et al., 1985b). Some success in culturing bovine embryos through the period of blocked development has also been achieved by coculture with bovine trophoblastic cells (Camous et al., 1984; Heyman, 1985).

Embryo transfer techniques are available for most mammalian species and most extensively commercialized for cattle where nonsurgical transfer procedures are used. The earliest stage at which uterine transfer can be accomplished differs for each species. For swine this is as early as the 2-cell stage and before the block in culture thereby allowing development of offspring from in vitro fertilization, gene transfer or other manipulations of early embryos (Polge, 1982). For the bovine, transfer to the oviduct requires considerable surgical effort and few or no pregnancies result (Newcomb, 1977; Sirard et al., 1985a). With uterine transfer of embryos earlier than the 16-cell stage, frequency of pregnancy is also low.

## CLONING EMBRYOS

There are two approaches to cloning mammalian embryos. One successful approach is to divide embryos into equal parts and derive a complete individual from each part. This can be done by separating individual blastomeres of early embryos or by cutting later preimplantation embryos into segments. This method is based on the fact that individual blastomeres of early embryos are totipotent. The number of clones that can be derived from an embryo by splitting is limited because the developmental schedule of the embryo is not altered by splitting but the number of cells in the embryo at a particular point in development is reduced (Tarkowski, 1965; Smith and McLaren, 1977; O'Brien et al., 1985). If embryos are split beyond halves or quarters the number of cells in each part is insufficient for proper differentiation of inner cell mass and trophectoderm at blastulation and the resulting embryos eventually die (Tarkowski and Wroblewska, 1967; Willadsen, 1982). Cloning by splitting, therefore, is of limited potential because only two to four clones can be produced from an embryo.

An alternative approach to cloning is the transplantation of nuclei from a multicellular donor tissue or embryo to oocytes or early (1 or 2 cell stage) embryos from which the nucleus has been removed. This has the potential for producing a new, complete embryo from each of the donor nuclei and if each of these clones could be recloned, an unlimited number of genetically identical individuals could be produced. Cloning by this method depends on the donor nuclei being capable of assuming the function of the recipient cell's nucleus; however, nuclei differentiate with development of the embryo and may not be able to dedifferentiate. Thus far, neither cloning from nuclei of adult mammals nor from embryonic cells has been satisfactorily developed to produce live cloned offspring. Research has demonstrated hopeful and promising leads as well as problems requiring solution.

Early enthusiasm for cloning mammals by nuclear transfer came from experiments in amphibians where donor nuclei from the multicellular blastula resulted in cloned offspring after these nuclei were transferred to a recently activated oocyte (Gurdon, 1964). Even donor cells from larval gut resulted in development (Reviewed by Gurdon, 1964 and DiBerardino, 1980). These studies were repeated by Illmensee and Hoppe (1981) with mice. They found that nuclei from the inner cell mass of the murine blastocyst were able to support development to live offspring when transplanted to enucleated zygotes. Others (McGrath and Solter, 1984; Robl et al., 1985) could not repeat the results of Illmensee and Hoppe (1981) and found the development of donor nuclei in enucleated zygotes to be much more restricted. When transplanted to the enucleated zygote, nuclei from 2-cell embryos form a few blastocysts whereas embryos with nuclei from later stages only cleave to the 2-cell stage.

There are several possible reasons why nuclei from blastulae or gastrulae of frogs are totipotent as donors for nuclear transfer, whereas cells from the blastocyst and earlier stages of mouse embryos are not. One reason may be that developmental events occur at different embryonic stages between these two species. Amphibians develop through 12 cell divisions under the control of genetic information transcribed during oogenesis before the embryonic genome becomes active (Newport and Kirschner, 1982). Mice develop under maternal control only as far as the first cleavage before the embryonic genome is activated (Johnson, 1981; Goddard and Pratt, 1983; Bolton et al., 1984). The stage of activation of the embryonic genome is indicative of a relatively late onset of nuclear differentiation in the frog and a very early onset of nuclear differentiation in the mouse. Because the differentiated state of a transplanted nucleus is likely to affect the extent of development in a recipient embryo it is not surprising that nuclear transplantation is more successful in frogs than in mice.

Because nuclear activity and differentiation begin so early in murine embryos, the mouse is a poor mammalian model for repetition of amphibian nuclear transfer experiments. Present evidence suggests the onset of nuclear activity is likely between the 4- and 8-cell stage in porcine embryos (Norberg, 1973; Polge, 1982) and 8- and 16-cell stage in ovine (Calarco and McLaren, 1976) and bovine embryos (King et al., 1985). In these species nuclei from 4- or 8-cell embryos may support development in enucleated zygotes or oocytes. We are presently testing these combinations in cattle.

Our method of transplanting nuclei or pronuclei in bovine embryos is based on a procedure developed by McGrath and Solter (1983a) for murine embryos. Briefly, this procedure entails inserting a micropipet of slightly smaller diameter than the nucleus through the zona pellucida but not through the plasma membrane of the embryo. The pipet is then moved adjacent to the nucleus and with gentle aspiration the nucleus is pulled into the pipet without rupturing the plasma membrane. As the pipet is pulled away from the embryo the zona pellucida pinches the membrane off between the enucleated blastomere and the plasma membrane bounded nucleus (Figs. 3 and 4). Nuclei or pronuclei are thereby removed without disrupting the plasma membrane. A plasma membrane bounded nucleus or pronucleus is inserted into an enucleated embryo by cell fusion (Fig. 5). Bovine embryos, in contrast to murine embryos, contain a large quantity of lipid granules that impede visualization of nuclei. This was resolved initially by labeling nuclei with a fluorescent stain (Critser and First., 1985), then, more satisfactorily, by centrifuging the lipid granules away from the nucleus (Fig. 2). The centrifugation method was adapted from a procedure by Wall et al. (1985) for porcine and bovine embryos. If the embryos are centrifuged at a sufficient time prior to cleavage the lipid granules become distributed uniformly throughout the cytoplasm and development progresses normally. For 2-cell and later stages nuclei are removed without centrifugation by aspirating the center of the blastomere (Fig. 4). Nuclear removal is confirmed by observing the nucleus in the micropipet. Another difficulty with bovine embryos is that Sendai virus which is a very effective fusigenic agent for murine embryos does not work well in bovine embryos. We have also tried without success polyethylene glycol and a bovid herpes virus, which fuses bovine tissue culture cells very effectively. We are successful with the dielectrophoretic method of fusion. Enucleated embryos with a membrane enclosed nucleus inserted in the perivitelline space are placed between two electrodes and a fusion pulse of 100 V for 40 µsec is applied. Approximately 80% of the nuclei fuse within 1 hour. If pronuclei are removed from an embryo and reinserted with this method, 30 to 40% develop to morulae after 5 days in a sheep oviduct and some of these are capable of developing at least to day 40 of gestation when transferred to recipient cows.

The development of a technique for transplanting nuclei allows us to test various combinations of donor nuclei and recipient cytoplasm. These experiments may lead to a method of cloning bovine embryos and certainly will lead to a greater understanding of early development and differentiation in cattle. The nuclear transfer technique has already provided an insight into several interesting problems in early murine embryonic development. Experiments in our laboratory show that enucleated 2-cell embryos with 8-cell nuclei develop 8 to 12 days in vivo in comparison to one or two cleavage divisions when the enucleated zygote is the recipient (Robl et al., 1985). This result is evidence for phases of differentiation and abrupt transitions between phases as proposed by Johnson (1981). Future experiments will likely be of importance in defining the mechanism of differentiation. In addition, the nuclear transplantation technique is useful for determining the nuclear or cytoplasmic origins of various antigens. As an example, McGrath and Solter (1983b) have determined that the stage-specific embryonic surface antigen, SSEA-3, is a cytoplasmic contribution of the unfertilized ovum.

In summary, amphibians can be cloned by nuclear transfer but only with nuclei from early stage embryos and not adult cells. Thus far, mammals have not been cloned, however, we are only beginning to understand early development in mammals sufficiently to design methods of cloning.

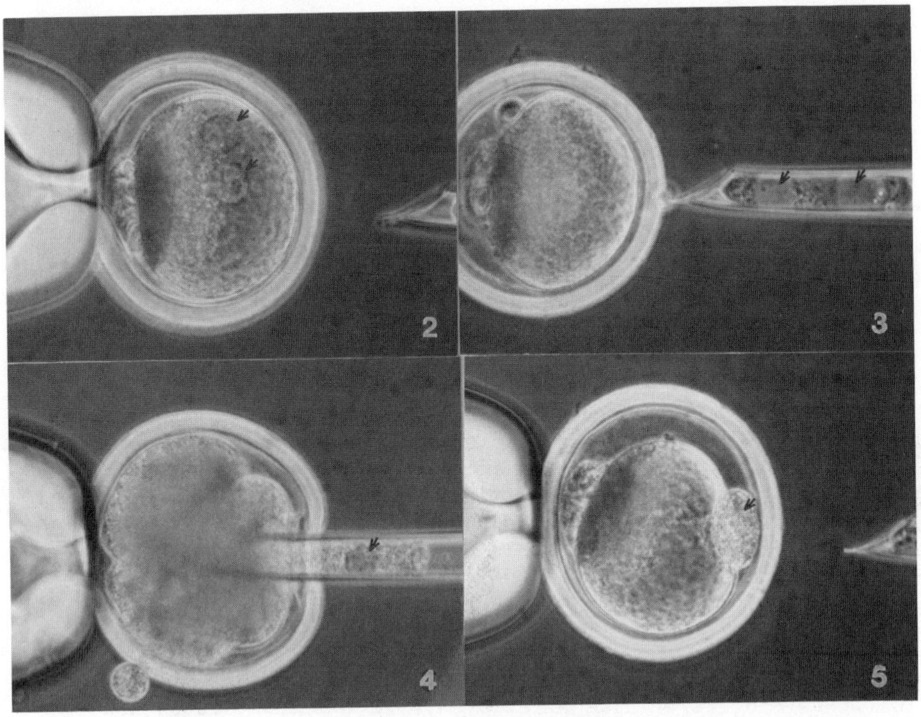


Fig. 2. Pronuclear stage bovine embryo centrifuged at 15,000 x g for 3 min to reveal two pronuclei (arrows). Lipid granules, which normally obscure the nuclei, are present in a pocket and dense area on the left edge of the embryo.

Fig. 3. Two pronuclei (arrows) after removal from a bovine embryo. The pronuclei are in a plasma membrane bounded vesicle in the nuclear transfer pipet.

Fig. 4. Removal of a nucleus (arrow) from one blastomere of a 4-cell stage bovine embryo. Nuclei are removed by blind aspiration in the center of the blastomere.

Fig. 5. Insertion of a membrane bounded nucleus (arrow) into the perivitelline space of an enucleated recipient embryo. The donor nucleus is then fused to the recipient by a high intensity electrical pulse.

## SEXING OF BOVINE EMBRYOS

Sexing of embryos before transfer is especially sought by the dairy cattle industry where females are the desired milk producing unit. To be useful sexing techniques must be accurate, efficient, rapid and without detrimental effects on the embryos. The two most successful approaches have been 1) cytogenetic karyotyping of the cells of the blastocyst and 2) immunological detection of the H-Y antigen on male embryos.

Sexing by Karyotyping. Cytogenetic methods are highly accurate and also allow identification of aberrant chromosomal alternatives such as XXY (King, 1984). However, this method requires a large number of colcemid arrested cells to insure a few readable metaphase chromosome displays (King 1984). Embryonic biopsies of sufficient size to yield sufficient cells may be damaging to the embryo. One approach to providing sufficient cells has been to bisect the embryo followed by cytogenetic analysis of the smaller half and transfer of the larger. In one experiment this resulted in a normal 60% pregnancy rate after transfer of the half embryo but sex could be determined for only 60% of the half embryos subjected to cytogenetic analysis. Sex when identified was predicted with 100% accuracy (Picard et al., 1985). Clearly further research on methods to increase the frequency of metaphase spreads or for culture of trophoblast cells to numbers sufficient for karyotyping is needed to increase the frequency of embryos which can be sexed. Nevertheless, cytogenetic analysis provides an accurate standard for quick evaluation of other methods.

Sexing by Immunological Methods. One of the first antigens expressed by the embryo is the male specific cell surface antigen designated H-Y. This antigen appears as early as the 8-cell stage on male murine embryos (Krco and Goldberg, 1976; Epstein et al., 1980; reviewed by Haseltine, 1983). The H-Y (histocompatibility-Y) antigen was originally defined as a cell surface antigen which was detected by skin graft rejection. In highly inbred strains of mice and rats females were shown to reject skin grafts from males (Eichwald and Silmser, 1955; Celada and Welshons, 1963; reviewed by Haseltine, 1983). Serum from females that have rejected male skin grafts contains antibodies which can identify male cells in serological systems and indeed male cells can be killed by female serum containing the H-Y antibody (Goldberg et al., 1971). There is evidence that the transplantation H-Y and the serological antigens may not be the same (Melvold et al., 1977; Puck et al., 1981; Haseltine et al., 1981; Haseltine and Ohno, 1981).

This antigen has been proposed to be a testicular organizing factor (Silvers, et al., 1968). Whether H-Y antigen is indeed the principal testicular organizer is still being questioned and studied (Haseltine, 1983; Wachtel, 1983, 1984). Nevertheless its male specificity and early expression make it a good candidate for recognition and identification of male embryos. The H-Y antigen is known to be highly conserved across species and present on cells of at least 70 species of vertebrates including male mice, rats, cattle, dogs, goats, donkeys, horses, pigs and humans as well as on cells of the female, the heterogametic sex of birds (Wachtel, 1984). Both polyclonal (Krco and Goldberg, 1976; Epstein et al., 1980; White et al., 1982) and monoclonal (Koo and Varano, 1981) antibodies have been prepared against the serological H-Y antigen.

The H-Y antigen has been detected on preimplantation murine embryos by incubation with H-Y antiserum and complement (Krco and Goldberg,

1976; Epstein et al., 1980; White et al., 1982; reviewed by Wachtel, 1984). Cell lysis occurred in approximately 50% of the embryos which were exposed to murine H-Y antiserum and complement for guinea pigs; but embryos cultured in medium with H-Y antiserum or complement alone were not damaged. Karyotypes of embryos that were unaffected by culture with antiserum and complement showed that 92% were female (Epstein et al., 1980). When unaffected embryos were transferred to pseudopregnant recipients, 86% of the pups born were female (White et al., 1983). The obvious disadvantage of this complement dependent cytolytic method for detection of H-Y antigen is that survival of male embryos is reduced. When a monoclonal H-Y antibody and fluorescent labeled second antibody were utilized together H-Y antigen and male embryos were identified without toxicity to embryos of either sex (White et al., 1983). These studies in mice suggest that it should be possible to sex embryos of bovine and other species by use of an antibody to H-Y antigen. Removal of complement and use of a fluorescent labeled second antibody for detection of binding of the first antibody should result in identification of both male and female embryos without cytotoxic death of the male embryos.

White et al. (1984) developed such an assay. The accuracy of predicting each sex from application of this assay to several species is shown in Table 1. In developing the assay antiserum was produced by repeated injection of spleen cells from male C57B1/6 mice into females of the same highly inbred strain. Blood was collected from immunized mice and antisera were absorbed twice with isolated bovine lymphocytes. Pooled antisera from six immunized mice were added to Ham's F10 culture medium at a 10% (v/v) concentration. Embryos at the 16-cell to early blastocyst stages were cultured for 90 minutes in the Ham's F10 antisera media. Embryos were then washed in Ham's F10 medium supplemented with 10% IgG-free fetal calf serum (FCS) and incubated for 90 minutes in drops of Ham's F10 medium containing 10% fluorescein isothiocyanate (FITC) - conjugated goat antimouse IgG antibody (Antibodies Inc., Davis, CA). After an additional wash embryos were transferred to fresh drops of Ham's F10 medium supplemented with IgG free fetal calf serum and individually evaluated at 200 x with an inverted fluorescent microscope equipped for FITC excitation. As indicated in Table 1 for bovine the assay was nearly perfect for identification of female embryos (93%). However, only 79% of male

TABLE 1. ACCURACY AND INDIRECT IMMUNOFLUORESCENT ASSAY IN SEXING EMBRYOS

| Species | Embryos Correctly Sexed | |
|---|---|---|
| | Fluorescing | Nonfluorescing |
| Mouse[a] | 18/23 (78%) | 19/23 (83%) |
| Cow[b] | 42/53 (79%) | 39/42 (93%) |
| Pig[c] | 23/30 (77%) | 25/29 (86%) |

Data based on young born or analysis of sex chromosomes.
[a]White et al., 1983.
[b]White et al., 1984.
[c]White et al., 1985.

embryos were identified. This reduced efficiency for males appeared to occur because dead cells of some embryos exhibited an autofluorescence at the same wave length as the FITC label. When these autofluroescing embryos were female the accuracy of male identification was reduced. It is likely that this problem could be eliminated by choosing a fluorescent label of a different wave length. While large scale testing of this antisera and second antibody system will be essential it would appear that with minor adjustments in the method such as indicated above, a method for determining the sex of bovine embryos is at hand and nearly ready for use.

## GENE TRANSFER

Strong interest in producing transgenic livestock occurred following the first production of transgenic mice by Gordon and Ruddle (1981). This interest was greatly enhanced by the experiments of Palmiter and Brinster and colleagues demonstrating that insertion of a linear fragment of a plasmid containing a metallothionein-I promoter and rat growth hormone (Palmiter et al., 1982) or human growth hormone (Palmiter et al., 1983) into the genome of murine embryos perturbed growth regulatory mechanisms sufficiently to cause as much as a two-fold increase in growth.

While most productivity traits are influenced by several genes, these experiments demonstrated that a gene coding for a product which perturbs a homeostatically maintained regulatory system or a gene coding for a rate limiting step in a process can cause significant change in the production of a product.

Several genes are of interest for insertion into the genome of livestock. These include growth hormone with its potential for increasing growth and lactation. In dairy cattle injection of growth hormone has resulted in an increase of approximately 15% to 40% in milk production (Bines et al., 1980; Peel et al., 1981, 1985; Gorewit et al., 1982; Bauman et al., 1985). The giant mouse gene identified by Bradford (1982) might also produce enhanced growth in livestock. Specific genes affecting components of reproduction have been identified. For example, the Booroola gene when present causes the Australian merino sheep to increase ovulation rate and to produce multiple births rather than single lambs (Davis et al., 1982). This gene is presently being cloned in Australia as well as two genes controlling wool growth. In mice Spearow (1984) has identified genes influencing ovulation rate which increase ovulation up to 6-fold. If the Booroola gene were inserted into cattle or the Spearow gene into swine it might be possible to reliably produce twins in cattle or increase litter size in swine. It may also be possible to impart resistance to specific diseases of animals or birds through transfer of genes. Resistance to some diseases of humans and mice (Bach, 1982) or Mareks disease in poultry (Payne, 1973) are known to be controlled by single gene loci. Cloned genes of the major histocompatibility complex and genes for interferon offer hope for enhancing immune protection from disease. One gene of the MHC complex, SLA-PD1, has been cloned (Singer et al., 1982) and shown to be expressed in transgenic mice (Frels et al., 1985). The MHC gene (SLA-PD1) has been introduced into the genome of swine, sheep and rabbits at the U.S.D.A. Beltsville laboratories but its effect on immune response is yet untested.

Gene transfer in domestic animals has been slower in development relative to mice for technological reasons, such as problems in visualizing pronuclei, and problems of injection and development of pronuclear embryos to a stage that can be transferred nonsurgically to recipient cows. As previously discussed these problems have been overcome and gene transfer can now be successfully performed in cattle (Fig. 6). The only report thus far of a gene expressed after transfer into bovine embryos is the transfer of the thymidine kinase gene and its assay in bovine embryos. Approximately 30% of bovine embryos derived from in vitro or in vivo fertilizations express the gene after transfer into a pronucleus (Lohse et al., 1985).

In swine, unlike cattle, the early 2-cell embryo can be transferred directly to the uterus and result in good survival. This and the fact that swine are a litter bearing species have allowed rapid adaptation of gene transfer technology developed for mice for use in swine. Offspring expressing an exogenous growth hormone gene have been produced in swine at U.S.D.A. Beltsville. These offspring exhibit increased levels of the exogenous growth hormone in their blood but thus far have not grown faster and are not larger than controls (Hammer et al., 1985). This fact suggests the need for research to understand the regulation of growth in swine. The production of transgenic livestock is of low efficiency. Based on experiments with mice and depending on the efficiencies of reproductive steps in each species, it is estimated that a gene must be injected into 50-200 pronuclei to produce one offspring which has integrated and expressed the gene. Additionally, experiments in mice indicate that one must generate individuals homozygous for the foreign gene to screen for insertional mutations. These are usually lethal and are caused by the disruption of a native gene. The frequency of insertional mutagenesis in mice is approximately 1 out of 7 to 1 out of 15 (Jenkins et al., 1981; Lacy et al., 1983: Jaenisch, 1980; Schnieke et al., 1983; Wagner et al., 1983; Palmiter et al., 1984).

More efficient methods for gene transfer and methods for transfer at a stage more compatible with commercial bovine embryo transfer are being sought. These explorations include the potential use of replication defective retroviral vectors to infect genes into late stage embryos (Mann et al., 1983; Emerman and Temin, 1984a,b; Bandyopadhyay and Temin, 1984a,b; Sorge et al., 1985).

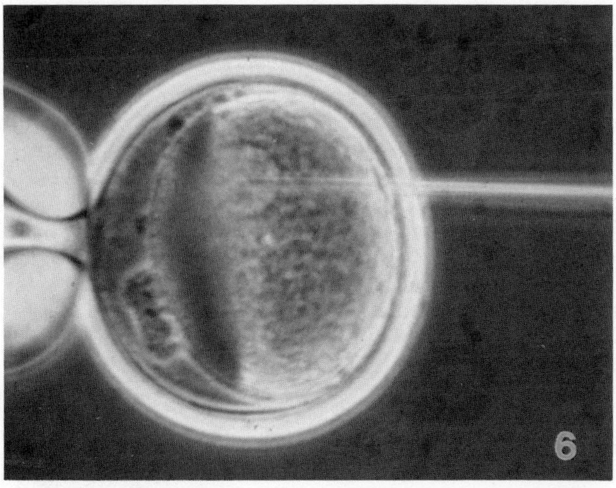


Fig. 6. Injection of a pronucleus in a bovine embryo.

## ACKNOWLEDGMENTS

Research supported in part by the College of Agricultural and Life Sciences, University of Wisconsin, Madison, WI, The W. R. Grace Company and NIH Grant HD 18345. This is Meat and Animal Science Department Paper No. 961. We are grateful to Julie Busby for typing and Lorraine Leibfried-Rutledge and John Parrish for reviewing this manuscript.

## REFERENCES

Bach, J. F., 1982, Genetic control of immune responses, in: "Immunology", J. F. Back, ed., John Wiley and Sons, New York.

Ball, G. D., Ax, R. L. and First, N. L., 1980, Mucopolysaccharide synthesis accompanies expansion of bovine cumulus-oocyte complex in vitro, in: "Functional Correlates of Hormone Receptors in Reproduction", ed., V. B. Mahesh and T. G. Muldoon, Elsevier, North Holland, New York.

Ball, G. D., Bellin, M. E., Ax, R. L. and First, N. L., 1982, Glycosaminoglycans in bovine cumulus-oocyte complexes: morphology and chemistry, Mol. Cell. Endocr., 28:113.

Ball, G. D., Leibfried, M. L., Lenz, R. W., Ax, R. L., Bavister, B. D. and First, N. L., 1983, Factors affecting successful in vitro fertilization of bovine follicular oocytes, Biol. Reprod., 28:717.

Bandyopadhyay, P. K. and Temin, H. M., 1984a, Expression of complete chicken thymidine kinase gene inserted in a retrovirus vector, Mol. Cell. Biol., 4:749.

Bandyopadhyay, P. K. and Temin, H. M., 1984b, Expression from an internal AUG codeon of herpes simplex thymidine gene in a retrovirus vector, Mol. Cell. Biol., 4:743.

Bauman, D. E., Eppard, P. J., DeGeeter, M. J. and Lanza, G. M., 1985, Responses of high producing dairy cows to long term treatment with pituitary- and recombinant-somatotropin. J. Diary Sci. 68.

Bines, J. A., Hart, I. C. and Morant, S. V., 1980, Endocrine control of energy metabolism in the cow: the effect on milk yield and levels of some blood constituents of injection growth hormone and growth hormone fragments, Br. J. Nutr., 43:179.

Boland, M. P., 1984, Use of the rabbit oviduct as a screening tool for the viability of mammalian eggs, Theriogenology, 21:126.

Bolton, V. N., Oades, P. J. and Johnson, M. H., 1984, The relationship between cleavage, DNA replication and gene expression in the mouse 2-cell embryo, J. Embryol. exp. Morph., 27:139.

Bradford, G. E., 1982, Evidence for a major gene for rapid growth in mice, J. Anim. Sci. (Suppl. 1):140) abstract, American and Canadian Meetings.

Bradley, M. P. and Garbers, D. L., 1983, The stimulation of bovine caudal epididymal sperm forward motility on bovine cumulus-egg complexes in vitro, Biochem. Biophys. Res. Comm., 115:777.

Braude, P., Pelham, H., Flach, G. and Lobatto, R., 1979, Post transcriptional control in the early mouse embryo, Nature 282:102-105.

Calarco, P. G. and McLaren, A., 1976, Ultrastructural observations of preimplantation stages of sheep, J. Embryol. exp. Morph., 36:609.

Camous, S., Heyman, Y., Meziou, W. and Menezo, Y., 1984, Cleavage beyond the block stage and survival after transfer of early bovine embryos cultured with trophoblastic vesicles. J. Reprod. Fert., 72:479.

Cascio, S. M. and Wasserman, P. M., 1982, Program of early development in the mammal: Post transcriptional control of a class of proteins synthesized by mouse oocytes and early embryos, Devel. Biol., 89:397.

Celada, F. and Welshons, W. J., 1963, An immunogenetic analysis of the

male antigen in mice utilizing animals with an exceptional chromosomal constitution. Genetics, 48:139.
Critser, E. S. and First, N. L., 1985, Use of a fluorescent stain for visualization of nuclear material in living oocytes and early embryos. Stain Tech. (accepted).
Davis, G. H., Montgomery, G. W., Allison, A. J., Kelley, R. W. and Bray, A. R., 1982, Segregation of a major gene influencing fecundity in progeny of Booroola sheep. N.Z.J. Agric. Res., 25:525.
DiBerardino, M. A., 1980, Genetic stability and modulation of metazoan nuclei into eggs and oocytes. Differentiation, 17:17.
Eichwald, E. J. and Silmser, C. R., 1955, untitled communication, Transplantation, 2:148.
Emerman, M. and Temin, H. M., 1984a, High frequency deletion in recovered retrovirus vectors containing exogenous DNA with promoters, J. Virol., 50:42.
Emerman, M. and Temin, H. M., 1984b, Genes with promoters and retrovirus vectors can be independently suppressed by an epigenetic mechanism, Cell, 39:459.
Epstein, C. J., Smith, S. and Travis, B., 1980, Expression of H-Y antigen on preimplantation mouse embryos, Tiss. Antigens, 15:63.
Eyestone, W. H., Northey, D. L. and Leibfried-Rutledge, M. L., 1985, Culture of 1-cell bovine embryos in the sheep oviduct, Biol. Reprod., 32:(Suppl 1)100 (abstract 125).
Fehilly, C. B., Willadsen, S. M. and Tucker, E. M., 1984, Interspecific chimaerism between sheep and goat, Nature 307:634.
Frels, W. I., Bluestone, J. A., Hodes, R. J., Capecchi, M. R. and Singer, D. S., 1985, Expression of microinjected porcine class I major histocompatibility gene in transgenic mice, Science 228:577.
Gold, M., 1985, "The Baby Makers", Science(85)6:26.
Goldberg, E. H., Boyse, E. A., Bennett, T., Shied, M. and Carswell, E. A., 1971, Serological demonstration of H-Y (male) antigen on mouse sperm, Nature 232:478.
Goddard, M. J. and Pratt, H. P. M., 1983, Control of events during early cleavage of the mouse embryo: an analysis of the "2-cell block", J. Embryol. exp. Morph., 73:111.
Gordon, J. W. and Ruddle, F. H., 1981, Integration and stable germ line transmission of genes injected into mouse pronuclei, Science 214:1244.
Gorewit, R. C., Bauman, D. E. and Peel, C. J., 1982, Improved animal efficiency using pituitary hormones, in: "Abstracts of, Biotechnology: Commercial and Industrial Applications and Opportunities Conference", Battelle Memorial Institute, Seattle, WA.
Gurdon, J. B., 1964, The transplantation of living cell nuclei, Advances in Morphogenesis 4:1.
Hammer, R. E., Pursel, V. G., Rexroad, C. E., Jr., Wall, R. J., Bolt, D. J., Ebert, K. M., Palmiter, R. D. and Brinster, R. L., 1985, Production of transgenic rabbits, sheep and pigs by microinjection, Nature 315:680.
Handrow, R. R., Lenz, R. W. and Ax, R. L., 1982, Structural comparisons among glycosaminoglycans to promote an acrosome reaction in bovine spermatozoa, Biochem. Biophys. Res. Comm. 197:1326.
Hansbrough, I. and Garbers, D. L., 1981, Purification and characterization of a peptide associated with eggs that activates spermatozoa, J. Biol. Chem. 256:1447.
Hansmann, I., Gebauer, J., Bihl, L. and Grimm, T., 1978, Onset of nucleolus organizer activity in early mouse embryogenesis and evidence of its regulation, Exp. Cell Res. 114:263.
Haseltine, F. P. and Ohno, S., 1981, Mechanisms of sex differentiation, Science 211:1272.
Haseltine, F. P., Genel, M., Crawford, J. D. and Berg, W. R., 1981, H-Y antigen negative patients with testicular tissue and 46 X-Y

karyotype, Hum. Genet. 57:265.
Haseltine, F. P., 1983, Sex differentiation, current concepts, in: "The Biological Basis of Reproductive and Developmental Medicine", J. B. Warshaw, ed., Elsevier Biomedical, Amsterdam.
Heyman, Y., 1985, Factors affecting the survival of transferred whole and half embryos in cattle, Theriogenology 23:63.
Hillman, N. and Tasch, R. J., 1969, Ultrastructural and autoradiographic studies of mouse cleavage stages, Am. J. Anat. 126:151.
Illmensee, K. and Hoppe, H. C., 1981, Nuclear transplantation in mus musculus: Developmental potential of nuclei from preimplantation embryos, Cell:23:9.
Jaenisch, R., 1980, Retroviruses and embryogenesis: microinjection of Moloney leukemia virus into midgestation mouse embryos, Cell 19:181.
Jenkins, N. A., Copeland, N. G., Taylor, B. A. and Lee, B. K., 1981, Dilute (d) coat colour mutation of DBA/2J mice is associated with the site of integration of an ecotropic MuLV genome, Nature 293:370.
Johnson, M. H., 1981, The molecular and cellular basis of preimplantation mouse development, Biol. Rev. 56:463.
King, W. A., 1984, Sexing embryos by cytological methods, Theriogenology 21:7.
King, W. A., Niar, A. and Betteridge, K. J., 1985, The nucleolus organizer regions of early bovine embryos, J. Dairy Sci. 68:(Suppl. 1)249 (abstract).
Knowland, J. and Graham, C., 1972, RNA synthesis at the 2-cell stage of mouse development, J. Embryol. Exp. Morphol. 27:167.
Koo, G. C. and Varano, A., 1981, Inhibition of H-Y cell mediated cytolysis by monoclonal H-Y specific antibody, Immunogenetics 14:183.
Krco, C. J. and Goldberg, E. H., 1976, H-Y (male) antigen: detection on 8-cell embryos, Science 193:1134.
Lacy, E., Roberts, S., Evans, E. P., Burtenshaw, M. D. and Constantini, F. D., 1983, A foreign ß-globin gene in transgenic mice: integration at abnormal chromosomal positions and expression in inappropriate tissues, Cell 34:343.
Lee, C. N. and Ax, R. L., 1984, Concentrations and composition of glycosaminoglycans in the female bovine reproductive tract, J. Dairy Sci. 67:2006.
Leibfried-Rutledge, M. L., Critser, E. S. and First, N. L., 1985, Fertilization potential of follicular oocytes classified by stage of cycle and size of follicle, Theriogenology (in press).
Leibfried, L. and First, N. L., 1979, Characterization of bovine follicular oocytes and their ability to mature in vitro, J. Anim. Sci. 48:76.
Lenz, R. W., Ball, G. D., Lohse, J. K., First, N. L. and Ax, R. L., 1983, Chondroitin sulfate facilitates an acrosome reaction in bovine spermatozoa as evidenced by light microscopy, electron microscopy and in vitro fertilization, Biol. Reprod. 28:683.
Lohse, J. K., Robl, J. M. and First, N. L., 1985, Progress towards transgenic cattle, Theriogenology 23:No. 1 (abstract).
Mahi-Brown, C. A. and Yanagimachi, R., 1983, Parameters influencing ovum pickup by oviductal fimbria in the golden hamster, Gamete Research 8:1-10.
Mann, R., Mulligan, R. and Baltimore, D., 1983, Construction of a retrovirus packaging mutant and its use to produce helper free defective retrovirus, Cell 33:153.
McGrath, J. and Solter, D., 1983a, Nuclear transplantation in the mouse embryo by microsurgery and cell fusion, Science 220:1300.
McGrath, J. and Solter, D., 1983b, Nuclear transplantation in mouse embryos, J. Exp. Zool. 228:355.
McGrath, J. and Solter, D., 1984, Inability of mouse blastomere nuclei

transferred to enucleated zygotes to support development in vitro, Science 226:1317.
Melvold, R. W., Kohn, H. I., Yerganian, G. and Fawcett, D. W., 1977, Evidence suggesting the existence of two H-Y antigens in the mouse, Immunogenetics 5:33.
Newcomb, R., 1977, Influence of synchrony and methods of synchrony on embryo transfer, in: "Embryo Transfer in Farm Animals" Betteridge, ed., Monograph 16, Agriculture Canada, Ottawa.
Newport, J. W. and Kirschner, M. W., 1982, A major developmental transition in early xenopus embryos: I. characterization and timing of cellular changes at the midblastula stage, Cell 30:675.
Norberg, H. S., 1973, Ultrastructural aspects of the preattached pig embryo: cleavage and early blastocyst stages, J. Anat. Entwickl.-Gesch. 143:95.
O'Brien, M. J., Critser, E. S. and First, N. L., 1985, Developmental potential of isolated blastomeres from early murine embryos, Theriogenology 22:601.
Palmiter, R. D., Brinster, R. L., Hammer, R. E., Trumbauer, M. E., Rosenfeld, M. G., Birnberg, N. C. and Evans, R. M., 1982, Dramatic growth of mice that develop from eggs microinjected with metallothionein-growth hormone fusion genes, Nature 300:611.
Palmiter, R. D., Norstedt, G., Gelinas, R. E., Hammer, R. E., Brinster, R. L., 1983, Metallothionein-human GH fusion genes stimulate growth of mice, Science 222:809.
Palmiter, R. D., Wilkie, T. M., Chin, H-Y. and Brinster, R. L., 1984, Transmission distortion and mosaicism in an unusual transgenic mouse pedigree, Cell 36:869.
Papaioannov, V. E., 1982, Lineage analysis of innercell mass and trophectoderm using microsurgically reconstituted mouse blastocysts, J. Embryol. exp. Morphol. 68:199.
Parrish, J. J., Parrish, J. L. and First, N. L., 1984, Effect of swimup separation and heparin pretreatment of frozen thawed spermatozoa on in vitro fertilization of bovine oocytes, Biol. Reprod. 30:(Suppl. 1):112.
Parrish, J. J., Susko-Parrish, J. L. and First, N. L., 1985, In vitro fertilization of bovine oocytes using heparin treated and swimup separated frozen thawed bovine sperm is repeatable and results in high frequencies of fertilization, Theriogenology 23:No. 1 (abstract).
Payne, L. N., 1973, Genetics and control of avian diseases, Avia Pathology 2:237.
Peel, C. J., Bauman, D. E., Gorewit, R. G. and Sniffen, C. J., 1981, Effect of exogenous growth hormone on lactation performance in high yielding dairy cows, J. Nutr. 111:1662.
Peel, C. J., Sandles, L. D., Quelch, K. J. and Herington, A. C., 1985, The effects of long term administration of bovine growth hormone on the lactational performance of identical twin dairy cows. Anim. Prod. (in press).
Picard, L., King, W. A. and Betteridge, K. J., Production of sexed calves from frozen-thawed embryos, Vet. Rec. (in press, 1985).
Polge, C., 1982, Embryo transplantation and preservation, in: "Control of Pig Reproduction", Cole and Foxcroft, ed., Buttersworth, London.
Puck, S. M., Haseltine, F. P. and Francke, U., 1981, Absence of H-Y antigen in an X-Y female with campomelic dysplasia, Hum. Genet. 817:1.
Robl, J. M., Gilligan, B., Critser, E. S. and First, N. L., 1985, Nuclear transplantation in mouse embryos: assessment of recipient cell stage, Biol. Reprod. (submitted).
Rossant, J., Vijh, M., Siracusa, L. D. and Chapman, V. M., 1983, Identification of embryonic cell lineages in histological sections of chimeras between mus-musculus and mus caroli, J. Embryol. Exp. Morph. 73:179.

Schnieke, A., Harbers, K. and Jaenisch, R., 1983, Embryonic lethal mutation in mice induced by retrovirus insertion in the α1 collagen gene, Nature 304:315.
Silvers, W. K., Billingham, R. E. and Sanford, B. H., 1968, H-Y antigen serological detectable male antigen and sex determination. Cell 28:439.
Singer, D. S., Otero, R. C. D., Sotz, M. L., Osborne, B., Socks, D. and Rudikoff, S., 1982, Characterization of a porcine genomic clone encoding a major histocompatibility antigen: Expression in mouse L cells, Proc. Natl. Acad. Sci. 79:1403.
Sirard, M. A., Lambert, R. D., Guoy, P., Menard, D. P. and Bedoya, M., 1985a, In vivo and in vitro development of in vitro fertilized bovine follicular oocytes obtained by laparoscopy, Theriogenology 23:230.
Sirard, M. A., Lambert, R. D., Menard, D. P. and Bedoya, M., 1985b, Pregnancies resulting from in vitro fertilization of bovine follicular oocytes following their incubation in rabbit oviduct and their transfer to the cows uterus, Biol. Reprod. 32:(Suppl. 1)99 (abstract 124).
Smith, R. S. and McLaren, A., 1977, Factors affecting the time of formation of the mouse blastocoele. J. Embryol. Exp. Morphol. 41:79.
Sorge, J., Wright, D., Erdman, V. D. and Cutting, A. E., 1985, Amphotrophic retrovirus vector system for human cell gene transfer. Mol. Cell. Biol. 4:1730.
Spearow, Jimmy L., 1984, Mechanism of action of genes controlling reproduction, in: "Genetics of Reproduction in Sheep", R. B. Land and D. W. Robinson, eds., Buttersworth, London.
Staigmiller, R. B. and Moor, R. M., 1984, Effect of follicle cells on the maturation and developmental competence of ovine oocytes matured outside the follicle, Gamete Research 9:221.
Tarkowski, A. K., 1965, Preimplantation Stages of Pregnancy, G. E. W. Walstenholme and M. O'Connor, eds., Churchille Livingston, London.
Tarkowski, A. K. and Wroblewska, J., 1967, Development of blastomeres of mouse eggs isolated at the 4 and 8 cell stage, J. Embryol. exp. Morph. 18:155.
Thibault, C., Gerard, M. and Menezo, Y., 1975, Acquisiton per l'oocyte de lapine et de veau du Facteur de decondensation du noyau du spermatozolde fecondant (MPGF), Ann. Biol. Anim. Bioch. Biophys. 15:705.
Tsafriri, A. and Channing, C. P., 1975, An inhibitory influence of granulosa cells and follicular fluid upon porcine oocyte meiosis in vitro, Endocrinology 96:922.
Wachtel, S. S., 1983, H-Y Antigen and the Biology of Sex Determination. Grune Stratton, NY.
Wachtel, S. S., 1984, H-Y antigen in a study of sex determination and control of sex ratio, Theriogenology 21:18.
Wagner, E. F., Covarrubias, L., Steward, T. A. and Mintz, B., 1983, Prenatal lethalities in mice homozygous for human growth hormone gene sequences integrated in the germ line, Cell 25:647.
Wall, R. J., Pursel, V. G., Hammer, R. E. and Brinster, R. L., 1985, Development of porcine ova that were centrifuged to permit visualization of pronuclei and nuclei, Biol. Reprod. 32:645.
Westergaard, L., Byskov, A. G., Andersen, C. Y., Grinsted, J. and McNatty, K. P., 1984, Is resumption of meiosis in the human preovulatory oocyte triggered by a meiosis-inducing substance (MIS) in the follicular fluid? Fertil. and Steril. 41:337.
White K. L., Lindner, G. M., Anderson, G. B. and Bon Durant, R. H., 1982, Survival after transfer of sexed mouse embryos exposed to H-Y antisera, Theriogenology 18:655.

White, K. L., Lindner, G. M., Anderson, G. B. and Bon Durant, R. H., 1983, Cytolytic and fluorescent detection of H-Y antigen on preimplantation mouse embryos, Theriogenology 19:701.

White, K. L., Bradbury, M. W., Anderson, G. B. and Bon Durant, R. H., 1984, Immunofluorescent detection of a male specific factor on preimplantation bovine embryos, Theriogenology 21:275(abstract).

White, K. L., Anderson, G. B., Berger, P. J., Bon Durant, R. H. and Pashen, R. L., 1985, Expression of a male-specific factor (H-Y antigen) on preimplantation porcine embryos. Proc. Amer. Soc. Anim. Sci. Aug. 1985

Willadsen, S. M., 1982, Micromanipulation of embryos of the large domestic species, in: "Mammalian Egg Transfer", C. E. Adams, ed., CRC Press, Boca Raton, FL.

# PREGNANCY OUTCOME IN HUMAN COUPLES WITH IDIOPATHIC RECURRENT ABORTIONS: THE ROLE(S) OF FEMALE SERUM, MIXED LYMPHOCYTE CULTURE BLOCKING FACTORS, POTENTIATING FACTORS, AND LOCAL UTERINE IMMUNITY BEFORE AND AFTER PATERNAL LEUKOCYTE IMMUNIZATION

Alan E. Beer, Zhu Xiaoyu[+], A.E. Semprini[*]
and James F. Quebbeman

University of Michigan
Department of Obstetrics and Gynecology
L5007-Women's Hospital
Ann Arbor, Michigan 48109
Tele: 313-763-2253
[+] W.H.O. Research Fellow, Maternal and Child Health Hospital, Hubei Province, China
[*]Senior Research Scholar, University of Milano, Italy

## ABSTRACT

Two hundred-fifty couples with 4.6 $\pm$ 2.2 recurrent spontaneous abortions were fully worked up to ensure the absence of medical, genetic, infectious, structural, or a combination of these etiologies known to be associated with recurrent abortion. In addition, all were evaluated immunogenetically. In 67 couples reported here, the female was immunized with paternal leukocytes on two occasions and post-immunization immune response parameters were evaluated. Pregnancy outcome post-immunization can be predicted by analyzing the normal female serum and heat inactivated female serum mixed lymphocyte culture (MLR) blocking factors and potentiating factors with specificity for the male spouse. Women who abort an additional time post-immunization develop leukocytotoxic antibodies with paternal specificity and do not develop MLR blocking factors with specificity for B lymphocytes. Women who deliver a live born child post-immunization develop leukocytotoxic antibodies with less frequency and all develop maternal/anti-paternal specific MLR blocking factors that are not heat inactivatable and are nearly 100% effective in blocking female stimulator/male responder mixed lymphocyte culture reactivity. A subset of women immunized with paternal leukocytes established pregnancies and delivered severely growth retarded infants. In these patients, lymphocytes in the decidua mantling the conceptus were isolated and were found to be cytotoxic and hyperresponsive in MLR to paternal as well as to third party alloantigens.

## INTRODUCTION

Recent investigations are directed toward studying the possibility of an immunogenetic basis for recurrent idiopathic spontaneous abortion in humans. One half of all couples with three or more spontaneous abortions who have been evaluated medically, genetically, microbiologically and structurally, as previously reported by us (1), are normal. We have evaluated 250 couples in this latter category immunogenetically as noted on Table 1. Couples who lacked an etiology for their pregnancy losses and who met immunogenetic criteria established by our group as outlined in Table 2 were offered intradermal immunization of the female spouse with paternal leukocytes on two occasions separated by six weeks as previously reported (2). Sixty-seven women were immunized and post-immunization immune response profiles were obtained six weeks following the second immunization. All couples in whom the female was immunized were advised to establish a pregnancy within two to three months post-immunization.

The purpose of this contribution is to present the sequential immune response profiles pre-immunization, post-immunization, during pregnancy and delivery or at the time of a repeat abortion in two groups of couples, 31 who delivered a child at term following leukocyte immunization and 17 women who aborted an additional time post-immunization. Nineteen women are currently pregnant and beyond 20 weeks gestation. The immunogenetic analyses were conducted in an attempt to establish the role(s) that the maternal immune response plays in the immunoprotection of the fetoplacental unit in utero (3). It is now well established that the critical features of the placental trophoblast for immune protection in the mother must be met to ensure survival of the infant to term. These are outlined in Table 4.

We have questioned if an inappropriate, inadequate, or absent immune response by the mother to paternally derived antigens or, an inefficient induction of this response by the fetoplacental unit may be a mechanism to ensure the maintenance of MHC genetic polymorphisms in humans. Earlier studies in inbred strains of animals have shown: 1) there are intense selective pressures operating during gestation against fetuses that are homozygous with their mothers with regard to MHC antigens; 2) there is decreased reproductive efficiency when MHC homozygous young are gestated in homozygous mothers; 3) there is selective elimination of MHC homozygotes either prenatally or early post-natally as the result of immunological responses to antigens not associated with the major histocompatibility complex but most likely linked to it; 4) recent studies in CBA/J female mice and DBA/2J

Table 1. Immunogenetic Workup of Couples With Three or More Recurrent Abortions of Unknown Etiology

1. HLA and ABO blood group antigen profiles
2. Maternal antipaternal leukocytotoxic antibodies
3. Mixed lymphocyte culture responses of maternal to paternal as compared to third party stimulator antigens
4. Immunoreactivity of lymphocytes harvested from lymph nodes of the uterine lymphatic drainage fields, and lymphocytes harvested from decidual tissue mantling the conceptus
5. Female serum complement independent/dependent mixed lymphocyte culture blocking factors
6. Analysis of maternal antibodies to T-cells, B-cells, and monocytes
7. Maternal serum antisperm antibodies by four assays

Table 2. Criteria Necessary in a Couple With Three or More Abortions for Immunization of the Female With Paternal Leukocytes

1. Share 3 or more HLA antigens
2. Maternal antipaternal immunological hyporesponsiveness in MLR compared to third party stimulators
3. Presence of cellular suppressors that block mixed lymphocyte culture reactions
4. No maternal antipaternal serum MLR blocking factors
5. No genetic, endocrine, structural, or infectious etiology found for pregnancy wastage

males provide a model that may allow definition of the gene products that incite a protective immune response toward the fetoplacental unit in the mother (5).

There is now recent scientific underpinning for this concept and Table 4 lists the best studied and documented mechanisms of the preferential production and maintenance in utero of fetuses MHC heterozygous with their mothers.

## MATERIALS AND METHODS

Two hundred and fifty caucasian couples from all parts of the United States, Canada, Great Britain and Europe with $4.6 \pm 2.2$ consecutive spontaneous abortions, each with a single partner, were evaluated by our medical and immunogenetic group as previously reported

Table 3. Critical Features of the Trophoblast for Immune Protection in the Mother

1. It is normally resistant to immune damage by lymphocytes, cytotoxic antibodies, or by antigen/antibody complexes.
2. It forms a physical barrier to most immune effectors except IgG antibody from reaching the fetus.
3. It signals and recruits the migration into the uterine decidua of lymphocytes that have suppressed activity or are functionally hyporesponsive to paternal antigens.
4. It produces steroid and protein hormones locally that are anti-inflammatory, immunosuppressive, and regulate gene expression of uterine cells.
5. It produces in the mother blocking factors that suppress maternal immune reactivity to paternal alloantigens in mixed lymphocyte cultures.
6. These blocking factors bind to the placenta on an antigen specific basis and achieve an immunological camouflage blocking the efferent limb of the immune reflex arc.

Table 4. Documented Mechanisms for the Preferential Production of MHC Heterozygotes

1. MATING PREFERENCES: male mice have been shown to exhibit a strong mating preference according to the MHC of their prospective mates (6).

2. SELECTIVE FERTILIZATION: preferential production of MHC heterozygotes due to selective fertilization (7).

3. SELECTIVE ABORTION: intrauterine selection against MHC homozygotes (8, 9).

4. HOMOZYGOUS LETHALS: recessive lethal MHC linked genes similar to the T/t complex in the mouse and the growth and reproduction (gr) complex in the rat (10, 9, 11).

5. ABERRANT MATERNAL IMMUNE RESPONSE: inability of MHC homozygous fetuses to initiate in the mother immunoprotection required for survival (12, 13, 14, 15, 16, 17).

6. MATERNAL/FETAL ALLELIC IDENTITY: with regard to the polymorphic antigen system TLX in man and the Pa antigen system in rats (8, 19).

(20). Female members of 67 couples were immunized with paternal leukocytes as previously reported (1). The post-immunization immune response profiles were followed sequentially during pregnancy, at delivery, or at the time of a repeat abortion. Laboratory testing relevant to this contribution included assays for maternal/anti-paternal leukocytotoxic antibodies and HLA A, B, C, and D/DR tissue typing (8). Mixed lymphocyte culture assays between spouses and an HLA incompatible third party were done sequentially to determine relative response ratios. Normal maternal serum and heat inactivated serum mixed lymphocyte culture blocking and potentiating assays were done post-immunization with paternal leukocytes during pregnancy, at delivery of a live born infant, or at the time of a repeat abortion. Some patients in both groups had lymphoid cells harvested from the uterine decidua mantling the conceptus and in vitro immune responses of these lymphocytes harvested and isolated by techniques developed by our laboratory were analyzed in mixed lymphocyte cultures involving mother, father, third party, and child when available.

## STATISTICS

These were performed by the Chi-square test with Yates' continuity when appropriate.

## RESULTS

### Complement Dependent Maternal Anti-paternal Lymphocytotoxic Antibodies

Sixteen percent of women studied by our group with 4.6 $\pm$ 2.2 consecutive abortions had detectable serum lymphocytotoxic antibodies with specificity for paternal HLA antigens in each case. This incidence is lower than that seen in primiparae, 20% or multiparae, 35 to 64% (20).

Figure 1 depicts the incidence of paternal specific complement dependent lymphocytotoxic antibodies in women immunized with paternal leukocytes who subsequently delivered a live born child or aborted an additional time post-immunization. Fifty-six percent of the women who delivered post-immunization became positive. All patients who aborted an additional time post-immunization developed paternal specific complement dependent lymphocytotoxic antibodies.

## SPECIFICITY OF THE LYMPHOCYTOTOXIC ANTIBODIES

All women who delivered a live born child at term developed lymphocytotoxic antibodies with B cell specificity. No woman who aborted an additional time post-immunization developed anti-B cell antibodies; however, all developed lymphocytotoxic anti-T cell antibodies (19).

## MIXED LYMPHOCYTE CULTURE RESPONSES

Genes within the D/DR locus are thought to determine mixed lymphocyte culture responses (MLR). The mixed lymphocyte culture responses of peripheral blood leukocytes were determined as we have previously reported (1). In all couples the relative response ratios of maternal lymphocytes to paternal and MHC unrelated third party individuals were tested. Figure 2 compares the relative reactivity of maternal lymphocytes to paternal lymphocytes as compared to an HLA incompatible third party stimulator in women immunized with paternal leukocytes who became pregnant post-immunization and delivered a child. Although there was a slight decrease in reactivity post-immunization,

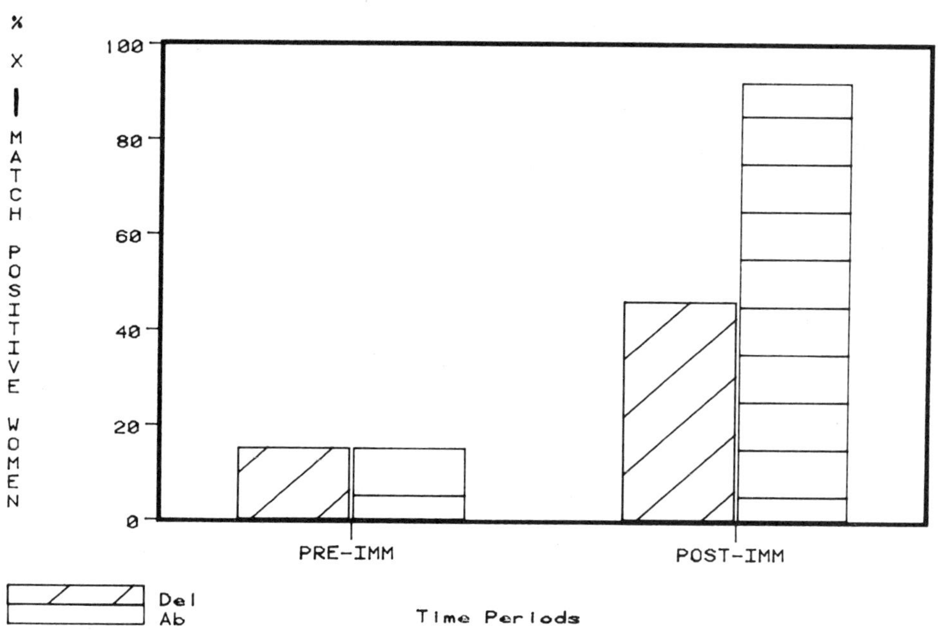


Figure 1. Incidence (%) of Maternal Antipaternal Anti-leukocytotoxic Antibodies in Women With Recurrent Abortions Immunized With Paternal Leukocytes Who Delivered a Live Born Child or Aborted an Additional Time Post-immunization

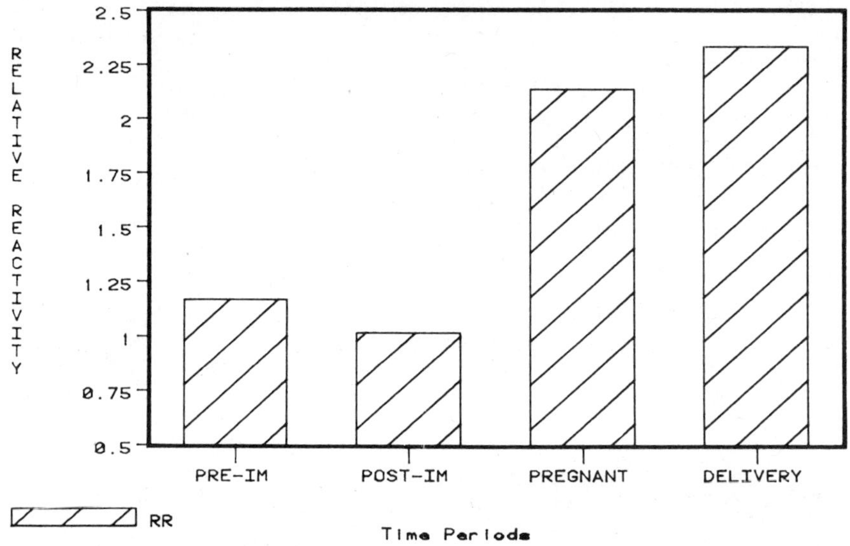


Figure 2. Comparing the Relative Reactivity in MLR of Lymphocytes From Women With Recurrent Abortion to Paternal and Third Party Lymphocytes Pre- and Post-Immunization With Paternal Leukocytes, During Pregnancy and at the Delivery of a Live Born Child at Term

this reactivity increased significantly during pregnancy and even further at the time of delivery, when testing of maternal reactivity to father/child/third party could be done (p less than 0.01).

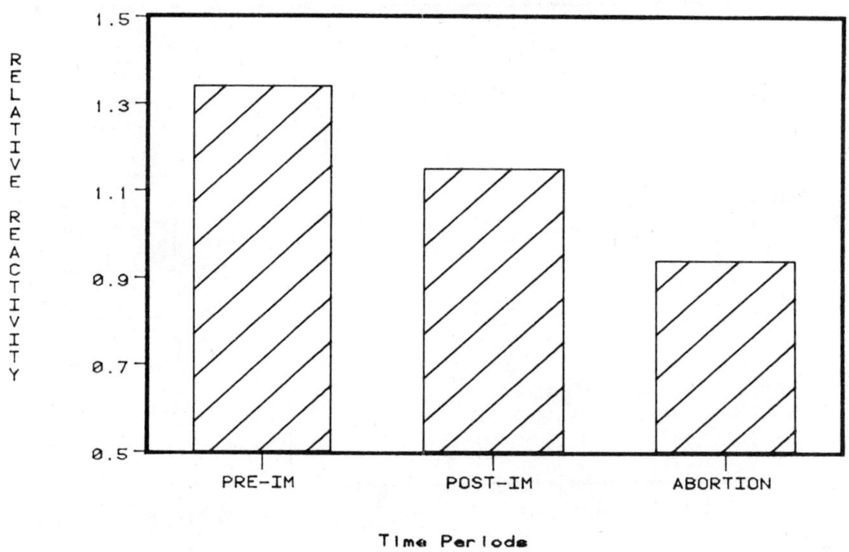


Figure 3. Comparing the Relative Reactivity of Lymphocytes From Women With Recurrent Abortions to Paternal and Third Party Lymphocytes Pre- and Post-Immunization With Paternal Leukocytes and at the Time of a Repeat Abortion

Figure 3 depicts the same type data in 17 couples who experienced a repeat abortion post-immunization. Although there were no differences in the pre-immunization relative reactivity in this group compared with the group who delivered a child there was a significant trend with a decrease in reactivity post-immunization and a further decrease at the time when assays were done on the day of the repeat abortion (p less than 0.05).

DYNAMICS OF SUPPRESSION BY NORMAL FEMALE SERUM AND HEAT INACTIVATED SERUM OF MLR IN WOMEN PRE- AND POST-IMMUNIZATION RELATIONSHIP WITH PREGNANCY OUTCOME

Patterns of humoral suppression by normal female serum and heat inactivated serum of MLR in women pre- and post-immunization with paternal leukocytes were studied. Suppression of greater than 20% was considered significant in that day to day variability of mixed lymphocyte culture assays done repeatedly is never more than 15%.

Figure 4 compares the patterns of suppression by normal female serum and heat inactivated serum of mixed lymphocyte culture reactivity (father stimulator, mother responder) pre- and post-immunization with paternal leukocytes, during pregnancy and at delivery. All 31 women in this category increased their paternal specific blocking activity in normal serum and heat inactivated serum to levels of 80 to 90% at delivery. This blocking activity was seen in all normal women with no history of repeated abortion who deliver a child at term (17).

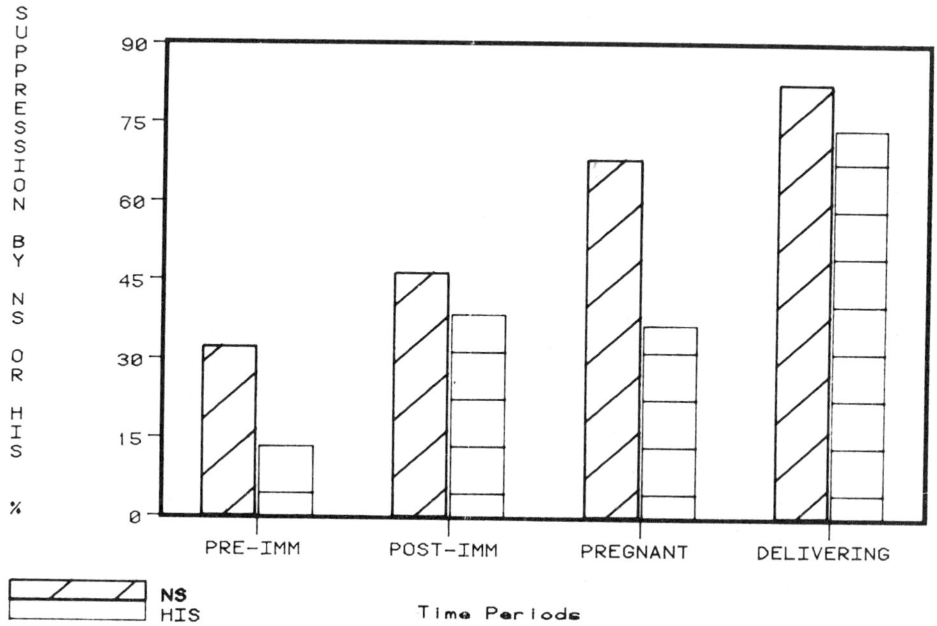


Figure 4. Patterns of Humoral Suppression by Normal Female Serum (NS) and Heat Inactivated Serum (HIS) of MLR (Male and Female) Pre-, Post-immunization With Paternal Leukocytes, During Pregnancy, and at Delivery of a Live Born Baby

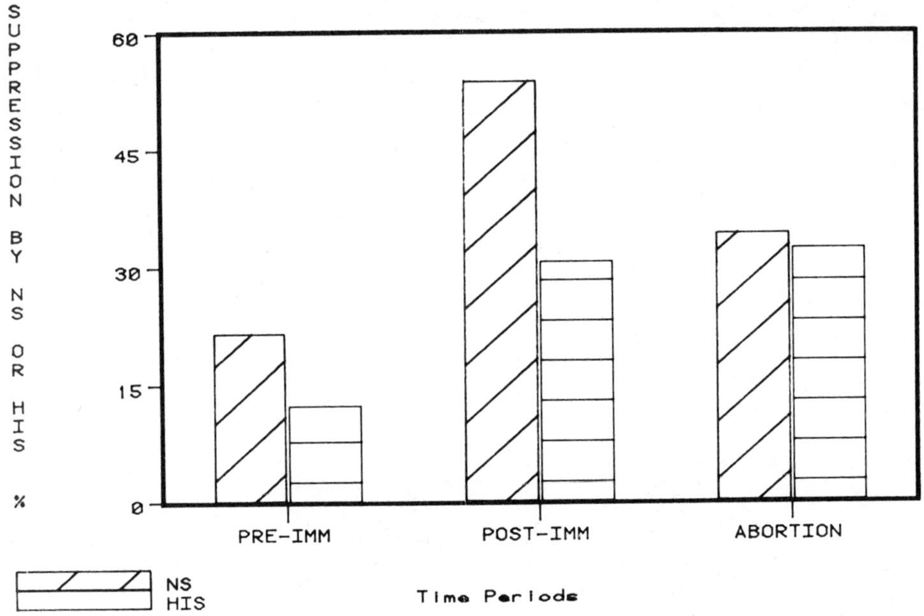


Figure 5. Patterns of Humoral Suppression by Normal Female Serum (NS) and Heat Inactivated Serum (HIS) of MLR (Female and Male) Pre-, Post-immunization With Paternal Leukocytes and After Subsequent Spontaneous Abortion

Figure 5 analyzes the same parameters sequentially in 17 women experiencing an abortion post-immunization. Post-immunization, the normal female serum blocking of MLR approached that seen in the group of patients that subsequently delivered; however, when the serum was heat inactivated MLR blocking dropped significantly. At the time of the abortion the MLR blocking was virtually absent (p less than 0.01). A more detailed analysis of this phenomenon has been reported previously (20).

The presence of female serum blocking activity post-immunization of 40% or greater that persists with heat inactivation of the female sera is predictive of a subsequent successful pregnancy outcome. Failure to see a significant rise in normal serum and heat inactivated serum MLR blocking early in pregnancy (6 to 8 weeks gestation) is associated with a subsequent abortion.

## POTENTIATION OR ENHANCEMENT OF MIXED LYMPHOCYTE CULTURE RESPONSES BY NORMAL FEMALE SERUM AND HEAT INACTIVATED SERUM: RELATIONSHIP TO PREGNANCY OUTCOME.

The addition of normal female serum to MLR involving paternal lymphocytes as stimulators and maternal lymphocytes as responders often enhances the stimulation index by 100% or greater. Figure 6 presents the percentage enhancement or potentiation by normal female serum compared with AB serum supplemented cultures sequentially from pre-immunization to delivery. Although significant enhancement by normal serum and heat inactivated serum is present to nearly 70% pre-immunization this phenomenon decreases totally in all patients who go to term delivery of a live born infant (p less than 0.05).

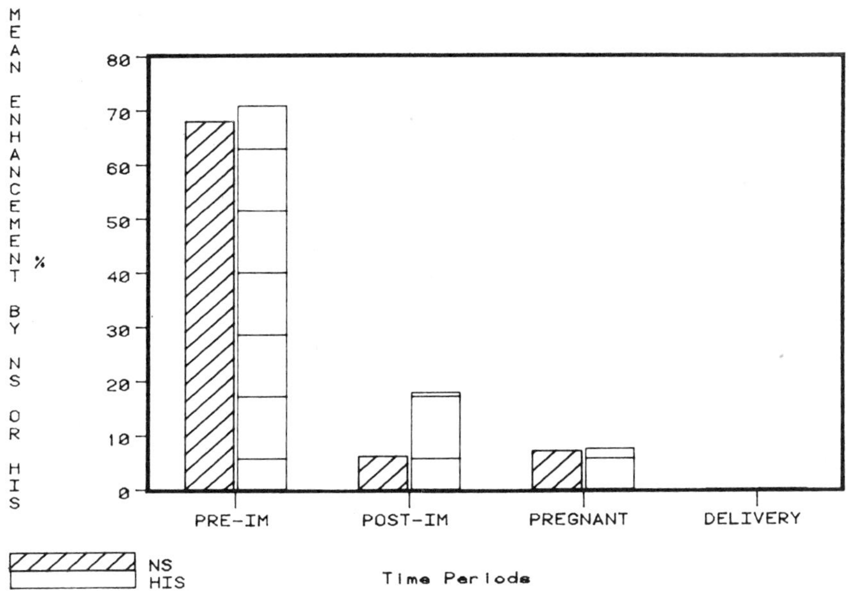


Figure 6. Patterns of Humoral Enhancement/Potentiation by Normal Female Serum (NS) and Heat Inactivated Serum (HIS) of MLR Pre- and Post-immunization With Paternal Leukocytes, During Pregnancy and at Delivery of a Live Born Child

Figure 7 compares the mean enhancement or potentiation by normal and heat inactivated serum pre-immunization, post-immunization and at

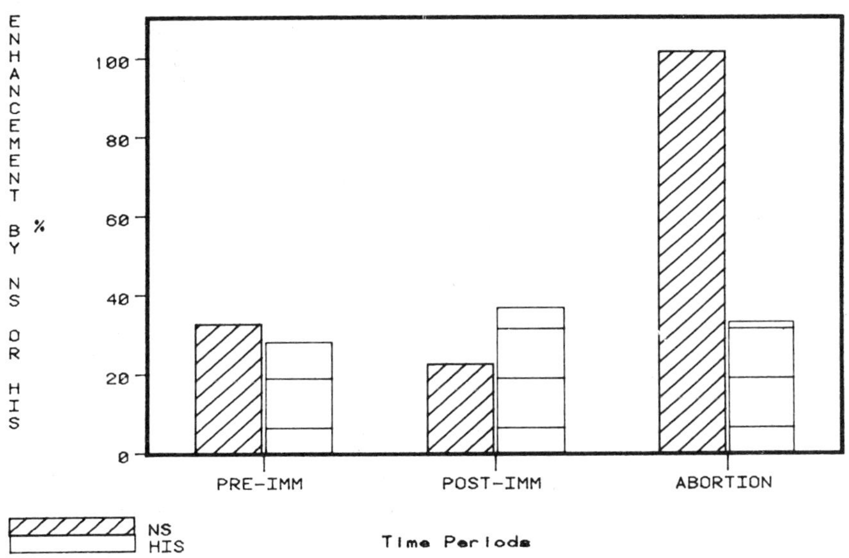


Figure 7. Patterns of Humoral Enhancement/Potentiation by Normal Female Serum (NS) and Heat Inactivated Serum (HIS) of MLR Pre- and Post-immunization With Paternal Leukocytes and at the Time of a Subsequent Abortion Post-immunization

the time of a repeat abortion. The addition of normal serum from the aborting female potentiates the reactivity of maternal cells responding to paternal cells significantly (p 0.01). The lack of normal female serum MLR blocking activity post-immunization and the presence of normal female serum potentiating or enhancing activity in MLR of 30% or greater is predictive of subsequent pregnancy loss. Studies utilizing immunoglobulin separation techniques are underway to determine what serum factor is responsible for promoting and/or suppressing the increase in the mixed lymphocyte culture reactivity in women with recurrent abortions.

## INTRAUTERINE FETAL GROWTH RETARDATION

We have seen a 10% incidence of severe symmetrical intrauterine growth retardation (IUGR) in recurrent aborting women subsequent to immunization with paternal leukocytes. Figure 8 compares a percentage of women in this IUGR group showing anti-T cell antibody pre- and post-immunization with the same parameters in women immunized with paternal leukocytes who subsequently delivered. No woman with an IUGR infant had T-cell antibodies prior to immunization, 50% developed anti-T cell antibodies at the time of delivery compared to 40% of those who delivered at term, P nonsignificant. As can be seen on Figure 9, no differences were detected in the two groups with regard to their production of anti-B cell antibodies. All women in both groups had anti-B cell antibodies.

## IMMUNODYNAMICS OF DECIDUAL LYMPHOCYTES

We have reported previously the immunoreactivity of maternal

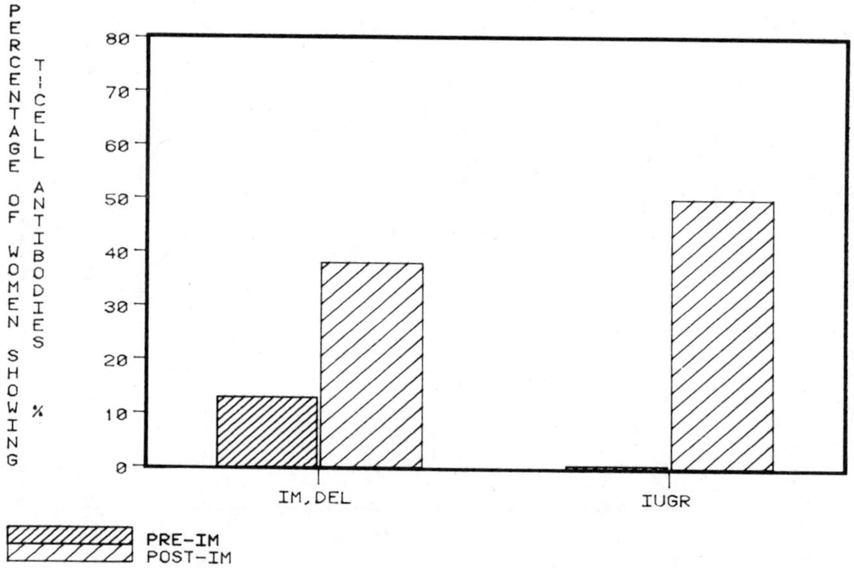


Figure 8. Comparing the Presence of Anti-T Cell Antibodies in Women Pre- and Post-immunization With Paternal Leukocytes Who Delivered a Normal Infant at Term (DEL) or a Severely Growth Retarded Infant (IUGR)

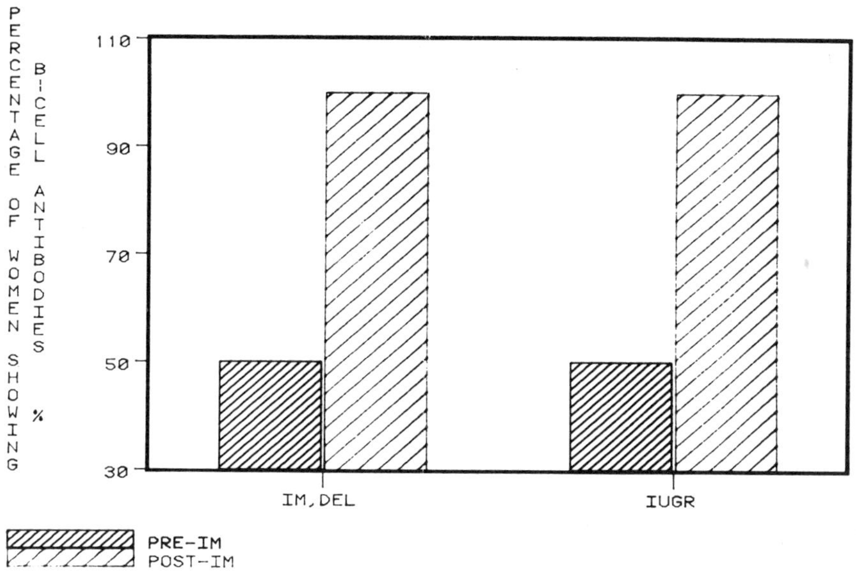


Figure 9. Comparing the Presence of Anti-B Cell Antibodies in Women Pre- and Post-Immunization With Paternal Leukocytes Who Delivered a Normal Infant at Term (DEL) or One Severely Growth Retarded (IUGR)

peripheral blood lymphocytes, iliac lymph node lymphocytes harvested from the uterine lymphatic drainage field, decidual lymphocytes and infants peripheral blood lymphocytes in one-way mixed lymphocyte culture reactions and have analyzed the patterns of suppression by AB, maternal and cord sera in women at the time of a normal delivery or at the time of an elective termination of a normal pregnancy (17). Lymphocytes from the uterine lymphatic drainage fields and lymphocytes from the decidua mantling the conceptus are nonresponsive, noncytotoxic to paternal or child's lymphocytes in MLR. They respond to PHA. Women at the time of a repeat abortion post-immunization have decidual lymphocytes surrounding the conceptus that are highly responsive to paternal and to third party alloantigens. The responses are significantly greater than peripheral blood lymphocytes in MLR and normal female serum does not block their reactivity (20). Table 5 compares the immunoreactivity of peripheral blood lymphocytes and decidual lymphocytes in a woman whose infant had severe IUGR, at delivery and the reactivity of uterine decidual lymphocytes three months post delivery on the 27th day of a normal menstrual cycle. At the time of the delivery of the growth retarded infant very strong proliferative responses of the maternal decidual lymphocytes to father and third party were seen. The same hyperreaction is seen in couples experiencing an abortion. Three months following delivery the lymphocytes harvested from the decidua of the same woman were functionally hyporesponsive. All patients with infants experiencing IUGR had strong serum MLR blocking factors with paternal specificity as well as antibodies with B cell specificity. Studies quantitating the blocking factors eluted from the placenta are in progress. Since dense accumulation of lymphoid cells are seen around and within the placentas of IUGR infants we must question whether idiopathic IUGR is a later manifestation of improper immunoprotection of the

Table 5. Proliferative Responses of Decidual Lymphocytes in MLR, at Delivery, and Three Months Post-Partum in a Woman With Recurrent Abortions, Immunized With Paternal Leukocytes Who Delivered a Severely Growth Retarded Male Infant Weighing 399 Grams at 32 Weeks Gestation

| Stimulator / Responder | Stimulation Index Delivery | 3 Months post partum |
|---|---|---|
| Unstimulated Decidual Cells | 0 | 0 |
| Decidual Cells + PHA | 664.6 | 4.1 |
| Mother(S) / Decidual(R) | 2.31 | 0.9 |
| Father(S) / Decidual(R) | 192.5 | 6.6 |
| 3rd Party(S) / Decidual(R) | 98.0 | 1.8 |

S = Stimulator
R = Responder

fetal placental unit or represents a breakdown of the trophoblast barrier function that excludes maternal lymphoid cells. Studies of this type are in progress. In addition, do MLR blocking factors known to be adsorbed to the placental trophoblast having a directive role(s) in recruiting suppressor cells and excluding other reactive cytotoxic cells at the trophoblast/decidual frontier? In addition, one must determine if the trophoblast of a child with intrauterine growth retardation (IUGR) is ineffective in expressing of gene products that are involved in immunoregulation and gene regulation locally.

## DISCUSSION AND CONCLUSIONS

There is now good evidence that the fetoplacental unit in all mammals studied expresses paternally derived antigens with determinants including Class I MHC alloantigens. These antigens are presented to the uterus and the maternal immune system in a manner that orchestrates an effective immune response systemically and locally that assists in the immunological camouflage of the fetoplacental unit. Immunogenetic studies in women with idiopathic recurrent abortions presented in this contribution has given insight regarding the elicitation of immune responses that are evoked in recurrently aborting women post-immunization with paternal leukocytes that eventually are associated with a normal pregnancy and delivery, a repeat abortion, or a pregnancy that results in a symmetrically growth retarded infant. The nature of the antigen stimulus that eventually confers protection on the fetoplacental unit is still unknown.

Taylor and Faulk suggest that spontaneous abortion can be attributed to maternal/fetal compatibility with regard to a polymorphic gene product(s) called trophoblast lymphocyte cross-reactive antigen-TLX. This results in the failure of the mother to produce anti-TLX antibodies that when present inhibit recognition or cytotoxicity to placental antigens (21). Our patients who have failed to mount an MLR blocking response post-immunization with paternal leukocytes and who have aborted again demonstrate hyperresponsive/cytotoxic lymphocytes in the decidua incapsulating the conceptus. These may be couples sharing the same TLX antigenic determinates. Three patients in this category are now successfully pregnant following immunization with HLA incompatible third party leukocytes and three are successfully pregnant following donor insemination with HLA incompatible semen.

Studies in progress of HLA identical twin sisters, one a recurrent aborter with her spouse and the other with children. These couples are providing much information relating to MLR blocking factors, local immune responses and recurrent abortion. Other experiments involving identical twin brothers one whose spouse is a recurrent aborter, the other whose spouse has born children has allowed us to address the question of extended haplotypes (some of which have been claimed the equivalent of the T/t locus in man) and their influence on reproduction (21).

The complexities of reproductive immunogenetics are beginning to come in to clear focus. It is quite certain that there is no singular simple explanation to explain successful viviparity. It nonetheless is equally clear that a successful pregnancy evokes in the mother measurable immune responses that have efferent paternal specificity and that the lack of these responses systemically or locally predicts a subsequent pregnancy failure. In summary: 1) MHC homozygosity between spouses is significantly greater in couples with recurrent abortion of unknown etiology (20); 2) couples with recurrent abortions may represent couples with extended HLA haplotypes that have been associated with other disease states (22); 3) women with recurrent abortion of unknown etiology immunized with paternal leukocytes who abort an additional time post-immunization have relative response ratios in MLR that decrease during pregnancy when compared with women who go on to deliver an infant at term; 4) these same women failed to develop antibodies with B-cell specificity but all develop antipaternal antileukocytotoxic antibodies; 5) a significant portion of these women lacking MLR blocking activity demonstrate enhancement or potentiation of MLR reactivity when maternal serum or maternal heat inactivated serum is added to culture; 6) immunization of women with recurrent abortion with paternal leukocytes that fails to result in paternal specific female serum MLR blocking factors or results in blocking factors that disappear with heat inactivation of the female sera is associated with an additional abortion post-immunization; 7) women with recurrent abortion of unknown etiology immunized with paternal leukocytes may become mothers of growth retarded infants.

## References


1. Beer A.E., Quebbeman J.F., Ayers J.W.T. and Haines, R.F.: Major Histocompatibility Complex Antigens, Maternal and Paternal Immune Responses, and Chronic Habitual Abortions in Humans. Am. J. Obstet. Gynecol. 141:987, 1981.

2. Beer A.E., Quebbeman J.F., Semprini A.E., Smouse P.E. and Haines R.F.: Recurrent Abortion: Analysis of the Roles of Parental Sharing of Histocompatibility Antigens and Maternal Immunological Responses to Paternal Antigens. Reproductive Immunology, Isojima S. and Billington W.D. (eds), Elsevier Science Publishers, Amsterdam, 1983.
3. Chaouat G., Kolb P.J., and Wegmann T.G.: The Murine Placenta as an Immunological Barrier Between the Mother and the Fetus, Immunological Reviews 75:31-60, 1984.
4. Chaouat G: The Riddle of the Fetal Allograft. Ann. Immunol (Inst. Pasteur) 135 D:301-351, 1984.
5. Chaouat G, Kiger N., Wegmann T.G.: Vaccination Against Spontaneous Abortion in Mice. J. Reprod. Immunol. 5:389-392, 1983.
6. Boyce E.A., Beauchamp G.K. and Yamakazi K.: The Sensory Perception of Genotypic Polymorphism of the Major Histocompatibility Complex and Other Genes: Some Physiological and Pylogenetic Implications. Hum. Immun. 6:177-183, 1983.
8. Beer A.E., Quebbeman J.F. and Semprini A.E.: Immunopathological Factors Contributing to Recurrent Spontaneous Abortion In Humans. Edmonds D.K. and Bennett M.J. (eds), Blackwell Scientific Publication, London, 1985, in press.
9. Gill T.J.: Immunogenetics of Spontaneous Abortions in Humans. Transplan. 35:1-6, 1983.
10. Bennett D.: The T Locus of the Mouse Cell. 6:441-454, 1975.
11. Thomas M.L., Harger J.H., Wagener D.K., Rabin B.S., and Gill T.J. III: Sharing and Spontaneous Abortion in Humans. Am. J. Obstet. Gynec., 1985, in press.
12. Palm J.: Association of Maternal Genotype and Excess Heterozygosity for Ag-B Histocompatibility Antigens Among Male Rats. Trans. Proc. 1(1):82-84, 1969.
13. Palm J.: Maternal-fetal Interactions and Histocompatibility Antigen Polymorphisms. Trans. Proc. 2:162-173, 1970.
14. Hings I.M. and Billingham R.E.: Splenectomy and Sensitization of Fischer Female Rats Favors Histoincompatibility of R2 Back-cross Progeny. Transplan. Proc. 13:1253-1255, 1981.
15. Michie D. and Anderson N.F.: A Strong Selective Effect Associated With a Histocompatibility Gene in the Rat. Ann. N.Y. Acad. Sci. 129:88-93.
16. Clark D.A.: Local Suppressor Cells and the Success or Failure of the Fetal Allograft. Ann. Immunol. (Inst. Pasteur) 135 D:321-324, 1984.
17. Beer, A.E.: How Did Your Mother Not Reject You? Ann. Immunol. (Inst. Pasteur) 135 D:315-318, 1984.
18. McIntrye J.A. and Faulk W.P.: Allotypic Trophoblast Lymphocyte Crossreactive (TLX) Cell Surface Antigens. Hum. Immunol. 4:27, 1982.
19. Johnson P.M., Barner R.M.R., Risk J.M., Mollay C.M. and Woodrow J.C.: Immunogenetic Studies of Recurrent Spontaneous Abortions in Humans. Expl. Clin. Immunogenet. 2:77-83, 1985.
20. Beer A.E., Semprini A.E., Xiaoyu Z. and Quebbeman J.F.: Pregnancy Outcome in Human Couples With Recurrent Spontaneous Abortions: 1) HLA Antigen Profiles; 2) HLA Antigen Sharing; 3) Female Serum MLR Blocking Factors; and, 4) Paternal Leukocyte Immunization. Exp. Clin. Immunogenet., 1985a, in press.
21. Taylor C. and Faulk W.P.: Prevention of Recurrent Abortions With Leukocyte Transfusions. Lancet II, 8237:68, 1981.
22. Alper C.A., Awdeh Z.L., Roum D.D., Yunis E.J.: Possible Human Analogs of the Murine T/t Complex: Expl. Clin. Immunogenet. 2:125-136, 1985.

# IMMUNOSTIMULATION AND THE PROMOTION OF FERTILITY

Irene Athanassakis and Thomas G. Wegmann

Department of Immunology
University of Alberta
Edmonton, Alberta, Canada T6G 2H7

## GENERAL INTRODUCTION

One fact emerging from a number of studies of the maternal-fetal relationship is that the trophoblast--which forms the interface between the maternal and fetal circulations (see Figure 1)--is a privileged tissue with respect to transplantation rejection. Classic studies of Simmons and Russell (1962) showed that it is almost impossible to elicit a destructive reaction using transplanted allogeneic trophoblast. Recent striking experiments by Rossant and her colleagues (Clark et al., 1984; Rossant et al., 1982) and others (Fehilly et al., 1984; Meinecke-Tillman and Meinecke, 1984) emphasize the role of the trophoblast in protecting the fetus *in situ*. They have been able to produce viable adult interspecies chimeras by the construction of "Trojan horse" embryos. These reconstructed preimplantation embryos consist of an outer layer of trophectoderm that is syngeneic to the foster mother whose uterus is used for gestation. Trophectoderm is the layer that gives rise to the fetal part of the fetal-maternal interface in the placenta. The inner cell mass--which gives rise to the embryo proper--is all, or in part, derived from a xenogeneic embryo so that the resultant animal is completely or partly derived from a different species. This is only possible when the trophoblast is of the same species as the mother, as demonstrated by various control experiments. Although these studies do not elucidate what mechanisms are responsible for the protective role of the trophoblast, they certainly call attention to its existence. Support for the privileged transplant status of trophoblast is provided by studying the immunological correlates of interspecies implantations and contrasting them with "Trojan horse" chimeras (Clark et al., 1984). Whenthe embryo is surrounded by trophoblast which is xenogeneic to the female, one sees a lack of the maternally derived decidual suppressor cells that routinely appear in ordinary decidua. In addition, there is an obvious penetration of the giant cell trophoblast layer by maternal lymphocytes. These experiments suggest, but do not provide direct evidence for, an immunoprotective role for the trophoblast, perhaps analogous to that seen with histoincompatibility in primitive marine invertebrates, such as sponges and sea anemones (Bigger et al., 1980, 1982, 1983; Francis, 1976). Here, histocompatibility-like reactions are thought to be involved in maintaining colonial integrity.

For a long time it was believed that paternally derived major histocompatibility complex (MHC) antigens were either not expressed or were covered up in fetal tissues in direct contact with maternal circulation. However, recent experiments using both murine and human placentas indicate that paternally derived MHC antigens are present on cells in direct contact with maternal circulation, albeit in low amounts (Singh et al., 1983; Kawata et al., 1984). This is especially clear for antigens of the Class I variety, and is the basis of the placenta's ability to serve as an immunoabsorbent barrier for antipaternal MHC antibodies (Chaouat et al., 1983). However, it is not clear what type of Class I antigens are expressed and recent unpublished observations indicate that the Class I antigens may be of an unusual type (T.J. Gill and P.M. Johnson, personal communication, 1985). There is also ample evidence that during the course of both murine and human pregnancy, maternal recognition of alloantigen takes place, even in the first pregnancy (Gill and Repetti, 1979; Wegmann and Gill, 1983). This is reflected in increased lymph node size and changes in lymphoid morphology in those nodes draining an allogeneically pregnant uterus, a concomitant decrease in the thymus of the allogeneically pregnant mother, and indications of lymphokine release into the serum of allogeneically pregnant rats (Chaouat et al., 1983; Gill and Repetti, 1979; Wegmann and Gill, 1983). In addition, there has been a longstanding awareness of alloantibody formation during first pregnancy in a variety of different species. A major question to be addressed is whether this immune recognition by the mother is merely without harmful consequences to the fetus or whether it in fact promotes placental growth and fetal viability. This is not a new question. The issue was first addressed clearly in the late 1960s by Clarke and Kirby, who postulated that maternal immune recognition led to improved fetal viability and was therefore a driving force leading to increased MHC polymorphism (Clarke and Kirby, 1966). The data on which this hypothesis was built, mainly involving increases in allogeneic placental and fetal weights and improved growth of trophoblast under conditions of immune stimulation, did not survive attempts to replicate the experiments in the hands of others. Therefore the idea did not survive critical review (McLaren, 1975). Nevertheless, the idea has not totally disappeared, as one continues to read claims in the literature of how immune responses can improve fetal viability and increase placental and fetal weights, although clearly this is not a universal phenomenon (Gill, 1983a; Zuckermann and Head, 1985).

The controversy brings to mind the concept of immunostimulation as a contributing factor to oncogenesis, which has been formulated by Prehn (1972, 1983). He has collected evidence that in certain phases of cancer growth, some types of antitumor immunity can promote rather than hinder tumor growth. The difference between this phenomenon and immunostimulation as applied to outbred pregnancy is that in the latter instance, it would occur as part of a centrally important physiological rather than pathological process, making it unique and therefore of great interest to confirm or deny.

## VACCINATION AGAINST ABORTION

Recent information compels a re-examination of these ideas as applied to pregnancy. There have been numerous reports of instances in which human couples with multiple spontaneous abortions show significantly more sharing of HLA specifities than do control couples (Amar et al., 1984; Beer et al., 1981; Gerencer et al., 1978, 1979; Gill, 1983b; Komlos et al., 1977; Lauritsen et al., 1976a, 1976b; Shaacter et al., 1979; Taylor and Faulk, 1981). Taken at face value, these data indicate that there could be merit to the idea that HLA polymorphism is driven by an increased viability among HLA incompatible offspring. Reinforcing this view are clinical observations in which mothers undergoing repeated spontaneous abortions can subsequently deliver live offspring following subcutaneous injection of either paternal lymphocytes or pooled allogeneic lymphocytes (Beer et al., 1981; Taylor and Fault, 1981). However, a correct interpretation of these clinical trials, which have been reported from a number of centers, awaits double-blind studies using maternal lymphocyte injection as a control (Gill, 1983b; see below). Even if the effect depends upon priming by alloantigens, ethical considerations will hinder an exact analysis of the primary immunological events behind the antiabortion effect. It is therefore fortunate that an animal model exists which simulates the clinical observations.

The model is based on the work of David Clark and his associates who observed that CBA/J females pregnant by DBA/2J male mice show an increased rate of spontaneous abortion when compared to other strains, or to the reciprocal strain combination. They also found that the cells of the decidua and draining lymph nodes in this strain combination have a lower immunosuppressive capacity than cells of other strains, thus providing an *in vivo* correlate to their previous observations of *in vitro* immunosuppression in the vicinity of the fetal-placental unit (Clark et al., 1980, 1984). While on sabbatical in Paris, French colleagues and I decided to see whether we could repeat these observations and alter the rate of spontaneous abortion by vaccination with spleen cells, in analogy to the human situation. We found that vaccination with spleen cells of maternal or paternal type seven days prior to pregnancy had no effect of the incidence of abortion. We still observed approximately a 25% resorption rate at day 12 of pregnancy. However, when the CBA/J females were vaccinated with Balb/c spleen cells, which share the H-2*d* haplotype with the paternal strain cell but differ in other parts of the genome, the resorption rate was brought down to less than 5% (Chaouat et al., 1983b). Additional studies indicate that congenic Balb.K and Balb.B spleen cells do not produce the antiresorption effect. These cells differ from the Balb/c cells only at the chromosomal region surrounding the MHC haplotype (Kiger et al., 1985). Since that time, we have been studying the immunological consequences of this vaccination (Chaouat et al., 1985). We have found that spleen cells from CBA/J females pregnant by DBA/2J males have a greater capacity to suppress immunological activity *in vitro* (MLR and CTL) if they are vaccinated with Balb/c cells, compared to vaccination with DBA/2J or CBA/J cells (Chaouat et al., 1983v, 1984). This active suppression has specificity, as shown by control experiments involving attempts to suppress third party reacitivity. However, as argued elsewhere in detail (Chaouat et al., 1983a), peripheral active suppression in the pregnant female is unlikely to be important in protecting the fetus. This is because it can easily be overridden by deliberate immunization with no harmful consequences to the fetus or placenta. Perhaps of more importance is the active suppression seen in the vicinity of the fetoplacental unit.

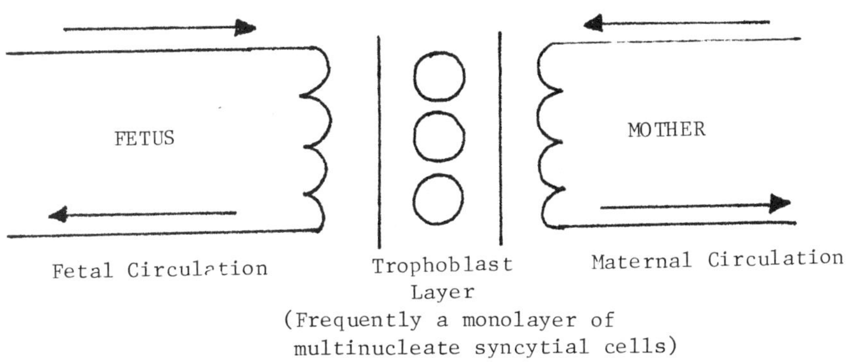


Figure 1. Circuit diagram of hemochorial placenta, found in rodents and primates, including the human species. Emphasis on trophoblast layer and the circulation.

Here one also sees an increase in active suppression (against natural killer cells) in CBA/J x DBA/2J placentas following immunization with Balb/c, but not in the controls. Successful vaccination (that is, Balb *versus* DBA spleen cells) also correlates with the appearance of antipaternal MHC antibody in maternal serum. This antibody is diminished if sampled at a time during pregnancy when the placenta has fetal MHC antigens expressed on it. A large number of experiments indicate that the placenta can serve as an immunoabsorbent for antipaternal MHC antibody, so the antibody undoubtedly binds to the placenta (Moller, 1983).

This set of observations may well be the key to understanding how vaccination protects the fetus, because one can adoptively transfer fetal protection in this strain combination with CBA/J anti-Balb/c immune serum. The adoptive transfer remains effective following *in vitro* absorption of the serum by Balb.K cells, but not by DBA/2 cells (see Table 1). This indicates that the antibody responsible for fetal protection is directed at some component of the MHC complex. These results also suggest that for some reason DBA/2J cells have the relevant MHC antigen, but they are not immunogenic when injected into the CBA/J female. Following adoptive transfer of the serum, the placentas yield increased numbers of suppressor cells (Chaouat et al., 1986). A straightforward (and perhaps simple-minded) interpretation of these results would be that vaccination simply stimulates the mother to produce antipaternal MHC antibodies. These antibodies, in turn, bind to the placenta and somehow trigger fetally derived cells to provide more effective immunosuppression, perhaps with signals from Fc-binding cells. Alternatively, this "immunostimulation" could cause, via growth factors, fetal cell proliferation which, in turn, might improve the general functional characteristics of the placenta, leading to increased fetal viability.

These recent findings, then, force a new look at the old concept that immune stimulation may promote fetal viability. Of course, new approaches will have to be devised to examine this concept rather than relying on crude placental and fetal weights as end points, as has been done in the past. For example, the placenta can be fractionated and fetal cells separated from maternal cells on the basis of surface markers and size. Proliferation by incorporation of nucleotide precursors rather than weight my turn out to be a more precise indicator of immunostimulation, in analogy to mixed lymphocyte culture reactivity. Such a protocol or a variation on it will allow a more accurate definition of what effect maternal immune recognition has on placental growth and immunoregulation. It will be worth the effort if we can come to some understanding of how fetal tissues and their malignant counterparts that bear paternally derived Class I MHC antigens can live in harmony with--if not be stimulated by--the otherwise destructive capabilities of the maternal transplantation reaction.

## PLACENTAL CELL PROLIFERATION *IN VITRO*

To this end, we have been examining how a number of defined T cell-derived lymphokines influence the proliferation of fetally derived cells from the placenta *in vitro*, under the assumption that the lymphokine(s) identified may be important in mediating the fetal protection effect. These experiments have been done in conjunction with Dr C. Bleakley of the Department of Biochemistry at the University of Alberta, who has been purifying these lymphokines in collaboration with Dr V. Paetkau (Paetkau et al., 1985). Our original experiments employed F3, a supernatant derived from EL-4 T-cell hybridoma (subline E1), stimulated by phorbol myristic acetate. We found that a combination of the F3 supernatant and monoclonal anti-Class I MHC antibody directed against maternal components of the placenta leads to the *in vitro* proliferation of cells derived from the fetus, as measured by tritiated thymidine incorporation. The fact that the cells are of fetal origin

Table 1. Effect of Active and Passive Immunity on Fetal Resorption in CBA/J Females Pregnant by DBA/2 Males.

| | Treatment on Day -7 Before Conception | Number of Live Fetuses (Day 12) | Number of Resorbed Fetuses (Day 12) | Per cent Resorption |
|---|---|---|---|---|
| 1. | Null | 121 | 60 | 33 |
| 2. | $10^7$ BALB/cJ spleen cells i.p. | 194 | 24 | 11 |
| 3. | $10^7$ DBA/2J spleen cells i.p. | 106 | 55 | 34 |
| 4. | 0.2 ml RPMI 1640 medium i.v. | 74 | 43 | 37 |
| 5. | 0.2 ml CBA/J serum i.v. | 153 | 64 | 29 |
| 6. | 0.2 ml CBA/J anti-BALB serum i.v. * | 365 | 39 | 10 |
| 7. | 0.2 ml CBA/J anti-BALB serum, * absorbed with BALB/K spleen cells, i.v. ** | 142 | 20 | 12 |
| 8. | 0.2 ml CBA/J anti-BALB serum, * absorbed with DBA/2J spleen cells, i.v. ** | 82 | 50 | 38 |

* CBA females immunized with $10^7$ BALB/cJ spleen cells and bled 21 days later.

** 1 ml of serum was absorbed for 1 hour at 4° C with $10^8$ spleen cells.

Table revised from Chaouat et al., 1986, in Gill and Wegmann, 1986.

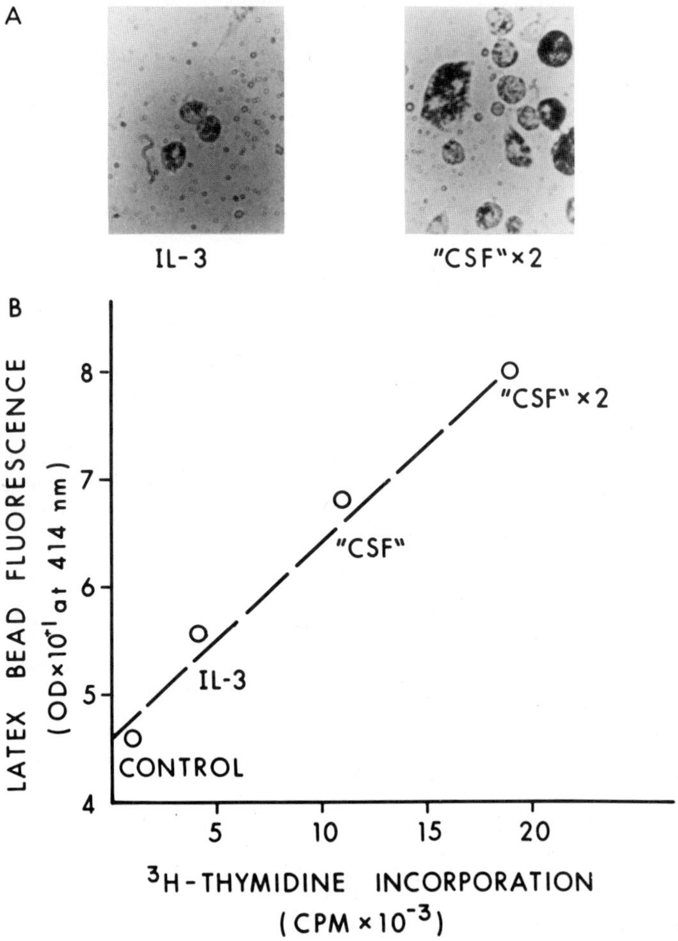


Figure 2. A. The left-hand panel shows a microscopic view of fetally derived placental cells under control lymphokine stimulation (IL-3) and the right-hand panel shows them after two additions, on day 0 and day 2, of CSF.GM. The dark material inside the cells represents latex bead incorporation. Notice the increased number and size of the CSF-stimulated cells.

B. Correlation between proliferation of fetally derived placental cells, as measured by tritiated thymidine uptake, and phagocytosis, as measured by latex bead incorporation.

OD optical density, read in a Titertech multiscan Elisa plate reader. All measurements were made at the end of culture, which is 48 hours in the control, IL-3, and CSF cultures, and 96 hours in the case of CFS x 2, in which CSF was added at 0 and 48 hours. Notice that a greater degree of lymphokine induced proliferation clearly correlate with an increased amount of phagocytosis (r 0.99). Thus, a T-cell-derived lymphokine can improve a critical function of fetally derived placental cells, namely phagocytosis, which is not doubt of importance in fetal survival.

was ascertained by a quantitative isozyme technique employing the dimeric genetic marker glucose phosphate isomerase that can distinguish between maternal and fetal cells (Hunziker et al., 1984)(discretely, in the present case, due to the use of interstrain blastocyst transfer, thus avoiding overlapping parental and $F_1$ hybrid bands). Further experiments indicate that the most effective lymphokine within the mixture represented by F3 is partially purified colony stimulating factor-granulocyte-macrophage ("CSF-GM"). For example, adding "CSF-GM" at times 0 and 48 hours to $10^6$ placental cells in culture gives an incorporation of $H^3T$ of 18,889 _ 1880 dpm/$10^6$ cells in culture, whereas IL-3 gives 3189 _ 366 dpm and placental cells alone as a control give 1078 _ 241 dpm. IL-1 and IL-2 show no significant effects. It is also of some interest to note that "CSF-GM" dramatically increased the ability of these fetally derived placental cells to phagocytose latex beads *in vitro*, in rough correlation with the amount of $H^3T$ incorporated (Figure 2) (Athanassakis et al., 1985). The cells that proliferate are large, phagocytic, esterase positive and are frequently multinucleate. We are actively working on their relation to trophoblast and ordinary tissue macrophages. At this stage, we do not know for certain the molecular identity of the "CSF-GM". This will require further purification and molecular cloning and is being actively pursued by Drs Bleackley and Paetkau.

These studies, albeit preliminary, indicate that fetally derived placental cells can respond by proliferation to well-defined T cell-derived lymphokines *in vitro*. They are reminiscent of work by Edidin and his colleagues, who have shown that peritoneal exudate cells from multiparous but not virgin female mice can induce proliferation of both teratocarcinoma cells and embryonic blastocysts *in vitro* (Fenderson et al., 1983). More recently, Mayumi and his colleagues have shown that supernatants from early mouse embryos are capable of immunosuppressive activities, a finding similar to the descriptions of early pregnancy factor over a number of years (Mayumi et al., 1985). The major question remaining is the physiological significance of these observations and their relation to immunostimulation of tumors.

## REFERENCES


Amar, A., J.R. Oksenberg, E. Persitz, et al. 1984. Specific depressed mixed lymphocyte reaction in couples with recurrent abortions. *Human Immunol.*

Athanassakis, I., C. Bleakley, V. Paetkau, and T.G. Wegmann. 1986. The immunostimulatory effect of T-cell-derived lymphokines on fetally derived murine placental cells. In preparation.

Beer, A.E., J.F. Quebbeman, J.W.T. Ayers, and R.F. Haines. 1981. Major histocompatibility antigens, maternal and paternal immune response, and chronic habitual abortions in humans. *Amer. J. Obstet. Gynecol.* 141:987.

Bigger, C.H. 1980. Interspecific and intraspecific acrochagial aggressive behavior among sea anemones: A recognition of self and non-self. *Biol. Bull.* 159:117.

Bigger, C.H., P.L. Jokiel, W.H. Hildemann, and I.S. Johnston. 1982. Characterization of alloimmune memory in a sponge. *J. Immunol.* 129:1570.

Bigger, C.H., P.L. Jokiel, and W.H. Hildemann. 1983. Cytotoxic transplantation immunity in the sponge *Toxadoria violacea*. *Transplantation* 35:239.

Chaouat, G., J.-P. Kolb, and T.G. Wegmann. 1983. The murine placenta as an immunological barrier between the mother and the fetus. *Immunol. Rev.* 75:31.

Chaouat, G., J.-P. Kolb, M. Stanislawski, and T.G. Wegmann. 1984. Immunological consequences of vaccination against abortion in mice. *J. Immunol.*

Chaouat, G., N. Kiger, and T.G. Wegmann. 1983. Vaccination against spontaneous abortion in mice. *J. Reprod. Immunol.* 5:389.

Chaouat, G., J.-P. Kolb, S. Chaffaux, M. Rivière, I. Athanassakis, D. Green, and T.G. Wegmann. 1986. The placenta and the survival of the fetal allograft. In *Immunoregulation and Fetal Survival*, T.J. Gill III and

T.G. Wegmann, eds. New York: Oxford University Press. In press.

Clark, D.S., M. McDermott, and M.R. Sczewzuk. 1980. Impairment of host vs graft reaction in pregnant mice. II. Selective suppression of cytotoxic cell generation correlates with soluble suppressor activity and with successful allogeneic pregnancy. *Cell. Immunol.* 52:106.

Clarke, D.A., R.M. Slapsys, B.A. Croy, and J. Rossant. 1984. Immunoregulation of host-versus-graft responses in the uterus. *Immunol. Today* 5:111.

Clarke, B. and D.R.S. Kirby. 1966. Maintenance of histocompatibility polymorphisms. *Nature* 211:999.

Fehilly, C.B., S.M. Willadsen, and E.M. Tucker. 1984. Interspecific chimerism between sheep and goat. *Nature* 307:637.

Fenderson, B.A., P.F. Bartlett, and M. Edidin. Maternal immunostimulation of a teratocarcinoma-derived cell line, TerCs. *J. Reprod. Immunol.* 5:287.

Francis, L. 1976. Social organization within clones of the sea anemone *Anthopleura elegantissima*. *Biol. Bull.* 150:361.

Gerencer, M., A. Kastelan, A. Drazancic, V. Kerhin-Brklacic, and M. Madjaric. 1978. The HLA antigens in women with recurrent abnormal pregnancies of unknown etiology. *Tissue Antigens* 12:223.

Gill, T.J. III. 1983. Immunogenetics of spontaneous abortion in humans. *Transplantation* 35:1.

Gill, T.J. III. 1983. Immunogenetic aspects of the maternal-fetal interaction. In *Immunology of Reproduction*, T.G. Wegmann and T.J. Gill III, eds. New York: Oxford University Press, p. 54.

Gill, T.J. III and C.F. Repetti. 1979. Immunologic and genetic factors influencing reproduction. *Amer. J. Pathol.* 95:463.

Hunziker, R.D., P. Gambel, and T.G. Wegmann. 1984. Placenta as a selective barrier to cellular traffic. *J. Immunol.* 133:667.

Kawata, K., J.R. Parkes, L.A. Herzenberg. 1984. Transcriptional control of HLA-A,B,C antigen in human placental cytotrophoblast isolated using trophoblast and HLA-specific monoclonal antibodies and the fluorescein-activated cell sorter. *J. Exp. Med.* 160:633.

Kiger, N., G. Chaouat, J.-P. Kolb, T.G. Wegmann, and J.-L. Guenet. 1985. Immunogenetic studies of spontaneous abortion in mice. I. Preimmunization of females with allogeneic cells. *J. Immunol.* In press.

Komlos, L., R. Zamir, H. Joshua, and I. Halbrecht. 1977. Common HLA antigens in couples with repeated abortions. *Clin. Immunol. Immunopathol.* 7:330.

Lauritsen, J.G., T. Kristensen, and N. Grunnet. 1976. Depressed mixed lymphocyte culture reactivity in mothers with recurrent spontaneous abortion. *Amer. J. Obstet. Gynecol.* 125:35.

Lauritsen, J.G., J. Jorgensen, and F. Kissmeyer-Nielson. 1976. Significance of HLA and blood-group incompatibility in spontaneous abortion. *Clin. Genet.* 9:575.

Mayumi, T., S. Bitoh, S. Anan, T. Hama, S. Fujimoto, and H. Yamamoto. Suppressor T lymphocyte induction by a factor released from cultured blastocysts. *J. Immunol.* 134:404.

McLaren, A. 1975. Antigenic disparity: Does it affect placental size, implantation, or population genetics? In *Immunobiology of Trophoblast*, R.G. Edwards, C.W.S. Howe, and M. Johnson, eds. Cambridge, U.K.: Cambridge University Press, p. 255.

Meinecke-Tillman, S., and B. Meinecke. 1984. Experimental chimeras: Removal of reproductive barrier between sheep and goat. *Nature* 307:637.

Prehn, R.T. 1972. The immune reaction as a stimulator of tumor growth. *Science* 176:170.

Prehn, R.T. 1983. The dose-response curve in tomor immunity. *Internat. J. Immunopharm.* 5:255.

Rossant, J. V.M. Mauro, and B.A. Croy. 1982. Importance of trophoblast genotype for survival of interspecific murine chimeras. *J. Embryol. Exp. Morphol.* 69:411.

Schaacter, B., A. Muir, M. Gyves, and M. Tasin. 1979. HLA-A,B compatibility in parents of offspring with neural-tube defects or couples experiencing involuntary fetal wastage. *Lancet* 1:796.

Simmons, R.L. and P.S. Russell. 1962. The antigenicity of mouse trophoblast. *Ann. N. Y. Acad. Sci.* 99:717.

Singh, B., R. Raghupathy, D.J. Anderson, and T.G. Wegmann. 1983. The placenta as an immunological barrier between mother and fetus. In *Immunology of Reproduction*, T.G. Wegmann and T.J. Gill III, eds. New York: Oxford University Press, p. 229.

Taylor, C. and W.P. Faulk. 1981. Prevention of recurrent abortion with leucocyte transfusions. *Lancet* 2:68.

Wegmann, T.G. and T.J. Gill III eds. 1983. *Immunology of Reproduction*, New York: Oxford University Press.

Zuckermann, F. and J.R. Head. 1985. Susceptibility of mouse trophoblast to antibody and complement-mediated damage. *Transplant. Proc.* 17:925.

# HISTOCOMPATIBILITY AND REPRODUCTION

Susan Heyner

Department of Obstetrics and Gynecology
Albert Einstein Medical Center, Northern Division
Philadelphia, PA

## INTRODUCTION

In all outbreeding populations, fetal and maternal tissues are in intimate juxtaposition, and there is ample evidence to show that the maternal organism responds immunologically to the paternally derived histocompatibility antigens of the fetus (reviewed by Head and Billingham, 1983). This situation has led a number of biologists to consider the fetus as an allograft, and to propose various mechanisms whereby the fetus evades immunological rejection (Medawar, 1953).

It is an oversimplification to compare the surgical exchange of tissue into a prepared vascular bed with the development of a fetus separated from the maternal circulation by an extraembryonic organ; nevertheless, there is a growing amount of evidence that implicates histocompatibility antigen expression with successful reproduction.

The arguments for a beneficial effect of immunological disparity between the maternal organism and the fetus are based on observations that litter sizes, and possibly also the fetal and placental weights are larger in allogeneic pregnancies than in syngeneic pregnancies (McLaren, 1976; Auerbach et al., 1980). Further, in the animal species studies, an increased reproductive capacity appears to be present in heterozygous pregnancies, in terms of litter size, and number of fetuses homozygous with the mother (Clarke and Kirby, 1966; Tofoski and Gill, 1977; Beer et al., 1975).

In humans, a number of investigators have reported that women suffering from recurrent spontaneous abortion can realize successful term pregnancies following immunization with white blood cells from either their husband, or a donor pool (Beer et al. 1981; Taylor and Faulk, 1981; Gill, 1983). A recent report indicates that treatment with the paternal lymphocytes is significantly superior, thus implicating the expression of paternally-derived alloantigens with successful pregnancy (Mowbray et al., 1985). Taken together the evidence from both animal studies and the clinical experience may provide insight not only into the mechanisms that operate to provide fetal protection from the maternal immune response, but have the potential also, to provide a means of modifying fertility.

## HISTOCOMPATIBILITY ANTIGENS

In most mammalian species that have been examined critically, there is a cluster of genes designated as the major histocompatibility complex (MHC). In the mouse this is designated H-2 and is located on chromosome 17. These genes code for proteins that enable T-lymphocytes to recognize antigens (Klein et al 1983). The MHC loci can be divided into two classes, designated class I and class II (Klein, 1977). Class I gene products are characteristically glycopeptides of molecular weight 44,000 with a chain length of approximately 350 amino acids, associated with $\beta_2$ microglobulin. Class II gene products are also glycoproteins with two different chains, $\alpha$ chains (28,000 mw) and $\beta$ chains (34,000 mw).

The K and D regions of the mouse H-2 system constitute the class I antigens or the classic histocompatibility antigens. These are the loci whose products were first demonstrated by alloantisera and are the source of much of the complexity of the H-2. Each individual possesses two haplotypes, a paternal and a maternal one.

Class II antigens, characteristic of the I regions are termed Ia antigens. The function of these genes is not entirely clear, but they are generally recognized to be involved with antigen recognition by T-helper and T-suppressor cells.

In addition to antigens of the MHC, other histocompatibility loci, termed non-H-2 loci, are found on other chromosomes as well as on chromosome 17. Although their precise number is not known, current estimates put their number in excess of 30. Very little is known of their biological function or their chemical structure, although it has been long recognized by transplantation biologists that they present an obstacle to tissue graft acceptance when the host and donor are compatible at the MHC.

## ALLOANTIGEN EXPRESSION ON GAMETES

Evidence for the expression of MHC antigens on gametes has been conflicting (Heyner, 1983). One of the problems with assaying MHC components on sperm is the presence of contaminating cells present in the ejaculate. However, a study by Anderson and her colleagues (Anderson et al., 1982) appears to have circumvented this problem. The use of a cell-binding radioimmunoassay in conjunction with a panel of highly specific monoclonal antibodies with well-defined reactivities against determinants on HLA Class I and Class II molecules revealed binding that was similar to that obtained with negative monoclonal controls. In contrast to the numerous studies on sperm, there have been relatively few studies of alloantigen expression on the surface of oocytes.

Studies in the mouse (see Table I) have utilized a number of different techniques; Edidin et al (1974) reported some positive results using complement-mediated cytotoxicity, but Billington et al (1977) were unable to detect MHC antigens on the oocyte membrane using an immunoperoxidase labelling technique. Studies on the mouse oocytes at the dictyate and metaphase II stages out using multispecific sera, raised in congenic strains of mice and rendered monospecific by absorptions, have shown serologically specific reactivity to H-2 antibody on the oocyte membrane. In contrast, zygotes were found to exhibit variable reactivity, and two-cell stages were found to be negative (Heyner and Hunziker, 1979). These findings suggested that fertilization results in altered expression of membrane components, a confirmation of the observations of Johnson and Edidin (1978) that there are marked changes in the lateral mobility of the mouse oocyte membrane following fertilization. Other studies from our laboratory, using monoclonal antibodies indicate that

Table I

Serological Detection of Antigens on Oocytes

| Antibody Directed Against | Results | Technique |
|---|---|---|
| H-2 | $\pm$ | Complement-mediated cytotoxicity |
| H-2 | - | Immunoperoxidase |
| H-2 | + | Indirect immunofluorescence |
| H-1, H-3, H-4<br>H-7, H-9, H-13 | + | Indirect immunofluorescence |

Positive results are indicated by +; inability to detect is indicated by -.

Class 1 antigens are distributed very sparsely on the surface of the oocyte, and consequently support the conclusion of Anderson et al. (1982) that these antigens are probably not involved in sperm-egg recognition events.

Table I shows that a number of non-H-2 antigens can also be detected on the surface of the unfertilized oocyte. These have been recognized using antisera elicited against a number of non-H-2 specificities, and subsequently rendered monospecific by the appropriate absorption (Heyner et al. 1980; Heyner and Giles-Komar 1983). Nothing is known of corresponding antigens on the membrane of sperm, so it is not clear whether or not these molecules may be involved in gamete recognition.

## ALLOANTIGEN EXPRESSION ON EMBRYOS

Early transplantation experiments showed that when mouse tubal embryos were placed under the kidney capsule of specifically sensitized recipients, the graft was destroyed, establishing the presence of alloantigens on the embryo (Simmons and Russell, 1966). Since this experiment, there has been extensive investigation of the expression of Class I antigenic determinants on early embryos. Early studies using indirect immunofluorescence (Palm et al. 1971; Muggleton-Harris and Johnson, 1976) indicated that MHC antigens could not be detected on tubal cleavage stages or blastocysts. The earliest detection of MHC antigens by indirect immunofluorescence on blastocyst outgrowths was around day 6, and that reactivity was restricted to the ICM (Heyner, 1973). These results were in agreement with transplantation studies by Patthey and Edidin (1973).

Most studies are in agreement that MHC antigens are first detected on the ICM of the blastocyst (see Table II); Webb et al. (1977) grew mouse embryos in media containing radiolabelled amino acids and used sensitive immunoprecipitation methods to show that H-2 synthesis could be detected in the cells of the ICM of the late blastocyst.

The expression of Class I antigens on trophectoderm is controversial. Although most investigators have been unable to detect MHC antigens on these cells, Searle et al (1976) used a sensitive immunoperoxidase assay to demonstrate transient expression of Class I antigens on early blastocyst trophectoderm. Trophectoderm of blastocysts undergoing delay of implantation showed variable expression of MHC antigens when examined with a sensitive antiglobulin technique, while those blastocysts released from delay were negative (Hakansson et al. 1975).

Table II

Detection of MHC Antigens on the Surface of Mouse Embryos

| | | Blastocyst | | Blastocyst Outgrowth | | |
|---|---|---|---|---|---|---|
| Zygote | Tubal Egg | ICM | TRP | Embryo | TRP | Technique |
| NT | - | NT | - | NT | NT | Cytotoxicity |
| + | - | - | - | + | - | Immunofluorescence |
| NT | NT | NT | NT | NT | + | Mixed hemadsorption |
| NT | NT | NT | + | + | - | Immunoperoxidase |
| NT | - | + | - | NT | NT | Immunoprecipitation |
| NT | NT | NT | -* | NT | NT | Isotope antiglobulin |

Positive results are indicated by +; inability to detect the antigen is indicated by - and NT means that the particular stage has not been examined.

*Blastocysts undergoing experimentally-induced delay of implantation were variably positive.

From the foregoing it is apparent that the majority of studies are in agreement that MHC antigens can be detected first on the ICM of the blastocyst, and are not present in significant amounts on the trophectoderm. An interesting aspect of many early studies is that antibodies were raised without considering the possibility that Class II antigens might have been involved. Indeed, analysis of most of the strain combinations used to raise the reagents shows that Class II antibodies were probably present. However, studies by Delovitch et al (1978) utilizing sensitive immunoprecipitation methods have revealed that Ia antigens appear first at day 11 of gestation and are restricted to the liver until day 16.

It is generally recognized from the experimental data that early mouse embryos are immunogenic, and this property has been ascribed to the expression of non-H-2 histocompatibility antigens on the surface of the early embryo. While there are a number of early reports describing the detection of non-H-2 antigens on the surface of the preimplantation embryo (reviewed in Heyner, 1983) the reagents used in these studies had the potential to contain a number of contaminating antibodies. In an attempt to circumvent these problems, Heyner et al (1980) and Heyner and Giles-Komar (1983) used alloantibodies elicited in mice compatible at the MHC but differing at multiple non-H-2 loci to map minor alloantigen expression during different stages of preimplantation development.

These authors showed that while the unfertilized ovum is weakly positive, the two cell stage is negative, although by the eight cell stage, a number of non-H-2 alloantigens could be detected. From the studies to date, it appears that embryos at the stage express alloantigens in a similar distribution to that found on adult tissues.

The blastocyst represents two cell lineages; the inner cell mass and the trophectoderm. Alloantigen expression on trophectoderm has been of particular interest since this tissue is in intimate contact with the maternal tissues during implantation. The detection of specific minor alloantigens on the surface of the trophectoderm comfirms the antigenicity of this tissue, as shown by studies utilizing indirect immunofluorescence (Muggleton-Harris and Johnson, 1976) mixed hemadsorption (Billington et al. 1977; Sellens 1977) and transplantation to specifically preimmunized hosts (Johnson 1975). After implantation, trophectoderm differentiates into a variety of cell types. Therefore studies of trophoblast immunogenicity are often difficult to intepret. This is particularly true of many *in vitro* studies in which the normal architecture of the tissue is lost. Interestingly, antigen expression on trophoblastic stages later in pregnancy is believed to be one mechanism whereby the fetus is able to evade immune rejection by the maternal organism due to the immobilization of maternal antibody (Wegmann et al 1979).

## DISCUSSION

In the context of immunoreproduction, the ontogeny of paternal Class I antigens is clearly of significant interest, and it is therefore of potential importance that although the early embryo expresses H-2 by the late blastocyst stage, Class II antigens have not been detected until almost midgestation. The role of Class II antigens in the rejection response has been well-documented (Bach et al. 1976) and the inability to detect such antigens on early developmental stages may indicate a mechanism whereby the embryo evades immunological surveillance.

It is of particular interest to note that the studies of Rossant and her colleagues (Croy et al. 1982) have shown that rejection of the fetal allograft begins to occur around 9.5 days of gestation; similarly, the studies of Clark et al. (1980) indicated that the fetal rejection they observed when CBA/J females were mated with DBA/2J males took place post implantation. In both these examples, reproductive failure occurred around mid-gestation, suggesting a failure in the maternal immune regulatory circuits.

Using this concept of altering the maternal immune responses, Tartakovsky (1985) has shown that mid-gestation abortions can be induced in C57BL/6J females with intravenous injection of fetal/placental cells of $F_1$ origin or in $C_3$H/HeN females following injection of syngeneic tumor cells. The females were immunized prior to mating with $BDF_1$ males, and an abortion rate of nearly 50% resulted.

On the other hand, the studies of Mowbray (1985) and of Beer (this volume) indicate that an appropriate immunization regimen may allow women who abort recurrently to carry a pregnancy to term. Of the greatest interest to reproductive immunologists, is an understanding of the mechanisms underlying rejection of the fetus in the human and mouse models. For example, the class of the target antigen(s) remains to be revealed, as does the nature of alterations in the maternal immunoregulatory circuits that permit rejection of the semiallogeneic fetus that is normally tolerated. When these mechanisms are more clearly revealed, investigations along the lines described by Beer and by Wegmann (this volume) should allow informed manipulation of fertility.

## REFERENCES


Anderson, D.J., Bach, D.L., Yunis, E.J., and DeWolf, W.C., 1982, Major histocompatibility antigens are not expressed on human epididyman sperm, J. Immunol. 129:452.

Auerbach, R., Hay, J.B., and Kubai, L., 1980, Feto-maternal histocompatibility and placental blood flow, J. Physiol. 307:465.

Bach, F.H., Bach, M.L., and Sondel, P.M., 1976, Differential function of major histocompatibility complex antigens in T-lymphocyte antigen activation, Nature (Lond) 259:273-281.

Beer, A.E., Scott, J.R., and Billingham, R.E., 1975, Histocompatibility and maternal immunological status as determinants of fetoplacental weight and litter size in rodents, J. Exp. Med. 142:180.

Beer, A.E., Quebbeman, J.F., Ayers, J.W.T., and Haines, R.F., 1981, Major histocompatibility complex antigens, maternal and paternal immune responses, and chronic habitual abortions in humans, Am. J. Obstet. Gynecol. 141:987-997.

Billington, W.D., Jenkinson, E.J., Searle, R.F., and Sellens, M.H., 1977, Alloantigen expression during early embryogenesis and placental ontogeny in the mouse. Immunoperoxidase and mixed hemadsorption studies, Transplant. Proc. IX:1371.

Clark, D.A., McDermott, M. and Sczewzuk, M.R., 1980, Impairment of host vs graft reaction in pregnant mice. II selective suppression of cytotoxic cell generation correlates with soluble suppressor activity and with successful allogeneic pregnancy, Cell. Immunol. 52: 106.

Clarke, B. and Kirby, D.R.S., 1966, Maintenance of histocompatibility polymorphisms, Nature (Lond.) 291:999.

Croy, B.A., Rossant, J. and Clark, D.A., 1982, Histological and immunological studies of post-implantation death of _Mus caroli_ embryos in the _Mus musculus_ uterus, J. Reprod. Immunol. 4:277.

Delovitch, T., Press, J.L., and McDevitt, H.O., 1978, Expression of murine Ia antigens during embryonic development, J. Immunol. 120:818-824.

Edidin, M., Gooding, L.R., and Johnson, M., 1974, In: Immunological Approaches to Fertility Control (E. Diczfalušy, ed.), Karolinska Institutet, Stockholm, pp 336-356.

Hakansson, S., Heyner, S., Sundqvist, K.G., and Bergstrom, S., 1975, The presence of paternal H-2 antigens on hybrid mouse blastocysts during experimental delay of implantation and the disappearance of these antigens after onset of implantation, Int. J. Fertil. 20:137-140.

Head, J.R., and Billingham, R.E., 1983, Transplantation biology revisited. In: Immunology of Reproduction (T.G. Wegmann and T.J. Gill eds.) Oxford University Press, pp 27.

Heyner, S., 1973, Detection of H-2 antigens on the surface of the early mouse embryo, Transplantation, 16:675.

Heyner, S., and Hunziker, R.D., 1979, Differential expression of alloantigens of the major histocompatibility complex on unfertilized and fertilized eggs, Dev. Genet. 1:69.

Heyner, S., Hunziker, R.D., and Zink, G.L., 1980, Differential expression of minor histocompatibility antigens on the surface of the mouse oocyte and preimplantation developmental stages, J. Reprod. Immunol. 2:269.

Heyner, S., 1983, Alloantigen expression on oocytes and embryos, In: Immunology of Reproduction (T.G. Wegmann, and T. Gill, eds.) Oxford University Press, pp 79-99.

Heyner S., and Giles-Komar, J., 1983, Differential expression of minor histocompatibility antigens on the surface of the early mouse embryo, J. Cell Biol. 97:38a.

Johnson, M.H., 1975, In: Immunobiology of Trophoblast, (R.G. Edwards, C.W.S. Howe, and M.H. Johnson, eds.) Cambridge University Press.

Johnson, M.H., and Edidin, M., 1978, Lateral diffusion in plasma membrane of mouse egg is restricted after fertilization, Nature (Lond.), 272:448.

Klein, J., 1977, In: The Major Histocompatibility System in Man and Animals (D. Gotze, ed.), New York: Springer-Verlag.

Klein, J., Figueroa, F. and Nagy, Z.A., 1983, Genetics of the major histocompatibility complex: the final act, Ann. Rev. Immunol. 1:119.

McLaren, A., 1976, Genetic and environmental effects on fetal and placental growth in mice. J. Reprod. Fertil., 9:79.

Mowbray, J.F., Liddel, H., Underwood, J.L., Gibbings, C., Reginald, P.W. and Beard, R.W., 1985, Controlled trial of treatment of recurrent spontaneous abortion by immunization with paternal cells, Lancet ii 941.

Medawar, P.B., 1953, Some immunological and endocrinological problems raised by the evolution of viviparity in vertebrates, Symp. Soc. Exp. Biol. 7:320.

Muggleton-Harris, A.L., and Johnson, M.H., 1976, The nature and distribution of serologically detectable alloantigens on the preimplantation mouse embryo, J. Embryol. Exp. Morph. 35:59.

Searle, R.F., Sellens, M.H., Elson, J., Jenkinson, E.J., and Billington, W.D., 1976, Detection of alloantigens during preimplantation development and early trophoblast differentiation in the mouse by immunoperoxidase labelling, J. Exp. Med. 143:348-359.

Sellens, M.H., 1977, Antigen expression on early mouse trophoblast, Nature (Lond.), 269:60-61.

Simmons, R.L., and Russell, P.S., 1966, The histocompatibility antigens of fertilized mouse eggs and trophoblast, Ann N.Y. Acad. Sci. 129:35-45.

Tartakovsky, B., 1985, A new approach to the immunologic disruption of pregnancy, Transplant. Proc. XVII:919.

Tofoski, J.G., and Gill, T.J., 1977, The production of migration inhibitory factor and reproductive capacity in allogeneic pregnancies. Am. J. Pathol., 88:333.

Webb, C.G., Gall, W.E., and Edelman, G.M., 1977, Synthesis and distribution of H-2 antigens in preimplantation embryos, J. Exp. Med. 146:923-932.

Wegmann, T.G., Singh, B., Carlson, G.A., 1979, Allogeneic placenta as a paternal strain antigen immunoabsorbant, J. Immunol. 122:270-274.

VALEDICTION

# IMMUNOCONTRACEPTION - FROM ROMANCE TO REALITY

V. Ramalingaswami

Director-General
Indian Council of Medical Research
New Delhi, India 110029

## PREAMBLE

One of Dr. G.P. Talwar's Dramatis Personnae is a male baboon by the name of Hanuman, who successfully inseminated a female baboon by the name of Radha soon after successful termination of a previous pregnancy induced by passive immunization with anti β-hCG antibody. Radha gave birth to a female offspring named Baby Radha, now thriving at 5 years of age. I have had the opportunity of visiting this family from time to time at the All India Institute of Medical Sciences. Hanuman in the great Indian Epic, Ramayana, is an embodiment of courage, strength and loyalty. He was not known to have had any children and is often seen in pictures carrying a mountain with a luxuriant growth of medicinal herbs on it. Radha in Indian mythology is a woman of beauty and grace in spiritual love with Krishna. Hanuman and Radha in the Indian tradition portray qualities of courage, daring, grace and beauty.

I am neither an immunologist nor a molecular biologist, nor a reproductive biologist. In the past I have studied, with Dr. M.G Deo, the cell proliferation kinetics of spermatogenesis in rhesus monkeys exposed to protein malnutrition. I am a general pathologist and have been following with interest the developments in the field of immuno-contraception ever since Dr. Talwar revealed his ideas to me in the 1970s at the All India Institute of Medical Sciences. Since then I have played some role, perhaps an adjuvant one, in giving impetus to this work in India.

What we witnessed in the last two and a half days is the romance and reality of birth control vaccines. We witnessed good science and a welcome interdisciplinarity between molecular biology, immunology and reproductive biology and much upstream work dealing with basic phenomena of the reproductive process. The whole scene is moving downstream towards the technology end and its application and soon we will enter the various phases of clinical trails. We are told that there are three vaccines ready to go into Phase-I clinical trials later this year. There will then follow work on product development, upscaling of manufacture technology, fit into the delivery system and varying socio-economic millieus and all the rest of it. Perhaps the next Fogarty Conference could possibly be on aspects dealing with the human application end.

The Symposium got off to a good start with rain and clouds which later in the evening ended in an electrical storm which blew out the bulb of the projector. I understand Fogarty Conferences usually start in this way but end up in bright sunshine! "Vaccines against unwanted pregnancies" was the theme of Dr. Craig Wallace's opening address in which he referred to the global problem of avoiding pregnancies, both in the developed and developing countries. This was followed by Dr. Duane Alexander telling the Symposium that in the United States of America 50 percent of pregnancies were unwanted, not to speak of the desperateness of the problem in much of the developing world.

The essence of the Symposium was manipulation of the body's defences to intercept the reproductive process. The cells of the reproductive system make unique molecules either secreted or on the surface which mediate steps involved in successful reproductive performance. Such molecules could serve as antigens. The gamete, the zygote and the early blastocyst are the targets of such a study together with the hormones GnRH, o-LH and o-FSH. The work on stage-specific surface antigens of gametes and zygotes is reminiscent of the current thrust in the immunobiology of parasitic disease, for example the work on circumsporozoite protein of *Plasmodium falciparum*.

## β-hCG

The *piece de resistans* was β-hCG - either the whole of the β subunit or the 109 to 145 aminoacid C-terminal fragment. Dr. Talwar gave an overview of the current status of the whole field of immunocontraception. He talked about first and second generation vaccines. By second generation he meant purer, highly specific candidate antigens produced either through the biological process route or the chemical synthetic route, whether they are glycosylated or non-glycosylated. This is again similar to trends in the development of vaccines against infectious disease agents; for example against rabies, the acellular pertussis vaccine and the recombinant anti-hepatitis B vaccine. Dr. Roy Hertz introduced the tantalizing question: Are we losing something in this search for specificity, for example, in the amplitude of the immune response? He also introduced a touch of history to the proceedings which humanized the entire symposium by referring to the great men and women who pioneered immunocontraception in the early days. Dr. N.A. Mitchison introduced a spark into the proceedings by referring to the opportunities offered by molecular genetics and cautioned that in our efforts at molecular cartography of the surface of gametes and zygotes, we should not fall into the trap of being attracted towards distracting surface molecules and miss the right ones.

Dr. Talwar's second generation vaccine concept includes not only purer and purer candidate vaccines but also multivalent vaccines by introducing different antigens to attack the host at different points - a multi-point attack. His concept includes further introducing carrier molecules other than diptheria and tetanus toxoids to include other large molecules such as the B subunit of the cholera toxin. In this connection, Dr. J.B. Biggers raised the question of multivalent vaccines using different antigens acting in an additive manner or in a synergistic manner or in an antagonistic manner. The work of Dr. B. Moss here at the NIH has opened the opportunity of incorporating on the vaccinia virus, DNA fragments that could code for a number of different antigens including the reproductive tract antigens.

A survey of the existing fertility regulating methods shows that they suffer from a number of limitations. We need safer, more effective and more acceptable methods of contraception. Indeed, considering the fact that contraceptive methods are used in people who are well and not ill, it is but right to insist on the highest possible levels of safety. We prefer these newer methods to be non-hormonal in nature, to have a compatibility with local logistic and outreach systems, and to be reversible especially in the context of their being given to young women in settings characterized by high childhood mortality rates. We need contraceptive methods that produce the least disturbance of menstrual cycles as these are culture-sensitive issues in many locations. They should not, if possible, interfere with ovulation, and they should be independent of the sexual act and not need genital manipulation. These methods should also be capable of being applied by paramedicals with training, and they should be able to provide at least one to two years of protection. The hope is that immunocontraception methods might be able to satisfy many if not most of these criteria. Vaccines are history's most cost-effective tools in health. Dr. Halfdan Mahler of W.H.O. said they are an "opportunistic marvel."

## Generic Problems

There are four generic problems that were thrown up during the course of the Symposium: 1. Reproductive antigens are generally weak immunogens and the problem is how to enhance their immunogenecity, as much the duration of the immune response as the height of it. There is still need to determine for each antigen how high is high enough for the immune response and the cut off points of antibody levels above which protection occurs. Work presented at the symposium indicates that good old alum has stood the test of time as an adjuvant to enlarge the immune response to reproductive antigens. Dr. H. Nash reviewed the current state of the art on adjuvants for fertility control vaccines including MDPs, lipopolysacchrides etc. 2. The second generic problem is individual variability in immune response. A great deal of work has been reported on adjuvants, vehicles and carriers as well as the need for conformational studies to overcome this problem. 3. The third issue is reversibility. This idea runs through most experiments presented involving a variety of animal species. In general it seems that reversibility is characteristic of current immunocontraception experiments except for the one bitch which, in Dr. Mahi-Brown's experiment, was immunized with porcine zona pellucida antigens. 4. The concern about teratogenic effects is universal with respect to any new products for human use. They are of particular concern in the area of immunoreproduction especially at a time when the antibody levels are declining and when conception may occur. There is a general impression that teratogenic effects are not observed in most of the experiments described except for a mention made in the discussion that still births and cranial defects were observed in some experiments with zona pellucida antigens.

Dr. V. Reddy and Dr. W. Chin presented work on the cloning and expression of subunits of hCG and other gonadotropins and their regulation respectively. Do we need to go into this modality of obtaining hCG and its subunits or can we depend as of now, upon its extraction and purification from the urine of pregnant women? Is there a shortage or will there be a shortage of urine from pregnant women?

## Sperm Antigens

The presentations by Drs. N. Alexander, R. Naz, P. Saling, D. Anderson, E. Goldberg, and A. Bellve demonstrated a speedily moving front in the area of stage-specific sperm antigens. It was recalled that this approach had its origins nearly 50 years ago. Recent experiments demonstrate that during capacitation, a remodeling of surface antigens takes place and if one blocked these antigens one would block capacitation. Sperm surface changes continuously, the plasma membrane acquiring domains. Acrosomal antigens are evolutionarily preserved and the goal here is to inhibit single epitope on sperm. Extensive work on monoclonal antibodies was presented in this section. The additive effect of two monoclonals was described by Dr. Saling. Dr. D. Anderson pleaded for greater interdisciplinary work. She said that we ought to identify the sperm specific antigens first and then call in the immunologist. I guess the immunologist would then step in with his "hubristic air" as Peter Medawar would say. The prima dona in this area continues to be immunosuppression of fertility by LDH-C4 - the 11 residue fragment of it. This work is a fine example of the reductionist approach in science.

The discussion raised by Dr. Madhwa Raj brought out the fact that the anti-fertility effect of sperm antigens in females would be dependent upon the levels of antibodies attained in the female reproductive tract. This reminded me of a reference made elsewhere by Drs. N. Alexander and E. Goldberg that the sperm will have to pass through the cervix, and the cervix for the sperm is what the fatal columns of Gibraltar (Pillars of Hercules) are to the ships passing through. Perhaps it is the level of antibodies in the Fallopian tubes that are really critical. Naz and Nancy's MA24 and Salings M29 and M42 monoclonals were described.

Dr. A. Bellve referred to the sperm area as a landscape of wonder and the Symposium showed this to be an area of great potential as well.

## From Sperm to the Ovum

Again it is the surface, the investment of the oocyte, that was the focus in a series of presentations including Dr. J. Dean's paper on Molecular Genetics. In fact in an area of waxing and weaning promise, the view emerged that the zona is fundamental in the reproductive process. Zona pellucida antigen-based immunocontraception is an appropriate target, it is affirmed.

Work in this area is bogged down unfortunately by the concommitant ovarian tissue damage accompanying immunization with zona antigens. Perhaps this problem could be overcome if one can get zona pellucida antigen in the late stage of development of the oocyte and thus it may be possible to avoid cross-reactivity with oocyte elements in the ovary. Dr. A. Sacco's 55 K macromolecule looked promising.

## Anti-hormonal contraception

We had a peep into the work of Drs K. Catt and C. Das on GnRH and apart from the expected localization of antibodies on the pituitary, placental localization of anti-GnRH monoclonals was intriguing. Work on immunization against LHRH was presented by Drs. H. Fraser and C. Shaha. There are problems of long term metabolic effects and side reactions.

Encouraging results were presented with o-FSH which seems to be back in the race. The Neischlag-Moudgal disparity in results may be attributable to the seasonality of rhesus monkeys; this seasonality disappears and uniform responses take place when one uses bonnet monkeys as Moudgal did. It looks as if o-FSH is a good immunogen; it does not disturb the production of testosterone but the problem of the significance of oligospermia-versus azoospermia still needs to be resolved. After all, attention should be focused on the quality of sperm and its ability to penetrate and fertilize the ovum, although their numbers cannot be ignored.

## Conclusion

So we come to the end of a memorable symposium and we should thank Dr. G.P. Talwar and the Fogarty International Center for this. I would like to extend my apologies to several speakers to whose work I made no reference in this presentation, especially the fine presentations on immunopromotion of fertility. The discussions ranged from molecular biology to barnyard environments. We are launched on a journey of immunocontraception. Many gaps in basic knowledge still exist. Increasing interdisciplinarity is evident. We have now reached the stage of being able to navigate in this area rather than drift, in the fulfillment of a daring concept, in the pursuit of a novel method, moving closer and closer to reality but not without a sense of romance.

# INDEX